COLORECTAL CANCER BIOLOGY – FROM GENES TO TUMOR

Edited by **Rajunor Ettarh**

Colorectal Cancer Biology – From Genes to Tumor
Edited by Rajunor Ettarh

Published by InTech

Janeza Trdine 9, 51000 Rijeka, Croatia

Publishing Process Manager Tajana Jevtic

Technical Editor Teodora Smiljanic

Cover Designer InTech Design Team

Additional hard copies can be obtained from orders@intechopen.com

Colorectal Cancer Biology – From Genes to Tumor, Edited by Rajunor Ettarh
p. cm.
978-953-51-0062-1

For EU product safety concerns:
IN TECH d.o.o., Prolaz Marije Krucifikse Kozulić 3, 51000 Rijeka, Croatia,
info@intechopen.com or visit our website at intechopen.com.

Meet the editor

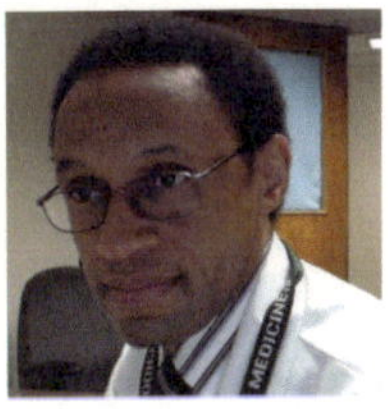

Dr Rajunor Ettarh is Professor and Associate Director of Anatomical Teaching at Tulane University School of Medicine and a Fellow of the Royal Society of Medicine in London. Previously he was a visiting professor at University of Perugia, Italy and investigator at the Conway Institute, University College Dublin. His research interests include enteric epithelial cell biology, non-steroidal anti-inflammatory agents, peroxisome proliferator-activated receptors and medical education. He is a member of the American Association of Anatomists, sits on the Council of the Anatomical Society (UK) and has reviewed for several journals including Carcinogenesis and Anatomical Sciences Education.

Contents

Preface

When a patient is diagnosed with colorectal cancer, the options available to that patient are determined by the current state of knowledge. That knowledge is dependent on a complex balance, between the advances in fundamental cell and tissue research in experimental environments on the one hand, and the advances in clinical management and treatment that result from better knowledge and application of the fundamental information about the disease.

Colorectal cancer is a major killer - that much is restated in many parts of this book. This underlies the drive in research efforts towards finding solutions to important questions about how the disease starts, how it progresses, and how it spreads. So what do we know? A lot has been discovered, but all of the answers are still not within reach. Great steps and strides forward in in vitro studies still defy translation to the patient and hospital bedside - more work needs to be done to find out how to safely and effectively apply what we have discovered to the patient's illness.

This book about colorectal cancer comes in two volumes - both of which address several aspects of the endeavors of the biomedical and clinical community to find resolutions and solutions to the disease and its complications. The first section of this volume (Volume 1) deals with genes and genetic background associated with colorectal cancer and explores roles of the gene polymorphisms that mediate some of the presentations of the disease, as well as the short single strand ribonucleic acid molecules (microRNA) that help to regulate the expression of these genes. The second section deals with many cellular and molecular aspects of the biochemical pathways involved in colorectal carcinogenesis and tumor progression. Section 3 examines the tumor microenvironment and the role of intestinal microbes and host-microbial interactions in colorectal cancer. Section 4 presents a collection of short reports from studies that explore aspects such as fluorescent biomarkers and tumor infiltrating lymphocytes. The chapters in this book represent some of the efforts of the thousands of workers involved in finding solutions and cures to colorectal cancer. This book is directed to clinicians and scientists who want to ask why, learn how and know more.

Dr Rajunor Ettarh
Professor & Associate Director of Anatomical Teaching,
Department of Structural and Cellular Biology,
Tulane University School of Medicine, New Orleans,
USA

Acknowledgements

The publication of this book would not have been possible without the support of my family. I am also especially indebted to Publishing Process Manager Tajana Jevtic whose infinite patience, timely reminders, and never-ending assistance and support made the task of editing this book easier.

Part 1

Introduction

1

Colorectal Cancer: It Starts and It Runs

Rajunor Ettarh
Department of Structural and Cellular Biology,
Tulane University School of Medicine, New Orleans,
USA

1. Introduction

An automobile starts and runs. In much the same way, colorectal cancer starts and runs but our understanding of how this happens is incomplete. The disease affects millions of men and women around the world, and is responsible for significant morbidity and mortality in patients. Increasing numbers of new cases continue to appear worldwide and there is little evidence of a decline in incidence of the disease. The necessity for improved management and treatment of colorectal cancer in patients continues to drive studies and investigations towards a better understanding of the origins of the disease. Much of the evidence suggests that the origins of colorectal cancer are multifactorial: genetic and environmental factors intertwine with risk factors. Figure 1 lays out various aspects of colorectal cancer that provide broad focal points for studies and research investigations. In vitro studies have helped to define the scientific knowledge base regarding initiation of colorectal cancer and the mechanisms that sustain progression and encourage spread of the disease. Clinical studies and trials have provided insights into disease management and patient care. Animal modeling provides an important bridge between in vitro studies and investigations in patients. So what is the current state of the evidence regarding the causes and biological mechanisms involved in colorectal cancer? While the chapters in this volume of the book deliver detailed overviews of various aspects of the basic science involved in our understanding of the disease, this introductory chapter offers a summary outline of some of the evidence.

2. Genes and heredity

Genetic and hereditary mechanisms have a significant influence on colorectal cancer. Studies indicate that familial history plays a role in up to 25% of patients who are diagnosed with colorectal cancer (Gala & Chung, 2011) and this helps to explain the origins of their disease. Several genes have been implicated in the process of colorectal carcinogenesis including adenomatous polyposis coli (APC), rat sarcoma oncogene K-ras, tumor suppressor TP53, DNA glycosylase gene MUTYH, and murine sarcoma oncogene BRAF. In many patients, the most frequently mutated gene is the APC gene (Bettstetter et al, 2007; Vasovcak et al, 2011). Some of the methods by which these genes are affected include hypermethylation of promoter sequences for tumor suppressor genes as well as the induction of microsatellite instability. About 15% of colorectal cancers show microsatellite instability from mutated mismatch repair genes (Pino & Chung, 2011).

A majority of colorectal cancers are associated with colonic polyposis. Familial adenomatous polyposis (FAP) confers a genetic predisposition to developing multiple benign polyps in the large intestine, a reflection of the inherited mutation in the APC gene. Polyps eventually progress to malignant colorectal cancer. Patients with Lynch Syndrome have a genetic predisposition that confers a high risk for developing early onset, right-sided colorectal cancer (Bellizzi & Frankel, 2009). More recently recognized syndromes also include MUTYH-associated polyposis (MAP), and hyperplastic polyposis syndromes which show mutations of K-ras and microsatellite instability - changes similar to those associated with colorectal cancer (Hawkins et al, 2000; Jass et al, 2000; Liljegren et al, 2003).

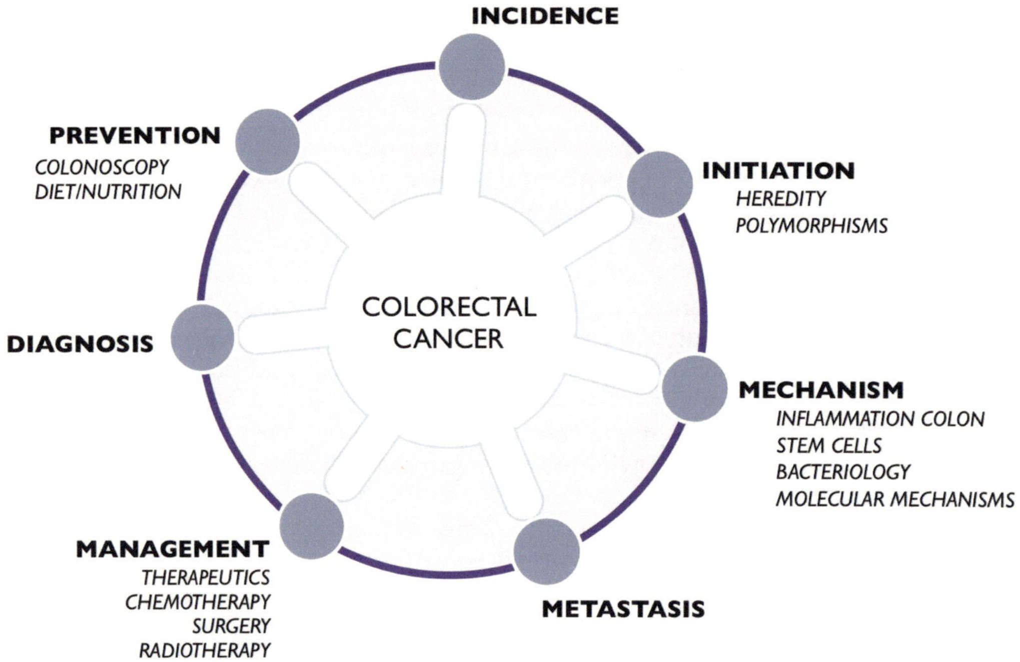

Fig. 1. The aspects of colorectal cancer that drive the quest for improved understanding, better management, effective therapies, and prevention. Aspects of initiation and mechanisms are considered in this volume of the book. Management, diagnosis and epidemiological considerations are dealt with in the second volume of the book.

Animal models of colorectal cancer have contributed to improving understanding of the disease. The APC min mouse model develops multiple intestinal polyps and illustrates the role of Wnt signaling and beta catenin regulation in the formation of these polyps (Kawahara et al, 2000; Senda et al, 2007). The model provides one avenue for testing and evaluating pharmacotherapeutic approaches in colorectal cancer.

3. Nutrition

The relationship between nutrition and colorectal cancer remains inconsistent and debatable. Some studies suggest variable colorectal cancer risk with ingestion of fruit and vegetables, other studies indicate a reduction in the risk (Millen et al, 2007; Koushik et al,

2007; Anemma et al, 2011). The evidence is just as conflicting even when specific food components such as folate are considered (Mason, 2011). Some of the published data supports the association between colorectal cancer and processed foods as well as with consumption of red meat: the risk of colorectal cancer increases in line with increasing intake (Fu et al, 2011; Gingras and Beliveau, 2011). In addition, the risk among heavy alcohol drinkers for developing colorectal cancer is considerably higher than the risk for those whose alcohol intake is low (Pelluchi et al, 2011).

4. Mechanisms

The role of inflammation in colorectal cancer is demonstrated by the increased risk of colorectal in patients with chronic inflammatory conditions: the risk in patients with ulcerative colitis is 2-fold higher than for the general population and up to 0.8% of patients with Crohn's disease develop colorectal cancer (Pohl et al, 2000; Rizzo et al, 2011). These inflammatory diseases also demonstrate genetic alterations in some of the same targets associated with colorectal cancer. In addition, anti-inflammatory therapy significantly reduces the risk of colorectal cancer (Trinchieri, 2011).

The intestine is colonized by great numbers of microbes in a symbiotic relationship with the gut epithelium, a relationship that affects digestion, absorption and nutrition. Nonetheless, there is increasing evidence of the association between intestinal streptococcal infection and colorectal cancer. However the precise mechanism by which these streptococcal strains are involved in the development or propagation of colorectal cancer remains unclear (Boleij et al, 2011). Enteric microbes are thought to alter normal regulatory mechanisms in epithelial cells to promote disruption and tumor growth (Wu et al, 2003; Sun et al, 2004; Franco et al, 2005; Ye et al, 2007; Suzuki et al, 2009; Gnad et al, 2010; Liu et al, 2010).

The idea that colorectal cancer is sustained by stem cells that continually supply new tumor cells continues to spur research investigations and generate new data. The idea however remains controversial despite several reports presenting data on putative cell surface markers for these stem cells. Isolated colorectal cancer stem cells (initiating cells) express a variety of cluster of differentiation proteins or markers that suggest a multipotent ability (Willis et al, 2008; Kemper et al, 2010; Davies et al, 2011; Zeki et al, 2011) but identification of a reliable stem cell biomarker is still elusive. These cells offer a potential target for cure of the disease in patients and for the control of metastatic spread that is thought to arise from residual stem cells that survive therapy for the primary tumor.

5. Conclusion

Our understanding of colorectal cancer in terms of origination, genesis, initiating causes and progression continues to improve. While multiple factors contribute to and influence the initiation and progression of the disease, the number of potential targets continues to increase. This targeting potential will ultimately lead to the development of effective strategies for management of the disease and translate into improved treatments for patients.

6. References

Annema N, Heyworth JS, McNaughton SA, Iacopetta B, Fritschi L. (2011). Fruit and vegetable consumption and the risk of proximal colon, distal colon, and rectal cancers in a case-control study in Western Australia. *J Am Diet Assoc*, Vol.111, No.10, pp. 1479-1490.

Bellizzi AM, Frankel WL. (2009). Colorectal cancer due to deficiency in DNA mismatch repair function: a review. *Adv Anat Pathol*, Vol.16, No.6, pp. 405-417.

Bettstetter M, Dechant S, Ruemmele P, Grabowski M, Keller G, Holinski-Feder E, Hartmann A, Hofstaedter F, Dietmaier W. (2007). Distinction of hereditary nonpolyposis colorectal cancer and sporadic microsatellite-unstable colorectal cancer through quantification of MLH1 methylation by real-time PCR. *Clin Cancer Res*, Vol.13. No.11, pp. 3221-3228.

Boleij A, van Gelder MM, Swinkels DW, Tjalsma H. (2011). Clinical Importance of Streptococcus gallolyticus Infection Among Colorectal Cancer Patients: Systematic Review and Meta-analysis. *Clin Infect Dis*, Vol.53, No.9, pp. 870-878.

Davies EJ, Marsh V, Clarke AR. (2011). Origin and maintenance of the intestinal cancer stem cell. *Mol Carcinog*, Vol.50, No.4, pp. 254-263.

Franco AT, Israel DA, Washington MK, Krishna U, Fox JG, Rogers AB, Neish AS, Collier-Hyams L, Perez-Perez GI, Hatakeyama M, Whitehead R, Gaus K, O'Brien DP, Romero-Gallo J, Peek RM Jr. (2005). Activation of beta-catenin by carcinogenic helicobacter pylori. *Proc Natl Acad Sci USA*, Vol.102, pp. 10646–10651.

Fu Z, Shrubsole MJ, Smalley WE, Wu H, Chen Z, Shyr Y, Ness RM, Zheng W. (2011) Association of meat intake and meat-derived mutagen exposure with the risk of colorectal polyps by histologic type. *Cancer Prev Res (Phila)*, Vol.4, No.10, pp. 1686-1697.

Gala M, Chung DC. (2011). Hereditary colon cancer syndromes. *Semin Oncol*, Vol.38, No.4, pp. 490-499.

Gingras D, Béliveau R. (2011) Colorectal cancer prevention through dietary and lifestyle modifications. *Cancer Microenviron*, Vol.4, No.2, pp. 133-139.

Gnad T, Feoktistova M, Leverkus M, Lendeckel U, Naumann M. (2010). Helicobacter pylori-induced activation of beta-catenin involves low density lipoprotein receptor-related protein 6 and dishevelled. *Mol Cancer*, Vol.9, pp.31

Hawkins NJ, Gorman P, Tomlinson IPM, Bullpitt P, Ward RL. (2000). Colorectal Carcinomas Arising in the Hyperplastic Polyposis Syndrome Progress through the Chromosomal Instability Pathway. *American Journal of Pathology*, Vol.157, pp. 385-392.

Jass JR, Lino H, Ruszkiewicz A, Painter D, Solomon MJ, Koorey DJ, Cohn D, Furlong KL, Walsh MD, Palazzo J, Edmonston TB, Fishel R, Young J, Leggett BA. (2000). Neoplastic progression occurs through mutator pathways in hyperplastic polyposis of the colorectum. *Gut*, Vol.47, pp. 43-49.

Kawahara K, Morishita T, Nakamura T, Hamada F, Toyoshima K, Akiyama T. (2000). Down-regulation of beta-catenin by the colorectal tumor suppressor APC requires association with Axin and beta-catenin. *J Biol Chem*, Vol.275, No.12, pp. 8369-8374.

Kemper K, Grandela C, Medema JP. (2010). Molecular identification and targeting of colorectal cancer stem cells. *Oncotarget*, Vol.1, No.6, pp. 387-395.

Koushik A, Hunter DJ, Spiegelman D, Beeson WL, van den Brandt PA, Buring JE, Calle EE, Cho E, Fraser GE, Freudenheim JL, Fuchs CS, Giovannucci EL, Goldbohm RA, Harnack L, Jacobs DR Jr, Kato I, Krogh V, Larsson SC, Leitzmann MF, Marshall JR,

McCullough ML, Miller AB, Pietinen P, Rohan TE, Schatzkin A, Sieri S, Virtanen MJ, Wolk A, Zeleniuch-Jacquotte A, Zhang SM, Smith-Warner SA. (2007). Fruits, vegetables, and colon cancer risk in a pooled analysis of 14 cohort studies. *J Natl Cancer Inst*, Vol.99, No.19, pp. 1471-1483.

Liljegren A, Lindblom A, Rotstein S, Nilsson B, Rubio C, Jaramillo E. (2003). Prevalence and incidence of hyperplastic polyps and adenomas in familial colorectal cancer: correlation between the two types of colon polyps. *Gut*, Vol.52, No.8, pp. 1140-1147.

Liu X, Lu R, Wu S, Sun J. (2010). Salmonella regulation of intestinal stem cells through the Wnt/beta-catenin pathway. *FEBS Lett*, Vol.584, pp. 911–916

Mason JB. (2011). Unraveling the complex relationship between folate and cancer risk. *Biofactors*, Vol.37, No.4, pp. 253-260.

Millen AE, Subar AF, Graubard BI, Peters U, Hayes RB, Weissfeld JL, Yokochi LA, Ziegler RG; PLCO Cancer Screening Trial Project Team. (2007). Fruit and vegetable intake and prevalence of colorectal adenoma in a cancer screening trial. *Am J Clin Nutr*, Vol.86, No.6, pp. 1754-1764.

Pelucchi C, Tramacere I, Boffetta P, Negri E, La Vecchia C. (2011) Alcohol consumption and cancer risk. *Nutr Cancer*, Vol.63, No.7, pp. 983-990.

Pino MS, Chung DC. (2011). Microsatellite instability in the management of colorectal cancer. *Expert Rev Gastroenterol Hepatol*, Vol.5, No.3, pp. 385-399.

Pohl C, Hombach A, Kruis W. (2000). Chronic inflammatory bowel disease and cancer. *Hepatogastroenterology*, Vol.47, No.31, pp. 57-70.

Rizzo A, Pallone F, Monteleone G, Fantini MC. (2011). Intestinal inflammation and colorectal cancer: A double-edged sword? World J Gastroenterol. 17(26):3092-100.

Senda T, Iizuka-Kogo A, Onouchi T, Shimomura A. (2007). Adenomatous polyposis coli (APC) plays multiple roles in the intestinal and colorectal epithelia. *Med Mol Morphol*, Vol.40, No.2, pp. 68-81.

Sun J, Hobert ME, Rao AS, Neish AS, Madara JL. (2004). Bacterial activation of beta-catenin signaling in human epithelia. *Am J Physiol Gastrointest Liver Physiol*, Vol.287, pp. G220–G227

Suzuki M, Mimuro H, Kiga K, Fukumatsu M, Ishijima N, Morikawa H, Nagai S, Koyasu S, Gilman RH, Kersulyte D, Berg DE, Sasakawa C. (2009). Helicobacter pylori CagA phosphorylation-independent function in epithelial proliferation and inflammation. *Cell Host Microbe*, Vol.5, pp. 23–34.

Trinchieri G. (2011) Innate inflammation and cancer: Is it time for cancer prevention? *F1000 Med Rep*, Vol.3, pp. 11.

Vasovcak P, Pavlikova K, Sedlacek Z, Skapa P, Kouda M, Hoch J, Krepelova A. (2011). Molecular genetic analysis of 103 sporadic colorectal tumours in czech patients. *PLoS One*, Vol.6, No.8, pp. e24114.

Willis ND, Przyborski SA, Hutchison CJ, Wilson RG. (2008) Colonic and colorectal cancer stem cells: progress in the search for putative biomarkers. *J Anat*, Vol.213, No.1, pp. 59-65.

Wu S, Morin PJ, Maouyo D, Sears CL. (2003). Bacteroides fragilis enterotoxin induces c-myc expression and cellular proliferation. *Gastroenterology*, Vol.124, pp. 392–400.

Ye Z, Petrof EO, Boone D, Claud EC, Sun J. (2007). Salmonella effector avra regulation of colonic epithelial cell inflammation by deubiquitination. *Am J Pathol*, Vol.171, pp. 882–892

Zeki SS, Graham TA, Wright NA. (2011). Stem cells and their implications for colorectal cancer. *Nat Rev Gastroenterol Hepatol*, Vol.8, No.2, pp. 90-100

Part 2

Genes and Polymorphisms

2

Germline Genetics in Colorectal Cancer Susceptibility and Prognosis

Amanda Ewart Toland
The Ohio State University, USA

1. Introduction

Population-based studies indicate that approximately 35% of an individual's risk of developing colorectal cancer (CRC) is due to inherited genetic factors (Lichtenstein et al. 2000). Indeed, approximately 50,000 individuals diagnosed with CRC in the United States each year will have at least one other family member with CRC (Kaz & Brenthall, 2006). Classically, genetic susceptibility to CRC is described as three types: Low, moderate and high risk. In reality, the risk of developing colorectal cancer due to genetic factors exists on a continuum from very low to very high risk (Figure 1). In addition to colon cancer susceptibility, genetic variants are likely to play a role in response to therapy and prognosis of colon cancer. This Chapter will provide an overview of the current knowledge in genetic susceptibility to hereditary and non-hereditary CRC, the complexities and issues around the identification of germline genetic risk factors, and the current and future use of genetic information in the clinic.

High penetrance risk includes inheritance of mutations in genes which segregate in a Mendelian fashion in families and confer a high lifetime risk of disease. Hereditary cancer syndromes are those in which a mutation confers a high lifetime risk of developing CRC. Several syndromes have been described. The two most familiar CRC syndromes are Familial Adenomatous Polyposis (FAP) and Lynch Syndrome (LS) (Table 1). Moderately-penetrant mutations are mutations or polymorphic variants which can manifest as colon cancer clustering in families but without a clear cancer syndrome or inheritance pattern. Low-penetrance variants are those which are present in a reasonably high frequency in the general population, but have small influences on risk and are not themselves sufficient for the development of colon cancer.

2. Hereditary colorectal cancer syndromes

Hereditary colorectal cancer syndromes are those in which an inherited or de novo germline mutation confers a high lifetime risk of developing CRC. Approximately 5% of all CRC diagnoses are thought to be due to highly penetrant mutations (Bodmer, 2006; de la Chapelle, 2004). These familial mutations were the first germline genetic alterations to be discovered to be important for CRC risk. Several syndromes have been described. They can be subdivided into syndromes with adenomatous polyps, those with hamartomatous polyps and syndromes with polyps of mixed histopathology (Table 1). Syndromes that present with a few or many adenomatous polyps include FAP, LS and MUTYH-associated polyposis (MAP) (Table 1). The hamartomatous polyp syndromes include Cowden Syndrome, Juvenile Polyposis and Peutz-Jeghers Syndrome. Not all genes contributing to hereditary CRC have been identified and characterized. It is likely as genome-wide and exonic sequencing become more common that additional rare mutations leading to hereditary colorectal cancer will be discovered.

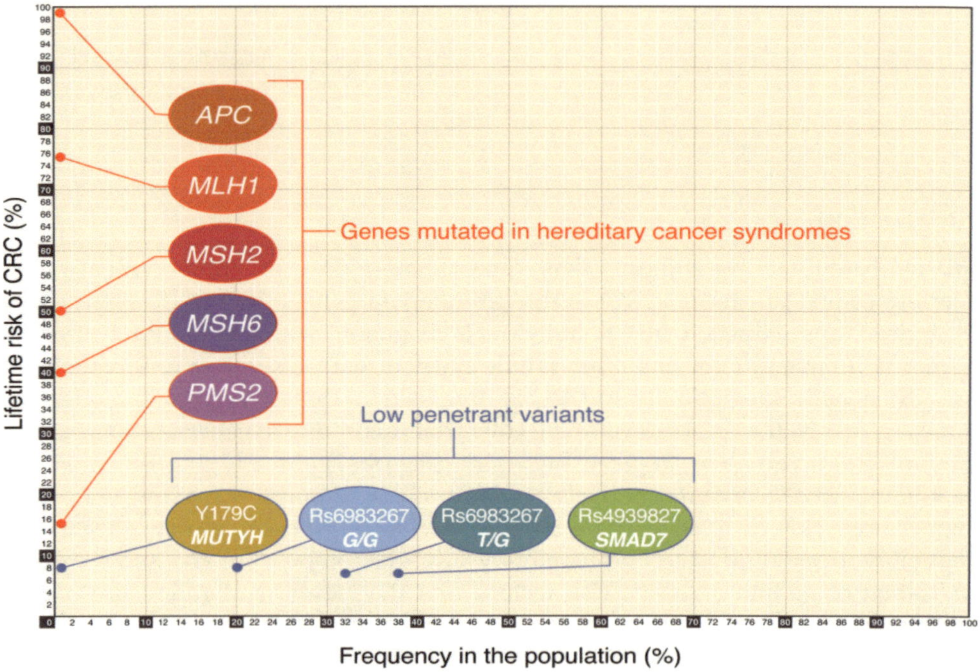

Fig. 1. Genes and variants associated with CRC risk. The allele frequency and lifetime risk of genes associated with familial colorectal cancer (red) and variants associated with a small increase in lifetime risk of CRC (blue) are illustrated. (The Y179C variant is associated with a low risk of CRC when individuals only carry one mutated *MUTYH* allele.)

One common feature of all of these CRC syndromes is that the age of diagnosis of cancer tends to be much earlier than that in the general population. Typically colorectal cancer occurs 10-20 years earlier in individuals with these syndromes than in the general population. In individuals who carry a mutation in one of these hereditary CRC genes there is also considerable increased risk, up to 99%, of developing colon cancer. Individuals with most of these syndromes have detectable polyps prior to the onset of colorectal cancer; however many probands that were not undergoing regular screening are brought to attention following a diagnosis of CRC.

A clinical diagnosis of a specific cancer syndrome can be made based on an extensive family history in combination with histological and pathological information about the number and type of polyps. More definitive diagnoses are made by genetic testing coordinated through a genetic counsellor or medical geneticist of an affected proband, or, in the case of LS, analysis of tumours for loss of one of the LS-related proteins. Even though individually these syndrome are rare, proper management and diagnoses can impact the incidence and mortality related to CRC. Because mutations leading to these genes confer a high lifetime risk of CRC, knowledge of one's family history and mutation status influences medical management and can significantly reduce the incidence of CRC.

Syndrome	CRC Risk	Unique characteristics	Other features	Gene(s)
HNPCC	20-75%*	Microsatellite instability of tumors	Endometrial, gastric, ovarian, small bowel, biliary & urothelial ca	*MSH1, MLH2, PMS2, MSH6 EPCAM*
FAP	99%	Hundreds of polyps	Desmoids, hepatoblastoma & papillary thyroid ca, CHRPE	*APC*
Peutz-Jeghers	39%	Hamartomatous polyps	Gastric, breast, & ovarian ca, sex cord tumors, mucocutaneous hyperpigmentation	*LKB1 (STK11)*
MAP	80%	Recessive inheritance, many adenomatous polyps	Two common mutations in individuals with Northern European ancestry: Y179C and G396D	*MUTYH (MYH)*
Hereditary Mixed Polyposis	ND	Inflammatory & metaplastic polyps		*BMPR1A*
Cowden	None	Hamartomatous polyps	Macrocephaly, benign & malignant thryoid, breast & uterine neoplasms	*PTEN*
Juvenile Polyposis	39%	Hamartomatous polyps	GI polyps, gastric ca	*SMAD4, BMPR1A,*

Table 1. Hereditary Colon Cancer and Polyposis Syndromes. ca, cancer; CHRPE, congenital hypertrophy of the retinal pigment epithelium; ND, not determined; GI, gastrointestinal; *CRC risk depends on which gene is mutated.

2.1 Hereditary non-polyposis colorectal cancer/lynch syndrome

Hereditary non-polyposis colorectal cancer (HNPCC), also known as Lynch syndrome (LS), is the most common hereditary CRC syndrome associated with a strong family history of colon cancer. Approximately 2-4% of all colon cancers are due to LS (Hampel et al., 2008). Although individuals with LS frequently have adenomatous polyps, individuals with this syndrome do not have polyposis. In addition to a lifetime risk of approximately 50-80% for colorectal cancer, there is an increased risk of ovarian, endometrial and gastric cancers (Jasperson et al., 2010). Since the genes have been identified, some conditions which were once thought to be distinct (e.g. Muir-Torre syndrome which is characterized by familial

CRC with sebaceous neoplasms and Turcot syndrome which is characterized by CRC with glioblastomas) are variants of LS. LS is inherited in an autosomal dominant fashion and is associated with mutations in four genes important in mismatch repair (MMR): *MLH1, MSH2, PMS2* and *MSH6*. Tumours arising in individuals with germline mutations in these genes, which are important for DNA repair, typically exhibit microsatellite instability which is sometimes used clinically to aid in a diagnosis. The most commonly mutated genes in LS are *MLH1* and *MSH2*. Recently, deletions of the 3'end of *EPCAM*, a gene mapping 5' of the *MSH2* gene, have been found to give rise to LS by causing methylation of the *MSH2* gene in about 6% of LS cases (Niessen et al., 2009a).

Criteria based on family history, Amsterdam I, Amsterdam II and Bethesda criteria, were developed in order to identify families for further evaluation of Lynch syndrome. Amsterdam I criteria, the first described, includes three first degree relatives with CRC, two or more generations affected, one family member with CRC diagnosed under the age of 50 and FAP must be ruled out (Vasen et al., 1991). Amsterdam II criteria are the same as Amsterdam I except that endometrial, small bowel or other LS-related cancers can be substituted for CRC (Vasen et al., 1999). Revised Bethesda criteria include one CRC diagnosed under the age of 50, one CRC under the age of 60 with evidence of microsatellite instability, CRC or LS-related cancer in at least one first degree relative under the age of fifty or CRC or LS-related cancers in at least two first or second degree relatives at any age (Umar et al., 2004). In addition, three online prediction programs MMRpredict, PREMM, and MMRpro have been developed to identify families with LS. Sensitivities of the online models and revised Bethesda criteria are about 75% with a range of specificity from 50-60%; the Amsterdam II criteria have a lower sensitivity of 37.5%, but a better specificity of 99% (Tresallet et al., 2011). Many hospitals have begun to screen all colon cancer cases by immunohistochemistry for loss of the four MMR proteins or for microsatellite instability regardless of family history which has a higher sensitivity than the family history based models (Hampel et al., 2008). Individuals whose tumours show absence of MLH1, MSH2, PMS2 and MSH6 and/or microsatellite instability are referred for genetic evaluation of LS and, in some cases, additional testing to rule out somatic events specific to the tumours which lead to loss of the proteins.

The risk and spectrum of cancer depends on which LS gene is mutated. The lifetime colon cancer risk is 97% for males and 53% for females with germline *MLH1* mutations. Endometrial cancer risk associated with *MLH1* mutations ranges from 25 to 33% (Ramsoekh et al., 2009; Stoffel et al., 2009). The lifetime risk of CRC in male *MSH2* mutation carriers is 52% and is 40% for females. There is a 44-49% risk of endometrial cancer for female *MSH2* mutation carriers (Stoffel et al., 2009). About 10% of Lynch syndrome families have a mutation in *MSH6* (Talseth-Palmer et al., 2010). The estimated risk of colorectal cancer in individuals with a *MLH6* mutation is lower than some of the other mutations at 30-61% and the risk of endometrial cancer is higher with 65-70% of females developing endometrial cancer by the age of 70 (Talseth-Palmer et al., 2010; Ramsoekh et al., 2009). *PMS2* mutations are less frequently the cause of LS accounting for only 2 to 14% of LS cases (Senter et al., 2008; Niessen et al., 2009b; Talseth-Palmer et al., 2010). The cumulative risk by the age of 70 of developing a colon cancer in mono-allelic *PMS2* mutation carriers is 15-20%, endometrial cancer is 15% and other Lynch-related cancers is from 25-32% (Senter et al., 2008). Bi-allelic mutations in the MMR genes have been observed and lead to a severe phenotype with childhood brain tumours, leukaemia, and LS-associated tumors known as Constitutional MMR Deficiency (Senter et al., 2008; Felton et al., 2007; Wimmer & Kratz, 2010). *EPCAM* deletions show a comparable risk of colon cancer to *MLH1* and *MSH2* mutation carriers, but a decreased risk of endometrial cancer. In families with *EPCAM* deletions there is a 75% risk of developing cancer by the age of 70 and a 12% risk of endometrial cancer (Kempers et al., 2011). As the risks of colon, endometrial and other cancers are high, regardless of the gene, individuals with LS are recommended to follow more intensive cancer screening guidelines.

2.2 Familial adenomatous polyposis

Familial adenomatous polyposis (FAP) is an autosomal dominant CRC syndrome that accounts for less than 1% of all CRC diagnoses (Burt, 2000). In classic FAP, individuals develop hundreds to thousands of adenomatous polyps beginning in the early to mid-teen years. By age 35, 95% of individuals with FAP have polyps and the penetrance of colorectal cancer associated with this disease is over 90% (Petersen et al., 1991) which is why prophylactic colectomy is recommended in individuals who have this syndrome. FAP is caused by mutations in the adenomatous polyposis coli (*APC*) gene, although a high percentage (12-20%) of individuals with a clinical diagnosis of classical FAP do not have identifiable mutations in *APC* or another polyposis gene, *MUTYH,* (de la Chapelle, 2004; Filipe et al., 2009). Other features of FAP include small bowel adenomas, gastric polyposis, congenital hypertrophy of the retinal pigment epithelium (CHRPE), and desmoids (Allen & Terdiman, 2003). Desmoids cause significant mortality in FAP despite their non-malignant nature. Attenuated FAP is a milder form of this disease in which there are fewer polyps and a later onset of disease. Two other variants of FAP are Turcot syndrome which includes FAP and central nervous syndrome tumors, primarily medulloblastomas, and Gardner syndrome which includes soft-tissue tumours, osteomas and dental abnormalities.

2.3 *MUTYH*-associated polyposis

MUTYH-associated polyposis (MAP) is an autosomal recessive syndrome conferring a 43 to nearly 100% lifetime risk of CRC (Farrington et al., 2005; Lubbe et al., 2009). Penetrance for cancer in bi-allelic mutation carriers is estimated to be 20% at 40 years and 43% at 50 years of age (Lubbe et al., 2009). Individuals typically present with 10-100 adenomatous polyps, although some bi-allelic mutation carriers do not have any polyps on screening (Farrington et al, 2005; Nielsen et al., 2007). Polyposis of the duodenum can also be observed. Between 24 and 56% of FAP and attenuated-FAP families lacking mutations in APC have been found to carry bi-allelic mutations in *MUTYH,* suggesting that mutations in the two genes account for a significant proportion of familial polyposis (Nielsen et al., 2007; Gomez-Fernandez et al., 2009). Two common *MUTYH* mutations comprising 80-85% of disease causing mutations in Caucasians of Northern European ancestry are Tyr179Cys and Gly396Asp (previously known as Y165C and G382D; Al-Tassan et al., 2002). Importantly, 4% of bi-allelic mutation carriers will not have either of the two common mutations (Goodenberger et al., 2011). The mutation frequency of these mutations varies between populations and other founder and relatively frequent mutations have been identified (Gomez-Fernandez et al., 2009).

2.4 Other adenomatous polyposis syndromes

A handful of case reports of mutations leading to unique or rare familial presentation of CRC exist which may explain a small proportion of polyposis families that do not have *APC* or *MUTYH* germline mutations. One recent description is of homozygous mutations in *BUB1B* leading to CRC (Rio Frio et al., 2010). This gene has not been extensively tested in polyposis families so it is unknown if it will contribute much to the overall risk of familial adenomatous polyposis. Mutations in the *AXIN2* gene are associated with tooth agenesis-colorectal cancer syndrome in a large Finnish family (Lammi et al., 2004), but mutations in this gene do not appear to account for a large proportion of hereditary CRC.

2.5 Familial Colorectal Cancer Type X

About half of the families that have a strong-family history of colorectal cancer suggestive of LS by Amsterdam or Bethesda criteria have no evidence of mismatch repair deficiency or loss of any of the HNPCC related proteins in tumours (de la Chapelle & Lynch, 2003). To be classified as Familial Colorectal Cancer Type X, families must meet Amsterdam I criteria and have no evidence of MMR deficiency. A closer look at these pedigrees shows that they tend to have fewer individuals diagnosed with cancer, their cancers are less likely to look like those in LS and their average age of diagnosis is older than those in families with MMR mutations (Jass et al., 1995; Lindor et al. 2005). The genes contributing to Familial Colorectal Cancer Type X are as yet unknown.

2.6 Peutz-Jeghers syndrome

Peutz-Jeghers syndrome is a rare autosomal dominant condition with an estimated incidence of 1 in 200,000 births first described by Peutz in 1921. It is characterized by childhood onset of hamartomatous polyps in the gastrointestinal tract and by mucocutaneous pigmentation of the lips and buccal mucosa. Mutations in *LKB1* (*STK11*) are the only known cause of Peutz-Jeghers syndrome. *LKB1* mutations have been found in 50-94% of individuals with classic features of this disorder indicating that there may be locus heterogeneity (Boardman et al. 2000; Volikos et al., 2006; Aretz et al., 2005). The penetrance for GI polyps in this syndrome is 100%. There is also a 76-85% lifetime risk of cancer which includes lifetime risks of 40% for colon cancer, 30-60% for gastric cancer, 15-30% for small intestinal cancer and 11-35% for pancreatic cancer (Hearle et al., 2006, van Lier et al., 2010; van Lier et al., 2011). Breast and gynaecological cancers can be seen at high frequencies. There is a high mortality associated with this syndrome with a median age of death at 45 years of life, mostly due to cancer or bowel intussusceptions (van Lier et al., 2011).

2.7 Cowden syndrome

Cowden syndrome is an autosomal dominant syndrome with features of skin lesions, macrocephaly, thyroid manifestations and hamartomatous polyps of the GI tract. It is caused by mutations in the *PTEN* gene. Although this disorder and an allelic disorder Bannayan-Ruvalcaba-Riley Syndrome are both characterized by many hamartomatous polyps, there is no clear increased risk of colon cancer associated with Cowden syndrome.

2.8 Juvenile Polyposis

Hereditary juvenile polyposis (JP) is defined as the presence of 10 or more juvenile polyps. These polyps are primarily hamartomatous. The typical age of diagnosis is between the ages of 5 and 15 years (Merg & Howe, 2004). Most children are brought to medical attention because of colorectal bleeding. The risk of CRC associated with JP varies from 20-50% depending on the study and the gene which is mutated. (Handra-Luca et al., 2005). In addition to CRC, there is a significant risk of upper GI cancers. JP is inherited as an autosomal dominant syndrome. Multiple genes have been implicated in this disorder. The majority of mutations in individuals with JP have been found in *SMAD4* and *BMPR1A*. Individuals with *BMPR1A* mutations have a higher risk of cancers including those of the stomach, pancreas and small bowel. Mutations have also been found in *PTEN*, but these may be misdiagnosed cases of Cowden syndrome. There have been reports of *SMAD4* mutations in families with features of both juvenile polyposis and hereditary hemorrhagic telangiectasia (Gallione et al., 2004). Not all individuals with features of JP have identifiable mutations implicating additional as yet unidentified genes (Handra-Luca et al., 2005).

2.9 Hereditary mixed polyposis

Hereditary mixed polyposis (HMP) is an autosomal dominant condition characterized by polyps of mixed histology including adenomatous, hyperplastic and atypical juvenile types. Mutations in *BMPR1A* have been found in a proportion of families presenting with polyps of mixed type (Cheah et al., 2009). Despite the observation that families with both juvenile polyps and hereditary mixed polyposis can have mutations in *BMPR1A*, families with HMP are less likely to have juvenile type polyps and have an older age of diagnosis in adulthood (Merg & Howe, 2004). A locus for HMP, called *CRAC1* or *HMPS*, has been mapped to chromosome 15q13-q14 in multiple in several Ashkenazi Jewish families, but the gene has not yet been identified (Jaeger et al., 2008).

2.10 Hyperplastic polyposis (HPP)

Hyperplastic polyposis syndrome (HPP) is not yet well defined, but is characterized by multiple or large hyperplastic or serrated polyps and an association with an increased risk of CRC. The range of polyps has been described from 5 to over 100 and the pathology of the polyps can be diverse. HPP is often diagnosed in the fifth through seventh decade of life. The frequency of CRC in individuals with HPP ranges from 25-50% (Lage et al., 2004; Kalady et al., 2011). About 30% of individuals with HPP have a family history of CRC. The inheritance pattern of HPP is not well defined, but a few characterized families show possible recessive inheritance (Young & Jass, 2006). A germline mutation in *EPHB2* was identified in an individual who had more than 100 hyperplastic polyps, but *EPHB2* mutations have not been observed in other HPP cases (Kokko et al., 2006). Thus, the causal genes for most individuals with HPP have yet to be identified.

2.11 Rare cancer predisposition syndromes and risk of colon cancer

Whereas many hereditary cancer syndromes have specific cancers which occur at greater frequency than the general population, a few syndromes have elevated risks of many different types of cancer. Li-Fraumeni syndrome (LFS) is a rare autosomal dominant inherited condition caused by germline mutations in *TP53*. The classical types of cancer seen in individuals with LFS include breast cancer, sarcomas, brain tumors, leukemia and adrenal cortical tumours; however, there is also an increased risk of colon cancer of 2.8-fold over the general population (Ruijs et al., 2010).

3. Moderate risk alleles

Familial clusters of colon cancer account for approximately 20% of all CRC cases, however, most of these cases will not be due to the known CRC syndromes (Burt et al., 1990). A familial cluster is multiple individuals within families who have a similar presentation, but no clear inheritance pattern of disease transmission. The risk of colon cancer is increased to individuals who have a relative with CRC or adenomas; first-degree relatives of affected individuals have a two- to three-fold increase in risk and when more than one first-degree relative is affected the risk increases to nearly four-fold (Butterworth et al., 2006; Taylor et al. 2010). To date, moderate-risk alleles (ORs of 3-5) have not been identified. It is possible that some families exhibiting clustering of CRC may have multiple low-penetrance alleles which work synergistically to increase risk.

4. Low-penetrance risk alleles

The majority of genetic risk for CRC in the population is likely to be due to low-penetrance susceptibility alleles which act with other low-pentrance variants and the environment. A debate in the field is whether most of the genetic risk will be due to common variants with low effects and allele frequencies greater than 1% or rare or unique variants with low to moderate effects (Bodmer, 2006). Historically, variants conferring an increased risk of CRC in the general population have been identified through cohort or population-based case/control studies looking at candidate genes, but recent genome-wide association studies (GWAS) have been quite successful in identifying well-replicated variants conferring risk. Whereas a great many studies have identified positive associations with some of these genes, the vast majority have not been consistently replicated. Lack of replication does not mean in all cases that the initial association is faulty, but could be due to differences in populations leading to differences in allele frequencies or linkage disquilibrium, environmental exposures, study design or underpowered replicate studies.

Whereas the low-penetrance variants identified to date are not particularly predictive for CRC risk on their own, several direct-to-consumer genetic testing companies include some of these variants in their analysis of genomic risks of common disease. We will highlight some of the different types of variants which have been identified through multiple types of studies as showing evidence of contribution to CRC risk.

4.1 Candidate-gene studies

The studies to assess the risk of DNA variants, mainly single nucleotide polymorphisms (SNPs), have been association case/control studies or cohort studies testing SNPs in genes with relevant biological function for CRC. Many such candidate gene studies for CRC risk have been completed. Some of these have been replicated in one or two studies, but few have stood up to repeated replication studies or meta-analyses. A meta-analysis of 50 published CRC association studies for common alleles in 13 genes found three variants: *APC* I1307K, a *HRAS1* repeat variant and *MTHFR* 677V were convincingly associated with modest CRC risk in the general population (Houlston & Tomlinson, 2001). Other genes with variants showing CRC risk in multiple studies include *NAT1*, *NAT2* and *TGFBRII* (Burt, 2010). It is possible that some of these are real associations, but are population-specific or depend upon gene-environment interactions present only in certain individuals.

Candidate genes for CRC case/control studies have been chosen in a variety of ways. Variants and genes studied include common variants in high-risk genes, genes in pathways believed to be important in CRC and genes in pathways linked to environmental factors associated with CRC. One strategy which has been under-utilized is to map loci for cancer susceptibility in the mouse and then test these genes/loci for cancer risk in human populations (Ruivenkamp et al., 2002; Ewart-Toland et al., 2005; Toland et al., 2008). A large number of cancer susceptibility and resistance loci for cancers of the lung, colon, skin, liver, and the hematopoetic system have been identified using mouse models. Two putative CRC susceptibility genes, *PTPRJ* and *AURKA,* were first identified from mouse studies (Ruivenkamp et al., 2002; Ewart-Toland et al., 2003). Variants in these genes show evidence of modest CRC risk in some human studies (Ewart-Toland et al., 2005; Toland et al., 2008).

4.2 Variants of high-risk genes

Once genes for hereditary cancer syndromes began to be identified, researchers hypothesized that common variants in these genes contribute to cancer risk in the general population. Studies on common variants of almost all hereditary CRC predisposition genes have been assessed, but only a handful of variants in these high risk genes have been determined to contribute to sporadic CRC risk.

4.2.1 Carriers of *MUTYH* mutations

Bi-allelic mutations in *MUTYH* lead to MAP as described above. Several studies have looked at the cancer risks associated with mono-allelic mutations in *MUTYH*. The range of cancer incidence associated with the Y179C allele is between 1.27 to 2-fold (Table 2, Jones et al., 2009; Tenesa et al., 2006; Theodoratou et al., 2010). As a result, colon adenomas or cancer cancer may be seen in multiple generations in families with MAP.

4.2.2 APC I1307K

One frequently described modest-risk allele is the I1307K variant in the *APC* gene. This variant is seen in approximately 6% of individuals of Ashkenazi jewish (AJ) ancestry and 28% of AJ individuals with a family history of CRC (Laken et al., 1997). Carriers of the I1307K allele have 1.5 to 2-fold increased risk of CRC compared to individuals who are non-carriers (Table 2, Dundar et al., 2007; Gryfe et al., 1999). The variant itself is not thought to change function of the APC gene, however, the change results in a stretch of eight consecutive adenosines. During replication this polyadenosine track is thought to have increased risk of somatic mutation due to polymerase slippage. Addition or loss of a single nucleotide then results in a frame-shift and non-functional *APC* gene (Laken et al., 1997). As the age of onset of CRC related to this polymorphism does not appear to differ from sporadic CRC, cancer screening beyond general population recommendations is not typically done (Petersen et al., 1999).

4.2.3 Bloom's syndrome mutation carriers

Bloom's syndrome is a rare autosomal recessive condition characterized by abnormal rates of sister chromatid exchange, growth deficiency and an increased incidence of multiple types of cancer. One in 107 individuals of AJ ancestry carries a founder mutation, designated as Blm^{Ash}, in the Bloom's syndrome gene, *BLM* (Li et al., 1998). Early studies suggested a 2-fold increase in colon cancer risk in Blm^{Ash} carriers, but this has not held up in subsequent studies (Gruber et al, 2002; Cleary et al., 2003).

4.2.4 *CHEK2*

CHEK2 is a gene important in response to DNA damage. Studies have demonstrated increased risk of breast cancer with an 1100delC polymorphism but have been inconclusive for the role of the 1100del C variant in CRC risk. However, another variant, I157T, has been associated with Lynch-syndrome like cancers and confers an increased risk of 1.4 to 2-fold of CRC (Kilpivaara et al., 2006).

4.3 Genome-wide association studies (GWAS)

With technological advances allowing the genotyping of up to millions of SNPs, the ability to interrogate the entire genome without bias has led to the identification of SNPs with reproducible, but small associations with cancer risk. The strength of these studies is that that very large numbers of samples were used, large independent replication studies have been completed and very low p-values were required to meet genome-wide significance. About 18 SNPs have been identified to date (Table 2). Interestingly, although many map near genes, none of them fall within coding regions of genes suggesting that these SNPs may play a role in gene regulation. Despite the confidence that these are "real", the variants identified through GWAS to date explain a very small percentage of the overall risk of CRC ascribed to genetics. One computational assessment estimates that there may be as many as 170 low-penetrance variants which contribute to CRC risk (Tenesa and Dunlop, 2009).

4.3.1 8q24 and rs6983267

Two of the first GWAS studies for CRC identified a variant, rs6983267, on chromosome 8q24 which was significantly associated with CRC risk (Tomlinson et al. 2007; Haiman et al. 2007). The effects were modest with ORs ranging from of 1.14 to 1.24. Additional variants on 8q24 including rs7014346, rs783728, and rs10505477 were also identified in subsequent screens (Tenesa et al. 2008; Poynter et al. 2007). Several groups have replicated these findings and show a consistent effect of the rs6983267 variant. This SNP falls into a gene-poor region on 8q24 with the closest gene, *cMYC*, 335 kb away. One study showed that the rs6983267 variant falls within an enhancer element and alleles differentially bind a WNT-related transcription-factor 7-like 2 (TCF7L2). However, correlation with expression of *MYC* has not been detected, and the exact role of this SNP in colon cancer development has yet to be definitively determined (Pomerantz et al. 2009; Tuupanen et al. 2009).

4.3.2 GWAS variants in the Bone Morphogenic Protein (BMP)/Transforming Growth Factor Beta (TGFβ) pathway

Multiple variants identified by GWAS (rs4444235, rs4939827, rs4779584, rs961253 rs10411210, rs4925386) are located near genes involved in BMP and/or TGFβ signalling (Tenesa & Dunlop, 2009). BMP proteins are positive regulators of the Wnt pathway which have long been known to be important in CRC tumorigenesis. TGFβ is a master signalling molecule controlling many processes important in cancer and cancer suppression. There is considerable overlap and interaction between the BMP and TGFβ pathways. Germline mutations in *SMAD4*, *BMPR1A* and *APC* are associated with specific hereditary colon cancer syndromes. Whereas the exact effect of these SNPs on the nearby BMP/TGFβ signalling genes is not determined, location and number of these SNPs suggest that perturbation of these pathways may be critical for CRC risk in the general population.

4.4 Population specific risk factors

One of the caveats to many of the candidate gene and GWAS studies for CRC risk to date is that they have been predominantly completed in Caucasian populations. The rs6983267

SNP	Locus	Nearby genes	OR	Type of Study	Reference
Rs6691170	1q41	*DUSP10*	1.06	GWAS	Houlston et al., 2010
Rs6687758	1q41	*DUSP10*	1.09	GWAS	Houlston et al., 2010
Rs10936599	3q26.2	*MYNN*	0.93	GWAS	Houlston et al., 2010
Rs16892766	8q23.3	*EIF3H*	1.27	GWAS	Tomlinson et al., 2008
Rs6983267	8q24	Gene desert	1.21-1.23	GWAS	Tomlinson et al. 2007; Xiong et al. 2011
Rs7014346	8q24	*POU5F1P1, DQ515897*	1.19	GWAS	Tenesa et al., 2008
Rs719725	9p24	Several	1.46	GWAS	Poynter et al. 2007
Rs10795668	10p14	*FLJ3802842*	1.23	GWAS	Tomlinson et al., 2008; Xiong et al., 2011
Rs3802842	11q23	Several	1.11-1.29	GWAS	Pittman et al., 2008; Tenesa et al., 2008; Xing et al., 2011
Rs11169552	12q13.13	*LARP4, DIP2B*	0.92*	GWAS	Houlston et al., 2010
Rs7136702	12q13.13	*LARP4, DIP2B*	1.06	GWAS	Houlston et al., 2010
Rs4444235	14q22.2	*BMP4*	1.11	GWAS	Houlston et al. 2008
Rs4779584	15q13.3	*CRAC1/ GREM1*	1.23	GWAS	Jaeger et al., 2008
Rs9929218	16q22.1	*CDH1*	0.91*	GWAS	Houlston et al. 2008
Rs4939827	18q21	*SMAD7*	1.17	GWAS	Tenesa et al., 2008; Xiong et al., 2011
Rs10411210	19q13.1	*RHPN2*	0.87*	GWAS	Houlston et al. 2008
Rs961253	20p12.3	*BMP2*	1.12-1.37	GWAS	Xiong et al., 2011
Rs4925386	20q13.3	*LAMA5*	0.93	GWAS	Houlston et al., 2010
I1307K	5q21-22	*APC*	1.5-2.0	Candidate	Dundar et al., 2007; Gryfe et al., 1999
Y179C (mono-allelic)	1p34.1	*MUTYH*	1.27-2.0	Candidate	Tenesa et al., 2006 Theodoratou et al., 2010

Table 2. Low-penetrance variants associated with CRC Risk
OR, odds ratio; *The common allele is the risk allele.

variant has been replicated in multiple ethnic groups including African-American and Chinese populations with fairly consistent results (Xiong et al., 2011; He et al. 2011). However, rs3802842 on chromosome 11q23 is associated with no increased risk in Japanese populations. A GWAS performed in Japanese CRC cases identified a novel variant, rs7758229 on chromosome 6 which has not been linked with risk in Caucasians (Cui et al.,

2011). These examples illustrate that specific variants identified by GWAS are often markers for the causal, as yet unidentified variant, which may be absent or in different linkage disquilibrium patterns with the identified SNP in other populations. Additional possibilities for the differential risk effects include different frequencies of important interacting variants or population specific gene-environment interactions. When low-penetrance variants become a part of determination of cancer risk, care should be taken to ensure that only variants which have been validated in the ethnic background of the patient be utilized.

4.5 Missing heritability: Additive effects, gene-gene and gene-environmental factors

When GWAS were first utilized they were hailed as the tool by which all low-penetrance variants for disease risk would be identified. While these screens have been successful, the variants identified to date explain less than 10% of the estimated genetic contributions to CRC which makes use of known variants for risk prediction difficult. Several possible explanations for the "missing heritability" exist. One is that much of the genetic risk of CRC will be due to rare or unique low-penetrance variants which are not detectible by population-based GWAS. A second is that synergistic or epistatic gene-gene interactions which are only detectible when taking into account interacting loci will account for the missing heritability. Gene-environmental interactions in which risk is dependent on both a variant and exposure to the environmental risk factor may also play a role. Transgenerational epigenetic effects, epigenetic alterations which are inherited through the germline and/or observed through multiple generations, may also account for some of the missing heritability (Fleming et al., 2008).

As the effects of single variants identified by candidate gene or genome-wide studies have been low, it is important to determine if there are combined effects of carrying multiple risk alleles. One study assessed three SNPs identified through GWAS (rs3802842, rs7014346, rs4939827) and found that carrying all six risk alleles confers a 2.6-fold increased risk of CRC (Tenesa et al., 2008). It is likely that CRC risk could increase if all 18 identified GWAS variants were included in the analysis. Animal models have been instrumental for demonstrating synergistic and epistatic interactions between genetic risk factors (Nagase et al. 2001). Mouse models led to the identification of several CRC susceptibility loci that interact synergistically or epistatically (van Wezel et al., 1996; van Wezel et al. 1999). Thus far, no synergistic or epistatic interactions for CRC risk have been definitively identified in human populations. As computational tools for assessing the data from GWAS studies improve, genetic interactions are likely to be identified as important factors for CRC risk in humans.

Several environmental factors including cigarette smoking, body mass index, polycyclic aromatic hydrocarbons, N-nitroso compounds, and diets high in red meat which increase exposure to heterocyclic amines have been associated with increased risk of CRC (Botteri et al. 2008; Norat et al. 2002; Pischon et al. 2006). Although many studies show contradictory results, interactions between genetic variations and environmental exposures can modify CRC risk. mEH is an enzyme important in xenobiotic activation of tobacco carcinogens. Two variants have been identified in the *mEH* gene which lead to low or high activity. A meta-analysis of several studies showed that smokers with the *mEH3* low metabolizer genotype had lower risk of colon cancer compared to smokers with a *mEH3* high metabolizer genotype suggesting that genetic variants can modify the cancer risk associated with smoking (Raimondi et al. 2009). Interactions between dietary factors and genotypes have also been observed for CRC. In one study, individuals who consumed browned red meat and had the 751Lys/Lys and 312 Asp/Asp genotypes in the *XPD* gene were at highest risk of developing CRC (Joshi et al., 2009). Much work remains to be done to fully assess gene-environment interactions for CRC.

4.6 Modifier genes for penetrance in high-risk syndromes

The risk of cancer does not reach 100% even for individuals with mutations leading to high-penetrance CRC syndromes like LS. Thus, it has been proposed that even in the context of a mutation, environmental factors and low-penetrance variants may impact cancer risk. To this end, modifier genes, alleles that modify the risk of a mutation, have been sought. Most of the studies to date have been for LS. A variant in *CHEK2*, 1100delC, has been established as a moderate risk allele for breast cancer. Some families with 1100delC mutations have CRC in addition to breast cancer. Several studies have tested this variant for risk in LS families and some found modest increases in risk in LS carriers who also have the 1100delC variant (Wasielewski et al., 2008) while others have found no increase in risk (Sanchez et al., 2005). Genes with variants conferring suggestive effects in some studies for age of diagnosis in HNPCC carriers include *CCND1, CDKN2A, AURKA, TP53, E2F2,* and *IGF1* (Talseth et al. 2008; Jones et al., 2004; Chen et al. 2009).

5. The use of genetic information for CRC treatment and prognosis

Currently, the use of germline genetic variants is not used routinely for making clinical decisions regarding colorectal cancer therapy. The bulk of research and clinical application has been with somatic tumour mutations. Despite this, germline mutations and variants have been associated with different tumor histopathology and survival outcomes.

5.1 Low-penetrance risk alleles and tumor histopathology

In addition to playing a role in overall CRC risk, studies indicate that SNPs may impact morphology and type of colon cancer. Some of the low-penetrance SNPs identified through GWAS (rs3802842, rs4939827) have higher risks for rectal cancer than colon cancer (Tanesa et al., 2008). Preliminary studies also suggest differences in risk of necrosis (rs719725), mucin production (rs96153), desmoplastic reaction (rs10411210), Crohn-like lymphocytic reaction (rs6983267, rs4444235) and moderate/well-differentiated histology (rs10795668)(Ghazi et al., 2010). The SNP rs4779584 is associated with reduced risk of death in a Chinese cohort (Xing et al. 2011), but thus far, none of the GWAS-identified variants assessed show an effect on overall survival in Caucasian populations (Tenesa et al., 2010). These studies suggest that variants may impact the development of certain subtypes of colon cancer which provide possible mechanistic insights into colon tumorigenesis and new therapeutic targets.

5.2 Variants to predict response to and off-target effects of cancer therapy

Targeted therapies for colorectal cancer have been developed based on somatic mutations occurring during tumorigenesis. In addition to targeted therapies to somatic mutations, germline variations in enzymes which process more standard chemotherapeutic agents impact prognosis and treatment response. Standard therapies for CRC include 5-fluorouracil and oxaliplatin (FOLFOX). One study looked at the role of germline variants of DNA repair pathways on metastatic CRC patients' response to FOLFOX (Lamas et al., 2011). One variant in *XPD,* Lys751Gln, was associated with longer survival, but the numbers in this study were small. Variants in *TS* and *GSTT1* have been found to be associated with response to both LV5FU2 and FOLFOX (Boige et al. 2010), and two variants in *MTHFR* (677C>T and 1298 C>A) were associated with better response to FOLFOX (Etienne-Grimaldi et al. 2010). A variant in *ERCC2*, K751Q was associated with FOLFOX-induced hematologic toxicity (Boige et al. 2010), suggesting that germline variations may also predict CRC treatment side-effects. Since the field of colon cancer pharmacogenomics is still new, it is likely that other variants important in metabolism of CRC therapeutics will be identified.

5.3 Prognosis in tumors with mismatch instability mutations

Colorectal cancers can be divided into different subtypes depending on histology and the presence or absence of specific molecular markers. Treatment and prognosis of these subtypes varies. About 15% of all CRC tumours show evidence of microsatellite instability of which a small proportion are germline mutations (Murphy et al., 2006; Salovaara et al., 2000). A meta-analysis of 32 studies correlating MSI status with clinical outcomes included patients with both germline LS mutations and sporadic MMR defects. Individuals with no evidence of MSI or with MSI-low tumours showed decreased survival (HR=0.67, 95%CI 0.53-0.83) compared to individuals with MSI-high tumours. Polymorphisms in MMR genes are also associated with specific phenotypes. In one study, individuals who carried one or more G alleles of the *MLH1* 655A>G SNP had a better outcome and less risk of vascular invasion, distant metastasis or recurrence (Nejda et al., 2009). Some studies have documented better survival in individuals with MUTYH-associated colorectal cancer compared to matched controls with colon cancer (Nielsen et al., 2010). Together these data suggest that tumours that have deficits in DNA repair capabilities through germline or somatic mutations show better survival than tumours competent in DNA repair.

6. Conclusion

In summary, just over a third of colorectal cancer risk is thought to be due to inherited genetic factors. A number of mutations in genes have been found to increase CRC in individuals with hereditary cancer syndromes. These syndromes confer a vastly increased risk of CRC over the general population and an earlier age of diagnosis. Individuals with a family history of CRC should be referred to genetics for evaluation of a genetic syndrome and for guidelines for risk-reducing strategies. In addition to highly-penetrant mutations, many variants of small effect sizes have been identified through family-based and genome-wide association based studies. Whereas many of the variants identified through GWAS have been replicated in many studies, the effect size is small, only a small part of the total genetic risk has been identified, and the clinical utility is not established. The use of germline genetic information may be of clinical utility in the prevention and treatment of CRC; yet there is much that remains to be discovered. Technological advances are yielding new insights into genetic susceptibility to CRC on the population level, but we have yet to find the aetiology of most of the genetic risk contributing to CRC.

7. Acknowledgments

This work was funded by the National Institutes of Health/National Cancer Institute (R01 CA-134461-01) and the Ohio State University Comprehensive Cancer Center. We thank Heather Hampel for thoughtful review of this manuscript.

8. References

Al-Tassan, N.; Chmiel, N.H.; Maynard, J.; Fleming, N.; Livingston, Al.L.; Williams, G.T.; Hodges, A,K.; Davies, D.R.; David, S.S.; Sampson, J.R. & Cheadle, J.P. (2002).Inherited mutations of MYH associated with somatic G:C>T:A mutations in colorectal tumors. *Nature Genetics*, Vol.30, No.2, pp.227-32, ISSN 1061-4036.

Allen, B. & Terdiman, J.P. (2003). Hereditary polyposis syndromes and hereditary non-polyposis colorectal cancer. *Best Practice & Research Clinical Gastroenterology*, Vol.17, No.2, pp.237-58, ISSN 1521-6981.

Aretz, S.; Stienen, D.; Uhlhaas, S.; Loff, S.; Back, W.; Pagenstecher, C.; McLeod, D.R.; Graham, G.E.; Mangold, E.; Santer, R.; Propping, P. & Friedl, W. (2005). High propotion of large genomic STK11 deletions in Peutz-Jeghers syndrome. *Human Mutation*, Vol.26, No.6, pp.513-9, ISSN 1098-1004.

Boardman, L.A.; Couch, F.J.; Burgart, L.J.; Schwartz, D.; Berry, R.; McDonnell, S.K.; Schaid, D.J.; Hartmann, L.C.; Schroeder, J.J.; Stratakis, C.A. & Thibodeau, S.N. (2000). Genetic heterogeneity in Peutz-Jeghers syndrome. *Human Mutation*, Vol.16, No.1, pp.23-30, ISSN 1098-1004.

Bodmer, W.F. (2006). Cancer genetics: colorectal cancer as a model. *Journal of Human Genetics*, Vol.51, No.5, pp.391-6, ISSN 1434-5161.

Boige, V.; Mendiboure, J.; Pignon, J.P, Loriot,M.A. Castaing, M.; Barrois, M.; Malka, D.; Tregouet, D.A.; Bouche, O.; Le Corre, D.; Miran, I.; Mulot, C.; Ducreux, M.; Beaune, P. & Laurent-Puig, P. (2010). Pharmacogenetic assessment of toxicity and outcome in patients with metastatic colorectal cancer treated with LV5FU2, FOLFOX and FOLFIR: FFDC 2000-05. *Journal of Clinical Oncology*, Vol.28, No.15, pp.2556-64. ISSN 0732-183X.

Botteri, E.; Iodice, S.; Bagnardi, V.; Raimondi, S.; Lowenfels, A.B. & Maisonneuve, P. (2008). Smokijng and colorectal cancer: a meta-analysis. *JAMA*, Vol.300, No.23, pp.2765-78, ISSN 0098-7484.

Burt, R.W., Bishop, D.T.; Lynch, H.T.; Rozen, P. & Winawer, S.J. (1990). Risk and surveillance of individuals with heritable factors for colorectal cancer: WHO collaborating centre for the prevention of colorectal cancer, *Bulletin of the World Health Organization*, Vol.68, No.5, pp.655-65, ISSN 0042-9686.

Burt, R.W. (2000). Colon cancer screening. *Gastoenterology*, Vol.119, No.3, pp.837-53, ISSN 0016-5085.

Butterworth, A.S.; Higgins, J.P. & Pharoah, P. (2006). Relative and absolute risk of colorectal cancer for individuals with a family history: a meta-analysis. *European Journal of Cancer*. Vol.42, No.2, pp.216-27, ISSN 0959-8049.

Cheah, P.Y.; Wong, Y.H.; Chau, Y.P.; Loi, C.; Lim, K.H.; Lim, J.F.; Koh, P.K. & Eu, K.W. (2009). Germline bone morphogenesis protein receptor 1A mutation causes colorectal tumorigenesis in hereditary mixed polyposis syndrome. *American Journal of Gastroenterology*, Vol.104, No.12, pp.3027-33, ISSN 0002-9270.

Cleary, S.P.; Zhang, W.; Di Nicola, N.; Aronson, M.; Aube, J.; Steinman, A.; Haddad, R.; Redston, M.; Gallinger, S.; Narod, S.A. & Gryfe, R. (2003). Heterozygosity for the BLM(Ash) mutation and cancer risk. *Cancer Research*, Vol.63, No.8, pp.1769-71, ISSN 1538-7445.

Chen, J.; Etzel, C.J.; Amos, C.I.; Zhang, Q.; Viscofsky, N.; Lindor, N.M.; Lynch, P.M. & Frazier, M.L. (2009). *Cancer Causes and Control*, Vol.20, No.9, pp.1769-77, ISSN 1573-7225.

Cui, R.; Okada, Y.; Jang, S.G.; Ku, J.L.; Park, J.G.; Kamatani, Y.; Hosono, N.; Tsunoda, T.; Kumar, V.; Tanikawa, C.; Kamatani, N.; Yamada, R.; Kubo, M.; Nakamura, Y.; Matsuda, K. (2011). Common variant in 6q26-q27 is associated with distal colon cancer in an Asian population. *Gut*, Vol.60, No.6, pp.799-805, ISSN 1468-3288.

de la Chapelle, A. (2004). Genetic predisposition to colorectal cancer. *Nature Reviews Cancer*, Vol.4, No.10, pp769-80, ISSN 1474-175X.

Des Guetz, G.; Mariani, P.; Cucherousset, J.; Benamoun, M.; Lagorce, C.; Sastre, X.; Le Toumelin, P.; Uzzan, B.; Perret, G.Y.; Morere, J.F.; Breau, J.L.; Fagard, R.; Schischmanoff, P.O. (2007). Microsatellite instability and sensitivitiy to FOLFOX treatment in metastatic colorectal cancer. *Anticancer Research*, Vol.27, No.4, pp.2715-9, ISSN 1791-7530.

Dundar, M.; Caglayan, A.O.; Saatci, C.; Karaca, H.; Baskol, M.; Tahiri, S. & Ozkul, Y. (2007). How the I1307K adenomatous polyposis coli gene variant contributes in the assessment of risk of colorectal cancer, but not stomach cancer in a Turkish population. *Cancer Genetics & Cytogenetics*, Vol.177, No.2, pp.95-77, ISSN 0165-4608.

Etienne-Grimaldi, M.C.; Milano, G.; Maindrault-Goebel, F.; Chibaudel, B.; Formento, J.L.; Francoual, M.; Lledo, G.; Andre, T.; Mabro, M.; Mineur, L.; Flesch, M.; Carola, E. & de Gramont, A. (2010). Methylenetetrahydrofolate reductase (MTHFR) gene polymorphisms and FOLFOX response in colorectal cancer patients. *British Journal of Clinical Pharmacology*, Vol.69, No.1, pp.58-66, ISSN 1365-2125.

Ewart-Toland, A.; Briassouli, P.; de Koning, J.P.; Mao, J.H.; Yuan, J.; Chan, F.; MacCarthy-Morrogh, L.; Ponder, B.A.; Nagase, H.; Burn, J.; Ball, S.; Almeida, M.; Linardopoulous, S. & Balmain, A. (2003). *Nature Genetics*, Vol.34, No.4, pp.403-12, ISSN 1061-4036.

Ewart-Toland, A.; Dai, Q.; Gao, Y.T.; Nagase, H.; Dunlop, M.G.; Farrington, S.M.; Barnetson, R.A.; Anton-Culver, H.; Peel, D.; Ziogas, A.; Lin, D.; Miao, X.; Sun, T.; Ostrander, E.A.; Stanford, J.L.; Langlois, M.; Chan, J.M.; Yuan, J.; Harris, C.C.; Bowman, E.D.; Clayman, G.L.; Lippman, S.M.; Lee, J.J.; Zheng, W. & Balmain, A. (2005). Aurora-A/STK15 T+91A is a general low penetrance cancer susceptibility gene: a meta-analysis of multiple cancer types. *Carcinogenesis*, Vol.26, No.8, pp1368-73, ISSN 1460-2180.

Farrington, S.M. Tenesa, A.; Barnetson, R.; Wiltshire, A.; Prendergast J.; Porteous, M.; Campbell, H. & Dunlop, M.G. (2005). Germline susceptibility to colorectal cancer due to base-excision repair gene defects. *American Journal of Human Genetics*, Vol.77, No.1, pp.112-9, ISSN 0002-9297.

Felton, K.E.; Gilchrist, D.M.; & Andrew, S.E. (2007). Constitutive deficiency in DNA mismatch repair: is it time for Lynch III? *Clinical Genetics*, Vol.71, No.6, pp.499-500, ISSN 1339-0004.

Filipe, B.; Baltazar, C.; Albuquerque, C.; Fragosi, S.; Lage, P.; Vitoriano, I.; Mao de Ferro, S.; Claro, I.; Rodrigues, P.; Fidalgo, P.; Chaves, P.; Cravo, M. & Nobre Leitao, C. (2009). APC or MUTYH mutations account for the majority of clinically well-characterized families with FAP or AFAP phenotype and patients with more than 30 adenomas. *Clinical Genetics*, Vol.76, No.3, pp.242-55. ISSN 1399-0004.

Fleming, J.L.; Huang, T.H. & Toland, A.E. (2008). The role of parental and grandparental epigenetic alterations in familial cancer risk. *Cancer Research*, Vol.68, No.22, pp.9116-21, ISSN 1538-7445.

Gallione, C.; Aylsworth, A.S.; Beis, J.; Berk, T.; Bernhardt, B.; Clark, R.D.; Clericuzio, C.; Danesino, C.; Drautz, J.; Fahl, J.; Fan, Z.; Faughman, M.E.; Ganguly, A.; Garvie, J.; Henderson, K.; Kini, U.; Leedom, T.; Ludman, M.; Luz, A.; Maisenbacher, M.; Mazzucco, S.; Olivieri, C.; van Amstel, J.K.Pl; Prigoda-Lee, N.; Pyeritz, R.E.; Reardon, W.; Vandezande, K.; Waldman, J.D.; White, R.I.; Williams, C.A. & Marchuck, D.A. (2010). Overlapping spectra of *SMAD4* mutations in juvenile polyposis (JP) and JP-HHT syndrome. *American Journal of Medical Genetics Part A*, Vol.152A, No.2, pp333-9, ISSN 1552-4833.

Ghazi, S.; von Holst, S.; Picelli, S.; Linforss, U.; Tenesa, A.; Farrington, S.M.; Campbell, H.; Dunlop, M.G.; Papadogiannakis, N.; Lindblom, A.; Low-Risk Colorectal Cancer Study Group. (2010). Colorectal cancer susceptibility loci in a population-based study:Associations with morphological parameters. *American Journal of Pathology*, Vol.177, No.6, pp.2688-93, ISSN 0002-9440.

Gomez-Fernandez, N.; Castellvi-Bel, S.; Fernandez-Rozadilla, C.; Balaguer, F.; Munoz, J.; Madrigal, I.; Mila, M.; Grana, B.; Vega, A.; Castells, A.; Carracedo, A. & Ruiz-Ponte, C. (2009). Molecular analysis of the APC and MUTYH genes in Galician and Catalonian FAP families: a different spectrum of mutations? *BMC Medical Genetics*, Vol.10, pp.57, ISSN 1471-2350.

Goodenberger, M. & Lindor, N. (2011). Lynch syndrome and MYH-associated polyposis: review and testing strategy. *Journal of Clinical Gastroenterology*, Vol.45, No.6, pp.488-500, ISSN 0192-0790.

Gruber, S.B.; Ellis, N.A.; Scott, K.K.; Almog, R.; Kolachana, P.; Bonner, J.D.; Kirchoff, T.; Tomsho, L.P; Nafa, K.; Pierce, H.; Low, M.; Satagopah, J.; Rennert, H.; Huang, H.; Greenson, J.K.; Groden, J.; Rapaport, B.; Shia, J.; Johnson, S.; Gergersen, P.K.; Harris, C.C.; Boyd, J.; Rennert, G. & Offit, K. (2002). BLM heterozygosity and the risk of colorectal cancer. *Science*, Vol.297, No.5589, ISSN 1095-9203.

Gryfe, R.; Di Nicola, N.; Lal, G.; Gallinger, S. & Redston, M. (1999). Inherited colorectal polyposis and cancer risk of the APC I1307K polymorphism. *American Journal of Human Genetics*, Vol.64, No.2, pp.378-84, ISSN 0002-9297.

Haiman, C.A.; Le Marchand, L.; Yamamato, J.; Stram, D.O.; Sheng, X.; Kolonel, L.N.; Wu, A.H.; Reich, D. & Henderson, B.E. (2007). A common genetic risk factor for colorectal and prostate cancer. *Nature Genetics*, Vol.39, No.8, pp.954-6, ISSN 1061-4036.

Hampel H.; Frankel, W.L.; Martin, E.; Arnold, M.; Khanduja, K.; Kuebler, P.; Clendenning, M.; Sotamaa, K.; Prior, T.; Westman, J.A.; Panescu, J.; Fix, D.; Lockman, J.; LaJeunesse, J, Comeras, I. & de la Chapelle, A. (2008). Feasibility of screening for Lynch syndrome among patients with colorectal cancer. *Journal of Clinical Oncology*, Vol.26, No.35 , pp.5783-8, ISSN 1527-7755.

Handra-Luca, A.; Condroyer, C.; de Moncuit, C.; Tepper, M.; Flejou, J.-F.; Thomas, G. & Olschwang, S. (2005). Vessels' morphology in SMAD4 and BMPR1A-related juvenile polyposis. *American Journal of Medical Genetics Part A*, Vol.138A, No.2, pp.113-117, ISSN 1552-4833.

He, J.; Wilkens, L.R.; Stram, D.O.; Kolonel, L.N.; Henderson, B.E.; Wu, A.H.; Le Marchand, L. & Haiman, C.A. (2011). Generalizability and epidemiologic characterization of eleven colorectal cancer GWAS hits in multiple populations. *Cancer Epidemiology, Biomarkers & Prevention*, Vol.20, No.1, pp.70-81, ISSN 1055-9965.

Hearle, N.; Schumacher, V.; Menko, F.H.; Olschwang, S.; Boardman, L.A.; Gille, J.J.P.; Keller, J.J.; Westerman, A.M.; Scott, R.J.; Lim, W.; Trimbath, J.D.; Giardiello, F.M.; Gruber, S.B.; Offerhaus, G.J.A.; de Rooij, F.W.M.; Wilson, J.H.P.; Hansmann, A.; Moslein, G.; Royer-Polora, B.; Voget, T.; Phillips, R.K.S.; Spigelman, A.D. & Houlston, R.S. (2006). Frequency and sprectrum of cancers in the Peutz-Jeghers syndrome. *Clinical Cancer Research*, Vol.12, No.10, pp.3209-15, ISSN 1557-3265.

Houlston, R.S; Webb, E.; Broderick, P.; Pittman, A.M.; Di Bernardo, M.C.; Lubbe, S.; Chandler, I.; Vijayakrishnan, J.; Sullivan, K.; Penegar, S.; Colorectal Cancer Association Study Consortium, Carvajal-Carmona, L.; Howarth, K.; Jaeger, E.; Spain, S.L.; Walther, A.; Barclay, E.; Martin, L.; Gorman, M.; Domingo, E.; Teixeira, A.S.; CoRGI Consortium, Kerr, D.; Cazier, J.B.; Nittymaki, I.; Tuupanen, S.; Karhu, A.; Aaltonen, L.A.; Tomlinson, I.P.; Farrington, S.M.; Tenesa, A.; Prendergast, J.G.; Barnetson, R.A.; Cetnarskyj, R.; Poretous, M.E.; Paroah, P.D.; Koessler, T.; Hampe, J.; Buch, S.; Schafmayer, C.; Tepel, J.; Schreiber, S.; Volzke, H.; Chang-Claude, J.; Hoffmeister, M.; Brenner, H.; Zanke, B.W.; Montpetit, A.; Hudson, T.J.; Gallinger, S.; International Colorectal Cancer Genetic Association Consortium, Campbell, H.; Dunlop, M.G. (2008). Meta-analysis of genome-wide association data identifies four new susceptibility loci for colorectal cancer. *Nature Genetics*, Vol. 40, No.12, pp.1426-35, ISSN 1061-4036.

Houlston, R.S.; Cheadle, J.; Dobbins, S.E.; Tenesa, A.; Jones, A.M.; Howarth, K.; Spain, S.L; Broderick, P.; Domingo, E.; Farrington, S.; Prendergast, J.G.; Pittman, A.M. Theodoratou, E.; Smith, C.G.; Olver, B.; Walther, A.; Barnetson, R.A.; Churchman, M.; Jaeger, E.E.; Penegar, S.; Barclay, E.; Martin, L.; Gorman, M.; Mager, R.; Johnstone, E.; Midgley, R.; Nittymaki, I. Tuupanen, S.; Colley, J.; Idziaszczyk, S.; COGENT Consortium; Thomas, H.J.; Lucassen, A.M.; Evans, D.G.; Maher, E.R.; CORGI Consortium; COIN Collaborative Group; COINB Collaborative Group, Maughan, T.; Dimas, A. Dermitzakis, E.; Cazier, J.B.; Aaltonen, L.A.; Pharoah, P.; Kerr, D.J.; Carvajal-Carmona, L.G.; Campbell, H.; Dunlop, M.G. & Tomlinson, I.P. (2010). Meta-analysis of three genome-wide association studies identifies loci for colorectal cancer at 1q41, 3q26.2, 12q13.13 and 20q13.33. *Nature Genetics*, Vol.42, No.11, pp.973-7, ISSN 1061-4036.

Houlston, R.S. & Tomlinson, I.P.M. (2001). Polymorphisms and colorectal cancer risk. *Gastroenterology*, Vol.121, No.2, pp.282-301, ISSN 0016-5085.

Jaeger, E.; Webb, E.; Howarth, K.; Carvajal-Carmona, L.; Rowan, A.; Broderick, P.; Walther, A.; Spain, S.; Pittman, A.; Kemp, Z.; Sullivan, K.; Heinimann, K.; Lubbe, S.; Domingo, E.; Barclay, E.; Martin, L.; Gorman, M.; Chandler, I.; Vijayakrishnan, J.; Wood, W.; Papaemmanuil, E.; Penegar, S.; Qureshi, M.; CORGI Consortium; Farrington, S.; Tenesa, A.; Cazier, J.B.; Kerr, D.; Gray, R.; Peto, J.; Dunlop, M.; Campbell, H.; Thomas, H.; Houlston, R.; & Tomlinson, I. (2008). Common genetic variants at the CRAC1 (HMPS) locus on chromosome 15q13.3 influence colorectal cancer risk. *Nature Genetics*, Vol.40, No.1, pp.26-8, ISSN 1061-4036.

Jasperson, K.W.; Tuohy, T.M.; Neklason, D.W. & Burt, R.W. (2010). Hereditary and familial colon cancer. *Gastroenterology*, Vol.138, No.6, pp.2044-58, ISSN 0016-5085.

Jass, J.R.; Cottier, D.S.; Jeevaratnam, P.; Pokos, V.; Holdaway, K.M.; Bowden, Ml.L. Van de Water, N.S. & Browett, P.J. (1995). Diagnostic use of microsatellite instability in hereditary non-polyposis colorectal cancer. *Lancet*, Vol.346, No.8984, pp.1200-1, ISSN 0140-6736.

Jones, J.S.; Chi, X.; Gu, X.; Lynch, P.M.; Amos, C.I. & Frazier, M.L. (2004). P53 polymorphism and age of onset of hereditary nonpolyposis colorectal cancer in a Caucasian population. *Clinical Cancer Research*, Vol.10, No.17, pp.5845-9, ISSN 1557-3265.

Jones, N.; Vogt, S.; Nielsen, M.; Christian, D.; Wark, P.A.; Ecceles, D.; Edwards, E.; Evans, D.G.; Maher, E.R.; Vasen, H.F.; Hes, F.J.; Aretz, S. & Sampson, J.R. (2009). Increeased colorectal cancer incidence in obligate carriers of heterozygous mutations in MUTYH. *Gastroenterology*, Vol.137, No.2, pp.489-94, ISSN 0016-5085.

Joshi, A.D.; Corral, R.; Siegmund, K.D.; Haile, R.W.; Le Marchard, L.; Martinez, M.E.; Ahnen, D.J.; Sandler, R.S.; Lance, P. & Stern, M.C. (2009). Red meat and poultry intake, polymorphisms in the nucleotide excision repair and mismatch repair pathways and colorectal cancer risk. *Carcinogenesis*, Vol.30, No.3, pp.472-9, ISSN 1460-2180.

Kalady, M.; Jarrar, A.; Leach, B.; LaGuardia, L.; O'Malley, M.; Eng, C. & Church, J. (2011). Defining phenotypes and cancer risk in hyperplastic polyposis syndrome. *Diseases of the Colon & Rectum*, Vol.54, No.2, ISSN 0012-3706.

Kaz, A.M. & Brentnall, T.A. (2006). Genetic testing for colon cancer. *Nature Clinical Practice Gastroenterology and Hepatology*, Vol.3, No.12, pp.670-9, ISSN 1743-4378.

Kempers, M.J.; Kuiper, R.P.; Ockeloen, C.W.; Chappuis, P.O.; Hutter, P.; Raner, N.; Schackert, H.K.; Steinke, V.; Holinski-Feder, E.; Morak, M.; Kloor, M.; Buttner, R.; Verwiel, E.T.; van Krieken, J.H.; Nagtegaal, I.D.; Goossens, M.; van der Post, R.S.; Niessen, R.C.; Sijmons, R.H.; Kluijt, I.; Hogervorst, F.B.; Leter, E.M.; Gille, J.J.; Aalfs, C.M.; Redkere, E.J.; Hes, F.J.; Tops, C.M.; van Nesselrooij, B.P.; van Gijn, M.E.; Gomez Garcia, E.B.; Eccles, D.M.; Bunyan, D.J.; Syngal, S.; Stoffel, E.M.; Culber, J.O.; Palomares, M.R.; Garham, T.; Velsher, L.; Papp, J.; Olah, E.; Chan, T.L.; Leung, S.Y.; van Kessel, A.G.; Kiemeney, L.A.; Hoogerbrugge, N. & Ligtenberg, M.J. (2011). Risk of colorectal and endometrial cancers in EPCAM deletion-positive Lynch syndrome: a cohort study. *Lancet Oncology*, Vol.12, No.1, pp.49-55, ISSN 1470-2045.

Kilpivaara, O.; Alhopuro, P.; Vaheristo, P.; Aaltonen, L.A. & Nevanlinna, H. (2006). CHEK2 I157T associates with familial and sporadic colorectal cancers. *Journal of Medical Genetics*, Vol.43, No.7, p.e34, ISSN 1468-6244.

Kokko, A.; Laiho, P.; Lehtonen, R.; Korja, S.; Carvajal-Carmona, L.G.; Jarvinen, H.; Mecklin, J.P.; Eng, C.; Schleutker, J.; Tomlinson, I.; Vahteristo, P. & Aaltonen, L.A. (2006). EPHB2 germline variants in patients with colorectal cancer or hyperplastic polyposis. *BMC Cancer*, Vol.6, pp.145. ISSN 1471-2407.

Lage, P.; Cravo, M.; Sousa, R.; Chaves, P.; Salazar, M.; Fonseca, R.; Claro, I.; Suspiro, A.; Rodrigues, P.; Raposo, H.; Fidalgo, P. & Nobre-Leitao, C. (2004). Management of Portugese patients with hyperplastic polyposis and screening of at-risk first-degree relatives: a contribution for future guidelines based on a clinical study. *American Journal of Gastroenterology*, Vol.99, No.9, pp.1779-84, ISSN 0002-9270.

Laken, S.J.; Petersen, G.M.; Gruber, S.B.; Oddoux, C.; Ostrer, H.; Giardiello, F.M.; Hamilton, S.R.; Hampel, H.; Markowitz, A.; Klimstra, D.; Jhanwar, S.; Winawer, S.; Offit, K.;Luce, M.C.; Kinzler, K.W. & Vogelstein, B. (1997). Familial colorectal cancer in Ashkenazim due to a hypermutable tract in APC. *Nature Genetics*, Vol.17, No., pp.79-83, ISSN 1061-4036.

Lamas, M.J.; Duran, G.; Balboa, E.; Bernardez, B.; Touris, M.; Vidal, Y.; Gallardo, E.; Lopez, R.; Carracedo, A. & Barros, F. (2011). Use of a comprehensive panel of biomarkers to predict response to a fluorouracil-oxaliplatin regimen in patients with metastatic colorectal cancer. *Pharmacogenomics*, Vol.12, No.3, pp. 433-442, ISSN 1462-2416.

Lammi, L.; Arte, S.; Somer, M.; Jarvinen, H.; Lahermo, P.; Thesleff, I.; Pirinen, S.; Nieminen, P. (2004). Mutations in AXIN2 cause familial tooth agenesis and predispose to colorectal cancer. *American Journal of Human Genetics*, Vol.74, No.5, pp.1043-50, ISSN 0002-9297.

Li, L.; Eng, C.; Desnick, R.J.; German, J. & Ellis, N.A. (1998). Carrier frequency of the Bloom syndrome blmAsh mutation in the Ashkenazi Jewish population. *Molecular Genetics and Metabolism*, Vol.64, No.4, pp.286-90, ISSN 1096-7192.

Lichtenstein, P.; Holm, N.V.; Verkasalo, N.V.; Iliadou, A. Kaprio, J.; Koskenvuo, M.; Pukkala, E.; Skytthe, A. & Hemminki, K. (2000). Environmental and heritablefactors in the causation of cancer: analyses of cohorts of twins from Sweden, Denmark, and Finland. *New England Journal of Medicine*, Vol.343, No.2, pp.78-84, ISSN 1533-4406.

Lim, W.; Hearle, N.; Shah, B.; Murday, V.; Hodgson, S.V.; Lucassen, A.; Eccles, D.; Talbot, I.; Neale, K.; Lim, A.G.; O'Donohue, J.; Donaldson, A.; Macdonald, R.C.; Young, I.D.; Robinson, M.H.; Lee, P.W.; Stoodley, B.J.; Tomlinson, I.; Alderson, D.; Holbrook, A.Gl.; Vyas, S.; Swarbrick, E.T.; Lewis, A.A.; Phillips, R.K. & Houlston, R.S. (2003). Further observations on LKB1/STK11 status and cancer risk in Peutz-Jeghers syndrome. *British Journal of Cancer*, Vol.98, No.2, pp.308-13, ISSN 0007-0920.

Lindor, N.M.; Rabe, K.; Petersen, G.M.; Haile, R.; Casey, G.; Baron, J.; Gallinger, S.; Bapat, S.; Aronson, M.; Hopper, J.; Jass, J.; LeMarchand, L.; Grove, J.; Potter, J.; Newcomb, P.; Terdiman, J.P.; Conrad, P.; Moslein, G.; Goldberg, R.; Ziogas, A.; Anton-Culver, H.; de Andrade, M.; Siegmund, K.; Thibodeau, S.N.; Boardman, L.A. & Seminara, D. (2005).Lower cancer incidence in Amsterdam-I criteria families without mismatch repair deficiency: familial colorectal cancer type X. *JAMA*, Vol.293, No.16, pp.1979-85, ISSN 0098-7484.

Lubbe, S.J.; Di Bernardo, M.C.; Chandler, I.P. & Houlston, R.S. (2009). Clinical implications of the colorectal cancer risk associated with MUTYH mutation. *Journal of Clinical Oncology*, Vol.27, No.23, pp.3975-80, ISSN 1527-7755.

Lynch, H. & de la Chapelle, A. (2003). Hereditary colorectal cancer, *New England Journal of Medicine*, Vol.348, No.10, pp.919-32, ISSN 1533-4406.

Merg, A. & Howe, J.R. (2004). Genetic conditions associated with intestinal juvenile polyps. *American Journal of Medical Genetics*, Vol.129c, No. 1, pp.44-55, ISSN 1552-4825.

Murphy, K.M.; Zhang, S.; Geiger, T.; Hafez, M.J.; Bacher, J.; Berg, K.D. & Eshleman, J.R. (2006). *Journal of Molecular Diagnostics*, Vol.8, No.3, pp.305-11, ISSN 1525-1578.

Nagase, H.; Mao, J.H.; de Koning, J.P. Minami, T. & Balmain. A. (2001). Epistatic interactions between skin tumor modifier loci in interspecific (spretus/musculus) backcross mice. *Cancer Research*, Vol.61, No.4, pp.1305-8, ISSN 1538-7445.

Nejda, N.; Iglesias, D.; Moreno Azcoita, M.; Medina Arana, V.; Gonzalez-Aguilera, J.J. & Prenandez-Peralta, A.M. (2009). A *MLH1* polymorphism that increase cancer risk is associated with better outcome in sporadic cancer. *Cancer Genetics & Cytogenetics*, Vol.193, No.2, pp.71-7, ISSN 0165-4608.

Nielsen, M.; Hes, F.J.; Nagengast, F.M.; Weiss, M.M.; Mathus-Vliegen, E.M.; Morreau, H.; Breuning, M.H.; Wijnen, J.T.; Tops, C.M.J.; Vasen, H.F.A. (2007). Germline mutations in APC and MUTYH are responsible for the majority of families with attenuated familial adenomatous polyposis. *Clinical Genetics*, Vol. 71, No.5, pp.427-33. ISSN 1399-0004.

Nielsen, M.; van Steenbergen, L.N.; Jones, N.; Vogt, S.; Vasen, H.F.A.; Morreau, H.; Aretz, S.; Sampson, J.R.; Dekkers, O.M.; Janssen-Heijnen, M.L.G. & Hes, F.J. (2010). Survival of MUTYH-associated polyposis patients with colorectal cancer and matched control colorectal cancer patients. *Journal of the National Cancer Institute*, Vol.102, No.22, pp.1724-1730, ISSN 1460-2105.

Niessen, R.C.; Hofstra, R.M.; Westers, H.; Ligtenberg, M.J.; Kooi, K.; Jager, P.O.; de Groote, M.L.; Dijkhuizen, T.; Olderode-Berends, M.J.; Hollema, H.; Kleibeuker, J.H.& Sijmons, R.H. (2009a). Germline hypermethylation of *MLH1* and *EPCAM* deletions are a frequent cause of Lynch syndrome. *Genes Chromosomes Cancer*, Vol.48, No.8, pp.737-44, ISSN 1098-2264.

Niessen, R.C.; Kleibeuker, J.H.; Westers, H.; Jager, P.O.; Roseveld, D.; Bos, K.K.; Boersma-van Ek, W.; Hollema, H.; Sijmons, R.H. & Hofstra, R.M. (2009b). PMS2 involement in patients suspected of Lynch syndrome. *Genes Chromosomes Cancer*, Vol.48, No.4, pp.322-9, ISSN 1098-2264.

Norat, T.; Lukanova, A.; Ferrari, P. & Riboli, E. (2002). Meat consumption and colorectal cancer risk: dose-dependent meta-analysis of epidemiological studies. *International Journal of Cancer*, Vol.98, No.2, pp.241-56, ISSN 1097-0215.

Peterson, G.M.; Slack, J.; Nakamura, Y. (1991). Screening guidelines and premorbid diagnosis of familial adenomatous polyposis using linkage. *Gastroenterology*, Vol.100, No.6, pp. 1658-64, ISSN 0016-5085.

Petersen, G.M.; Brensinger, J.D.; Johnson, K.A. & Giardiello, F.M. (1999). Genetic testing and counseling for hereditary forms of colorectal cancer. *Cancer*, Vol.86, No. 11Suppl, pp.2450-50, ISSN 1097-0142.

Pischon, T.; Lahmann, P.H.; Boening, H.; Friedenreich, C.; Norat, T, Tjonneland, A.; Halkjaer, J.; Overvad, K.; Clavel-Chapelon, F.; Boutron-Rualut, M.C.; Guernec, G.; Bergmann, M.M.; Linseisen, J.; Becker, N.; Trichopoulou, A.; Trichopoulos, D.; Sieri, S.; Palli, D.; Tumino, R.; Vineis, P., Panico, S.; Peeters, P.H.; Bueno-de-Mesquita, H.B.; Boshuizen, H.C.; Van Guelpen, B.; Palmqvist, R.; Berglund, G.; Gonzalez, C.A.; Dorronsoro, M.; Barricarte, A.; Navarro, C.; Martinez, C.; Quiros, J.R.; roddam, A.; Allen, N.; Bingham, S.; Khaw, K.T.; Ferrari, P.; Kaaks, R.; Slimani, N. & Riboli, E. (2006). Body size and risk of colon and rectal cancer in the European Prospective Investigation into cancer and nutrition (EPIC). *Journal of the National Cancer Institute*, Vol.98, No.13, pp.320-31, ISSN 1460-2105.

Pittman, A.M.; Webb, E.; Carvajal-Carmona, L.; Howarth, K.; Di Bernardo, M.C.; Broderick, P.; Spain, S.; Walther, A.; Price, A.; Sullivan, K.; Twiss, P.; Fielding, S.; Rowan, A.; Jaeger, E.; Vijayakrishnan, J.; Chandler, I.; Penegar, S.; Qureshi, M.; Lubbe, S.; Domingo, E.; Kemp, Z.; Barclay, E.; Wood, W.; Martin, L.; Gorman, M.; Thomas,

H.; Peto, J.; Bishop, T.; Gray, R.; Maher, E.R.; Lucassen, A.; Kerr, D.; Evans, G.R.; CORGI Consortium; van Wezel, T.; Morreau, H.; Wijnen, J.T.; Hopper, J.L.; Southey, M.C.; Giles, G.G.; Severi, G.; Castellví-Bel, S.; Ruiz-Ponte, C.; Carracedo, A.; Castells, A.; EPICOLON Consortium; Försti, A.; Hemminki, K.; Vodicka, P.; Naccarati, A.; Lipton, L.; Ho, J.W.; Cheng, K.K.; Sham, P.C.; Luk, J.; Agúndez, J.A.; Ladero, J.M.; de la Hoya, M.; Caldés, T.; Niittymäki, I.; Tuupanen, S.; Karhu, A.; Aaltonen, L.A.; Cazier, J.B.; Tomlinson, I.P. & Houlston, R.S. (2008). Refinement of the basis and impact of common 11q23.1 variation to the risk of developing colorectal cancer. *Human Molecular Genetics*, Vol.17, No.23, pp.3720-7, ISSN 1460-2083.

Pomerantz, M.M., Ahmadiyeh, N.; Jia, L.; Herman, P.; Verzi, M.P.; Doddapaneni, H.; Beckwith, C.A.; Chan, J.A.; Hills, A.; Davis, M.; Yao, K.; Kehoe, S.M.; Lenz, H.J.; Haiman, C.A.; Yan, C.; Henderson, B.E.; Frenkel, B.; Barretina, J.; Bass, A.; Tabernero, J.; Baselga, J.; Regan, M.M.; Manak, J.R.; Shivdasani, R.; Coetzee, G.A. & Freedman, M.L. (2009). The 8q24 cancer risk variant rs6983267 shows long-range interaction with MYC in colorectal cancer. *Nature Genetics*, Vol.41, No.8, pp.882-4, ISSN 1061-4036.

Poynter, J.N.; Figueiredo, J.C.; Conti, D.V.; Kennedy, K.; Gallinger, S.; Siegmund, K.D.; Casey, G.; Thibodeau, S.N.; Jenkins, M.A.; Hopper, J.L.; Byrnes, G.B.; Baron, J.A.; Goode, E.L.; Tiirikainen, M.; Lindor, N.; Grove, J.; Newcomb, P.; Jass, J.; Young, J.; Potter, J.D.; Haile, R.W.; Duggan, D.J.; Le Marchand, L. & Colon C.F.R. (2007). Variants on 9p24 and 8q24 are associated with risk of colorectal cancer: results from the Colon Cancer Family Registry. *Cancer Research*, Vol.63, No.23, pp.11128-32, ISSN 1538-7445.

Raimondi, S.; Botteri, E.; Iodice, S.; Lowenfels, A.B.; & Maisonneuve, P. (2009). Gene-smoking interaction on colorectal adenoma and cancer risk: review and meta-analysis. *Mutation Research*, Vol.670, No.1-2, pp.6-14, ISSN 0921-8262.

Ramsoekh, D.; Wagner, A.; van Leerdam, M.E.; Dooijes, D.; Tops, C.M>; Steyerberg, E.W.; Kuipers, E.J. (2009). Cancer risk in MLH1, MSH2, and MSH6 mutation carriers; different risk profiles may influence clinical management. *Hereditary Cancer in Clinical Practice*, Vol.23, No.1, pp.17, ISSN 1897-4287.

Ribic, C.M.; Sargent, D.J.; Moore, M.J.; Thibodeau, S.N.; French, A.J.; Goldberg, R.M.; Hamilton, S.R.; Laurent-Puig, P.; Gryfe, R.; Shepherd, L.E.; Tu, D.; Redston, M. & Gallinger, S. (2003). Tumor microsatellite-instability status as a predictor of benefit from flurouracil-based adjuvant chemotherapy for colon cancer. *New England Journal of Medicine*, Vol.349, No.3, pp.247-57, ISSN 1533-4406.

Rio Frio, T.; Lavoie, J.; Hamel, N.; Geyer, F.C.; Kushner, Y.B.; Novak, D.J.; Wark, L.: Capelli, C.; Reis-Filho, J.S.; Mai, S.; Pastinen, T.; Tischlowitz, M.D.; Marcus, V.A.& Foulkes, W.D. (2010). Homozygous BUB1B Mutation and Susceptibility to Gastrointestinal Neoplasia. *New England Journal of Medicine*, Vol.363, No.27, pp.2628-37, ISSN 1533-4406.

Ruijs, M.W.G.; Verhoef, S.; Rookus, M.A.; Pruntel, R.; van der Hout, A.H.; Hogervorst, F.B.L.; Kluijt, I.; Sijmons, R.H.; Aalfs, C.M.; Wagner, A.; Ausems, M.G.E.M.; Hoogerbrugge, N.; van Asperen, C.J.; Gomez Garcia, E.B.; Meijers-Heijboer, H.; ten Kate, L.P.; Menko, F.H. & van't Veer, L. (2010). TP53 germline mutation testing in 180 families suspected of Li-Fraumeni syndrome: mutation detection rate and relative frequency of cancers in different familial phenotypes. *Journal of Medical Genetics*, Vol. 47, No.6, pp.421-428, ISSN 1468-6244.

Ruivenkamp, C.A.; van Wezel, T.; Zanon, C.; Stassen, A.P.; Vlcek, C.; Csikos, T.; Klous, A.M.; Tripodis, N.; Perrakis, A.; Beorrigter, L.; Groot, P.C.; Lindeman, J.; Mooi, W.J.; Meijer, G.A.; Scholten, G.; Dauwerse, H.; Paces, V.; van Zandwijk, N.; van Ommen, G.J. & Demant, P. (2002). Ptprj is a candidate for the mosue colon-cancer susceptibility locus Scc1 and is frequently deleted in human cancers. *Nature Genetics*, Vol.31, No.3, pp.295-300, ISSN 1061-4036.

Salovaara, R.; Loukola, A.; Kristo, P.; Kaariainen, H.; Ahtola, H.; Eskelinen, M.; Harkonen, N.; Julkunen, R.; Kangas, E.; Ojala, S.; Tulikoura, J.; Valkamo, E.; Jarvinen, H.; Mecklin, J.P.; Aaltonen, L.A. & de la Chapelle, A. (2000). Population-based molecular detection of hereditary nonpolyposis colorectal cancer. *Journal of Clinical Oncology*, Vol.18, No.11, pp.2193-200, ISSN 1527-7755.

Sanchez de Abajo, A.; de la Hoya, M.; Fodrino, J.; Furio, V.; Tosar, A.; Perez-Segura, P.; Diaz-Ruibo, E. & Caldes T. (2005). The CHEK2 1100delC allele is not relevant for risk assessment in HNPCC and HBCC Spanish Families. *Familial Cancer*, Vol.4, No.2., pp.183-6, ISSN 1573-7292.

Senter, L.; Clendenning, M.; Sotamaa, K.; Hampel, H.; Green, J.; Potter, J.D.; Lindblom, A.; Lagerstedt, K.; Thibodeau, S.N.; Lindor, N.M.; Young, J.; Winship, I.; Dowty, J.G., White, D.M.; Hopper, J.L.; Baglietto, L.; Jenkins, M.A. & de la Chapelle, A. (2008). The clinical phenotype of Lynch syndrome due to germl-line PMS mutations. *Gastroenterology*, Vol.135, No.2, pp.419-28, ISSN 0016-5085.

Talseth, B.A.; Ashton, K.A.; Meldrum, C.; Suchy, J.; Kurzawski, G.; Lubinski, J. & Scott, R.J. (2008). Aurora-A and Cyclin D1 polymorphisms and the age of onset of colorectal cancer in hereditary nonpolyposis colorectal cancer. *International Journal of Cancer*, Vol.122, No.6, pp.1273-7, ISSN 1097-0215.

Talseth-Palmer, B.A.; McPhillips, M.; Groombridge, C.; Spigelman, A. & Scott, R.J. (2010). MSH6 and PMS2 mutation positive Australian Lynch syndrome families: novel mutations, cancer risk and age of diagnosis of colorectal cancer. *Hereditary Cancer in Clinical Practice*, Vol.8, No.1, p.5. ISSN 1897-4287.

Tenesa, A.; Campbell, H.; Barnetson, R.; Porteous, M.; Dunlop, M. & Farrington, S.M. (2006). Association of MUTYH and colorectal cancer. *British Journal of Cancer*, Vol.95, No.2, pp.239-42, ISSN 0007-0920.

Taylor, D.P.; Burt, R.W.; Williams, M.S.; Haug, P.J. & Cannon-Albright, L.A. (2010). Population-based family history specific risks for colorectal cancer: a constellation approach. *Gastroenterology*, Vol.138, No.3, pp.877-85, ISSN 0016-5085.

Tenesa, A.; Farrington, S.M.; Prendergast, J.G.; Porteous, M.E.; Walker, M.; Haq, N.; Barnetson, R.A.; Theodoratou, E.; Cetnarskyj, R.; Cartwright, N.;, Semple, C.; Clark, A.J.; Reid, F.J.; Smith, L.A.; Kavoussanakis, K.; Koessler, T.; Pharoah, P.D.; Buch, S.; Schafmayer, C.; Tepel, J., Schreiber, S; Völzke, H.; Schmidt, C.O.;Hampe, J.; Chang-Claude, J.; Hoffmeister, M.; Brenner, H.; Wilkening, S.; Canzian, F.; Capella, G.; Moreno, V.; Deary, I.J.; Starr, J.M.; Tomlinson, I.P.; Kemp, Z.; Howarth, K.; Carvajal-Carmona, L.; Webb, E.; Broderick, P.; Vijayakrishnan, J.; Houlston, R.S.; Rennert, G.; Ballinger, D.; Rozek, L.; Gruber, S.B.; Matsuda, K.; Kidokoro, T.; Nakamura, Y.; Zanke, B.W.; Greenwood, C.M.; Rangrej, J.; Kustra, R.; Montpetit, A.; Hudson, T.J.; Gallinger, S.; Campbell, H. & Dunlop, M.G. (2008). Genome-wide association scan identifies a colorectal cancer susceptibility locus on 11q23 and replicates risk loci at 8q24 and 18q21. *Nature Genetics*, Vol.40, No.5, pp.631-7, ISSN 1061-4036.

Tenesa, A. & Dunlop, M.G. (2009). New insights into the aetiology of colorectal cancer from genome-wide association studies. *Nature Reviews in Genetics*, Vol.10, No.6, pp.353-8, ISSN 1471-0056.

Tenesa, A.; Theodoratou, E.; Din, F.V.N.; Farrington, S.M.; Cetnarskyj, R.; Barnetson, R.A.; Porteous, M.E.; Campbell, H. & Dunlop, M.G. (2010). Ten common genetic variants associated with colorectal cancer risk are not associated with survival after diagnosis. *Clinical Cancer Research*, Vol.16, No.10, pp.3754-9, ISSN 1557-3265.

Theodoratou, E.; Campbell, H.; Tenesa, A.; Houlston, R.; Webb, E.; Lubbe, S.; Broderick, P.; Gallinger, S.; Croitoru, E.M.; Jenkins, M.A.; Win, A.K.; Cleary, S.P.; Koessler, T.; Pharoah, P.D.; Küry, S.; Bézieau, S.; Buecher, B.; Ellis, N.A.; Peterlongo, P.; Offit, K.; Aaltonen, L.A.; Enholm, S; Lindblom, A.; Zhou, X.L.; Tomlinson, I.P.; Moreno, V.; Blanco, I.; Capellà, G.; Barnetson, R.; Porteous, M.E.; Dunlop, M.G. & Farrington, S.M. (2010). A large-scale meta-analysis to refine colorectal cancer risk associated with MUTHY variants. *British Journal of Cancer*, Vol.103, No.12, pp.1875-84, ISSN 0007-0920.

Toland, A.E.; Rozek, L.S.; Presswala, S.; Rennert, G.; Gruber, S.B. PTPRJ haplotypes and colorectal cancer risk. (2008). *Cancer Epidemiology, Biomarkers & Prevention*, Vol.17, No.10, pp.2782-5, ISSN 1055-9965.

Tomlinson, I.; Webb, E.; Carvajal-Carmona, L.; Broderick, P.; Kemp, Z., Spain, S.; Penegar, S.; Chandler, I.; Gorman, M.; Wood, W.; Barclay, E.; Lubbe, S.; Martin, L.; Sellick, G.; Jaeger, E.; Hubner, R.; Wild, R.; Rowan, A.; Fielding, S.; Howarth, K.; CORGI Consortium; Silver, A.; Atkin, W.; Muir, K.; Logan, R.; Kerr, D.; Johnstone, E.; Sieber, O.; Gray, R.; Thomas, H.; Peto, J.; Cazier, J.B. & Houlston, R. (2007). A genome-wide association scan of tag SNPs identifies a susceptibility variant for colorectal cancer at 8q24.21. *Nature Genetics*, Vol.39, No.8, pp.984-8, ISSN 1061-4036.

Tomlinson, I.P.; Webb, E.; Carvajal-Carmona, L.; Broderick, P.; Howarth, K.; Pittman, A.M.; Spain, S.; Lubbe, S.; Walther, A.; Sullivan, K.; Jaeger, E.; Fielding, S.; Rowan, A.; Vijayakrishnan, J.; Domingo, E.; Chandler, I.; Kemp, Z.; Qureshi, M.; Farrington, S.M.; Tenesa, A.; Prendergast, J.G.; Barnetson, R.A.; Penegar, S.; Barclay, E.; Wood, W.; Martin, L.; Gorman, M.; Thomas, H.; Peto, J.; Bishop, D.T.; Gray, R.; Maher, E.R.; Lucassen, A.; Kerr, D.; Evans, D.G.; CORGI Consortium; Schafmayer, C.; Buch, S.; Völzke, H.; Hampe, J.; Schreiber, S.; John, U.; Koessler, T.; Pharoah, P.; van Wezel, T.; Morreau, H.; Wijnen, J.T.; Hopper, J.L.; Southey, M.C.; Giles, G.G.; Severi, G.; Castellví-Bel, S.; Ruiz-Ponte, C.; Carracedo, A.; Castells, A.; EPICOLON Consortium; Försti, A.; Hemminki, K.; Vodicka, P.; Naccarati, A.; Lipton, L.; Ho, J.W.; Cheng, K.K.; Sham, P.C.; Luk, J.; Agúndez, J.A.; Ladero, J.M.; de la Hoya, M.; Caldés, T.; Niittymäki, I.; Tuupanen, S.; Karhu, A.; Aaltonen, L.; Cazier, J.B.; Campbell, H.; Dunlop, M.G. & Houlston, R.S. (2008). A genome-wide association study identifies colorectal cancer susceptibility loci on chromosomes 10p14 and 8q23.3. *Nature Genetics*, Vol.40, No.5, pp.623-30, ISSN 1061-4036.

Tresallet C.; Brouquet, A.; Julie, C.; Beauchet, A.; Vallot, C.; Menegaux, F.; Mitry, E.; Radvanyi, F.; Malafosse, R.; Rougier, P.; Nordlinger, B.; Laurent-Puig, P.; Boileau, C.; Emile, J.-F.; Muti, C.; Penna, C.; Hofmann-Radvanyi, H. (2011). Evaluation of predictive models for the identification in daily practice of patients with Lynch syndrome. *International Journal of Cancer*, E-pub ahead of print, ISSN 1097-0215.

Tuupanen, S.; Turunen, M.; Lehtonen, R.; Hallikas, O.; Vanharanta, S.; Kivioja, T.; Bjorklund, M.; Wei, G.; Yan, J.; Nittymaki, I.; Mecklin, J.P.; Jarvinen, H.; Ristimaki, A.; Di-Bernardo, M.; East, P.; Carvajal-Carmona, L.; Houlston, R.S.; Tomlinson, I.; Palin, K.; Ukkonen, E.; Karhu, A.; Taipale, J.; Aaltonen, L.A. (2009). The common colorectal cancer predisposition SNP rs6983267 at chromosome 8q24 confers potential to enhanced Wnt signaling. *Nature Genetics*, Vol.41, No.8, pp.885-90, ISSN 1061-4036.

Umar, A.; Boland, C.R.; Terdiman, J.P.; Syngal, S.; de la Chapelle, A.; Ruschoff, J.; Fishel, R.; Lindor, N.M.; Burgart, L.J.; Hamelin, R.; Hamilton, S.R.; Hiatt, R.A.; Jass, J.;Lindblom, A.; Lynch, H.T.; Peltomaki, P.; Ramsey, S.D.; Rodriguez-Bigas, M.A.; Vasen, H.F.; Hawk, E.T.; Barrett, J.C.; Freedman, A.N. & Srivastava, S. (2004). Revised Bethesda guidelines for hereditary nonpolyposis colorectal cancer (Lynch syndrome) and microsatellite instability. *Journal of the National Cancer Institute*, Vol.96, No.4, pp.261-8, ISSN 1460-2105.

Van Lier, M.G.; Wagner, A.; Mathus-Vliegen, E.M.; Kuipers, E.J.; Steyerberg, E.W.; van Leerdam, M.E. (2010). High cancer risk in Peutz-Jeghers syndrome: a systematic review and surveillance recommendations. *American Journal of Gastroenterology*, Vol.105, No.6, pp.1258-1264, ISSN 0002-9270.

Van Lier, M.G.F.; Westerman, A.M.; Wagner, A.; Looman, C.W.N.; Wilson, J.H.P. de Rooij, F.W.M.; Lemmens, V.E.P.P.; Kuipers, E.J.; Mathus-Vliegen, E.M.H. & van Leerdam, M.E. (2011). High cancer risk and increased mortality in patients with Peutz-Jeghers syndrome. *Gut*, Vol. 60, No. pp.141-7, ISSN 1468-3288.

Van Wezel, T.; Stassen, A.P.; Moen, C.J.; Hart, A.A. van der Val, M.A. & Demant, P. (1996). Gene interaction and single gene effects in colon tumour susceptibility in mice. *Nature Genetics*, Vol.14, No.4, pp.468-70, ISSN 1061-4036.

Van Wezel, T.; Ruivenkamp, C.A.; Stassen, A.P.; Moen, C.J. & Demant, P. (1999). Four new colon cancer susceptibility loci, Scc6 to Scc9 in the mouse. *Cancer Research*, Vol.59, No.17, pp.4216-8, ISSN 1538-7445.

Vasen, H.F.; Mecklin, J.P.; Khan, P.M. & Lynch, H.T. (1991). The international collaborative group on Hereditary Non-Polyposis Colorectal Cancer (ICG-HNPCC). *Diseases of the Colon & Rectum*, Vol.34, No.5, pp.424-5, ISSN 1530-0358.

Vasen, H.F.; Watson, P.; Mecklin, J.P.; Lynch, H.T. (1999). New clinical criteria for hereditary nonpolyposis colorectal cancer (HNPCC, Lynch syndrome) proposed by the International Collaborative group on HNPCC. *Gastroenterology*, Vol.116, No.15, pp.1453-6, ISSN 0016-5085.

Volikos, E.; Robinson, J.; Aittomaki, K.; Mecklin, J.P.; Jarvinen, H.; Westerman, A.M.; de Rooji, F.W.; Vogel, T.; Moeslein, G.; Launonen, V.; Tomlinson, I.P.; Silver, A.R. & Aaltonen, L.A. (2006). LKB1 exonic and whole gene deletions are a common cause of Peutz-Jeghers syndrome. *Journal of Medical Genetics*, Vol.43, No.5, pp.e18, ISSN 1468-6244.

Wasielelewski, M.; Vasen, H.; Wijnen, J.; Hooning, M.; Dooijes, D.; Tops, C.; Klign, J.G.; Meijers-Heijboer, H. & Schutte, M. (2008). CHEK2 1100delC is a susceptibility allele for HNPCC-related colorectal cancer. *Clinical Cancer Research*, Vol.14, No.15, pp. 4989-94, ISSN 1557-3265.

Wimmer, K. & Kratz, C.P. (2010). Constitutional mismatch repair-deficiency syndrome. *Haematologica*, Vol.95, No.5, pp.699-701, ISSN 1592-8721.

Xing, J.; Myers, R.; He, X.; Qu, F.; Zhou, F.; Ma, X.; Hylsop, T.; Bao, G.; Wan, S.; Yang, H.; Chen, Z. (2011). GWAS-identified colorectal cancer susceptibility locus associates with disease prognosis. *European Journal of Cancer*, Vol.47, No.11, pp.1699-707, ISSN 0959-8049.

Xiong, F.; Wu, C.; Bi, X.; Yu, D.; Huang, L.; Xu, J.; Zhang, T.; Zhai, K.; Chang, J.; Tan, W.; Cai, J. & Lin D. (2011). Risk of Genome-Wide Association Study-Identified Genetic Variants for Colorectal Cancer in a Chinese Population. *Cancer Epidemiology, Biomarkers &Prevention*, Vol.19, No.7, pp.1855-61, ISSN 1538-775.

Young, J. & Jass, J.R. (2006). The case for a genetic predisposition to serrated neoplasia in the colorectum: hypothesis and review of the literature. *Cancer Epidemiology, Biomarkers & Prevention*, Vol.15, No.10, pp.1778-84, ISSN 1538-7755.

3

The Role of Modifier Genes in Lynch Syndrome

Rodney J. Scott[1,2,3], Stuart Reeves[1] and Bente Talseth-Palmer[1,3]
[1]*The Centre for Information Based Medicine, The School of Biomedical Sciences and Pharmacy, University of Newcastle,*
[2]*Division of Genetics, Hunter Area Pathology Service,*
[3]*Hunter Medical Research Institute,*
United Kingdom

1. Introduction

There are a number of inherited predispositions to colorectal cancer (CRC) which can be broadly categorized into two groups; those with associated polyposis, such as familial adenomatous polyposis and the hamartomatous polyposis syndromes; and those that are linked to the non-polyposis syndromes, such as hereditary non polyposis colorectal cancer (HNPCC). The genetic basis of both the polyposis and non-polyposis syndromes are reflected in the CRC population who have no apparent family history of disease. Approximately 80% of all cases of CRC are associated with chromosomal instability [1] and are likely to have mutations in the Adenomatous Polyposis Coli (APC) gene whereas the remaining 20% with microsatellite instability appears to be due primarily to epigenetic inactivation of the DNA mismatch repair (MMR) gene *MLH1* [2].

The disease HNPCC accounts for somewhere between 2% and 5% of all CRCs diagnosed and is associated with a younger age of disease onset compared to the general population [3,4]. HNPCC is a disease by definition based on the Amsterdam Criteria where there need to be three cases of CRC, one of which must be diagnosed under the age of 50 years, one patient must be a first degree relative of the other two, span two generations and familial adenomatous polyposis should be excluded [5]. Modification of the Amsterdam Criteria has been ongoing since its original inception due to an increasing awareness of what constitutes this disease. HNPCC used to be known as either the Cancer Family Syndrome or Lynch Syndrome [6]. It is now accepted that families where a mutation in the DNA mismatch repair genes (MMR) *MSH2, MLH1, MSH6* or *PMS2* has been identified are now termed Lynch Syndrome families whereas those with no mutation are termed HNPCC [7]. The primary function of MMR genes is to eliminate base-base mismatches and insertion-deletion loops which arise as a consequence of DNA polymerase slippage during DNA replication [8]. MMR confers several genetic stabilisation functions; it corrects DNA biosynthesis errors, ensures the fidelity of genetic recombination and participates in the earliest steps of cell cycle checkpoint control and apoptotic responses [9,10]. MMR gene defects increases the risk of malignant transformation of cells, which ultimately results in the disruption of one or several genes associated with epithelial integrity. The identification of germline mutations in families with Lynch Syndrome accounts for only ~50% of all families that fulfil the clinical diagnosis defined by the Amsterdam criteria [11]. The remaining families have no identifiable genetic predisposition yet fulfil the diagnostic criteria for the disease and are referred to as HNPCC families.

DNA MMR is a housekeeping function of all nucleated cells and as such any breakdown in the fidelity of this process is likely to result in disease irrespective of which gene is affected. Unlike other predispositions to colorectal cancer such as familial adenomatous polyposis, there are no obvious genotype/phenotype correlations in Lynch syndrome. Mutations that result in the loss of MSH2 or MLH1 irrespective of where they occur in the respective gene alter the risk of developing malignancy. Furthermore, mutations in DNA MMR genes do not predict a phenotype since any breakdown in the fidelity of this process results in a "mutator phenotype". It has been obvious from the first MSH2 and MLH1 mutation reports that differences in the ages of cancer diagnosis in patients harbouring germline mutations in DNA MMR genes do occur both within and between families. Furthermore, unrelated families harbouring the same mutation present with different disease profiles as do patients from within the same family [12-14]. The differences in disease expression both within and between families harbouring the same mutation are most likely a result of environmental, genetic or a mixture of both influences.

Identification of environmental factors that could account for differences in the age of colorectal cancer diagnosis of Lynch Syndrome is almost intractable when undertaken as a retrospective study and is best undertaken prospectively to include as many environmental variables as possible. Notwithstanding, knowledge about environmental factors and disease risk in Lynch Syndrome is important and studies are required to identify those which protect or promote disease.

Conversely, as genetic factors can be assessed after the fact they lend themselves more readily to retrospective interrogation and consequently identification. Identifying genetic factors that could explain differential disease expression in Lynch syndrome is now achievable due to the development of appropriate technology that allows for the rapid screening of large numbers of patients in conjunction with the accumulation of large cohorts of patients that allow for robust statistical analysis.

The search for modifier genes has been ongoing ever since the first groups of Lynch syndrome families were identified. Initial studies focused on genes associated with xenobiotic metabolism which have been followed by genes involved in the immune response, DNA repair, cell cycle control and as yet undefined genomic regions identified as a result of large genome wide association studies searching for genetic risk factors for colorectal cancer. This review will focus on "modifiable" (those that can be altered by manipulation) candidate modifier genes and those that have been chosen as a result of biological plausibility (which may or may not be modifiable), as shown in Table 1.

Biological plausibility and pathways of published "positive" results have been questioned [15], indicating that the functional significance of single nucleotide polymorphisms (SNPs) should be known before they are linked to disease [16]. A few published reports linking SNPs without known functional significance [17,18] or studies have failed to confirm a reported associations [19]. Known genetic variation has significantly impacted on the early detection and diagnosis of inherited cancer [20, 21], indicating that the search for genetic variation in cancer should continue.

Modifier Genes and polymorphisms studied in Lynch Syndrome			
Candidate Genes	Type of Polymorphisms	Effect	Publication indicating association or not
IGF1	CA-repeat	promoter function	[22, 23]
MTHFR	SNP	enzyme activity	[24]
HFE	SNP	protein function	[25]
NAT2	SNP	enzyme activity	[26, 27]
GSTM1	null allele	enzyme activity	[26, 27]
GSTT1	null allele	enzyme activity	[26, 27]
ATM	SNP	protein function	[28]
IL6	SNP	cytokine activity	[29]
IL4	SNP	cytokine activity	[29]
IL1β	SNP	receptor binding	[29]
IL10	SNP	cytokine activity	[29]
IL1Rn	SNP	null receptor	[29]
TNF-α	SNP	cytokine activity	[29]
IFN-γ	SNP	cytokine activity	[29]
TP53	SNP	protein function	[32, 39, 40]
MDM2	SNP	promoter function	[42]
Aurora-A	SNP	protein function	[44, 45, 48]
Cyclin D1	SNP	protein function	[44, 45, 48]

Table. 1. Candidate modifier genes and their respective types of polymorphism that have been studied in cohorts of Lynch syndrome patients.

2. Cell cycle control gene polymorphisms: TP53. MDM2, Aurora-A and CyclinD1

The TP53 gene isa tumour suppressor gene that regulates the transcription of genes necessary for the maintenance of genomic integrity by blocking cell proliferation after DNA damage and initiating apoptosis if it is too extensive [30, 31]. In 2004 the R72P polymorphism in TP53 was found to be associated with age of diagnosis of colorectal cancer (CRC) in an American Lynch syndrome study [32]. The R72P SNP in TP53 has been shown to result in two forms of the protein, which are not functionally equivalent [33, 34], and has been widely studied in a variety of malignancies [35 - 38]. Subsequent studies, including one Finnish and a collaborative Australian and Polish study, of the TP53 polymorphism and age of diagnosis of CRC in Lynch syndrome failed to confirm the reported association [39, 40]. The lack of an association was suggested to be related to a polymorphism in MDM2, which results in increased levels of MDM2 that culminates in the inability to properly stabilise TP53's response to cellular stress [40]. Evidence supporting this notion in HNPCC however, could not be found in other studies [39, 41]. The failure to corroborate the role of TP53 as a modifier gene between the different studies could be due to differences in the mutation spectrum of the various study populations; number of relatives included, population stratification and/or type 1 statistical error. Population stratification is unlikely to account for differences between the study populations as it has been shown that for most of the common disease associated polymorphisms, ethnicity is likely to be a poor predictor of an individuals' genotype [43]. Type 1 statistical error seems to be the most likely explanation since the population sizes differ significantly in size with a range between 86 cases through to a maximum number of 220. In the larger studies reported to date (encompassing 193 and 220 patients, respectively), no association was observed thereby providing evidence against an association.

Aurora-A and Cyclin D1, genes both involved in cell cycle control, have also been associated with the age of onset of CRC in Lynch syndrome patients from North America [44, 45]. After the initial studies suggesting Aurora-A polymorphisms were linked to the average age of disease diagnosis follow-up reports in larger patient populations consistently failed to replicate this finding. In contrast, studies of Cyclin D1 polymorphisms and their association with the age of disease onset in Lynch syndrome resulted in contradictory results when studied in populations from North America, Germany, Finland and a combined study of Australian and Polish patients [44, 46 – 48]. A potential explanation for the association between Cyclin D1 and hMSH2 mutation carriers observed in the Australian and Polish Lynch syndrome patients was the relative paucity of MSH2 mutation carriers in the German and Finnish populations [47]. With the expansion of the study population from the Australian/Polish patient cohort the original report of an association with Cyclin D1 could not be replicated (See Fig. 1). In conclusion, the evidence now suggests that there is no association between Cyclin D1, MSH2 and disease risk in Lynch syndrome, such that overall Cyclin D1 does not appear to be associated with the age of disease diagnosis.

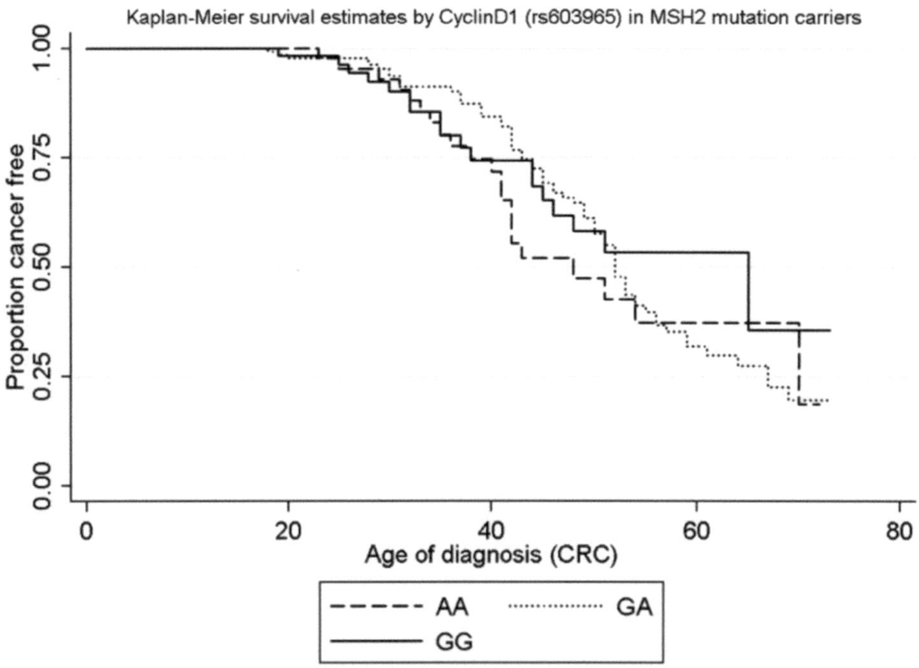

Fig. 1. Kaplan-Meier analysis of Cyclin D1 polymorphism and the age of disease onset in Australian and Polish Lynch syndrome patients. 276 MSH2 mutation positive patients were included in this study of which 107 were diagnosed with colorectal cancer. Log-rank, Wilcoxon and Tarone-Ware tests were not significant.

3. Xenobiotic clearance gene polymorphisms: NAT1, NAT2, GST, CYP1A1

Genes involved in xenobiotic metabolism, which include N-acetyl transferase 1 (NAT1), N-acetyl transferase 2 (NAT2), glutathione-S-transferase (GST) and cytochrome P450, have the ability to influence an individual's susceptibility to environmental and occupational carcinogens and predisposition to cancer [49]. The detoxification and elimination of foreign chemicals is controlled by complex mechanisms involving phase I enzymes that include cytochrome P450, and phase II enzymes such as GSTs and NATs [50]. Because of the significance of xenobiotics in the environment, perturbations in the ability to remove them are likely to alter disease risk. Polymorphisms in the genes mentioned above have been associated with colorectal cancer but the roles that the different SNPs have on cancer risk are controversial [26, 27, 51 - 61].

In 1999 an association between polymorphisms in NAT2 and the age of diagnosis of CRC in Lynch syndrome patients was reported, and the association was later replicated in a second independent report [26, 54]. Both studies had relatively small sample sizes (78 and 86 cases). Re-investigation of the association in a smaller study (69 cases) and a more appropriately sized one (220 cases) failed to confirm the association [58, 26]. The failure to confirm the association could be due to population stratification, but this is unlikely since if there is a functional difference in the gene in question,so its effects should be observed in all subjects, although not necessarily statistically significant in all populations. The most likely explanation for the failure to replicate initial findings is the small study population sizes that were used in assessing the potential association. This is further confirmed in a review by Brockton *et al.* 2000 [62] concluding that in 10 of 11 studies of invasive CRC and NAT2 acetylator genotype, no association was observed.

Similar results are reported for the polymorphisms in GST and cytochrome p450 genes and Lynch syndrome. Several research groups reported an association, while others failed to confirm them [25, 26, 51, 52, 53, 53, 63]. In on study the Msp1 wildtype allele of cytochrome P450 1A1 gene (CYP1A1) was associated with a decreased risk of CRC [26] which could have been due to it not being in Hardy-Weinberg equilibrium. The identification of an allele that is not in Hardy-Weinberg equilibrium suggests that either a genotyping error has occurred thereby skewing the results or it can be taken as supporting evidence for a correlation with disease [64]. The CYP1A1 gene has previously been associated with CRC and two SNPs in the CYP1A1 gene have been associated with CRC [65], which taken together with the report of Talseth et al. 2006 [26] supports the notion that variation in this gene is involved in the some aspect of CRC development.

Studies examining variation in xenobiotic clearance are likely to be subject to strong environmental influence and this is supported by findings from different countries. Studies examining patients of European descent for polymorphisms in GST genes seems to find no obvious relationship between the SNPs and cancer risk, while a study from Korea reports an association [25, 26, 63]. Taken together, these results suggest a complex relationship between the environment and individual genotypes that add to other more obvious problems associated with searching for modifier genes. Additional studies are required to determine the relationship between GST and CYP1A1 polymorphisms and disease risk in Lynch syndrome.

4. Immune response gene polymorphisms: IL6, IL4, IL1β, IL10, IL1Rn, TNF-α, IFN-γ

Cytokine mediated events may play a role in tumour development within inflammatory cells by producing an environment that supports tumour growth by promoting angiogenesis and facilitating genomic instability. The quintessential example is that of Crohn's disease where there is an increased risk of developing CRC if left untreated [66]. Inflammatory responses can also increase DNA damage, growth stimulation and enhanced survival of damaged cells [66, 67]. SNPs in cytokine genes can have an effect on the transcription levels of the respective genes and resulting in differences in both pro- and anti-inflammatory response activity. A series of polymorphisms in a number of cytokines has been investigated in relation to CRC risk and other cancer types but not for Lynch syndrome [68 - 77]. In addition, genetic variation in pro- and anti-inflammatory cytokine genes has been shown to influence individual response to carcinogen exposure [69], but no association has been identified in the one report focusing on a series of SNPs in cytokine genes and disease expression in Lynch syndrome [28]. Given the complexity of the inflammatory response and the limited number of SNPs utilised in that study, it cannot be ruled out that a relationship between SNPs influencing the immune response and Lynch syndrome exits.

5. Insulin like Growth Factor IGF-1 Gene polymorphisms

The *IGF-1* gene was first reported as a potential modifying gene in Lynch syndrome disease expression in 2006. The CA-repeat polymorphism located near the *IGF-1* promoter region was described as having an association with the age of disease onset in a cohort of 121 Lynch syndrome patients originating from the United States [22]. Certainly this is not the first time that a repeat region has been implicated in disease; with numerous studies reporting a link between DNA repeat regions significantly altering risk of prostate cancer [78 - 80] breast cancer, squamous cell carcinoma, bladder and lung cancers [81 - 84]. DNA microsatellite repeat regions are also strongly associated with Lynch Syndrome by virtue of their instability in tumours which is a consequence of the loss in the fidelity of DNA MMR [8].

IGF-1 is important for cellular proliferation and differentiation however, elevated levels of IGF-1 have been reported to have significant links to diseases such as CRC which is thought to be a result of the mitogenic and anti-apoptotic effects elicited by this protein [22, 85]. Several environmental and physiological reasons have been proposed that influence IGF-1 expression; however there is now evidence to suggest that a genetic role is significant. Rosen *et al.* was the first to report that the length of the CA repeat region in *IGF-1* may be associated with circulating IGF-1 levels [86]. In a similar growth factor related gene, Epidermal Growth Factor Receptor (EGFR), a CA repeat region is located in intron 1. A study of this *EGFR* polymorphic repeat region revealed lower transcriptional activity with increasing numbers of polymorphic CA repeats coinciding with lower levels of gene expression [87]. In 2007, a similar result was reported for the *IGF-1* gene in swine where the length of the CA repeat region was clearly associated with circulating levels of IGF-1 [88]. More recently, additional human data has been published which supports the notion that this polymorphism is linked to serum levels of IGF-1 [89]. From this data a trend is emerging that CA repeat polymorphisms in growth factor related genes, such as *IGF-1,* are related to overall gene expression, which is reflected in the circulating serum levels of the respective proteins. Accumulating evidence suggests that serum IGF-1 levels appear to be linked to disease with recent reports indicating that elevated levels of IGF-1 are observed in breast, prostate and CRC [90 - 93]. There have been estimates that higher circulating levels of IGF-1 result in a 15% increase in the risk of developing disease, insinuating the importance of circulating IGF-1 in disease progression [94].

As CRC involves the accrual of a number of specific molecular alterations [95, 96], consistently high IGF-1 serum levels may increase cellular proliferation, thereby enhancing the rate by which genetic alterations accumulate. Both normal colonic epithelial and transformed cells are IGF-1 responsive; thus, IGF-1 can influence not only the likelihood of disease initiation but also disease progression. This overall process provides some insight into how intracellular serum levels of IGF-1 may have a significant influence in accelerating the accumulation of genetic errors leading to disease, especially in persons who have inherited a predisposition to develop malignancy characterized by a mutator phenotype as observed in Lynch syndrome.

An equally important facet to disease risk as a result of increased levels of IGF-1 is its link with obesity. Obesity and physical inactivity are strong independent determinants of insulin resistance and hyperinsulinaemia [97 - 104] and this is associated with an increased risk of CRC [101, 102]. Increased blood insulin lowers IGF-1 binding protein levels, which often results in an increase of free IGF-1 [105]. As IGF-1 is associated with both percentage body fat and general overall obesity [106], an increased level of IGF-1 expression as a result of shorter CA repeat lengths may have an enhanced effect in persons who are obese where IGF-1 serum levels are already elevated.

In addition to the IGF-1 effect, CRC risk is also increased in obese patients through oxidative stress in adipose tissue. This is caused by increased lipid peroxidation leading to the production of reactive oxygen species. In regards to cancer, reactive oxygen species can damage DNA by several methods including DNA base modification, deletions, frame shifts, strand breaks, DNA-protein cross-links, and chromosomal rearrangements [107]. Both lipid peroxidation and increased DNA damage are likely to promote tumour development by generating reactive oxygen species, increasing hormone production/bioavailability of IGF-1 and providing an energy-rich environment. This combined mechanism is potentially a risk factor for all types of CRC, however in Lynch syndrome this may be of greater significance in a deficient DNA repair environment where enhanced levels of IGF-1 inhibit cell death and encourage cellular proliferation. Together, the relationship between obesity and *IGF-1* CA repeat length may be of particular importance in obese Lynch syndrome cases as these may be at greatest risk of developing disease at a younger age.

The role of inherited factors in circulating IGF1 serum levels is likely to be substantial with estimates of the proportion of variance in IGF-1 that is genetically determined varying somewhere between 38% to over 80% [108]. A substantial amount of data has been reported revealing differences in IGF levels across ethnic groups [109 - 111], however this is suggestive of dietary and lifestyle factors having a more modifiable effect on serum levels when combined with genetic ancestry. One such study has shown that the impact of several nutritional factors such as calcium, dairy products and vegetables on IGF1 levels is quite different in racially stratified models as reported between African-American and European American males [112]. This is strongly suggestive of there being population differences that differentially modify the effect of several nutrients on IGF levels. Together this information is suggestive that environmental factors such as calorific intake, lifestyle and demographic factors are probably playing a substantial role in ethnic variation in disease risk in regards to serum IGF levels. This is intriguing as it may also be contributing to the differences in relative disease risk observed between the Polish and Australian cohorts as reported [22].

The data reported to date [21] indicate a significant interaction between the CA repeat polymorphism length and disease expression in Lynch syndrome which is likely to be linked to circulating levels of IGF-1. The data suggest a significant correlation for earlier onset CRC in participants who carry 17 or less IGF-1 CA repeats in over 400 Lynch syndrome patients. An encouraging aspect of the results of this study is that significance is retained across two different populations where variance in IGF-1 allele size frequencies occur [22]. A limitation however in defining the exact relationship between IGF-1 expression and cancer incidence in Lynch syndrome patients is the genotype-phenotype correlation between the *IGF-1* CA-repeat number and the corresponding serum levels. Assessment of serum IGF-1 concentration, however, has the inherent problem of serum IGF-I measurement, which is typically assessed at only one time point yet for accurate analysis should be performed multiple times from any single patient. Whether it would be feasible to monitor IGF-1 serum levels in families with Lynch syndrome is an area which needs further investigation. Future work should also include additional candidate polymorphisms located within *IGF-1* or *IGFBP-3* that interact with the IGF-1 pathway and may provide further insight into the overall IGF-1 effect. At present, however the IGF-1 pathway remains largely under-investigated, and there is now a requirement for further work to develop a more thorough understanding of the relationship between *IGF-1* genotype, expression and its implication in disease risk.

6. Methylenetetrahydrofolate reductase (MTHFR) gene polymorphisms

There have been tantalizing reports in the literature that polymorphisms in the *MTHFR* gene are associated with altered CRC risk. These polymorphisms occur in relatively high frequency in the general population and the two that promote special attention are both associated with altered enzymatic function. MTHFR is a key folate-metabolizing enzyme involved in both DNA methylation and DNA synthesis. The enzyme catalyses the irreversible conversion of 5,10-methylenetetrahydrofolate (5,10-MTHF), needed for purine and thymidine synthesis, to 5-methyltetrahydrofolate (5-MTHF), which is necessary for methionine production. Insufficient thymidine results in uracil misincorporation into DNA, leading to single-strand and double-strand breaks. This can increase the incidence of DNA damage, thereby increasing the risk of genetic instability. The understanding that folate metabolism can both equally influence DNA synthesis and methylation has made the study of environmental and genetic variants associated with MTHFR particularly attractive as a candidate genetic factor that influences cancer susceptibility. Two common polymorphisms, *C677T* and *A1298C* are located within the MTHFR gene and have been linked to altering the function of the encoded protein. This has lead to these variants being the focus of numerous studies into CRC risk outside the context of an inherited predisposition to disease. Both polymorphisms result in a substitution of an amino acid and have previously been shown to significantly influence MTHFR enzyme activity [113]. *C677T* is located within the coding region for the catalytic domain, resulting in an amino acid substitution from alanine to valine that is associated with a reduction of enzyme activity. The *A1298C* polymorphism, located in the regulatory region of MTHFR, substitutes an amino acid change from glutamine to alanine. Evidence suggests that *A1298C* also reduces MTHFR activity, however it is reported to be less influential than *C677T* [114]. This modifying effect incurred by the presence of one or both polymorphisms in a pivotal folate metabolism pathway and its association with sporadic disease suggests that these polymorphisms are of particular interest with respect to modifying disease risk in Lynch syndrome.

Both *A1298C* and *C677T* are in strong linkage disequilibrium with no evidence of the existence of a *MTHFR* allele that carries both the homozygote (*C1298C/T677T*) variants of these polymorphisms [115 - 117]. Owing to this linkage disequilibrium, no studies have been reported where patients have inherited both homozygote variants. Nevertheless, heterozygote carriers of 1298C and 677T have been reported. The effect of inheriting both alleles in trans (i.e. one allele with the 677T polymorphism and the other with the 1298C polymorphism) effectively reduces overall MTHFR activity, thereby significantly altering the kinetics of folate metabolism. Data reported from an Australian and Polish study on the effects of MTHFR variants and disease expression in Lynch syndrome revealed that heterozygote forms of the *MTHFR* variants were required for a significant protective effect to occur [23]. The Kaplan-Meier survival estimates reported in this study predicted a median age gap of 10 years later for CRC onset in patients carrying the combined heterozygote *MTHFR* genotype which was supported by multi variable regression modelling statistics. The data also suggested this effect was significant in both *hMLH1* and *hMSH2* carriers, where previously only a significant association had been described in *hMLH1* for *C677T* only [118]. The most likely cause for this discrepancy between the Australian/Polish study and those by reported by Pande *et al* (2007) [119] is likely to be due to a type 1 statistical error as the reported association in *hMLH1* carriers were in a considerable smaller sample size, although differences in the ethnicity of Lynch syndrome cohorts cannot be ruled out as a contributing factor.

The mechanism by which *C677T* and *A1298C* appears to influence disease risk can be explained by the functional effects that these polymorphisms have on MTHFR and consequently folate metabolism. Previous reports have demonstrated a reduction of up to 60% in the activity of MTHFR when both *C677T* and *A1298C* heterozygote alleles were present in the gene. The reduction of *MTHFR* activity leads to an increased concentration of its substrate 5,10-MTHF. The increased pool of 5,10-MTHF pushes folate metabolism towards DNA synthesis, in turn reducing the pool of uracil. A reduced quantity of uracil potentially reduces the overall risk of uracil misincorporation as a result of its limited availability. For individuals with a MMR deficiency, the effect of reduced MTHFR enzyme activity may be advantageous since uracil misincorporation could be particularly deleterious in conjunction with an impaired DNA repair pathway. The subsequent lower levels of 5-MTHF may also be beneficial due to a potential reduction in DNA methylation. Hypermethylation of the promoter of tumour suppressor or MMR genes may lead to gene silencing, therefore a reduction in methylation through decreased MTHFR activity could lead to lower probability of this type of gene silencing occurring.

Numerous case control and cohort studies have investigated the relationship between folate intake and CRC risk with the majority reporting a reduction in CRC incidence with higher levels of folate [116]. The outcome of one meta-analysis suggested that CRC risk could be reduced by up to 25% with a high level of dietary folate compared to a low level one [117]. Further studies are required to clarify to what extent total folate has on disease risk; however it is generally accepted that there is an association and that a number of common genetic variants alter either the cellular levels or functioning of folate metabolism enzymes and are likely to have an important role in determining an individual's response to changes in dietary folate. With this in mind further studies into functional polymorphisms in the folate metabolism pathway would benefit significantly by including total folate levels so that a more exact assessment its role could be made. Using this approach a more precise view of the relationship between folate intake and disease risk may become apparent where Lynch syndrome patients could be stratified by *MTHFR* genotype. Accurately estimating dietary folate intake however may prove difficult and therefore the analysis of plasma folate levels may be a more viable alternative. Future studies would benefit by including other dietary factors including alcohol, choline, and methionine intake which are known to effect folate metabolism besides folate and folic acid [119]. An accurate level of plasma folate combined with *MTHFR C677T* and *A1298C* genotypes is an interesting prospect and may provide an indicator of individual risk of developing a Lynch syndrome related CRC.

The identification of *MTHFR* polymorphisms being associated with divergence in disease risk in Lynch syndrome provides the basis for targeted intervention measures that could be used to reduce the risk of disease development. Dietary supplementation of folate/folic acid in Lynch syndrome families may prove to be beneficial in decreasing disease risk or prolonging the time before the diagnosis of malignancy. Dietary supplementation and a change in disease risk however, are more complex than previously thought. Folic acid supplementation has been proven to be beneficial in decreasing neural tube defects (NTD's), [120] and was the catalyst for the United States and Canada introducing the compulsory supplementation of folic acid in flour in 1996 with the aim to reduce the incidence of NTD's. Despite proving successful for this purpose an unexpected trend was observed in both countries as described by Mason et al. (2007) [121] who investigated the relationship between the onset of folic acid fortification and rises in the incidence of CRC. This analysis indicated that in the early part of the 1990's the age-adjusted incidence of CRC had declined gradually in both countries. Between 1995 and 1996 however, the incidence rate in the United States showed a slight increase followed by more marked increases in 1997 and 1998. A similar finding was observed in the Canadian population, which also corresponded to the mandatory supplementation of folic acid. In both populations the increase in CRC incidence was highly significant when compared to pre-existing trends in both men and women. These observations have lead to a hypothesis that mandatory folic acid supplementation was responsible for the spike in CRC rates which after peaking approximately 2-3 years after its introduction have begun to decline once again [121].

The association of increased CRC incidence with folate supplementation has been supported by the results of two large-scale studies which have recently emerged from both the United States and United Kingdom. In both these phase III studies a common trend was observed in participants who supplemented their diets for three years with a daily dose of 1000ug and 500ug folic acid respectively, and an increased risk of developing a colorectal adenoma, with the greater risk in those participants consuming the higher 1000ug dose [122, 123]. Studies in mismatch repair or tumour suppressor gene deficient mice have demonstrated that the timing of folate supplementation is important in the association it may have on disease risk. In the first few months of folate supplementation a threefold decrease in colorectal adenomas has been observed when compared to mice with a moderate folate deficient diet. Dietary folate treatment after the development of carcinomas had the opposite effect however, with folate deficiency significantly decreasing the number of adenomas compared with supplementation [124, 125]. Together, this evidence suggests that as long as an individual is healthy, folate supplementation is protective whereas if a tumour has been initiated folate restriction is more important. This dual modulatory role of folate may be of even greater influence in an impaired DNA mismatch repair pathway as found in Lynch syndrome patients. In this case folate supplementation may be particularly beneficial or deleterious depending upon any early tumour development.

7. Haemochromatosis HFE gene polymorphisms

The role of high body iron levels in modifying the risk of colorectal cancer has been investigated by several groups but remains unclear [126 - 130]. The genetic iron overload disorder hereditary haemochromatosis (HH) is characterised by high iron indices and progressive parenchymal iron overload and occurs due to a problem in restricting iron uptake (reviewed in [131- 133]. While clear associations have been established between haemochromatosis and liver disease, studies investigating the correlation between haemochromatosis and other pathologies have yielded conflicting results [134 - 137].

The primary cause of classical HH has been ascribed to SNPs in the *HFE* gene, in particular the 845G>A SNP which results in the substitution of a tyrosine residue for a cysteine at position 282 (C282Y) and is present in 10-15% of individuals of northern European descent. The more common but less penetrant 163C>G SNP (H63D) is present in 15-30% of individuals [131, 136 - 142]. A longitudinal also study has demonstrated that up to 30% of men and 1% of women homozygous for the C282Y polymorphism develop iron overload that subsequently manifests as a disease phenotype [143]. The risk of developing colorectal cancer increased 3-fold in C282Y homozygotes when compared to matched controls without the mutation [144].

A number of other epidemiological studies have also investigated the impact of *HFE* genotype on colorectal cancer risk, with mixed results [145 -148]. Most studies exploring the link between *HFE* genotype and the risk of developing colorectal cancer have approached the problem by selecting subjects diagnosed with colorectal cancer and comparing the frequency of *HFE* polymorphisms to matched controls.

In regards to Lynch syndrome and the potential influence of disease risk one study has been reported suggesting that homozygosity of the *HFE* H63D mutation may act as a modifier, increasing the risk of developing CRC. In addition, there was evidence for earlier CRC onset age in H63D homozygotes [24]. The results of this study suggest that the median age of disease onset could be as much as 6 years earlier in H63D homozygotes (who represent around 2.5% of the Australian and Polish general populations).

While these findings will require substantiation in other populations, they support a possible relationship between iron dysregulation and colorectal cancer risk. While mechanisms cannot be established by a genetic epidemiological study of this nature, it appears likely that iron is involved, in view of the roles of the HFE gene in iron metabolism, the previously reported effects of H63D homozygosity on iron status [149] and existing evidence that iron status can modify CRC. Since iron levels in haemochromatosis patients can usually be maintained at normal levels through phlebotomy and regulating factors such as diet, this might have the potential to substantially reduce colorectal cancer risks or delay onset by several years in people with HNPCC-associated MMR gene mutations.

However the possibility of other mechanisms not directly reflecting abnormal body iron status cannot be ruled out. Homozygosity of the H63D polymorphism increases the risk of the neurodegenerative brain disease amyotrophic lateral sclerosis in the absence of apparent effects of C282Y polymorphism [150 - 152], suggesting that in some tissues the H63D mutation might have pathological consequences that are not directly related to whole body iron status. It will be important to validate the findings on H63D and also to investigate the effects of C282Y homozygosity in larger HNPCC samples, preferably in conjunction with information on patient iron status, to determine the mechanisms involved and the role of iron.

While this is the first time that the H63D polymorphism has been specifically associated with HNPCC, there is some previous evidence for association of both the H63D and the C282Y polymorphism with colorectal cancer in general [147, 148]. Power has limited past studies, as the homozygous and compound heterozygous mutations that have been associated with the greatest increases in iron loading and potentially the highest disease risks, are relatively rare. For this reason, some studies have analysed all *HFE* mutation genotypes as a single group, which may dilute observed effects. Although past epidemiological studies of *HFE* genotype and colorectal cancer risk have had mixed results, an American study of 475 colorectal cancer case patients and 833 control subjects found an odds ratio of 1.4 for participants with any *HFE* mutation after adjustment for a range of factors including age, gender and total iron intake [148]. The increased risk predominantly occurred in the quartile with greatest dietary iron intakes. In addition, a recent study of a large Australian sample has found that homozygosity for the C282Y SNP is associated with a three-fold increase in the risk of developing colorectal cancer in men [144]. This suggests that the effects of *HFE* on colorectal cancer may not be limited only to MMR gene mutation carriers, although such effects may be stronger when both types of mutation are present simultaneously.

Heterozygosity for either the H63D or C282Y SNP does not appear to have any modifying effect in either the Australian or Polish samples, although it is possible that small effects may be detectable with very large samples. While heterozygosity for C282Y or H63D has been reported to have a range of effects in other diseases, reviewed in [153], these genotypes are not usually associated with significant changes in iron parameters [26, 154 - 156]. For these reasons, for our final analyses it was considered more appropriate to compare mutant homozygotes to combined heterozygotes and wildtype homozygotes, as is usually done in most studies of *HFE* gene SNPs. However, while this was effective in revealing the potential modifying effect of H63D homozygosity on HNPCC development, we were not able to do this for the C282Y SNP, due to its relative rarity and the lack of C282Y homozygotes in the samples. Stronger modifying effects may occur in C282Y homozygotes or C282Y/H63D compound heterozygotes, as it is well established that iron indices are increased most in individuals with these genotypes, reviewed in [131, 132, 157].

Gender affects both the onset age and site of first tumour manifestation in HNPCC. In females, the age of onset of colorectal cancer is delayed 5 to 10 years when compared to males [158]. Gender is also a factor in the manifestation of iron loading as a result of *HFE* genotype, affecting males much earlier in life than females [159]. In a larger sample it is possible that *HFE* genotype may show a contribution to the earlier onset of CRC in males when compared to females.

8. Candidate polymorphisms not associated with disease risk

Not all polymorphisms which have been associated with hereditary disease have remained consistently significant across cohorts. An example is the delta *DNMT3b* SNP which was reported to have a significant association in a cohort of participants in the United States [160]. *DNMT3B* has been identified as a candidate in disease modifying risk due to its role in methylation. DNA methylation is regulated by a family of DNA methyltransferases (DNMTs), of which three active forms (DNMT1, DNMT3A and DNMT3B) have been identified in mammalian cells [161]. It has been reported that an increase in DNA methyltransferase enzyme activity of the DNA methyltransferases DNMT1, and DNMT3A and DNMT3B, is elevated in several types of disease including leukemia, prostate, lung, breast and endometrial cancers [162 -165]. A polymorphism located within *DNMT3b* has been reported to influence enzyme expression through altering promoter activity. It has been suggested that in *in vitro* assays the C>T variant could lead to an increase of promoter activity of up to 30% [161]. Using a study group of over 400 individuals, no association was observed between age of onset and *DNMT3b* genotype in an Australian and Polish Lynch syndrome cohort. The failure to confirm the potential modifying influence of a polymorphism in one population compared to another could be simply due to insufficient numbers of test subjects. If a polymorphism is an effect modifier its response should be similar no matter what population is examined even though it may not reach statistical significance. In the case of the delta *DNMT3b* SNP no such trend was observed. The Australian/Polish study group was approximately three times larger than the participants of a previous study [160] and the most likely explanation for the difference in results is a type 1 error. Notwithstanding, it is worth noting that it does not rule out the possibility that *DNMT3b* expression may be associated with Lynch syndrome disease expression. Different isoforms of DNMT3b exist therefore expression levels of these may vary influencing disease risk. Numerous other polymorphisms have also been reported in the functional domains of DNMT3b which could also alter methylation status and thereby alter disease risk.

Genes involved in DNA repair have also been prime candidates in the search for modifying effects due to their important role in the cell cycle. Polymorphisms located within genes involved in this process have been widely reported to be associated with cancer susceptibility in an extensive range of malignancies that include CRC. For one combined cohort (Australian and Polish Lynch syndrome patients), eight common polymorphisms were selected across several genes involved in the DNA repair pathway including *BRCA2, hMSH3, Lig4, hOGG1* and *XRCC* 1, 2 and 3, which had not previously been assessed for disease risk in Lynch syndrome. When considered separately conflicting data were identified in the two populations. Cox regression modelling indicated a significant protective effect in Polish participants for both polymorphisms *hMSH3* A>G (rs26279) and *XRCC2* G>A (rs1799793). This finding was somewhat contradictory as the homozygote form of both rs26279 and rs1799793 have been previously weakly associated with an increased risk of CRC and bladder cancer respectively [166, 167]. Two points need to be taken into account in interpreting this data. First, since multiple tests were undertaken in evaluating the possible influence of DNA repair gene polymorphisms a correction for multiple testing must be undertaken to ensure that any observed result is not due to a chance association; second, population stratification may adversely affect result outcome but is less likely (Reeves et al. 2011 [168]. Differences in the probabilities of an association with the age of disease onset in relation to DNA repair gene polymorphisms occurring in small study groups is more likely to be a result of a type 1 or 2 statistical error and can be overcome by undertaking an appropriate power calculation to determine the expected power to detect an association. Furthermore, statistical correction (such as Bonferroni) is required especially where multiple testing is undertaken although some types of correction are somewhat conservative and could remove an association where one exists.

9. Summary

There have been a number of studies that demonstrate the role of modifying genes that influence disease risk in Lynch Syndrome. Many studies have been undertaken that have failed to identify a range of candidate modifying genes as a result of studies being too small in size to provide robust statistical results. Nevertheless, there is a growing body of evidence that suggests modifying genes do influence disease risk in Lynch Syndrome and some of these are of particular interest as they suggest potential avenues by which disease risk can be modulated.

The role of genome wide association studies in identifying new agnostic modifier genes is currently generating special interest and at this point two studies have reported intriguing associations that correlate well with disease risk. It remains to be seen if such associations can be verified in larger populations. The use of genome wide data or even target assessment of several thousand potential modifiers is fraught with difficulties not the least of which is the available population size and the number of individual SNPs analysed.

Despite the difficulties encountered in identifying polymorphic modifier genes, their role in improving disease risk assessment is becoming clearer and the search for those that can make for individualised patient care will continue.

10. References

[1] Lengauer, C., et al. Genetic instabilities in human cancers. Nature 1998; 396:643-649.

[2] Boland, C.R. and Goel, A. Clearing the air on smoking and colorectal cancer. J. Natl Cancer Inst. 2010; 102:996-997.

[3] Lynch, H. T. and A. de la Chapelle (1999). Genetic susceptibility to non-polyposis colorectal cancer. Journal of medical genetics 1999; 36:801-818.

[4] Boland, C. R., et al. The biochemical basis of microsatellite instability and abnormal immunohistochemistry and clinical behavior in Lynch syndrome: from bench to bedside." Familial cancer 2008; 7:41-52.

[5] Vasen, H. F.,, et al. New clinical criteria for hereditary nonpolyposis colorectal cancer (HNPCC, Lynch syndrome) proposed by the International Collaborative group on HNPCC. Gastroenterology 1999;116: 1453-1456.

[6] Lynch H.T., et al. Hereditary factors in cancer. Study of two large Mid-Western kindreds. Arch. Intern. Med. 1996; 117:206-212.

[7] Lindor NM. Familial colorectal cancer type X: the other half of hereditary nonpolyposis colon cancer syndrome. Surg Oncol Clin N Am. 2009;18:637-645.

[8] Peltomaki, P. Deficient DNA mismatch repair: a common etiologic factor for colon cancer. Hum Mol Genet 2001; 10:735-740.

[9] Kunkel, T. A. and D. A. Erie. DNA mismatch repair. Annu Rev Biochem 2001; 74: 681-710.

[10] Jiricny, J. The multifaceted mismatch-repair system. Nat Rev Mol Cell Biol 2006; 7: 335-346.

[11] Bonis, P. A., et al. (2007). Hereditary nonpolyposis colorectal cancer: diagnostic strategies and their implications. Evid Rep Technol Assess 2007; 150: 1-180.

[12] Lynch, H. T., et al. Phenotypic variation in colorectal adenoma/cancer expression in two families. Hereditary flat adenoma syndrome. Cancer 1990; 66: 909-915.

[13] Lynch, H. T., et al. Genetics, natural history, tumor spectrum, and pathology of hereditary nonpolyposis colorectal cancer: an updated review. Gastroenterology 1993; 104:1535-1549.

[14] Scott, R. J., et al. (2001). Hereditary nonpolyposis colorectal cancer in 95 families: differences and similarities between mutation-positive and mutation-negative kindreds. Am J Hum Genet 2001; 68: 118-127.

[15] Rebbeck T.R., et al. Genetic variation and cancer: improving the environment for publication of association studies. Cancer Epidemiol. Biomarkers Prev. 2004; 13:1985-1986.

[16] Pharoah P.D., et al. The reliable identification of disease-gene associations. Cancer Epidemiol. Biomarkers Prev. 2005; 14:1362.

[17] Ross J.A., et al. Genetic variation in the leptin receptor gene and obesity in survivors of childhood acute lymphoblastic leukaemia: a report from the Childhood Cancer Survivor Study. J. Clin. Oncol. 2004; 22:3558-3562.

[18] Terry, K.L., et al. Genetic variation in the progesterone receptor gne and ovarian cancer risk. Am J. Epidemiol. 2005;161:442-451.

[19] Freedman, M.L., et al. Systematic evaluation of genetic variation at the androgen receptor locus and risk of prostate cancer in a multiethnic cohort study. Am. J. Hum. Genet. 2005; 76:82-90.

[20] Eerola, H., et al. Hereditary breast cancer and hanlding of patients risk. Scand J. Surg. 2002; 91:280-287.

[21] Stormorken, A.T., et al. Prevention of colorectal cancer by colonoscopic surveillance in families with hereditary colorectal cancer. Scand. J. Gastroenterol. 2007; 42:611-617.

[22] Zecevic, M., et al. (2006). IGF1 gene polymorphism and risk for hereditary nonpolyposis colorectal cancer. J National Cancer Inst 2006; 98: 139-143.

[23] Reeves, S. G., et al. IGF1 is a modifier of disease risk in hereditary non-polyposis colorectal cancer. International journal of cancer. Journal international du cancer 2008; 123: 1339-1343.

[24] Reeves, S.G., et al., MTHFR 677 C>T and 1298 A>C polymorphisms and the age of onset of colorectal cancer in hereditary nonpolyposis colorectal cancer. Eur J Hum Genet, 2009. 17: 629-635.

[25] Shi, Z., et al. Haemochromatosis HFE gene polymorphisms as potential modifiers of hereditary nonpolyposis colorectal cancer risk and onset age. Int. J. Cancer. 2009; 125: 78-83.

[26] Heinimann, K., et al. N-acetyltransferase 2 influences cancer prevalence in hMLH1/hMSH2 mutation carriers. Cancer research 1999; 59: 3038-3040.

[27] Talseth, B. A., et al. Genetic polymorphisms in xenobiotic clearance genes and their influence on disease expression in hereditary nonpolyposis colorectal cancer patients. Cancer Epidem. Biomarkers & Prevention 2006;15: 2307-2310.

[28] Jones, J. S., et al. ATM polymorphism and hereditary nonpolyposis colorectal cancer (HNPCC) age of onset (United States). Cancer causes & control : 2005; 6: 749-753.

[29] Talseth, B. A., et al. Lack of association between genetic polymorphisms in cytokine genes and disease expression in patients with hereditary non-polyposis colorectal cancer. Scandinavian journal of gastroenterology 2007; 42: 628-632.

[30] Levine, A. J. P53, the cellular gatekeeper for growth and division. Cell 1997; 88(3): 323-331.

[31] Xu, H. and M. R. el-Gewely. P53-responsive genes and the potential for cancer diagnostics and therapeutics development." Biotechnology Ann Rev 2001; 7:131-164.

[32] Jones, J. S., et al. P53 polymorphism and age of onset of hereditary nonpolyposis colorectal cancer in a Caucasian population. Clin. Cancer Res. 2004; 10:5845-5849.
[33] Thomas, M., et al. Two polymorphic variants of wild-type p53 differ biochemically and biologically. Molecular and cellular biology 1999; 19:1092-1100.
[34] Pim, D. and L. Banks. P53 polymorphic variants at codon 72 exert different effects on cell cycle progression." Int. J. Cancer. 2004 108: 196-199.
[35] Storey, A., et al. Role of a p53 polymorphism in the development of human papillomavirus-associated cancer. Nature 1998; 393: 229-234.
[36] Wang, Y. C., et al. (1999). "p53 codon 72 polymorphism in Taiwanese lung cancer patients: association with lung cancer susceptibility and prognosis." Clin. Can Res. 1999; 5:129-134.
[37] Bergamaschi, G., et al. TP53 codon 72 polymorphism in patients with chronic myeloid leukemia. Haematologica 2004; 89:868-869.
[38] Cortezzi, S. S., et al. Analysis of human papillomavirus prevalence and TP53 polymorphism in head and neck squamous cell carcinomas. Cancer Genet and Cytogenet. 2004; 150: 44-49.
[39] Sotamaa, K., et al. P53 codon 72 and MDM2 SNP309 polymorphisms and age of colorectal cancer onset in Lynch syndrome." Clin. Cancer Res 2005; 11: 6840-6844.
[40] Talseth, B. A., et al. Age of diagnosis of colorectal cancer in HNPCC patients is more complex than that predicted by R72P polymorphism in TP53. Int. J. Cancer. 2006; 118:2479-2484.
[41] Bond, G. L., et al. A single nucleotide polymorphism in the MDM2 promoter attenuates the p53 tumor suppressor pathway and accelerates tumor formation in humans. Cell 2004; 119:591-602.
[42] Talseth, B. A., et al. MDM2 SNP309 T>G alone or in combination with the TP53 R72P polymorphism does not appear to influence disease expression and age of diagnosis of colorectal cancer in HNPCC patients. Int. J. Cancer. 2007; 120: 563-565.
[43] Lohmueller, K. E., et al. Variants associated with common disease are not unusually differentiated in frequency across populations. Am J. Hum. Genet. 2006; 78:130-136.
[44] Kong, S., et al. Effects of cyclin D1 polymorphism on age of onset of hereditary nonpolyposis colorectal cancer. Cancer Res. 2000; 60: 249-252.
[45] Chen, J., et al. Association between Aurora-A kinase polymorphisms and age of onset of hereditary nonpolyposis colorectal cancer in a Caucasian population." Mol. Carcinogenesis 2007; 46: 249-256.
[46] Bala, S. and P. Peltomaki. CYCLIN D1 as a genetic modifier in hereditarynonpolyposis colorectal cancer. Cancer Res 2001; 61: 6042-6045.
[47] Kruger, S., et al. Absence of association between cyclin D1 (CCND1) G870A polymorphism and age of onset in hereditary nonpolyposis colorectal cancer. Cancer Letts 2006; 236:191-197.
[48] Talseth, B. A., et al. Aurora-A and Cyclin D1 polymorphisms and the age of onset of colorectal cancer in hereditary nonpolyposis colorectal cancer." Int J. Cancer 2008; 122: 1273-1277.
[49] Ferraz, J. M., et al. Impact of GSTT1, GSTM1, GSTP1 and NAT2 genotypes on KRAS2 and TP53 gene mutations in colorectal cancer. Int. J. Cancer 2004; 110:183-187.
[50] Smith G., et al. Metabolic polymorphisms and cancer susceptibility. Cancer Surv. 1995; 25:27-65.

[51] Campbell, P. T., et al. Cytochrome P450 17A1 and catechol O-methyltransferase polymorphisms and age at Lynch syndrome colon cancer onset in Newfoundland. Clin Cancer Res. 2007; 13:3783-3788.
[52] Esteller, M., et al. Germline polymorphisms in cytochrome-P4501A1 (C4887 CYP1A1) and methylenetetrahydrofolate reductase (MTHFR) genes and endometrial cancer susceptibility. Carcinogenesis 1997; 18:2307-2311.
[53] Felix, R., et al. GSTM1 and GSTT1 polymorphisms as modifiers of age at diagnosis of hereditary nonpolyposis colorectal cancer (HNPCC) in a homogeneous cohort of individuals carrying a single predisposing mutation. Mut. Research 2006; 602:175-181.
[54] Frazier, M. L., et al. Age-associated risk of cancer among individuals with N-acetyltransferase 2 (NAT2) mutations and mutations in DNA mismatch repair genes. Cancer Res. 2001; 61:1269-1271.
[55] He, L.J., et al. Genetic polymorphisms of N-acetyltransferase 2 and colorectal cancer risk. World J Gastroenterol. 2005; 11:4268-4271.
[56] Loktionov, A., et al. Glutathione-S-transferase gene polymorphisms in colorectal cancer patients: interaction between GSTM1 and GSTM3 allele variants as a risk-modulating factor. Carcinogenesis 2001; 22:1053-1060.
[57] Moisio, A. L., et al. Genetic polymorphisms in carcinogen metabolism and their association to hereditary nonpolyposis colon cancer. Gastroenterology 1998; 115: 1387-1394.
[58] Pistorius, S., et al. N-acetyltransferase (NAT) 2 acetylator status and age of onset in patients with hereditary nonpolyposis colorectal cancer (HNPCC). Cancer letters 2006; 241:150-157.
[59] Sivaraman, L., et al. CYP1A1 genetic polymorphisms and in situ colorectal cancer. Cancer Res. 1994; 54:3692-3695
[60] Slattery, M.L., et al. NAT2, GSTM-1, cigarette smoking and risk for colon cancer. Cancer Epidemiol. Biomarkers Prev. 1998; 7:1079-1084.
[61] Ye, Z. and Parry, J.M. Genetic polymorphisms in the cytochrome P4501A1, glutathione S-transferase M1 and T1, and susceptibility to colon cancer. Teratog. Carcinog. Mutagen 2002; 22:385-392.
[62] Brockton, N., et al. N-acetyltransferase polymorphisms and colorectal cancer: A HuGE review. Am. J. Epidemiol. 2000; 151, 846-861.
[63] Shin, J. H., et al. Glutathione S-transferase M1 associated with cancer occurrence in Korean HNPCC families carrying the hMLH1/hMSH2 mutation. Oncology Reports 2003;10: 483-486.
[64] Gyorffy B., Kocsis, I., Vasarhelyi, B. Biallelic genotype distributions in papers publidhed in Gut between 1998 and 2003: altered conclusions after recalculating the Hardy-Weinberg equilibrium. Gut 2004; 53:614-615.
[65] Landi, S., et al. A comprehensive analysis of phase I and phase II metabolism gene polymorphisms and risk of colrectal cancer. Pharmacogenet. Genomics 2005; 15:535-546
[66] Balkwill, F. and Mantovani, A. Inflammation and cancer: back to Virchow? Lancet 2001; 357:539-545
[67] Coussens, L.M. and Webb, Z. Inflammation and cancer. Nature 2002; 420:860-867
[68] Duarte, I., et al. G-308A TNF-alpha polymorphism is associated with an increased risk of invasive cervical cancer. Biochem. Biophys Res Commun. 2005; 334:588-592

[69] El-Omar, E.M., et al Increased risk of noncardia gastric cancaer associated with proinflammatory cytokine gene polymorphisms. Gastroenterology 2003; 124:1193-1201.

[70] Giordani, L., et al. Association of breast cancer and polymorphisms of interleukin-10 and tumor necrosis factor-alpha genes. Clin. Chem. 2003; 49:1664-1667.

[71] Graziano, F. et al. Prognostic role of interleukin-1beta gene and interleukin-1 receptor antagonist gene polymorphisms in patients with advance gastric cancer. J. Clin. Oncol. 2005; 23:2339-2345.

[72] Hefler, L.A., et al. An interleukin-6 gene promotor polymorphism influences the biological phenotype of ovarian cancer. Cancer Res. 2003; 63:3066-3068.

[73] Iacopetta, B., Grieu, F. and Joseph, D. The -174 G/C gene polymorphism in interleukin-6 is associated with an aggressive breast cancer phenotype. Br. J. Cancer 2004; 90: 419-422.

[74] Ikeda, H., Old, L.J., and Schreiber, R.D. The roles of IFN gamma in protection against tumor developmen and cacner immunoediing. Cytokine Growth Factor Res. 2002; 13:95-109.

[75] Landi, S., et al. association of common polymorphisms in inflammatroy genes interleukin (IL)6, IL8, tumor necrosis factor alpha, NFKB1, and peroxisome proliferator-activated recpetor gamma wtih colorectal cancer. Cancer Res. 2003; 3:3560-3566.

[76] Sugaya, K., et al. Molecular analysis of adrenergic receptor genes and interleukin-4/interleukin-4 receptor genes in patients with interstitial cystitis. J. Urol. 2002; 168:26768-2671.

[77] Tsai, F.J., et al. Interleukin-4 gene intron-3 polymorphism is associated with transitional cell carcinoma of the urinary bladder. BJU Int. 2005; 95:432-435

[78] Balic, I., et al., Androgen receptor length polymorphism associated with prostate cancer risk in Hispanic men. J Urol, 2002. 168: 2245-2248.

[79] Beilin, J., et al., A case-control study of the androgen receptor gene CAG repeat polymorphism in Australian prostate carcinoma subjects. Cancer, 2001. 92: 941-949.

[80] Bennett, C.L., et al., Racial variation in CAG repeat lengths within the androgen receptor gene among prostate cancer patients of lower socioeconomic status. J Clin Oncol, 2002. 20: 3599-3604.

[81] Nowacka-Zawisza, M., et al., Dinucleotide repeat polymorphisms of RAD51, BRCA1, BRCA2 gene regions in breast cancer. Pathol Int, 2008. 58: 275-281.

[82] Vashist, Y.K., et al., Microsatellite GTn-repeat polymorphism in the promoter of heme oxygenase-1 gene is an independent predictor of tumor recurrence in male oral squamous cell carcinoma patients. J Oral Pathol Med, 2008. 37: 480-484.

[83] Wang, L., et al., Association of a functional tandem repeats in the downstream of human telomerase gene and lung cancer. Oncogene, 2003. 22: 7123-7129.

[84] Wang, S., et al., A novel variable number of tandem repeats (VNTR) polymorphism containing Sp1 binding elements in the promoter of XRCC5 is a risk factor for human bladder cancer. Mutat Res, 2008. 638: 26-36.

[85] Giovannucci, E., Insulin, insulin-like growth factors and colon cancer: a review of the evidence. J Nutr, 2001. 131(Suppl): 3109S-3120S.

[86] Rosen, C.J., et al., Association between serum insulin growth factor-I (IGF-I) and a simple sequence repeat in IGF-I gene: implications for genetic studies of bone mineral density. J Clin Endocrinol Metab, 1998. 83: 2286-2290.

[87] Gebhardt, F., K.S. Zanker, and B. Brandt, Modulation of epidermal growth factor receptor gene transcription by a polymorphic dinucleotide repeat in intron 1. J Biol Chem, 1999. 274: 13176-13180.
[88] Estany, J., et al., Association of CA repeat polymorphism at intron 1 of insulin-like growth factor (IGF-I) gene with circulating IGF-I concentration, growth, and fatness in swine. Physiol Genomics, 2007. 31: 236-243.
[89] Hoyo, C., et al., Predictors of variation in serum IGF1 and IGFBP3 levels in healthy African American and white men. J Natl Med Assoc, 2009. 101: 711-716.
[90] Chen, W., et al., Phenotypes and genotypes of insulin-like growth factor 1, IGF-binding protein-3 and cancer risk: evidence from 96 studies. Eur J Hum Genet, 2009. 17: 1668-1675.
[91] Espelund, U., et al., Elevated free IGF2 levels in localized, early-stage breast cancer in women. Eur J Endocrinol, 2008. 159: 595-601.
[92] Renehan, A.G., et al., Insulin-like growth factor (IGF)-I, IGF binding protein-3, and cancer risk: systematic review and meta-regression analysis. Lancet, 2004. 363: 1346-1353.
[93] Shi, R., et al., IGF-I and breast cancer: a meta-analysis. Int J Cancer, 2004. 111: 418-423.
[94] Warren, R.S., et al., Induction of vascular endothelial growth factor by insulin-like growth factor 1 in colorectal carcinoma. J Biol Chem, 1996. 271: 29483-29488.
[95] Baserga, R., The insulin-like growth factor I receptor: a key to tumor growth? Cancer Res, 1995. 55: 249-252.
[96] Kaulfuss, S., et al., Dual silencing of insulin-like growth factor-I receptor and epidermal growth factor receptor in colorectal cancer cells is associated with decreased proliferation and enhanced apoptosis. Mol Cancer Ther, 2009. 8: 821-833.
[97] Bjorntorp, P., Metabolic implications of body fat distribution. Diabetes Care, 1991. 14: 1132-1143.
[98] Donahue, R.P. and R.D. Abbott, Central obesity and coronary heart disease in men. Lancet, 1987. 2: 1215.
[99] Kissebah, A.H., et al., Relation of body fat distribution to metabolic complications of obesity. J Clin Endocrinol Metab, 1982. 54: 254-260.
[100] Koivisto, V.A., H. Yki-Jarvinen, and R.A. DeFronzo, Physical training and insulin sensitivity. Diabetes Metab Rev, 1986. 1: 445-481.
[101] Krotkiewski, M., et al., Impact of obesity on metabolism in men and women. Importance of regional adipose tissue distribution. J Clin Invest, 1983. 72: 1150-1162.
[102] Regensteiner, J.G., et al., Relationship between habitual physical activity and insulin levels among nondiabetic men and women. San Luis Valley Diabetes Study. Diabetes Care, 1991. 14: 1066-1074.
[103] Potter, J.D., et al., Colon cancer: a review of the epidemiology. Epidemiol Rev, 1993. 15: 499-545.
[104] Riccardi, G. and A.A. Rivellese, Effects of dietary fiber and carbohydrate on glucose and lipoprotein metabolism in diabetic patients. Diabetes Care, 1991. 14: 1115-1125.
[105] Powell, D.R., et al., Insulin inhibits transcription of the human gene for insulin-like growth factor-binding protein-1. J Biol Chem, 1991. 266: 18868-18876.
[106] Kajantie, E., et al., Serum insulin-like growth factor (IGF)-I and IGF-binding protein-1 in elderly people: relationships with cardiovascular risk factors, body composition, size at birth, and childhood growth. J Clin Endocrinol Metab, 2003. 88: 1059-1065.
[107] Valko, M., et al., Role of oxygen radicals in DNA damage and cancer incidence. Mol Cell Biochem, 2004. 266: 37-56.

[108] Palles, C., et al., Identification of genetic variants that influence circulating IGF1 levels: a targeted search strategy. Hum Mol Genet, 2008. 17: 1457-1464.
[109] Colangelo, L.A., et al., IGF-1, IGFBP-3, and nutritional factors in young black and white men: the CARDIA Male Hormone Study. Nutr Cancer, 2005. 53: 57-64.
[110] Cruickshank, J.K., et al., Epidemiology of the insulin-like growth factor system in three ethnic groups. Am J Epidemiol, 2001. 154: 504-513.
[111] Platz, E.A., et al., Racial variation in insulin-like growth factor-1 and binding protein-3 concentrations in middle-aged men. Cancer Epidemiol Biomarkers Prev, 1999. 8: 1107-1110.
[112] McGreevy, K.M., et al., Impact of nutrients on insulin-like growth factor-I, insulin-like growth factor binding protein-3 and their ratio in African American and white males. Public Health Nutr, 2007. 10: 97-105.
[113] Weisberg, I., et al., A second genetic polymorphism in methylenetetrahydrofolate reductase (MTHFR) associated with decreased enzyme activity. Mol Genet Metab, 1998. 64: 169-172.
[114] Chen, J., et al., Linkage disequilibrium between the 677C>T and 1298A>C polymorphisms in human methylenetetrahydrofolate reductase gene and their contributions to risk of colorectal cancer. Pharmacogenetics, 2002. 12: 339-342.
[115] Yin, G., et al., Methylenetetrahydrofolate reductase C677T and A1298C polymorphisms and colorectal cancer: the Fukuoka Colorectal Cancer Study. Cancer Sci, 2004. 95: 908-913.
[116] Sharp, L. and J. Little, Polymorphisms in genes involved in folate metabolism and colorectal neoplasia: a HuGE review. Am J Epidemiol, 2004. 159: 423-443.
[117] Giovannucci, E., Epidemiologic studies of folate and colorectal neoplasia: a review. J Nutr, 2002. 132(Suppl): 2350S-2355S.
[118] Pande, M., et al., Influence of methylenetetrahydrofolate reductase gene polymorphisms C677T and A1298C on age-associated risk for colorectal cancer in a caucasian lynch syndrome population. Cancer Epidemiol Biomarkers Prev, 2007. 16: 1753-1759.
[119] Sanjoaquin, M.A., et al., Folate intake and colorectal cancer risk: a meta-analytical approach. Int J Cancer, 2005. 113: 825-828.
[120] Hubner, R.A. and R.S. Houlston, Folate and colorectal cancer prevention. Br J Cancer, 2009. 100: 233-239.
[121] Mason, J.B., et al., A temporal association between folic acid fortification and an increase in colorectal cancer rates may be illuminating important biological principles: a hypothesis. Cancer Epidemiol Biomarkers Prev, 2007. 16: 1325-1329.
[122] Cole, B.F., et al., Folic acid for the prevention of colorectal adenomas: a andomized clinical trial. Jama, 2007. 297: 2351-2359.
[123] Logan, R.F., et al., Aspirin and folic acid for the prevention of recurrent colorectal adenomas. Gastroenterology, 2008. 134: 29-38.
[124] Song, J., et al., Effects of dietary folate on intestinal tumorigenesis in the apcMin mouse. Cancer Res, 2000. 60: 5434-5440.
[125] Song, J., et al., Chemopreventive effects of dietary folate on intestinal polyps in Apc+/-Msh2-/- mice. Cancer Res, 2000. 60: 3191-3199.
[126] Kabat GC, et al. A cohort study of dietary iron and heme iron intake and risk of colorectal cancer in women. *British journal of cancer* 2007;97:118-22.
[127] Kato I, et al. Iron intake, body iron stores and colorectal cancer risk in women: a nested case-control study. *International journal of cancer* 1999;80:693-8.

[128] Larsson SC, et al. Red meat consumption and risk of cancers of the proximal colon, distal colon and rectum: the Swedish Mammography Cohort. *International journal of cancer* 2005;113:829-34.
[129] Nelson RL. Iron and colorectal cancer risk: human studies. *Nutrition reviews* 2001;59:140-8.
[130] Norat T, Riboli E. Meat consumption and colorectal cancer: a review of epidemiologic evidence. *Nutrition reviews* 2001;59:37-47.
[131] Beutler E. Hemochromatosis: genetics and pathophysiology. *Annu Rev Med* 2006;57:331-347.
[132] Camaschella C. Understanding iron homeostasis through genetic analysis of hemochromatosis and related disorders. *Blood* 2005;106:3710-7.
[133] Pietrangelo A. Hereditary hemochromatosis. *Annual review of nutrition* 2006;26;251-270.
[134] Adams PC, et al. Hemochromatosis and iron-overload screening in a racially diverse population. *The New England journal of medicine* 2005;352:1769-78.
[135] Ellervik C, et al. Hemochromatosis genotypes and risk of 31 disease endpoints: meta-analyses including 66,000 cases and 226,000 controls. *Hepatology (Baltimore, Md* 2007;46:1071-80.
[136] Olynyk JK, et al. A population-based study of the clinical expression of the hemochromatosis gene. *The New England journal of medicine* 1999;341:718-24.
[137] Whitlock EP, et al. Screening for hereditary hemochromatosis: a systematic review for the U.S. Preventive Services Task Force. *Annals of internal medicine* 2006;145:209-23.
[138] Chua AC, et al. The regulation of cellular iron metabolism. *Critical reviews in clinical laboratory sciences* 2007;44:413-59.
[139] Gochee PA, et al.. A population-based study of the biochemical and clinical expression of the H63D hemochromatosis mutation. *Gastroenterology* 2002;122:646-51.
[140] Jackson HA, et al.. HFE mutations, iron deficiency and overload in 10,500 blood donors. *Brit J Haematol* 2001;114:474-484.
[141] Milman N, et al. Frequency of the C282Y and H63D mutations of the hemochromatosis gene (HFE) in 2501 ethnic Danes. *Annals of hematology* 2004;83:654-7.
[142] Steinberg KK, et al. Prevalence of C282Y and H63D mutations in the hemochromatosis (HFE) gene in the United States. *Jama* 2001;285:2216-22.
[143] Allen KJ, et al. Iron-overload-related disease in HFE hereditary hemochromatosis. *The New England journal of medicine* 2008;358:221-30.
[144] Osborne NJ, et al. Homozygosity for the C282Y mutation in the HFE gene is associated with increased risk of colorectal and breast cancer in Australian population. *Am J Hematol.* 2007;82:575.
[145] Chan AT, et al. Hemochromatosis gene mutations, body iron stores, dietary iron, and risk of colorectal adenoma in women. *Journal of the National Cancer Institute* 2005;97:917-926.
[146] Macdonald GA, et al. No evidence of increased risk of colorectal cancer in individuals heterozygous for the Cys282Tyr haemochromatosis mutation. *Journal of gastroenterology and hepatology* 1999;14:1188-1191.
[147] Robinson JP, et al. Evidence for an association between compound heterozygosity for germ line mutations in the hemochromatosis (HFE) gene and increased risk of colorectal cancer. *Cancer Epidemiol Biomarkers Prev* 2005;14:1460-1463.
[148] Shaheen NJ, et al. Association between hemochromatosis (HFE) gene mutation carrier status and the risk of colon cancer. *Journal of the National Cancer Institute* 2003;95:154-159.

[149] Barton JC, et al. Initial screening transferrin saturation values, serum ferritin concentrations, and HFE genotypes in Native Americans and whites in the Hemochromatosis and Iron Overload Screening Study. *Clinical genetics* 2006;69(1):48-57.
[150] Goodall EF, et al. Association of the H63D polymorphism in the hemochromatosis gene with sporadic ALS. *Neurology* 2005;65:934-7.
[151] Sutedja NA, et al. The association between H63D mutations in HFE and amyotrophic lateral sclerosis in a Dutch population. *Archives of neurology* 2007;64:63-7.
[152] Wang XS, et al. Increased incidence of the Hfe mutation in amyotrophic lateral sclerosis and related cellular consequences. *Journal of the neurological sciences* 2004;227:27-33.
[153] Weinberg ED. Do some carriers of hemochromatosis gene mutations have higher than normal rates of disease and death? *Biometals* 2002;15:347-50.
[154] Beutler E, et al.. Penetrance of 845G--> A (C282Y) HFE hereditary haemochromatosis mutation in the USA. *Lancet* 2002;359:211-8.
[155] Hunt JR, Zeng H. Iron absorption by heterozygous carriers of the HFE C282Y mutation associated with hemochromatosis. *The American journal of clinical nutrition* 2004;80:924-31.
[156] Singh M, et al. Risk of iron overload in carriers of genetic mutations associated with hereditary haemochromatosis: UK Food Standards Agency workshop. *The British journal of nutrition* 2006;96:770-3.
[157] Pietrangelo A. Hereditary hemochromatosis. *Biochim Biophys Acta* 2006;1763:700-10.
[158] Parc Y, et al.. Cancer risk in 348 French MSH2 or MLH1 gene carriers. *Journal of medical genetics* 2003;40:208-13.
[159] Ayonrinde OT, et al. Clinical perspectives on hereditary hemochomatosis. *Critical reviews in clinical laboratory sciences* 2008; 45; 451-458.
[160] Jones, J.S., et al., DNMT3b polymorphism and hereditary nonpolyposis colorectal cancer age of onset. Cancer Epidemiol Biomarkers Prev, 2006. 15: 886-891.
[161] Shen, H., et al., A novel polymorphism in human cytosine DNA-methyltransferase-3B promoter is associated with an increased risk of lung cancer. Cancer Res, 2002. 62: 4992-4995.
[162] Jin, F., et al., Up-regulation of DNA methyltransferase 3B expression in endometrial cancers. Gynecol Oncol, 2005. 96: 531-538.
[163] Mizuno, S., et al., Expression of DNA methyltransferases DNMT1, 3A, and 3B in normal hematopoiesis and in acute and chronic myelogenous leukemia. Blood, 2001. 97: 1172-1179.
[164] Montgomery, K.G., et al., The DNMT3B C-->T promoter polymorphism and risk of breast cancer in a British population: a case-control study. Breast Cancer Res, 2004. 6: 390-394.
[165] Patra, S.K., et al., DNA methyltransferase and demethylase in human prostate cancer. Mol Carcinog, 2002. 33: 163-171.
[166] Chang, C.H., et al., Significant association of XPD codon 312 single nucleotide polymorphism with bladder cancer susceptibility in Taiwan. Anticancer Res, 2009. 29: 3903-3907.
[167] Koessler, T., et al., Common variants in mismatch repair genes and risk of colorectal cancer. Gut, 2008. 57: 1097-1101.
[168] Reeves S.G. et al. DNA repair gene polymorphisms and risk of early onset colorectal cancer in Lynch syndrome. 2011. doi:10.1016/j.canep.2011.09.003

4

Cytokine Gene Polymorphisms in Colorectal Cancer

Spaska Stanilova
Trakia University, Medical Faculty,
Department of Molecular Biology, Immunology and Medical Genetics,
Bulgaria

1. Introduction

Colorectal cancer is the second-leading cause of cancer-related deaths in Europe and the United States (Parkin DM, 2001). Although the primary therapy of CRC is surgical, the elucidation of different novel prognostic markers may prove to serve as future therapeutic options and contribute to the overall understanding of this cancer entity, as well as to improver disease outcome. Inflammation has been known to be a key factor of development and progression of cancer, and this is particularly notable in colorectal. At the cellular level, the colonic epithelium is exposed to a range of toxic and pathogenic challenges, including the balance between intestinal microflora. In turn, a shift can result in a change in immune response, leading to the induction of inflammation. Interactions between tumor and immune cells at the site of inflammation either enhance or inhibit cancer progression. The epidemiological data available are very impressive and show a clear association between chronic inflammatory conditions and subsequent malignant transformation in the inflamed tissue (Macarthur et al., 2004). New evidence suggests that up to 25% of all cancers are due to chronic infection or other types of chronic inflammation (Hussain SP, et al., 2007). Inflammation is mediated by an array of cytokines, which are synthesized by activated immune cells and exert their biological activities upon binding to specific receptors and activate the NF-κB transcription factor signal pathway in the epithelial cells. The ubiquitous transcription factor family NF-κB is a central regulator of the transcriptional activation of a number of genes involved in cell adhesion, immune and proinflammatory responses, apoptosis, differentiation, and growth. Induction of these genes in intestinal epithelial cells by activated NF-κB profoundly influences mucosal inflammation and repair (Jobin and Sartor, 2000).

There is strong evidence to suggest that cytokines are involved in the control of cancer development and also promote tumorigenesis, invasion, propagation, and metastasis of tumors, and that they may be relevant for gastrointestinal tumors. More recently, the molecular mechanism whereby the inflammation regulates the antitumor immune responses has been elucidated. In many tumors, signal transducers and activator of transcription (STAT)3 are activated, and thereby antitumor immune surveillance is suppressed (H. Yu and R. Jove, 2004).

In general the genes that encode cytokines involved in regulation of inflammatory conditions are genetically polymorphic and different genotypes are responsible for level of protein expression.

Genetic polymorphisms have emerged in recent years as important determinants of disease susceptibility and severity. Polymorphisms are naturally occurring DNA sequence variations, which differ from gene mutations in that they occur in the normal healthy population and have a frequency of at least 1%. Approximately 90% of DNA polymorphisms are single nucleotide polymorphisms (SNPs) due to single base substitutions. Others include insertion/deletion polymorphisms, minisatellite and microsatellite polymorphisms. Although most polymorphisms are functionally neutral, some have effects on regulation of gene expression or on the function of the coded protein. These functional polymorphisms, despite being of low penetrance, could contribute to the differences between individuals in susceptibility to and severity of disease. Many studies have examined the relationship between certain cytokine gene polymorphism, cytokine gene expression in vitro, and the susceptibility to and clinical severity of diseases (Bidwell et al., 1999; Hollegaard and Bidwell, 2006). SNPs are the most common sources of human genetic variation, and they may contribute to an individual's susceptibility to cancer. Cytokine gene polymorphisms have emerged in recent years as important determinants of susceptibility and severity of colorectal cancer. Cytokine polymorphisms directly influence interindividual variation in the magnitude of cytokine response, and this clearly contributes to an individual's ultimate clinical outcome. Dysregulation of cytokine production strongly influenced both tumor progression and host anti-tumor immunity. Cytokines secreted by activated immune and inflammatory cells can either promote tumor cell survival and growth or exert antitumor effects. In addition, some tumor cells may evade the immune system by secreting cytokines which may induce regulatory cells particularly the immunosuppressive CD4+CD25+ FoxP3+ T regulatory cells. In this chapter the polymorphisms of selected candidate genes for susceptibility to and/or severity of CRC are reviewed. Special attention is paid to studies concerning the genes of inflammatory related cytokines.

2. Cytokine gene polymorphisms of proinflammatory cytokines: IL-1; TNF-α and IL-6

The most compelling evidence for the role of inflammation in CRC comes from studies showing that proinflammatory cytokine gene polymorphisms increase the risk of cancer and its precursors.

IL-1β is a prominent proinflammatory cytokine, which together with tumor necrosis factor-α (TNF-α) serve as primary initiators of the complex inflammatory response and they are classical activators of NFkB signaling pathway. IL-1β and TNF-α genes have a number of functional polymorphisms. The IL-1B-31T/C and TNF-A-308G/A SNPs have been shown to be functionally significant with the C allele of IL-1B-31T/C and A allele of TNF-A-308G/A being associated with increased production of their respective cytokines (Hwang et al., 2002; Abraham and Kroeger, 1999). IL-1 gene cluster polymorphisms suspected of enhancing production of IL-1β have been shown to be relevant in the development of H. pylori-associated gastric adenocarcinoma. A study published in Nature showed for the first time that polymorphisms in interleukin-1B (IL-1B) were associated with gastric cancer risk (El Omar et al, 2000). Two of these polymorphisms are in near-complete linkage disequilibrium and one is a TATA-box polymorphism that markedly affects DNA–protein interactions in vitro. These linked IL-1B single nucleotide polymorphisms that increase IL-1β expression

(−511 C>T and −31 T>C) were associated with a 2- to 3-fold increased risk of gastric cancer. Heterozygosity at the IL1B −31T/C locus has also been associated with colorectal adenoma, a precursor of colorectal cancer (Gunter et al., 2006). However, Macarthur et al., 2005 did not reveal significant associations between the cytokine polymorphisms of IL-1B-31T/C and risk of colorectal cancer. In the same directions are results obtained by Ito et al., 2007 for the same SNP in IL-1B. Simultaneously they found that IL-1B-511 heterozygotes and T carriers had a significantly low risk for gastric and colorectal carcinoma in the Japanese population.

The TNF cytokines are well known for their cytotoxic and antitumor activity. TNF-α is a proinflammatory cytokine secreted mainly by activated monocytes/ macrophages. TNF-α mediates the early inflammatory response and regulates the production of other cytokines, including IL-1 and IL-6. TNF-α gene is transcriptionally silent in unstimulated monocytes and is rapidly transcribed in response to a variety of signals, such as bacterial endotoxin (LPS) and other stimuli. The signaling cascades leading to TNF-α production bifurcates to control both transcription of TNF-α gene and translation of TNF-α m RNA (Swantek et al., 1997). Transcriptional control of the TNF-α gene is mediated primarily by NF-kB binding sites present within the TNF-α gene promoter (Sweet and Hume, 1996; Yao et al., 1997). One microsatellite polymorphism in the vicinity of the TNF-α gene (TNF-A) has 14 different alleles (a1–a14). The a6 allele was associated with lower TNF-α secretion from activated monocytes (Pociot et al., 1993). For this TNF-α polymorphism, one allele was associated with an increased risk (a2 allele) and two other TNF-A alleles with decreased risks (a5 and a13 allele) of CRC (Gallagher, G et al., 1997; De Jong et al., 2002).

Among the other investigated polymorphisms of the TNF-α gene, the promoter -308G/A SNP was intensively studied. The presence of TNF-α -308A allele involved in gene transcription is associated with higher levels of TNF-α. Park et al., investigated TNF-A and Ncol RFLP of TNF-B genes and the risk of CRC (Park et al., 1998). The first intron of TNFB and the -308 promoter region of TNFA SNP polymorphisms were determined in 136 colorectal cancer patients and 325 healthy controls in an Asian population. Their results indicated that homozygous TNF-B*1/TNF-B*1 genotypes showed an increased risk for colorectal cancer, although no association in tumor susceptibility was found for the −308 G/A polymorphism of the TNF-α gene when comparing colorectal cancer patients and healthy controls. Landi et al., 2003 found a trend of reduced risk for CRC in TNF -308A allele carriers, but Theodoropoulos et al., 2006 found no effect of this SNP and the risk of CRC in Greek population.

For another SNP in TNF-α gene promoter, the −238 G > A site, has been reported that the A allele decreases the risk of developing colorectal cancer (Jang et al., 2001). Up to now, however, most studies have focused more on other cancer entities, such as melanoma and breast cancer, than on colorectal cancer.

The TNF-α pro-cancerous effect has recently been established. It's binding to specific receptors sets up signal transduction pathways, leading to cell apoptosis and gene regulation, via the MAPKinase and NF-kB pathways (Waterston A, and Bower, 2004).

Interleukin-6 (IL-6) is a pleiotropic cytokine that is participates in physiological and pathological processes for a variety of human malignancies including colorectal cancer. In particular, a preoperative IL-6 level is correlated with tumor stage, survival rate, and liver metastasis in CRC (Nakagoe et al., 2003). A significant association between serum IL-6 level and staging of the tumor ($P<0.001$), tumoral tissue IL-6 level ($r=0.95$, $P<0.001$) in the patients was founded (Esfandi F et al, 2006). IL-6 amount of the serum and tumoral tissue in the patients with colorectal cancer correlate significantly with the staging of the tumor and with each other. It has been demonstrated that IL-6 acts as a colorectal growth factor and as an autocrine growth factor for colorectal cancer cells (Chung and Chang, 2003).

A common G/C polymorphism located within the IL-6 gene promoter (chromosome 7p21) at position 174 bp, upstream from the start site of transcription (−174 G/C locus), has been reported (Fishman D et al, 1998). This promoter SNP affects the transcription of the gene, and altering the final levels of IL-6 released (Terry et al., 2000, Bonafe et al., 2001). The G allele increases IL-6 expression, both in stimulated and non stimulated conditions, the highest IL-6 levels being found in subjects homozygous for the G allele. In the same line are data of Belluco at al., 2003 for increased serum levels of IL-6 in colorectal cancer patients with genotype GG, regardless of the tumor stage, grade and location. Moreover, they also found a close correlation between high levels of circulating IL-6 and the presence of hepatic metastasis. The association between IL-6 serum level and CRC hepatic metastasis may depend on IL-6 properties to up-regulating the expression of adhesion receptors on endothelial cells and inducing the production of growth factors, such as hepatocyte growth factor and vascular endothelial growth factor, both of which may stimulate tumor metastasis. IL-6 promoter activation involves synergism between the transcription factors NF-IL-6 and NF-κB (Huang et al, 2000), and this may explain increased IL-6 serum levels in the CRC patients with hepatic metastasis. The first report, for investigation the promoter polymorphism in IL-6 gene with sporadic colorectal cancer risk has been the study of Landi et al., 2003. They found that the allele IL6 −174C is associated with increased risk of CRC. This association was seen both under a codominant model as well as when genotypes were grouped for both cancer of the colon and cancer of the rectum. A possible explanation of this effect is that the -174C allele could cause increased inflammation for colorectal cells in response to activated neutrophils (Nusrat et al., 2001). Slattery and colleagues reported that the GG genotype of the −174 G/C IL-6 polymorphism was associated with a significantly reduced risk of colon, but not rectal, cancers (Slattery et al., 2007). The IL6 −174C allele's role in CRC risk could not be replicated in the studies of others collectives (Theodopoulos et al., 2006; Cacev et al., 2010).

A possible cause for the conflicts and mismatches, like those observed here and the earlier study in allele and genotype distributions, may be the differences in racial or ethnical backgrounds. Duch et al. analyzed 52 patients with multiple myeloma and found that the G allele frequency was higher in the Brazilian population than in the European population (Duch C et al., 2007). Nowadays Yeh et al. observations on the allele and genotype distribution of the IL-6 −174 G/C polymorphism demonstrated that there are low frequencies of the G allele and GG genotype in the Taiwanese CRC population compared to the Western counterpart (Yeh et al., 2009).

Experimental data suggest that IL-6 plays an important role not only in developed but also in the progression of metastasis from colorectal cancer. In CRC patients, high expression of IL-6 has been correlated with poor survival and IL-6 -174 genotype CC was also significantly associated with shorter survival time when compared with the heterozygous genotype CG (Chung YC et al., 2006; Wilkening et al., 2008). Also, Belluco and colleagues analyzed 62 CRC patients and observed that patients with the C allele had lower serum IL-6 levels than those without the C allele, particularly in the presence of hepatic metastasis (Belluco C et al., 2003).

Specifically, IL-6/IL-6R complexes initiate homodimerization of gp 130, activate a cytoplasmic tyrosine kinase, and trigger signaling cascades through the JAK/STAT, Ras/MAPK and PI3-K/AKT pathways (Su et al., 2005; Chung YC et al., 2006). It has been shown that activation of signal transducers and activators of transcription 3 (STAT3) a member of a family of six different transcription factors is constitutively active in CRC cells (Corvinus et al., 2005). Ones of main activators of these signal transducers are proinflamatory cytokines such as IL-6, TNF-α and growth factors. STAT3 activity in CRC cells triggered through interleukins was found to be abundant in dedifferentiated cancer cells and infiltrating lymphocytes of CRC samples. These actions regulate inflammatory reactions, immune responses, and several other pathophysiological processes of malignancy including cell growth and survival, differentiation, cell mobility and angiogenesis. Thus, the presence of proinflammatory cytokine polymorphisms in colorectal cancer development remains a pertinent question and one that we are not aware of other investigators having considered.

3. Cytokine gene polymorphisms of antiinflamatory cytokines: TGF-β and IL-10

Anti-inflammatory cytokines play an important role in downregulation of inflammation and the prevention of neoplastic disorders. Genetic variations of anti-inflammatory cytokines are assumed to influence such responses. Typical anti-inflamatory cytokines (TGF-beta and IL-10) with immunosuppressive effect are secreted mainly from T regulatory cells (Tregs).

Transforming growth factor-beta (TGF-β or TGFB) is an immunoregulatory cytokine that plays an important role in tumor immune response within the gastrointestinal tract and this is shown in TGFB gene knockout mice, which proceed to develop uncontrolled inflammatory response and early death (Kulkarni et al., 1993). In mammalian cells, there are three isoforms described TGFB1, TGFB2, and TGFB3. Among them TGFB1 is the most abundant subtype.

TGF β1 is involved in many critical cellular processes, including cell growth, extracellular matrix formation, cell motility, angiogenesis, hematopoiesis, apoptosis, and immune function (Moustakas et al., 2002; Schuster & Krieglstein, 2002). All immune cell lineages, including B, T and dendritic cells as well as macrophages, secrete TGF-β, which negatively regulates their proliferation, differentiation and activation by other cytokines.

The TGF-β signaling pathway plays an important role in controlling cell proliferation and differentiation involved in colorectal carcinogenesis. Binding of cytokine to the TGF-β receptor complex leads to phosphorylation of Smad proteins and triggers Smads intracellular signaling mediators to modulate gene transcription, mainly by transcription factor Sp1. Xu and Pasche, 2007 shown that TGF-β signaling alterations have been implicated in susceptibility to colorectal cancer.

In normal intestinal epithelium TGF-β1 acts as a growth inhibitor, however loss of TGF-β1 - mediated growth restraint has been shown to be associated with the transformation of colorectal adenoma to cancer. In addition, there is evidence that excess production and/or activation of TGF-β by cancer cells can contributed to the tumor progression by paracrine mechanisms involving neoangiogenesis, production of stroma and proteases, and subversion of immune surveillance mechanisms in tumor hosts (Muraoka-Cook et al., 2005). Moreover, TGF-β is the most frequently up-regulated in tumor cells (Elliott and Blobe, 2005).

TGF-β1 is also a potent effector within the tumor microenvironment. It exerts a predominantly immunosuppressive effect on CD8+ cytotoxic T-lymphocytes and has been shown an active player in tumor immune evasion (Li et al., 2006). Friedman et al. reported that high levels of transforming growth factor β1 correlate with disease progression in human colon cancer (Friedman et al. 1995). In light of these finding TGF-β1 gene is a functional candidate gene for genetic predisposition in CRC.

The TGF-β1 gene is located on chromosome 19 and several SNPs were described in promoter region, in the non-translated region (introns), in the coding region (exons), and in the 3'-UTR region of the gene (Watanabe et al., 2002). Certain inherited variants in the promoter region of the TGF-β gene (-800G/A and -509C/T) have been associated with higher cytokine circulating concentrations. The -800G/A SNP is located in a consensus cyclic AMP response element binding protein (CREB) half site and may cause reduced affinity for CREB transcription factors whose binding is important for transcription control (Grainger D et al., 1999). The -509C/T is located within a YY1 consensus binding site and -509T allele has been associated with increased TGF-β1 plasma level (Grainger D et al., 1999) and reduced T-cell proliferation (Meng et al., 2005). Moreover these two SNPs of the TGF-β gene are in linkage disequilibrium. The 509 C/T polymorphism has been implicated in both colorectal adenoma and cancer risk. However, published data remains conflicting.

In the study of Macarthur et al., 2005 no association was found between -509C/T SNP in TGF-β1 promoter and colorectal cancer. Authors investigated also association between cytokine polymorphisms of IL-1, IL-10 and TNF-α genes in a population based case-control study of 264 CRC patients and 408 controls in the Northeast of Scotland and analyzed their interaction with regular aspirin use. The beneficial association between nonsteroidal anti-inflammatory drugs use, such as aspirin and decreased risk of colorectal cancer provided further evidence to suggest a role for chronic inflammation in the pathogenesis of sporadic colorectal cancer. Whereas a statistically significant association was not found between any of the SNPs and CRC alone, the authors observed a significant interaction between the IL-10-592 genotype and aspirin use. The effect of aspirin on CRC risk was limited to carriers of low producing A allele (AA and AC) compared with CC genotype. The authors postulated that individuals who are genetically prone to producing reduced levels of the anti-inflammatory IL-10 (i.e., carriers of the variant A allele) are more likely to benefit from the anti-inflammatory properties of aspirin in decreasing risk of CRC development.

Berndt et al., 2007 examined two SNPs in the promoter region of the TGFB1 (-800G/A; -509C/T) and two in exon 1 (Leu10Pro; Arg25Pro) and one in exon 5 (Thr263Ile) in association with advanced colorectal adenoma in population consisted primarily of Caucasians, living in the USA. The Leu10Pro and Arg25Pro SNPs encoded non synonymous amino acid substitution located in signal peptide sequence of the TGF-β1 pro-peptide.

Dunning et al., 2003 revealed that the 10Pro variant lead to increased TGF-β secretion compared with the 10Leu allele. Similarly, the 25Arg allele has been associated with increased TGF-β production upon stimulation in vitro (Awad MR et al., 1998).

Berndt et al., reported that the high TGF-β produced genotypes, *−509TT* and *10Pro/Pro* genotypes were associated with an increased risk of advanced colorectal adenoma compared with other genotypes. These increased risks, particularly for -509TT association were greater for the subsets of participant with multiple adenomas and those with rectal adenomas. Risk factors for hyperplastic and adenomatous polyps were generally similar to those for colorectal cancer. Another study investigated the same Leu10Pro polymorphism in association with colorectal adenoma and hyperplastic polyps. In this study no association was found with this SNP and adenoma, but a lower risk of hyperplastic polyps was suggested for Pro allele carriers who were current or past smokers (Sparks et al, 2004).

Together these studies give support to the possible role of TGFB1 in the adenoma-carcinoma sequence and suggest that high TGFB1 produced genotypes may modulate the risk in this transformation.

To characterize association of genetic variation at the TGFB1 gene with circulating cytokine levels of TGF-β and risk of colorectal adenoma and adenocarcinoma, Saltzman et al., 2008 conducted two case-control studies (including 271 colorectal adenoma cases and 544 controls, and 535 colorectal adenocarcinoma cases and 656 controls) among Japanese Americans, Caucasians, and Native Hawaiians in Hawaii. The authors investigated 26 SNPs, spanning 39.8 kb region of the TGFB1 gene, distributed in two haplotype blocks of linkage disequilibrium named as tagSNPs, including all previously commented SNPs. They found that the variant A allele for tagSNP in 3'UTR A/G (rs6957) was associated with an increased serum level of TGF-β, and no association with promoter -509C/T and Leu10Pro polymorphisms was found. However, published data remains conflicting. In the recent study the association between -509 C/T and -800 G/A SNPs of the TGFB1 gene, and susceptibility to colorectal cancer in Iranian patients was investigated (Amighofran Z et al., 2009). They found a statistically significant lower frequency of 509T allele and TT genotype in patients than in control subjects. At position 800, no significant differences in genotype distribution and allele frequencies between the patients and healthy controls were found. The authors concluded that the genotype distributions and allele frequencies of the TGFB1 gene polymorphism at -509 C/T were significantly related to colorectal carcinoma in Iranian subjects. In the same directions are the results of Chung et al., 2007, that -509T variant allele reduced risk of colorectal cancer, but not adenoma in Koreans. A possible explanation for discrepancy in above commented results for involvement of -509 C/T SNP in colorectal cancer susceptibility occurs in the investigation of Fang et al., 2010. To derive a more precise estimation of the relationship, a meta-analysis of 994 colorectal cases and 2,335 controls from five published paper was performed. Overall, significantly increased colorectal cancer risks were found for CC versus TT in the subgroup analysis by ethnicity. Fang et al., 2010 concluded that TGFB1 -509 C/T substitution has a role in genetic predisposition for developing colorectal cancer in Asians, but no significant associations were found among Europeans.

Thus far, TGF-β1 −509 T/C gene polymorphisms have been also relevant to Crohn's disease development (Schulte et al., 2001). In the same time patients with Crohn's disease are at increased risk for developing colorectal cancer. Several lines of evidence implicate chronic inflammation in inflammatory bowel disease (ulcerative colitis and Crohn's disease) as a key predisposing factor to distinct subset of colorectal tumors. (Itzkowitz and Yio, 2004).

IL-10 is an immuno-regulatory cytokine that plays a crucial role in modulating gastrointestinal tract inflammation (Moore et al, 2001; Lin and Karin, 2007). IL-10 is produced mainly by regulatory T cell and antigen presenting cells. It is pivotal in inhibiting inflammation and interrupting carcinogenesis. In cancer patients, the production of immune suppressive cytokines: IL-10 and TGF is accelerated, and IL-10-producing type I T-regulatory (Tr1) cells are highly infiltrated in tumor microenvironment. Thus, tumor cells might escape from the immune surveillance. That is the way the IL-10 gene might be involved in genetically predisposition and severity of CRC.

Large interindividual differences in the IL-10 inducibility have been observed, which has shown to have a genetic component of over 70%. The IL-10 gene comprises 5 exons, and it has been mapped to chromosome 1q31-32. To date, at least 49 *IL10*-associated polymorphisms have been reported, and an even larger number of polymorphisms are recorded in SNP databases (Ensembl Genome Browser, 2006). Promoter polymorphisms have been subject to the most studies, particularly with regard to possible influences on gene transcription and protein production. Three SNPs at -1082(A/G), -819(C/T), -592(C/A) upstream from the transcription start site (D'Alfonso S et al., 1995; Turner D et al., 1997) have been described as well as additional two microsatellite (CA)n repeats, termed IL-10G and IL-10R and located at -1151 and -3978 respectively (Eskdale J and Galager G, 1995; Eskdale J et al., 1997). In particular, SNP at position -1082A/G of IL-10 gene was associated with IL-10 production alone or in haplotypes with other distal SNPs. Turner et al.,1997 have shown that -1082A allele is associated with lower in vitro IL-10 production by Con A-stimulated PBMC from normal subjects. Crawley et al., 1999 have reported that GCC haplotype was associated with higher IL-10 level compared to ATA in whole blood cultures after LPS stimulation. In our studies, the functional effect of -1082 A/G polymorphism was demonstrated among the Bulgarian population in both healthy volunteers and in patients with sepsis (Stanilova et al., 2006).

Positive associations between IL-10 genotype or haplotype and cancer susceptibility, progression, or both were reported (Howell and Rose-Zerilli, 2007). The IL-10-1082/-819/-592 genotype status was associated with an increased risk for gastric cancer in Japan. The presence of the ATA/GCC haplotype of IL-10-1082/-819/-592 polymorphisms significantly increased the risk of gastric cancer development compared with presence of the ATA/ATA haplotype. (Sugimoto et al, 2007). The AA genotype of the -1082 A/G polymorphism in the interleukin-10 gene promoter was associated with lower IL-10 production in LPS, PHA or PWM stimulated healthy PBMC (Stanilova et al, 2006). This cytokine possess anti-inflammatory and immunoregulatory role and it is no wonder that IL-10 play a dual role in tumor development and progression (Mocellin et al., 2003; Mocellin et al, 2004; Dranoff 2004; Lin and Karin, 2007). Contradictory results are present in the literature concerning IL-10 systemic or tissue levels and survival of cancer patients. For instance, Mocellin et al. found that IL-10 overexpression within the tumour microenvironment was implicated in cancer immune rejection.

Although IL-10 suppression of pro-inflammatory cytokines synthesis favors its anti-tumor immunity, it might also promote tumor growth by stimulating cell proliferation and inhibiting cell apoptosis. A high systemic level of IL-10 has been reported for advanced colorectal cancer patients (O'Hara et al., 1998; Galizia et al., 2002). Increased level of IL-10 might better control inflammatory responses and cancer development. Results from our study demonstrated a stage dependent association between IL-10 serum level and severity of CRC (Stanilov et al., 2010). The highest IL-10 serum level was found in stage-IV CRC patients, suggesting a pro-tumorigenic activity of systemic IL-10 in CRC progression and play a role in tumor-induced immunosupression in CRC patients. In addition, we determined a significantly increased mRNA in tumor tissue compared to normal mucosa (Stanilov et al., 2009). Moreover expression of IL-10 mRNA correlated positively with increased Foxp3 mRNA expression detected in tumor tissue. These results confirm the role of Foxp3 transcription factor in induction of IL-10 production and differentiation of Treg-1 cells in tumor microenvironment.

Cacev et al, 2008 reported a statistically significant decrease in IL-10 mRNA expression in tumor tissue then normal mucous depending on IL-10 SNPs. IL-10 promoter genotypes −819 TT and −592 AA associated with low IL-10 mRNA expression in tumor and corresponding normal mucosa. The 'low-producer genotypes' were present more frequently in colon cancer patients and this difference in genotype distribution was statistically significant. In the same study IL-10 -1082AA genotype was associated with lower IL-10 mRNA expression, whereas -1082GG genotype was associated with higher IL-10 mRNA expression in tumor tissue. In a group of colon cancer patients, an increased frequency of the -1082AA genotype compared with control group was observed without statistical significance. The authors conclude that IL-10-1082G/A SNP did not influence sporadic colon cancer susceptibility.

No associations were observed among colorectal cancer patients and controls for IL-10 -1082G/A and -592C/A genotype frequencies in a case–control study of 62 patients and 124 matched controls (Crivello et al., 2006). A possible reason for these contradictory results might be a small number of patients.

A recent study of Tsilidis K et al., 2009 investigated the association of 17 candidate SNPs in IL-10 with colorectal cancer in 208 patients. The authors established that -1082 promoter SNP is implicated. Compared with the AA genotype at the candidate IL10-1082 locus (rs1800896), carrying one or two G alleles, a known higher producer of the anti-inflammatory cytokine IL-10 was associated with lower risk of colorectal cancer ($p = 0.03$). Statistically significant associations with colorectal cancer were observed for three tagSNPs in IL10 (rs1800890, rs3024496, rs3024498) and one common haplotype, but these associations were due to high linkage disequilibrium with IL10-1082.

Associations between IL-10 genotypes and cancer chemopreventive strategies and survival were also published. Results of Macarthur et al. suggest that IL-10 SNPs may play a role in predicting response to chemopreventive strategies. Carriers of the *IL-10-592*A allele, had a statistically significant 50% reduced risk of colorectal cancer when taking regular aspirin, whereas risk was not reduced in carriers of the A allele who did not use aspirin, or among aspirin users with the CC genotype. It is possible that carriers of the *IL-10-592C* allele are more likely to derive chemopreventive benefits from aspirin in the presence of a lower production of their own endogenous anti-inflammatory interleukin-10 (Macarthur et al, 2005).

In particular proinflammatory genotypes characterized by a low IL-10 producer seem to be associated with a worse clinical outcome. Sharma et al. investigated the prognostic value of an inflammation-based Glasgow Prognostic Score in advanced colorectal cancer to explore a predictive pattern of cytokine gene polymorphisms for clinical outcome (Sharma et al., 2008). They found that IL-10–592A/C and IL-10 –1082A/G were predictive for overall survival. Patients homozygous for IL-10–592 CC had improved overall survival compared with those patients with ≥ 1 A allele (median survival, 12.2 ± 0.7 months vs. 8.6 ± 1.6 months). In contrast, patients homozygous for IL-10–1082 AA had poorer overall survival compared with patients with ≥ 1 G allele (median survival, 8.8 months ± 3.2 months vs. 11.2 ± 2.1 months).

Although the functional effects of polymorphisms in immunosuppressive genes TGFB and IL-10 have not yet been elucidated, obviously that they may play a significant role in modulating susceptibility, development and survival of colorectal cancer (Fig.1). The observation of increased circulating levels of IL-10 in colorectal cancer patients may have important implications for future investigations, immunological monitoring and therapeutic intervention on neoplastic patients, and suggests a mechanism for tumour cells escaping from immune surveillance.

Gene/ polymorphism	Genotype or allele associated with			
	Succeptibility - increased risk of CRC	Protection – decreased risk of CRC	Survival rate - Shorter survival	References
PROINFLAMMATORY				
IL-1B -511 C>T		TT ; CT		Ito et al., 2007
TNF-B	TNF-B*1/TNF-B*1			Park et al.,1998
TNF-A microsatellite	a2 allele	a5 and a13 allele		Gallager et al., 1997 ; DeJong et al, 2002
TNF-A- 238 G >A		AA and AG		Jang et al., 2001
IL6 −174G>C	C allele			Landi et al., 2003
			CC	Chung YC et al., 2006
		GG		Slattery M et al., 2007
ANTIINFLAMATORY				
TGFB1 -509C>T	−509TT			Berndt et al., 2007
TGFB1 Leu10Pro	10Pro/Pro			Berndt et al., 2007
TGFB1 -509C>T		−509TT		Amighofran Z et al., 2009
TGFB1 -509C>T		−509T allele		Chung et al., 2007
TGFB1 -509C>T		−509TT		Fang et al., 2010
IL-10 -1082 A>G		G allele		Tsilidis K et al., 2009
IL-10 -592 C> A	−592 AA			Cacev et al, 2008
IL-10 -819 C>T	−819 TT			Cacev et al, 2008
IL-10 -1082 A>G ; -592 C> A			IL-10 - 1082AA IL-10 - 592 AA	Sharma et al., 2008

Table 1. Involvement of IL-1; TNF, IL-6, IL-10 and TGF-β gene polymorphisms into colorectal cancer.

4. Role of IL-12-related cytokines

Human interleukin (IL)-12 (IL-12p70) is a disulfide-linked heterodimer composed of two subunits p40 and p35. IL-12p40 subunit can be secreted as monomer, which can also form IL-23, a heterodimeric pro-inflammatory cytokine composed of p40 and p19 subunits, and a homodimer, IL-12p80, which can act as an IL-12 and IL-23 antagonist by competing at their receptors (Hoelscher, 2004). The IL-12 family cytokines are produced by antigen-presenting cells such as macrophages and dendritic cells and play critical roles in the regulation of Th cell differentiation. IL-12 induces IFN-γ production by NK and T cells and differentiation to Th1 cells. IL-23 induces IL-17 production by memory T cells and expands and maintains inflammatory Th17 cells. IL-27 induces the early Th1 differentiation and generation of IL-10-producing regulatory T cells. Although IL-12p70 is one of the most powerful antitumor cytokine (Colombo and Trinchieri, 2002), accumulating evidence revealed that the individual members of the IL-12 family play distinct roles in the regulation of antitumor immune responses.

Several polymorphisms have been described in the IL12B gene, encoding IL-12p40 subunit, including a single-nucleotide polymorphism in 3'-untranslated region (UTR) of IL12B with number rs3212227 and a complex polymorphism in promoter region of the IL12B (IL12Bpro), resulting from 4bp microinsertion combined with an AA/GC transition (rs17860508). Moreover, several studies have demonstrated that these two polymorphisms affect gene expression and IL-12 production (Morahan et al., 2001; Seegers et al., 2002; Muller-Berghaus et al., 2004; Stanilova and Miteva, 2005; Stanilova et al., 2008; Dobreva et al., 2009) and consequently could influence the pathogenesis of CRC. To test this hypothesis, we performed a case-control study to investigate the association between these gene polymorphisms and the risk of colorectal cancer. The paper of Miteva et al., 2009 was the first study which investigated the distribution of *IL12Bpro* polymorphism and the +16974A/C SNP in 3'UTR of *IL12B* among 85 Bulgarian patients with colorectal cancer. No differences in genotype and allelic frequencies of the *IL12B* polymorphisms in the promoter and 3'UTR regions between patients with CRC and controls were found, either when patients were analyzed as a whole group or when they were separated according to the TNM classification or clinical characteristics such as tumor location, differentiation degree, lymph node and metastases status. These data are in principal agreement with other studies, where no association with SNP in 3'UTR of *IL12B* was found in pathogenesis of other related gastrointestinal diseases. Navaglia et al. have reported that none of the studied *IL12B* gene polymorphisms, including SNP in 3'UTR, was correlated with Helicobacter pylori infection and intestinal metaplasia (Navaglia et al., 2005). There was no statistically significant association between the SNPs investigated in IL-12A gene ((+7506 A>T, +8707 A>G, +9177 T>A, +9508 G>A) and colorectal cancer risk in the study of Landi et al., 2006. The lack of association suggests that the role of both investigated polymorphisms in IL12B in susceptibility of sporadic colorectal cancer can be excluded. However, these findings do not exclude a key role for IL-12p40 in development and progression of the CRC. In our investigations, we have demonstrated that serum levels for IL-12p40 and IL-23 were significantly higher in patients compared to healthy donors. Additionally, we found the highest level of IL-12p40 in sera from patients with I stage of CRC and significantly lower in patients with more advanced stages. (Miteva et al., 2009; Stanilov et al., 2009; Stanilov et al., 2010). In respect to recent findings regarding different proteins in IL-12 related family which share the p40 subunit, we could attribute the relationship of decreased serum level of IL-

12p40 and severity of CRC to the action of Th1-promoting form of IL-12, such as IL-12p70, or free IL-12p40 in monomeric and homodimeric form.

In a recent study there were significant differences in the genotype and allele frequencies of the IL-12 gene 16974 A/C polymorphism between the group of patients with glioma and the control group (Zhao et al., 2009). Moreover, genotypes carrying the IL-12 16974 C variant allele were associated with decreased serum IL-12p40 and IL-27p28 levels compared to the homozygous wild-type genotype in patients with glioma.

The promoter polymorphisms in the human IL12B gene could influence JNK and p38 MAPKs control of IL-12p40 expression in human PBMC in response to mitogens and proinflammatory stimuli. The study of Dobreva et al., revealed that JNK and p38 MAPK inhibition in PBMC stimulated with C3bgp and LPS, significantly upregulated the IL-12p40 production from IL12Bpro-1 homozygotes and did not influence the IL-12p40 production from 1.2/2.2 genotypes (Dobreva et al., 2009). Also, the p38 inhibition led to significant increase of IL-12p40 production in IL12Bpro-1 homozygous PBMC stimulated with PHA. IL-12p40 is secreted at a 50-fold excess compared with IL-12p70 in a murine shock model (Wysocka et al., 1995) and at a 10-20-fold excess by stimulated human peripheral blood mononuclear cells (D'Andrea et al., 1992). IL-12p40 chain may form also a homodimer IL-12p80 that serves as an IL-12p70 and IL-23 antagonist by competing for binding at the receptor complexes of both cytokines (Cooper & Khader, 2006). The proper balance between IL-12p40-related cytokines play a key immunoregulatory role and control the appearance of protective Th1-mediated immune response. Current results demonstrated an opposite effect of JNK and p38 MAPKs inhibition on the IL-12p70 and IL-23 production in LPS and C3bgp-stimulated PBMC (Dobreva et al., 2008).Our results demonstrated that p38 MAPK inhibition down regulates IL-23 and up regulates IL-12p40/p70 inducible expression suggesting the benefit of p38 control in the treatment of inflammatory conditions.

IL-12 related cytokines (IL-12p70; IL-12p40 and IL-23) produced locally or systemic exhibit a significant role in progression of CRC. Accumulating evidence revealed that the individual members of the IL-12 family play distinct roles in progression of CRC. Studies have defined IL-12p70 as an important factor for the differentiation of naive T cells into IFN-γ producing Th1 cells and exhibits anti-tumor activity (Brunda et al., 1995; Gri et al., 2002). Although the antitumor activities of IL-12p70 are well characterized, studies of the role of IL-23 in development of CRC in humans are contradictory. Some authors reported that IL-23, as well as IL-12p70, have anti-tumor activity in murine tumor models (Wang et al., 2003; Lo et al., 2003; Shan et al.,2006). Contradictory results have been reported in studies of Langowski et al., 2006 which showed data that IL-23 promotes tumor incidence and growth in various human cancers. In this respect our results for enhanced serum levels of IL-23 in cancer patients regardless of severity supported the hypothesis that IL-23 promotes tumor development unlike IL-12p70 (Stanilov et al., 2010). Besides, the highest increase in transcriptional activity in tumor samples for IL-23p19 mRNA has been also reported in our study (Stanilov et al., 2009). IL-23p19 mRNA was approximately 29 fold upregulated ($p=0.0009$), whereas IL-12p35 mRNA was not significantly upregulated, when compared to their adjacent normal tissue. This difference indicated that IL-23 could be synthesized many times more than IL-12p70 in tumor tissue. Based on our and others data, we could assume that increased serum and locally produced IL-23 indicates impaired anti-tumor immune response and could be associated with poor prognosis of CRC. A molecular mechanism involved in IL-23 activities includes STAT3 activation. STAT3 signaling within the tumor microenvironment was recently elucidated to induce a protumor cytokine, IL-17 and IL-22, while inhibiting a central antitumor cytokine, IL-12p70, thereby shifting the balance of tumor immunity toward tumorigenesis. Interestingly, unlike spleen Treg cells, tumor-associated Treg cells express IL-23R and activate STAT3 in response to IL-23, leading to upregulation of the Treg-specific transcription factor Foxp3 and the immunosuppressive cytokine IL-10 (Xu M et al., 2010). Collectively, IL-12 and IL-23 play critical roles in the regulation of antitumor or protumor response in respective situation.

5. Conclusion

In recent years, efforts have been made to identify genes involved in the genetic predisposition or progression of colorectal cancer. During the last two decades, many of the 'candidate' cytokine genes implicated in colorectal tumorigenesis have been identified and were summarized in this review. As cancer is a complex genetic disease, it is probable that besides oncogenes and tumor suppressor genes a number of cytokine genes also contribute to cancer susceptibility and development. Moreover cytokines are a key-player in inflammation, which have protumoral effect and mediated anti-tumor immune response. Cytokines present in tumor microenvironment have gained much attention due to their influence on cell activation, growth, differentiation or cell migration and they are increasingly recognized as potential cancer modifying genes. While numerous factors influence the inflammatory response in cancer, the role of an individual's genetic background has recently received increasing attention.

Cytokines and their receptors are often encoded by highly polymorphic genes. Single-nucleotide polymorphisms in cytokine genes potentially affect their production by either creating or eliminating key binding motifs within promoter and other regulatory sequences. In investigating disease–gene associations, there is a strong argument for focusing on polymorphisms of functional significance. Up to date contradictory results from case-control study have been published concerning cytokine gene polymorphisms and colorectal cancer development. Obviously reasons for such results included different numbers of patients; their ethnicity and differences in clinical and pathological data. In any case-control study, there are potential limitations. Despite the limitations of most published studies, the preliminary literature indicates that selected cytokine polymorphisms, particularly in IL-10; TGF-β; IL-6 and TNF-α are required in colorectal cancer. Data included in this review summarized in table1 suggest that functional cytokine polymorphisms participate more in the onset of colorectal cancer progression rather than in its initial development. Due to the strong evidence concerning the biological significance of these SNPs further studies and meta analysis are needed to evaluate the significance in the clinic. Careful selection of SNPs to cover the whole length of a candidate gene sequence so that areas of association can be defined and informative haplotypes constructed. Emerging genotyping technologies will facilitate such definitive, comprehensive studies.

The preliminary data indicate that larger studies are required to confirm or reject existing results, extend studies to include more detailed genotype and haplotype analysis, and combine genotype and gene expression studies in the same subjects. Even larger numbers of cases and controls would be required to demonstrate more modest odds ratios with higher statistical power. Collection of definitive clinical and pathological data for all cases must be an integral part of such an approach.

Such studies will contribute significantly to our understanding of the biological role of cytokine polymorphisms in colorectal cancer development.

6. References

Abraham LJ, & Kroeger KM. (1999) Impact of the −308 TNF promoter polymorphism on the transcriptional regulation of the TNF gene: relevance to disease. *J Leukoc Biol*, 66:pp562–566.

Amirghofran Z., Jalali SA, Ghaderi A, & Hosseini SV. (2009) Genetic polymorphism in the transforming growth factor β1 gene (-509 C/T and -800G/A) and colorectal cancer. *Cancer genetics and cytogenetics*, 190:pp21-25

Belluco C, Olivieri F, Bonafe M, Giovagnetti S, Mammano E, Scalerta R, Ambrosi A, Franceschi C, Nitti D, & Lise M. (2003) −174 G>C polymorphism of interleukin 6 gene promoter affects interleukin 6 serum level in patients with colorectal cancer. *Clin Cancer Res*; 9:pp2173–2176.

Berndt S, Huang WY, Chatterjee N, Yeager M, Welch R, Chanock S, Weissfeld J, Schoen R &. Hayes R. (2007) Transforming growth factor beta 1 (TGFB1) gene polymorphisms and risk of advanced colorectal adenoma, *Carcinogenesis*, 28 pp.1965–1970,

Bidwell J, Keen L, Gallagher G, Kimberly R, Huizinga T, McDermott MF, Oksenberg J, McNicholl J, Pociot F, Hardt C & D'Alfonso S. (1999) Cytokine gene polymorphism in human disease: on-line databases. *Genes and immunity* 1:3-19

Bonafe M., Olivieri F., & Cavallone L., Giovagnetti S., Marchegiani F., Cardelli M., Pieri C., Marra M., Antonicelli R., Lisa R., Rizzo M. R., Paolisso G., Monti D., Franceschi C. (2001) A. gender-dependent genetic predisposition to produce high levels of IL-6 is detrimental for longevity. Eur. J. Immunol., 31: pp2357-2361.

Brunda MJ, Luistro L, Hendrzak JA, Fountoulakis M, Garotta G, & Gately MK (1995) Role of interferon-γ in mediating the antitumor efficacy of interleukin-12. *J Immunother*, 17: pp71-77.

Cacev T, Jokić M, Loncar B, Krizanac S, & Kapitanović S. (2010) Interleukin-6-174 G/C polymorphism is not associated with IL-6 expression and susceptibility to sporadic colon cancer. *DNA Cell Biol.*; 29(4):177-82.

Cacev T, Radosevic S, Krizanac S, & Kapitanovic S. (2008) Influence of interleukin-8 and interleukin-10 on sporadic colon cancer development and progression. *Carcinogenesis*; 29:pp1572-1580

Chung Y.C. & Y.F. Chang, (2003), Serum interleukin-6 levels reflect the disease status of colorectal cancer, *J. Surg. Oncol.* 83: pp. 222–226.

Chung YC., Chaen YL & Hsu CP. (2006) Clinical significance of tissue expression of interleukin-6 in colorectal carcinoma. *Anticancer Res.* 26:pp3905-3911.

Chung SJ, Kim JS, Jung HC, & Song IS. (2007) Transforming growth factor-β1 509T reduces risk of colorectal cancer, but not adenoma in Koreans. *Cancer Sci.* 98:pp401–404

Colombo M. P. & G. Trinchieri. (2002) Interleukin-12 in anti-tumor immunity and immunotherapy. *Cytokine and growth factor Reviews*, 13: pp155-168,

Cooper, A.M. & Khader, S.A. (2006) IL-12p40: an inherently agonistic cytokine. Trends Immunol. 28, pp33-38.

Corvinus FM, Orth C, Moriggl R, Tsareva SA, Wagner S, Pfitzner EB, Baus D, Kaufmann R, Huber LA, Zatloukal K, Beug H, Ohlschläger P, Schütz A, Halbhuber KJ, & Friedrich K. (2005) Persistent STAT3 activation in colon cancer is associated with enhanced cell proliferation and tumor growth. *Neoplasia*. 7:pp545-55.

Crawley E, Kay R, Sillibourne J, Patel P, Hutchinson I, & Woo P. (1999) Polymorphic haplotypes of the interleukin-10 5'flanking region determine variable interleukin-10 transcription and are associated with particular phenotypes of juvenile rheumatoid arthritis. *Arthritis Rheum*; 42, pp1101-1108.

Crivello A, Giacalone A, Vaglica M, Scola L, Forte GI, Macaluso MC, Raimondi C, Di Noto L, Bongiovanni A, Accardo A, Candore G, Palmeri L, Verna R, Caruso C, Lio D, & Palmeri S. (2006) Regulatory cytokine gene polymorphisms and risk of colorectal carcinoma. *Ann N Y* Acad Sci., 1089:pp98–103

D'Andrea, A., Rengaraju, M., Valiante, N.M., Chehimi, J., Kubin, M., Aste, M., Chan, S.H., Kobayashi, M., Young, D., Nickbarg, E., Chizzonite, R., Wolf, S.F., & Trinchieri, G. (1992) Production of natural killer cell stimulatory factor (NKSF/IL-12) by peripheral blood mononuclear cells. *J. Exp. Med.* 176,pp 1387-1398.

D'Alfonso S, Rampi M, Rolando V, Giordano M, & Momigliano-Richiardi P (2000) New polymorphisms in the IL-10 promoter region. *Genes Immun* 1:pp231-233.

De Jong MM, Nolte IM, te Meerman GJ, van der Graaf WT, de Vries EG, Sijmons RH, Hofstra RM, & Kleibeuker JH. (2002) Low-penetrance genes and their involvement in colorectal cancer susceptibility. *Cancer Epidemiol Biomarkers Prev* 11:pp1332-1352

Dobreva Z. Stanilova S. & Miteva L. (2008) Differences in the inducible gene expression and protein production of IL-12p40, Il-12p70 and IL-23: involvement of p38 and JNK kinase pathways. *Cytokine*, 43:pp76-82

Dobreva Z., Stanilova S, & Miteva L. (2009) Influence of JNK and p38 MAPKs inhibition on IL-12p40 and IL-23 production depending on IL12B promoter polymorphism. *Cell Mol Biol Lett*, , 14: pp609-621

Dranoff G (2004) Cytokines in cancer pathogenesis and cancer therapy. *Nat Rev Cancer*, 4: pp11-22.

Duch CR, Figueiredo MS, Ribas C, Almeida MS, Colleoni GW, & Bordin JO. (2007) Analysis of polymorphism at site −174 G/C of interleukin-6 promoter region in multiple myeloma. *Braz J Med Biol Res*. 40:pp265-267.

Elliott RL, Blobe GC. (2005) Role of transforming growth factor h in human cancer. *J Clin Oncol*; 23: pp2078–93.

El-Omar EM, Carrington M, Chow WH, McColl KE, Bream JH, Young HA, Herrera J, Lissowska J, Yuan CC, Rothman N, Lanyon G, Martin M, Fraumeni JF Jr, & Rabkin CS. (2000) Interleukin-1 polymorphisms associated with increased risk of gastric cancer. *Nature* 404: pp398-402,

El-Omar EM, Rabkin CS, Gammon MD, Vaughan TL, Risch HA, Schoenberg JB, Stanford JL, Mayne ST, Goedert J, Blot WJ, Fraumeni JF Jr, & Chow WH. (2003) Increased risk of noncardia gastric cancer associated with proinflammatory cytokine gene polymorphisms. *Gastroenterology*; 124: pp1193–1201.

Esfandi F, Mohammadzadeh Ghobadloo S, & Basati G. (2006) Interleukin-6 level in patients with colorectal cancer. *Cancer Lett*. 244: pp76-78

Eskdale J & Galager G (1995) A polymorphic dinucleotide repeat in the human IL- 10 promoter region. *Immunogenetics* 42: pp444-445.

Eskdale J, Kube D, Tesch H, & Gallagher G (1997) Mapping of the human IL10 gene and further characterization of the 5' flanking sequence. *Immunogenetics* 46:pp120-128

European Bioinformatics Institute, Sanger Institute. SNP database: Ensembl Genome Browser. 2006. Available at: http://www.ensembl.org/index.html.

Fang F, Yu L, Zhong Y, & Yao L. (2010) TGFB1 509 C/T polymorphism and colorectal cancer risk: a meta-analysis. *Med Oncol. Dec*; 27: pp1324-1328.

Fishman D, Faulds G, Jeffery R, Mohamed-Ali V, Yudkin JS, Humphries S, & Woo P. (1998) The effect of novel polymorphisms in the interleukin-6 (IL-6) gene on IL-6 transcription and plasma IL-6 levels, and an association with systemic-onset juvenile chronic arthritis. *J Clin Invest.*; 102:pp1369-1376

Friedman E, Gold LI, Klimstra D, Zeng ZS, Winawer S, & Cohen A. (1995) High levels of transforming growth factor β1 correlate with disease progression in human colon cancer. *Cancer Epidemiol Biomarkers Prev*, 4:pp549–554

Galizia G, Orditura M, Romano C, Lieto E, Castellano P, Pelosio L, Imperatore V, Catalano G, Pignatelli C, & De Vita F. (2002) Prognostic significance of circulating IL-10 and IL-6 serum levels in colon cancer patients undergoing surgery. *Clin Immunol*, 102: pp169–178,.

Gallagher, G., Lindemann, M., Oh, H. H., Ferencik, S., Walz, M. K.,Schmitz, A., Richards, S., Eskdale, J., Field, M., & Grosse-Wilde, H. (1997) Association of the TNFa2 microsatellite allele with the presence of colorectal cancer. *Tissue Antigens*, 50: pp47–51,.

Grainger DJ, Heathcote K, Chiano M, Snieder H, Kemp PR, Metcalfe JC, (1999) Genetic control of the circulating concentration of transforming growth factor type β1. *Hum Mol Genet.*; 8:pp93–97

Gri G, Chiodoni C, Gallo E, Stoppacciaro A, Liew F, & Colombo M (2002) Antitumor effect of Interleukin (IL)-12 in the absence of endogeneous IFN-γ: a role for intrinsic tumor immunogenicity and IL-15. *Cancer Res*, 62: pp4390-4397.

GunterM, Canzian F, Landi S, Chanock S, Sinha R, & Rothman N. (2006) Inflammation-Related Gene Polymorphisms and Colorectal Adenoma. *Cancer Epidemiol Biomarkers Prev*, 15: pp1126-1131

Hoelscher, C. (2004) The power of combinatorial immunology: IL-12 and IL-12-related dimeric cytokines in infectious diseases. *Med Microbiol Immunol.*, 193, pp1-17.

Hollegaard MV & Bidwell JL, (2006) Cytokine gene polymorphism in human disease: on-line databases, Supplement 3. *Genes Immun.*, 7:pp269-76.

Howell,W.M & Matthew J. Rose-Zerilli. (2007) Cytokine gene polymorphisms, cancer susceptibility, and prognosis. *J. Nutr.*, 137, pp194–199.

Huang 5., DeGuzman A., Bucana C. D., & Fidler I. J. (2000) Nuclear factor-kB activity correlates with growth, angiogenesis, and metastasis of human melanoma cells in nude mice. *Clin. Cancer. Res.*, 6: pp2573-2578.

Hussain SP, Harris CC, Inflammation and cancer: an ancient link with novel potentials. *Int. J. Cancer* 2007;121:pp2373-2380.

Hwang IR, Kodama T, Kikuchi S, Sakai K, Peterson LE, Graham DY, &Yamaoka Y. (2002) Effect of interleukin 1 polymorphisms on gastric mucosal interleukin 1β production in Helicobacter pylori infection. *Gastroenterology*; 123:pp1793–803.

Ito H, Kaneko K, Makino R, Konishi K, Kurahashi T, Yamamoto T, Katagiri A, Kumekawa Y, Kubota Y, Muramoto T, Mitamura K, & Imawari M (2007) Interleukin-1beta gene in esophageal, gastric and colorectal carcinomas. *Oncol Rep.* 18:pp473-81.

Jang WH, Yang YI, Yea SS et al (2001) The −238 tumor necrosis factor-alpha promoter polymorphism is associated with decreased susceptibility to cancers. *Cancer Lett* 166:pp41–46

Jobin C & Sartor B, (2000) The IκB/NF-κB system: a key determinant of mucosal inflammation and protection. *Am J Physiol Cell Physiol*, 278 ppC451-C462

Landi S, Gemignani F., Bottari F., Gioia-Patricola L, Guino E, Cambray M, Biondo S, Capella G, Boldrini L, Canzian F & Moreno V. (2006) Polymorphisms within inflammatory genes and colorectal cancer. *Journal of Negative Results in BioMedicine*, 5:pp5-15

Landi S, Moreno V, Gioia-Patricola L, Guino E, Navarro M, de Oca J, Capella G, & Canzian F; Bellvitge Colorectal Cancer Study Group (2003). Association of common polymorphisms in inflammatory genes interleukin (IL)6, IL8, tumor necrosis factor alpha, NFKB1, and peroxisome proliferator-activated receptor gamma with colorectal cancer. *Cancer Res*, 63:pp3560–3566.

Langowski JL, Zhang X, Wu L, Mattson JD, Chen T, Smith K, Basham B, McClanahan T, Kastelein RA, & Oft M (2006) IL-23 promotes tumor incidence and growth. *Nature*, 442: pp461-465.

Lin W, & Karin M (2007) A cytokine-mediated link between innate immunity, inflammation and cancer. *J Clin Invest*, 117: pp1175-1183.

Lo CH, Lee SC, Wu PY, Pan WY, Su J, Cheng CW, Roffler SR, Chiang BL, Lee CN, Wu CW, & Tao MH (2003) Antitumor and antimetastatic activity of IL-23. *J Immunol*, 171: pp600-607.

Macarthur M., Georgina L. Hold, & Emad M. El-Omar (2004) Inflammation and Cancer II. Role of chronic inflammation and cytokine gene polymorphisms in the pathogenesis of gastrointestinal malignancy. *Am J Physiol Gastrointest Liver Physiol* 286: ppG515–G520

Macarthur M, Sharp L, Hold GL, Little J, & El-Omar EM. (2005) The role of cytokine gene polymorphisms in colorectal cancer and their interaction with aspirin use in northeast of Scotland. *Cancer Epidemiol Biomarkers Prev.*;14:pp1623–1628.

Miteva L, Stanilov N, Deliysky T, Mintchev N, & Stanilova S. (2009) Association of polymorphisms in regulatory regions of interleukin-12p40 gene and cytokine serum level with colorectal cancer. *Cancer Investigation*, , 27:pp924-931

Mocellin S, Maricola FM, & Young HA: (2004) Interleukin-10 and the immune response against cancer: a counterpoint. *J Leukoc Biol*, 78: pp1043-1051.

Mocellin S, Panelli MC, Wang E, Nagorsen D, & Marincola FM (2003) The dual role of IL-10. *Trends Immunol*, 24: pp36-43.

Moore KW, de Waal MR, Coffman RL, & O'Garra A. (2001) Interleukin-10 and the interleukin-10 receptor. *Annu Rev Immunol*, 19:pp683–765.

Morahan, G.; Huang, D.; Wu, M.; Holt, B.J.; White, G.P.; Kendall, G.E.; Sly, P.D.; Holt, P.G. (2002) Association of IL12B promoter polymorphism with severity of atopic and non-atopic asthma in children. *Lancet.*, 360, pp455–459.

Morahan, G.; Huang, D.; Ymer, S.I.; Cancilla, M.R.; Stephen, K.; Dabadghao, P.; Werther, G.; Tait, B.D.; Harrison, L.C.; & Colman, P.G. (2001) Linkage disequilibrium of a type 1 diabetes susceptibility locus with a regulatory IL12B allele. *Nat Genet.*, 27, pp218-221.

Moustakas A, Pardali K, Gaal A, & Heldin CH. (2002) Mechanisms of TGF-β signaling in regulation of cell growth and differentiation. *Immunol Lett*, 82:pp85–91

Muller-Berghaus, J.; Kern, K.; Paschen, A.; Nguyen, X.D.; Klüter, H.; Morahan, G. & Schadendorf, D. (2004) Deficient IL-12p70 secretion by dendritic cells based on IL12B promoter genotype. *Genes Immun.*, 5, pp 431-434.

Nakagoe T., Tsuji T., Sawai T., Tanaka K., Hidaka S. & S. Shibasaki. (2003) Increased serum levels of interleukin-6 in malnourished patients with colorectal cancer, Cancer Lett. 202: pp. 109–115.

Navaglia, F.; Basso, D.; Zambon, C.F.; Ponzano, E.; Caenazzo, L.; Gallo, N.; Falda, A.; Belluco, C.; Fogar, P.; Greco, E.; Di Mario, F.; Rugge, M.; & Plebani, M. (2005) Interleukin 12 gene polymorphisms enhance gastric cancer risk in H pylori infected individuals. *J Med Genet.*, 42, pp 503-510.

Nusrat A., Sitaraman S. V., & Neish A. (2001) Interaction of bacteria and bacterial toxins with intestinal epithelial cells. *Curr. Gastroenterol. Rep.*, 3: pp392-398.

O'Hara RJ, Greenman J, MacDonald AW, Gaskell KM, Topping KP, Duthie GS, Kerin MJ, Lee PW, & Monson JR (1998) Advanced colorectal cancer is associated with impared interleukin 12 and enhanced interleukin 10 production. *Clin Cancer Res*, 4: pp1943-1948,.

Park KS, Mok JW, Rho SA & Kim JC (1998) Analysis of TNFB and TNFA Ncol RFLP in colorectal cancer. *Mol Cells* 8:pp246–249

Parkin DM (2001) Global cancer statistics in the year 2000. *Lancet Oncol* 2:533–543

Pociot, F., Briant, L., Jongeneel, C. V., Molvig, J., Worsaae, H., Abbal, M., Thomsen, M., Nerup, J., & Cambon-Thomsen, A. (1993) Association of tumor necrosis factor (TNF) and class II major histocompatibility complex alleles with the secretion of TNF-α and TNF-β by human mononuclear cells: a possible link to insulin-dependent diabetes mellitus. *Eur. J. Immunol.*, 23: pp224–231.

Schulte CM, Goebell H, & Roher HD (2001) C-509T polymorphism in the TGF-β1 gene promoter: impact on Crohn's disease susceptibility and clinical course? *Immunogenetics* 53:pp178–182

Schuster N, & Krieglstein K. (2002) Mechanisms of TGF-hmediated apoptosis. *Cell Tissue Res*; 307:pp1–14.

Seegers, D.; Zwiers, A.; Strober, W.; Pena, A.S.; & Bouma, G. (2002) A TaqI polymorphism in the 3' UTR of the IL-12 p40 gene correlates with increased IL-12 secretion. Genes Immun., 3, pp 419-423.

Shan B, Hao J, & Li Q, & Tagawa M (2006) Antitumor activity and immune enhancement of murine interleukin-23 expressed in murine colon carcinoma cells. *Cell Mol Immunol*, 3: pp47-52.

Sharma R, Zucknick M, London R, Kacevska M, Liddle C, & Clarke SJ. (2008) Systemic inflammatory response predicts prognosis in patients with advanced-stage colorectal cancer. *Clin Colorectal Cancer.*, 7:pp331–337

Slattery ML, Wolff RK, Herrick JS, Caan BJ, & Potter JD (2007) IL6 genotypes and colon and rectal cancer. *Cancer Causes Control.*; 18:pp1095-1105.

Stanilov N, Miteva L, Mintchev N, & Stanilova S. (2009) High expression of Foxp3, IL-23p19 and surviving mRNA in colorectal carcinoma. *International Journal of Colorectal Disease*, 24: pp151-157.

Stanilov N., Miteva L, Deliyski T, Jovchev J, & Stanilova S. (2010) Advanced colorectal cancer is assosiated with enhanced Interleukin-23 and Interleukin -10 serum level. *LabMedicine*, 41 :pp 159-163

Stanilova, S. & Miteva, L. (2005) Taq-I polymorphism in 3'UTR of the IL-12 and association with IL-12p40 production from human PBMC. *Genes Immun.*, 6, pp364-366.

Stanilova, S.; Miteva, L.; & Prakova, G. (2008) IL-12Bpro and GSTP1 polymorphisms in association with silicosis. *Tissue Antigens.*, 71, pp 169-174.

Steven H. Itzkowitz & Xianyang Yio. (2004) Inflammation and Cancer IV. Colorectal cancer in inflammatory bowel disease: the role of inflammation . *Am J Physiol Gastrointest Liver Physiol* 287: ppG7–G17.

Su JL, Lai KP, Chen CA, Yang CY, Chen PS, Chang C, Chou CH, Hu CL, Kuo ML, Hsieh CY & Wei LH (2005) A novel peptide specifically binding to interleukin-6 receptor (gp 80) inhibits angiogenesis and tumor growth. *Cancer Res,* 65: pp 4827-4835.

Sugimoto M, Furuta T, Shira N, Nakamura A, Kajimura M, Sugimura H, & Hishida A. (2007) Effects of interleukin-10 gene polymorphism on the development of gastric cancer and peptic ulcer in Japanese subjects. *Journal of Gastroenterology and Hepatology.*, 22: pp1443-1449.

Swantek JL, Cobb MH, & Gepperd DT. (1997) Jun N-Terminal Kinase/Stress - Activated Protein Kinase (JNK/SAPK) Is Required for Lipopolysaccharide Stimulation of Tumor necrosis factor alpha (TNF-α) Translation: Glucocorticoids Inhibit TNF-α Translation by blocking JNK/SAPK. *Mol Cell Biol.;* 17: pp6274-6282.

Sweet MJ, & Hume DA. (1996) Endotoxin signal transduction in macrophages. *J. Leukoc. Biol.;* 60:8-26.

Terry C. F., Loukaci V., & Green F. R. (2000) Cooperative influence of genetic polymorphisms on interleukin 6 transcriptional regulation. *J. Biol. Chem.,* 275: pp18138-18144.

Theodoropoulos G, Papaconstantinou I, Felekouras E, Nikiteas N, Karakitsos P, Panoussopoulos D, Ch Lazaris A, Patsouris E, Bramis J, & Gazouli M. (2006) Relation between common polymorphisms in genes related to inflammatory response and colorectal cancer. *World J Gastroenterol;* 12: pp5037-5043

Tsilidis KK, Helzlsouer KJ, Smith MW, Grinberg V, Hoffman-Bolton J, Clipp SL, Visvanathan K, & Platz EA. (2009) Association of common polymorphisms in IL10, and in other genes related to inflammatory response and obesity with colorectal cancer. *Cancer Causes Control.* 20:pp1739-51.

Turner DM, Williams DM, Sankaran D, Lazarus M, Sinnott PJ, & Hutchinson IV. (1997) An investigation of polymorphism in the interleukin-10 gene promoter. *Eur J Immunogenetics;* 24:pp1-8.

Wang YQ, Ugai S, Shimozato O, Yu L, Kawamura K, Yamamoto H, Yamaguchi T, Saisho H, & Tagawa M (2003) Induction of systemic immunity by expression of interleukin-23 in murine colon carcinoma cells. *Int J Cancer,* 105: pp820-824.

Watanabe Y, Kinoshita A, Yamada T, Ohta T, Kishino T, Matsumoto N, Ishikawa M, Niikawa N, & Yoshiura K. (2002) A catalog of 106 single nucleotide polymorphisms (SNPs) and 11 other types of variations in genes for transforming growth factor- 1 (TGF- 1) and its signaling pathway. *J Hum Genet* 47:pp 478-483.

Waterston A, & Bower M. (2004) TNF and cancer: good or bad? *Cancer therapy;* 2: pp131-148.

Wilkening S, Tavelin B, Canzian F, Enquist K, Palmqvist R, Altieri A, Hallmans G, Hemminki K, Lenner P, & Försti A. (2008) Interleukin promoter polymorphisms and prognosis in colorectal cancer. *Carcinogenesis;* 29:pp1202–6.

Wong SF,& Lai LC. (2001) The role of TGFβ in human cancers. *Pathology;* 33:85–92

Wysocka, M., Kubin, M., Vieira, L.Q., Ozmen, L., Garotta, G., Scott, P. & Trinchieri, G. (1995) Interleukin 12 is required for interferon-γ production and lethality in lipopolysaccharide-induced shock in mice. *Eur. J. Immunol.* 25,pp 672-676

Xu M, Mizoguchi I, Morishima N, Chiba Y, Mizuguchi J, & Yoshimoto T, Regulation of Antitumor Immune Responses by the IL-12 Family Cytokines, IL-12, IL-23, and IL-27. (2010) *Clinical and Developmental Immunology*. Volume 2010, Article ID 832454, doi:10.1155/2010/832454

Xu Y, & Pasche B. (2007) TGF-β signaling alterations and susceptibility to colorectal cancer. *Hum Mol Genet*, 15:ppR14–R2016

Yao, J.; Mackman, N.; Edgington, T. S., & Fan, S. T. (1997) Lipopolysaccharide induction of the tumor necrosis factor - alpha promoter in human monocytic cells. Regulation by Egr-1, c-Jun and NF-kappa B transcription factors. *J. Biol. Chem.*, 272: pp17795-17801.

Yu H. & R. Jove. The stats of cancer—new molecular targets come of age, (2004) *Nature Reviews Cancer*, vol. 4, pp. 97–105.

Zhao B, Meng LQ, Huang HN, Pan Y & Xu Q. A (2009) Novel Functional Polymorphism, 16974 A/C, in the Interleukin-12-3' Untranslated Region Is Associated with Risk of Glioma. DNA and Cell Biology. 28: pp335-341.

Part 3

Cell and Molecular Biology

5

Glutathione-S-Transferases in Development, Progression and Therapy of Colorectal Cancer

Tatyana Vlaykova[1], Maya Gulubova[2], Yovcho Yovchev[3], Dimo Dimov[4], Denitsa Vlaykova[1,6], Petjo Chilingirov[5] and Nikolai Zhelev[7]

[1]*Dept. Chemistry and Biochemistry, Medical Faculty, Trakia University, Stara Zagora,*
[2]*Dept. General and Clinical Pathology, Medical Faculty, Trakia University, Stara Zagora,*
[3]*Dept. General Surgery, Medical Faculty, Trakia University, Stara Zagora,*
[4]*Dept. Internal Medicine, Medical Faculty, Trakia University, Stara Zagora,*
[5]*Oncology Center, Stara Zagora,*
[6]*Regional Hospital, Burgass,*
[7]*University of Abertay Dundee,*
[1,2,3,4,5,6]*Bulgaria*
[7]*UK*

1. Introduction

Etiologically, sporadic colorectal cancer (CRC) is a complex, multifactorial disease that is linked to both exogenic and endogenic factors. Accumulating evidence indicates that susceptibility to cancer in general, and to CRC in particular, is mediated by genetically determined differences in the effectiveness of detoxification of potential carcinogens and reactive oxygen species. The antioxidant enzymes and phase I and II biotransformation enzymes are important candidates for involvement in susceptibility to sporadic CRC, due to their ability to regulate the metabolism of a wide range of environmental exposures (Perera, 1997; Potter, 1999; McIlwain et al., 2006; Di Pietro et al., 2010). In addition to carcinogens and reactive oxygen species, the majority of anticancer drugs applied in the chemotherapy are also substrates and are biotransformed by xenobiotic-metabolizing enzymes, leading to their activation and/or detoxification (O'Brien &Tew, 1996; Eaton &Bammler, 1999; Townsend &Tew, 2003; Hayes et al., 2005; Michael &Doherty, 2005; Townsend et al., 2005). In this respect, great efforts have been focused to clarify the effects of genetic variations, expression and activity of xenobiotic-metabolizing enzymes in development, progression and therapy of cancers with different histological origin, including CRC (Ranganathan &Tew, 1991; Tew &Ronai, 1999; Welfare et al., 1999; Cotton et al., 2000; de Jong et al., 2002; Dogru-Abbasoglu et al., 2002; Stoehlmacher et al., 2002; Ates et al., 2005; Romero et al., 2006; Liao et al., 2007; Pistorius et al., 2007; Koutros et al., 2009; Di Pietro et al., 2010; Economopoulos & Sergentanis, 2010).

2. Role of GSTs in cell processes

Glutathione-S-transferase (GST, EC. 2.5.1.18) isoemzymes are involved in phase II xenobiotic biotransformation. GSTs belong to a large superfamily of dimeric enzymes, which play an important role in cell defense system. So far, 24 isoenzymes have been described in humans, classified into 11 classes: 7 cytosolic - alpha (α, A), mu (μ, M), pi (π, P), sigma (σ, S), theta (θ, T), zeta (ζ, Z), and omega (ω, O), one mitochondrial - kappa (κ, K), and three microsomal classes, also referred to as membrane-associated proteins in eicosanoid and glutathione metabolism (MAPEG) (Sheehan et al., 2001; Hayes et al., 2005; McIlwain et al., 2006; Laborde, 2010) The most abundant mammalian GST enzymes belong to cytosolic classes alpha, mu, and pi, and their regulation has been studied in details (Hayes &Pulford, 1995). Most of the cytosolic GST classes are coded by several genes, gathered in clusters and thus these enzymes have several subunits, which form a number of homo- and/or heterodimeric isoenzymes (Table 1) (McIlwain et al., 2006; Laborde, 2010).

GST classes	Subunits	Gene (locus) designation	Chromosome location of the genes/gene clusters
		Cytosolic	
GST-alpha (GSTα, GSTA)	1,2,3,4,5	GSTA1, GSTA2, GSTA3, GSTA4, GSTA5	6p12
GST-mu (GSTμ, GSTM)	1,2,3,4,5	GSTM1, GSTM2, GSTM3, GSTM4, GSTM5	1p13
GST-omega (GSTω, GSTO)	1,2	GSTO1, GSTO2,	10q25.1
GST-pi (GSTπ, GSTP)	1	GSTP1	11q13
GST-sigma (GSTσ, GSTS)	1	GSTS ([a] HPGDS; PGDS)	4q22.3
GST-theta (GSTθ, GSTT)	1,2	GSTT1, GSTT2	22q11.2
GST-zeta (GSTξ, GSTZ)	1	GSTZ1	14q24.3
		Mitochondrial	
GST-kappa (GSTκ, GSTK)	1	GSTK1	7q34
		Microsomal	
[b]MAPEG		[c] MGST1, [c] MGST2, [d] ALOX5AP (FLAP) [e] LTC_4S [c] MGST3 [f] PGES (PTGES)	12p12.3-p12.1 4q28.3 13q12 5q35 1q23 9q34.3

[a]HPGDS - hematopoietic prostaglandin D synthase (PGDS - prostaglandin D synthase)
[b]MAPEG - membrane-associated proteins in eicosanoid and glutathione metabolism
[c]MGST - microsomal glutathione S-transferase
[d]ALOX5AP (FLAP) - arachidonate 5-lipoxygenase-activating protein
[e]LTC4S - leukotriene C4 synthase
[f]PGES - prostaglandin E synthase

Table 1. Classes, subunits and gene location of human GSTs

GSTs catalyze the conjugation of reduced glutathione with a variety of endogenic and exogenic electrophilic compounds, including several carcinogens and antineoplastics (Hayes &Strange, 1995; Hayes et al., 2005; Michael &Doherty, 2005). This process results in alteration, usually a reduction, of the reactivity of the compounds and makes them more water soluble and favors their elimination.

GSTs can also function as peroxidases and isomerases (Hayes &Pulford, 1995; Cho et al., 2001). Thus GSTA1-1 and GSTA2-2 efficiently catalyze the reduction of fatty acid and phospholipid hydroperoxides (Zhao et al., 1999). Moreover, it has been shown that GSTA3-3 is essential in obligatory double-bond isomerizations of precursors of testosterone and progesterone in steroid hormone biosynthesis (Johansson &Mannervik, 2001). Although the exact physiological function of omega-class GSTs remains undefined (Board et al., 2000; Board, 2011), it has been demonstrated that they can catalyze a range of thiol transferase and reduction reactions that are not catalyzed by members of the other classes: GSTO1 has GSH-dependent reductive activity to dehydroascorbate and to monomethylarsenic acid (V) (Board, 2011). GSTZ1 has isomerase activity and catalyzes the conversion of maleylacetoacetate to fumarylacetoacetate in the catabolic pathway of phenylalanine and tyrosine and also catalyzes the GSH-dependent transformation of α-halogenated acids (McIlwain et al., 2006).

There are six MAPEG (membrane associated proteins in eicosanoid and glutathione metabolism) subfamily members localized to the endoplasmic reticulum and outer mitochondrial membrane. Three of them are involved in the production of leukotrienes and prostaglandin E, whereas the other three have glutathione S-transferase and peroxidase activities, thus implicated in the protection of membranes from oxidative stress (Morgenstern et al., 2011).

In addition to their catalytic functions GSTs have several complementary functions. Some of the GSTs can serve as nonenzymatic binding proteins (known as ligandins) interacting with various lipophilic compounds including steroid and thyroid hormones (Litwack et al., 1971; Ishigaki et al., 1989; Cho et al., 2001; Vasieva, 2011). Moreover, GST isoenzymes can play a regulatory role in cellular signaling by forming protein:protein interactions with key signaling tyrosine kinases, involved in controlling stress response, apoptosis, inflammation, cellular differentiation and proliferation (Adler et al., 1999; Cho et al., 2001; Wang et al., 2001; Townsend &Tew, 2003; Townsend et al., 2005; McIlwain et al., 2006; Laborde, 2010; Vasieva, 2011).

There is strong evidence that GST-pi can bind by protein:protein interaction, sequester and inhibit c-Jun N-terminal kinase (JNK)/stress-activated protein kinases (SAPKs). JNK is a MAP kinase that phosphorylates c-Jun, a component of the activator protein-1 (AP-1) transcriptional factor, resulting in the induction of AP-1-dependent target genes which play role in cell survival and apoptosis. Thus JNK is implicated in pro-apoptotic/survival signaling pathways and may be required for induced cytotoxicity of a variety of antitumor drugs (Adler et al., 1999; Wang et al., 2001; Townsend &Tew, 2003; Townsend et al., 2005; McIlwain et al., 2006; Laborde, 2010; Vasieva, 2011).

Recently, GST-pi was shown to affect the apoptosis pathways also by physical association with TNF receptor associated factor 2 (TRAF2), an adaptor protein which mediates the signal transduction of different receptors and is required for the activation of ASK1 (apoptosis signal-regulating kinase 1) (Wu et al., 2006; Laborde, 2010; Sau et al., 2010;

Vasieva, 2011). ASK1 is a MAP kinase kinase kinase (MAP3 kinase, MAPKKK) that can phosphorylate MKK4/7 and MKK3/6 (MAP kinase kinases, MAP2Ks, MAPKK) which are involved in stress-induced activation of JNK- and p38 signaling pathways, respectively (Dorion et al., 2002; Wu et al., 2006; Sau et al., 2010).

Isoenzymes of the alpha and mu classes have also been shown in vitro to bind to JNK-Jun complexes and inhibit the activation of c-Jun by JNK, however their inhibitory activity was weaker than GST-pi (Villafania et al., 2000; Laborde, 2010). In addition, it has been noted that GST-mu interacts physically with N-terminal portion of ASK1, thus inhibiting its activity and the ASK1-elicited MKK4/7–JNK and MKK3/6–p38 signaling pathways (Dorion et al., 2002).

Another binding partner of GST-pi is the antioxidant enzyme 1-cys peroxiredoxin (1-cysPrx, Prx VI), which is a member of the peroxiredoxin superfamily and is able to protect cells from membrane peroxidation via GSH-dependent peroxidase activity on phospholipid hydroperoxides. The process of heterodimerization of 1-cysPrx with GST-pi leads to activation involving also the S-glutathionylation of 1-cysPrx (Manevich et al., 2004; Vasieva, 2011).

GST-pi has also been found to function in the S-glutathionylation of oxidized cysteine residues of several target proteins following oxidative and nitrosative stress thus playing a direct role in the control of posttranslational S-glutathionylation reactions (McIlwain et al., 2006; Townsend et al., 2006; Townsend et al., 2009; Tew et al., 2011). S-glutathionylation occurs on cysteine moieties located in relatively basic environment in response to oxidative (ROS) or nitrosative stress (RNS) signaling events. Glutathiolylation is reversible process that can occur spontaneously by GSH or catalytically by thioredoxin (Trx), glutaredoxin (Grx) or sylphoredoxin (Srx). Thus besides the phosphorylation/dephosphorylation, the cells are provided with additional dynamic system of controlling the protein activity (Townsend et al., 2009). Proteins sensitive to modification by S-glutathionylation are variety of enzymes with thiols in the active centers, cytoskeleton proteins, signaling proteins – particularly kinases and phosphatases, transcriptional factors, Ras oncogenic proteins, heat shock proteins, ion channels, and calcium pumps (Tew et al., 2011). Since a number of proteins that are S-glutathionylated are involved in growth regulatory pathways, the over-expression of GST-pi in cancers may account for the impaired balance between cell death, proliferation and differentiation and could contribute to tumor development, progression and treatment response (Townsend et al., 2009; Tew et al., 2011).

GST-pi was also shown to bind proteins and compounds containing iron and nitric oxide and thus may influence the NO metabolism and NO signaling (Vasieva, 2011). It has been shown that the natural low molecular mass NO carriers, dinitrosyl-iron complexes (DNIC) and S-nitrosoglutathion (GSNO) bind with high affinity to one active site of the dimeric GST-pi enzyme, while the enzyme maintains its detoxification activity (Lo Bello et al., 2001; Townsend et al., 2006; Vasieva, 2011). Hence, GST-pi (GSTP1-1) may act as a NO carrier, which determines it as a player of a number of processes as formation of nitrothiols, nitrosylation of proteins, NO mediated iron mobilization from cells, and Zn-homeostasis (Vasieva, 2011).

It has also been reported that certain GSTs play novel roles implicated in cell defense: GST-theta was suggested to inhibit the pro-apoptotic action of Bax (Kampranis et al., 2000), and GST-omega (GSTO1-1) was shown to modulate ryanodine receptors (RyR), which are calcium release channels in skeletal and cardiac sarcoplasmic reticulum, suggesting protective functions of GSTO1-1 in mammalian cells from radiation damage and Ca^{2+} induced apoptosis (Dulhunty et al., 2001)

Thereby, these multiple functionalities of the members of GST family, in addition to the well-characterized catalytic activities, could contribute and be of importance in GST-highly expressing tumors for development and progression of cancers and for acquisition of resistance to applied chemotherapeutics.

3. Polymorphic variants of GSTs

Numerous polymorphisms have been described in the genes encoding GSTs as most of them have been associated with a lack or an alteration of enzymatic activity toward several substrates (Ali-Osman et al., 1997; Whyatt et al., 2000; Hayes et al., 2005; McIlwain et al., 2006).

3.1 *GSTP* class

The GST-pi class is encoded by a single gene spanning approximately 3 kb and located on chromosome 11 (11q13). Two *GSTP1* single nucleotide polymorphisms (SNPs) have been identified. They are characterized by transitions at $A^{1578}G$ (exon 5, $A^{313}G$) and $C^{2293}T$ (exon 6, $C^{341}T$), resulting in amino acid substitutions $Ile^{105}Val$ and $Ala^{114}Val$, respectively, which appear to be within the active site of the GST-pi protein (Ali-Osman et al., 1997; Watson et al., 1998; Hayes et al., 2005; McIlwain et al., 2006). These two SNPs lead to the following four alleles: *GSTP1*A* (105Ile, 114Ala), *GSTP1*B* (105Val, 114Ala), *GSTP1*C* (105Val, 114Val), and *GSTP1*D* (105Ile, 114Val).

It has been proven that the substitutions due to SNPs in *GSTP1* are functional: the substitution of Ile to Val at position 105 (*GSTP1* $Ile^{105}Val$) results in altered enzyme activity to variety of electrophilic molecules (Hayes et al., 2005; McIlwain et al., 2006). Thus, there is a strong experimental evidence that the two proteins, encoded by the allelic variants, 105Ile and 105Val of the human *GSTP1* gene, differ significantly in their catalytic activities toward a model substrate; the GST-pi 105Val variant has lower activity toward 1-chloro-2,4-dinitrobenzene, a standard substrate, than its 105Ile counterpart (Ali-Osman et al., 1997; Townsend &Tew, 2003, Coles, 2000 #47). On the other hand, the same variant (105Val) displays greater activity toward polycyclic aromatic hydrocarbon (PAH) diol epoxides (Sundberg et al., 1998; Coles et al., 2000; Bostrom et al., 2002). The GST-pi 105Val enzyme variant is found to be more active than 105Ile variant in conjugation reactions with the bulky diol epoxides of PAHs, being up to 3-fold as active toward the *anti*- and *syn*-diol epoxide enantiomers with R-absolute configuration at the benzylic oxiranyl carbon (Sundberg et al., 1998; Coles et al., 2000). The bay-region diol epoxides of PAHs are known to be ultimate mutagenic and carcinogenic metabolites (Sundberg et al., 1998; Bostrom et al., 2002).

The frequency of *GSTP1* 105Ile allele in different Caucasian groups varied from 0.63 to 0.77, whereas the frequency of the variant *GSTP1* 105Val allele ranged between 0.23 and 0.37 (Table 2) (Katoh et al., 2008). In our previous study we determined the frequency of $Ile^{105}Val$ *GSTP1* genotypes in 126 ethnic Bulgarian individuals from the region of Stara Zagora (0.54 for Ile/Ile, 0.39 for Ile/Val and 0.07 for Val/Val) (Vlaykova et al., 2007). The obtained figures are consistent with those published for the controls in the case-control study of Bulgarian patients with Balkan endemic nephropathy (Andonova et al., 2004), and for other Caucasian type control cohorts in Finland (Mitrunen et al., 2001), Edinburgh area, Scotland (Harries et al., 1997), Newcastle and North Tyneside, England (Welfare et al., 1999), East Anglia region (Loktionov et al., 2001), etc. (Table 2). Based on these similarities we can conclude that despite the heterogeneous origin ethnic Bulgarians do not differ from other Caucasians in frequency of Ile^{105}Val *GSTP1* genotypes and could be included in larger interinstitutional case-control studies for investigation of the effect of this polymorphism on the susceptibility to different diseases, including cancers.

Country/racial origin	Allele frequencies			Genotype frequencies			
	105Ile (%)	105Val (%)	p-value	105 Ile/Ile (%)	105 Ile/Val (%)	105Val/ Val (%)	p-value
Bulgaria/Caucasian (Vlaykova et al., 2007)	73	27		54	39	7	
Bulgaria/Caucasian (Andonova et al., 2004)	66	34	0.284	47	38	15	0.182
Finland/Caucasian (Mitrunen et al., 2001)	74	26	0.873	55	38	7	0.989
Scotland (UK)/Caucasian (Harries et al., 1997)	72.2	27.8	0.899	51	42.5	6.5	0.906
Surrey, UK/Caucasian (Kote-Jarai et al., 2001)	70.4	29.6	0.684	51.2	38.5	10.3	0.702
Newcastle, UK/Caucasian (Welfare et al., 1999)	66.5	33.5	0.318	45	43	12	0.312
East Anglia, UK/Caucasian (Loktionov et al., 2001)	65.5	34.5	0.252	40	49	11	0.128
Germany/ Caucasian (Steinhoff et al., 2000)	73	27	1.00	55	36	9	0.827
Sweden/ Caucasian (Sorensen et al., 2007)	69	31	0.534	49	40	11	0.564
Austria/ Caucasian (Gsur et al., 2001)	63.3	36.7	0.142	39.2	48.2	12.6	0.085
Portugal/ Caucasian (Jeronimo et al., 2002)	67	33	0.356	43.3	47.5	9.2	0.315
American non-Hispanic/ Caucasian (Agalliu et al., 2006)	66	34	0.284	43	46	11	0.258

Table 2. Allele and genotype frequencies of the *GSTP1* Ile^{105}Val gene polymorphism in Bulgarians compared to other Caucasian populations.

3.2 *GSTM* class

GSTM1 together with the other four *GSTM* class members (*GSTM2, GSTM3, GSTM4* and *GSTM5*) are mapped to 1p13.3 (Pearson et al., 1993; McIlwain et al., 2006; Laborde, 2010). The close proximity of *GSTM1* and *GSTM2*, as well as the presence of two almost identical 4.2-kb regions flanking the *GSTM1* gene have been suggested to be the reasons for the observed entire *GSTM1* gene deletion resulting in a null *GSTM1* allele (*GSTM1*0*) (Pearson et al., 1993; Bolt &Thier, 2006). Furthermore, a transversion of G with C at position 534 (534G>C, formerly noted as 519G>C) was described leading to a substitution of 172Lys with 172Asn (formerly Lys^{173}Asn) (McLellan et al., 1997; Bolt &Thier, 2006; McIlwain et al., 2006; Gao et al., 2010). This SNP results in two new alleles - *GSTM1*A* and *GSTM1*B*, which were reported to be functionally identical (McLellan et al., 1997). In addition, a duplication of *GSTM1* gene has been identified and characterized (*GSTM1*1x2* allele) in people who displayed ultrarapid GSTM1 activity (McLellan et al., 1997).
Thus, four allele loci have been described in the human *GSTM1* - *GSTM1*A, GSTM1*B, GSTM1*0* and *GSTM1*1x2*, which determine several phenotypes. The frequencies of *GSTM1* alleles and genotypes display race and ethnic variations: 42% to 60% of Caucasians, 41% to 63% of Asians and only 16% to 36% of Africans are homozygous for *GSTM1*0* (null *GSTM1* genotype) (O'Brien &Tew, 1996; Cotton et al., 2000; He et al., 2004; Hayes et al., 2005; Bolt &Thier, 2006; McIlwain et al., 2006; Katoh et al., 2008; Gao et al., 2010). Our results showed that the frequency of *GSTM1* genotype in Bulgarian control individuals (36% and 42%) (Figure 1A) (Dimov et al., 2008; Emin et al., 2009; Vlaykova et al., 2009) is commensurable to that reported for some other European populations (Cotton et al., 2000; Ates et al., 2005; Katoh et al., 2008; Gao et al., 2010).
Polymorphic variants have been described for the other GSTM members: *GSTM2, GSTM3, GSTM4* and *GSTM5* (Inskip et al., 1995; Mitrunen et al., 2001; Reszka &Wasowicz, 2001; Hayes et al., 2005; Reszka et al., 2007; Yu et al., 2009; Moyer et al., 2010). The most extensive studies have been performed on *GSTM3* polymorphisms. This gene has an insertion/deletion polymorphism (rs1799735, *GSTM3*A/*B*) with a wild-type *GSTM3*A* allele and a variant one, *GSTM3*B*, which differ in the rate of expression. The variant *GSTM3*B* allele has 3 bp deletion in intron 6, which introduces a recognition site for YY1 transcriptional factor and results in enhanced expression of the enzyme protein. (Inskip et al., 1995; Loktionov et al., 2001; McIlwain et al., 2006; Reszka et al., 2007). Recently, several SNPs in *GSTM3* have been identified and studied for their functional activity and in association with variety of diseases. These are the rare Gln^{174}Trp (G^{174}W), the more common Val^{224}Ile (V^{224}I) substitutions, and the transversion of A with C at -63 position in promoter region of *GSTM3* (-62A>C) (Liu et al., 2005; McIlwain et al., 2006). The variant 174Trp allele, as well as the wild-type 224Val allele, were reported to exhibit decreased catalytic activity, whereas the variant -63C allele was associated with increased expression of the gene (Liu et al., 2005; McIlwain et al., 2006).

3.3 *GSTT* class

A null polymorphism has also been described in *T1* locus of *GSTT* cluster at 22q11.2. Analogously to *GSTM1, GSTT1* consisting of 5 exons, is flanked by two highly homologous 18 kb regions (HA3 and HA5). The null *GSTT1*0* allele is possibly caused by a homologous recombination resulting in 54 kb deletion containing the entire *GSTT1* gene (Sprenger et al.,

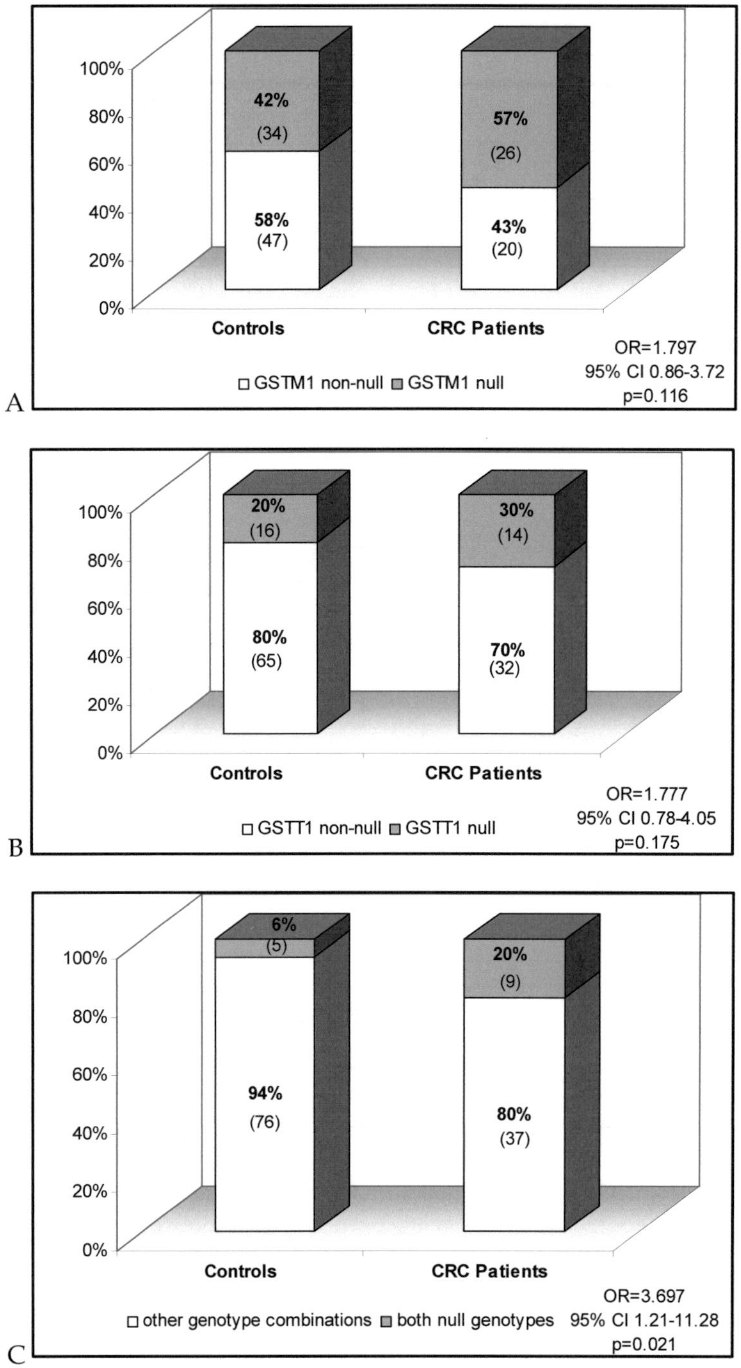

Fig. 1. Distribution of GSTM1 (A) and GSTT1 (B) null and non-null genotypes in Bulgarian patients with CRC and control individuals. Frequency of carriers of GSTM1 and GSTT1 double null genotype among the patients and controls (C). Data are presented in percentages and in real numbers (in brackets); the ORs and the 95% CI are also given.

2000; Bolt &Thier, 2006). A SNP (310A>C) in exon 3 of *GSTT1* is the reason for substitution of Tre104 with Pro104 ($Tre^{104}Pro$) in GST-theta protein, which was associated with a decrease in the catalytic activity possibly due to a conformational changes of the protein molecule (Alexandrie et al., 2002). The frequency of the null *GSTT1* genotype has also been found to vary significantly between different races and ethnic groups: between 13% and 31% (with some exceptions) in Caucasians in Europe and USA and between 35% and 48% in Asians (O'Brien &Tew, 1996; Cotton et al., 2000; He et al., 2004; Hayes et al., 2005; Bolt &Thier, 2006; McIlwain et al., 2006; Katoh et al., 2008). Our preliminary results concerning a small Bulgarian control group showed homozygosity for *GSTT1*0* (*GSTT1* null genotype) in a rate of only 7% (Dimov et al., 2008; Vlaykova et al., 2009). However, when the control group was extended the frequency of *GSTT1* null genotype turned out to be 20% (Figure 1B) (Emin et al., 2009) which is comparable to other Caucasian populations (Bolt &Thier, 2006; Katoh et al., 2008).

Polymorphic variants have been described also in the second theta-class GST gene, *GSTT2*. Coggan et al. reported a pseudogene (*GSTT2P*), which rises from G to T transition at nt 841 (841G>T) in intron 2 of *GSTT2* and C to T transition at nt 3255 (3255C>T) in exon 5 of *GSTT2P* changing 196Arg to a stop codon. In addition a G to A transition at nt 2732 (2732G>A) in exon 4 of *GSTT2* was defined that results in substitution of 139Met to 139Ile ($Met^{139}Ile$) (Coggan et al., 1998). However, there is still no clear evidence that the latter SNP may have influence on the enzyme function. In the meantime, the defined promoter polymorphisms in *GSTT2* (-537G>A, -277T>C, -158G>A, and -129T>C) were shown to affect the gene expression (Guy et al., 2004; Jang et al., 2007).

3.4 *GSTA* class

Although, variety of polymorphisms of alpha-class GST genes has been defined, their functional activity has not yet been comprehensively investigated. Nevertheless, it is already proven that the SNPs in the promoter (5′-regulatory) region of *GSTA1* (-567, -69, and -52) and specifically the substitution at -69C>T (determining a variant *GSTA1*B* allele), result in enhanced promoter activity and increased expression (Coles et al., 2001; Sweeney et al., 2002; McIlwain et al., 2006). However, for 10 SNPs in the coding regions (exons) of *GSTA1* and *GSTA2* was shown to have no significant functional effects (Tetlow et al., 2001). In a later study, the new $Pro^{110}Ser$ polymorphism in *GSTA2* was found to affect the catalysis with several substrates, as the Ser containing isoform has significantly diminished enzyme activity (Tetlow &Board, 2004). Similar decrease in the glutathione-conjugating activity was also shown for the Leu containing isoform of $Ile^{71}Leu$ ($I^{71}L$) polymorphism of *GSTA3* (Tetlow et al., 2004).

3.5 *GSTO* class

The omega-class GSTs are coded by 2 genes (*GSTO1* and *GSTO2*) both composed of six exons and spread by 7.5 kb on chromosome 10q25.1 (Whitbread et al., 2003; Whitbread et al., 2005). A total of 26 putative variants have been identified in the coding region of *GSTO1* in different databases. Among them only 10 have been confirmed candidates and only one GSTO1*A140D ($A^{140}D$, $Ala^{140}Asp$, 419C>T) has been found in the ethnic group studies (Whitbread et al., 2003). In addition a 3-bp deletion polymorphism (AGg from the final GAG codone [155E, 155Glu]) has been identified in the boundary of *GSTO1* exon4 and intron 4.

This deletion has the potential to alter the existing splice site, may reform a new splice donor site and causes the deletion of 155Glu (*GSTO1*E155del*) resulting in a loss of heat stability and increased enzyme activity toward 2-hydroxyethyl disulphide (HEDS) and CDNB (Whitbread et al., 2003). Only one variant in GSTO2 has been confirmed and identified in the population studies: this variation results from an A>G transition at nt 424 (424A>G) and causes a substitution of 142Asn to 142Asp ($Asn^{142}Asp$, $N^{142}D$) (Whitbread et al., 2003).

3.6 *GSTZ* class

A number of genetic polymorphisms in the gene encoding glutathione S-transferase-zeta (*GSTZ1*) have been defined: G-1002A, $Glu^{32}Lys$, $Gly^{42}Arg$, $Thr^{82}Met$. The latter three SNPs are functional and determine four *GSTZ1* alleles referred to as *GSTZ1*A* (32Lys, 42Arg, 82Thr), *GSTZ1*B* (32Lys, 42Gly, 82Thr), *GSTZ1*C* (32Glu, 42Gly, 82Thr), and *GSTZ1*D* (32Glu, 42Gly, 82Met) (Blackburn et al., 2001). The *B, C* and *D* alleles have been associated with a lower activity to dichloroacetic acid compared to *GSTZ1A* (Blackburn et al., 2001), but non of these SNPs affect significantly the risk of bladder cancer in Spain (Cantor et al., 2010) and breast cancer in Germany (Andonova et al., 2009).

4. Role of GSTs polymorphisms as risk factors for development, progression and therapeutic response of CRC

4.1 *GSTP1*

Epidemiological studies of *GSTP1* (*GSTP1 $Ile^{105}Val$*) and colorectal cancer risk have suggested a deleterious effect of the low activity genotypes, but findings have been inconsistent (Harries et al., 1997; Welfare et al., 1999; Kiyohara, 2000; Ates et al., 2005; Gao et al., 2009; Economopoulos &Sergentanis, 2010).

The results of our case-control study (Vlaykova et al., 2007) based on 80 patients with primary sporadic CRC and 98 unaffected control individuals showed that the genotype distribution is consistent with those published for other Caucasian type control cohorts. We also found a statistically significant prevalence of heterozygous *GSTP1* genotype by itself (*105Ile/Val* - co-dominant model) and the prevalence of variant allele-containing *GSTP1* genotypes (*105Ile/Val* or *105Val/Val* - dominant model) in control group compared to the CRC cases. This suggests a protective effect of the variant 105*Val* allele lowering the risk for developing of CRC. Based on our observations and on the experimental evidence reported by other research groups for greater activity of the enzyme encoded by the valiant *105Val* allele toward polycyclic aromatic hydrocarbon (PAH) diol epoxides (Sundberg et al., 1998; Coles et al., 2000; Bostrom et al., 2002), we suggest that the heterozygous *GSTP1* genotype may determine a better protection toward GST-pi-metabolized chemical toxins and reactive oxygen species (Vlaykova et al., 2007). This genotype may provide enzyme with an adequate detoxification of some and relatively weak activation of other carcinogens, depending on their characteristics.

Two recent large meta-analyses summarized the results focused on the role of *GSTP1 $Ile^{105}Val$* from 16 published case-control studies involving a total of 4386 colorectal cancer patients and 7127 controls (Gao et al., 2009) and 19 studies with altogether 5421 cases and 7671 controls (Economopoulos &Sergentanis, 2010) .The results of the meta-analysis performed by Gao et al. (Gao et al., 2009) sowed no strong evidence that the *105Val* allele conferred increased susceptibility to colorectal cancer compared to *105Ile* allele either in the whole pooled case-controls groups or in the stratified one: by race - Caucasian and Asian descent; by the type of controls - in healthy and hospital controls. They also did not find evidence for an association with colorectal cancer in dominant (OR= 1.02, 95% CI:0.94, 1.10) and co-dominant (OR= 0.88 , 95% CI: 0.77, 1.01) models for the effect of Val. Only a slight, but significant, protective effect of Val allele was observed in the recessive model 0.86 (95% CI: 0.76–0.98). The final conclusion of this large meta-analysis was that *GSTP1 Ile^{105}Val* polymorphism is unlikely to increase considerably the risk of sporadic colorectal cancer (Gao et al., 2009).

Similar are the results and final conclusion of the recent meta-analysis performed by Economopoulos et al. (Economopoulos &Sergentanis, 2010): there were no significant effects of *105Val* allele on the risk of colorectal cancer either in dominant model (OR=1.025, 95% CI: 0.922–1.138), co-dominant model (OR=1.050, 95% CI: 0.945–1.166), or in the recessive model (OR=0.936, 95% CI: 0.823–1.065). Hence, the conclusions confirmed that the *GSTP1 Ile^{105}Val* status did not seem to confer additional risk for colorectal cancer (Economopoulos &Sergentanis, 2010).

4.2 *GSTM1* and *GSTT1*

Because GST-mu and GST-theta are important in the detoxification of carcinogens implicated in colorectal cancer, the absence of these enzymes is assumed to increase the risk of this common malignancy. In this regard a number of epidemiological studies have investigated the association of *GSTM1* and *GSTT1* genetic polymorphisms with colorectal cancer risk, however the results from these studies have also been with quite controversial conclusions (Cotton et al., 2000; Economopoulos &Sergentanis, 2010; Gao et al., 2010). The preliminary results from our study including very limited number of patients and controls (45 and 42), showed a statistically significant case-control difference in the presence of *GSTT1* null genotype (0.30 vs. 0.07, p=0.006), and only a tendency for prevalence of *GSTM1* null genotype in CRC patient (0.57 vs. 0.36, p=0.052) (Vlaykova et al., 2009). The combined null genotypes were determined only in patients (0.20), whereas none of the control individual was with such genotype (p<0.0001). We found a 5.69-fold (95% CI, 1.59-20.00) and 2.34-fold (95% CI, 0.99-5.49) increased risk associated with *GSTT1* and *GSTM1* null genotypes, respectively and 21.533-fold (95% CI, 3.56-128.71) increased risk associated with the combined null genotypes. The colorectal cancer was diagnosed earlier in patients with *GSTM1* null genotype and those patients had tumors in more advanced stage (III or IV) (p=0.033) and were with more aggressive phenotype, such as presence of lymph vessel invasion (p=0.042) than the patients with non-null genotype.

A slight difference was obtained when the control group was extended to 81 persons (Figure 1A, 1B and 1C): the null *GSTT1* and *GSTM1* genotypes turned out only to tend to associate with an increased risk of colorectal cancer (OR=1.797, 95% CI 0.86-3.72, p=0.116 for *GSTM1*, and OR=1.777, 95% CI 0.78-4.05, p=0.175 for *GSTT1*), however the carriers of *GSTM1* and *GSTT1* double null genotype had significantly higher risk of development of the disease (OR=3.697, 95% CI 1.21-11.28, p=0.021) (Figure 1C). As a conclusion, we suggested that the inherited simultaneous lack of GST-theta and GST-mu detoxifying enzymes due to the presence of homozygous null genotypes may be associated with development of sporadic colorectal cancer (Vlaykova et al., 2009).

Our findings are analogous to the one of meta-analyses performed on a large number of published case-control studies. The results of these meta-analyses support the suggestion that *GSTM1* and *GSTT1* null polymorphisms are associated with increased risk of CRC, especially in the Caucasian population (Economopoulos &Sergentanis, 2010; Gao et al., 2010). Economopoulos et al. have summarized the results from 44 studies for *GSTM1* and 34 for *GSTT1* null polymorphisms and concluded that *GSTM1* null genotype carriers exhibited increased colorectal cancer risk in Caucasian population (OR=1.15, 95% CI: 1.06-1.25), but not in Chinese subjects (OR=1.03, 95% CI: 0.90-1.16). They reported similar results for *GSTT1* null polymorphism: OR=1.31, 95% CI:1.12-1.54 for Caucasian population and OR=1.07, 95% CI:0.79-1.45 for Chinese subjects (Economopoulos &Sergentanis, 2010). Gao at al., carried out a meta-analysis of *GSTM1* genotype data from 36 studied including 9149 patients with CRC and 13 916 control individuals (Gao et al., 2010). The results indicated that *GSTM1* null genotype was associated with CRC (OR=1.13, 95% CI: 1.03–1.23) in the pooled cases and controls from a number of different ethnics groups. However, the significance of this association remained for Caucasians, but not for Asians (Gao et al., 2010).

4.3 *GSTA1*, *GSTM3*, *GSTO2*

According to our knowledge there are only a limited number of studies aiming to evaluate the possible role of polymorphisms in the genes encoding other GST isoforms as predisposing factors for colorectal cancer. The polymorphisms in *GSTA1* have been explored in colorectal cancer only by four research teams (Sweeney et al., 2002; van der Logt et al., 2004; Martinez et al., 2006; Kury et al., 2008) . The Sweeney at al. have found that the *GSTA1*B/*B* (promoter polymorphisms) genotype is associated with an increased risk of colorectal cancer, particularly among consumers of well-done meat and have suggested that *GSTA1* genotype, in addition to the CYP2A6 phenotype should be evaluated as markers for susceptibility to dietary carcinogens (Sweeney et al., 2002). However, other studies did not find any associations between the *GSTA1* polymorphisms and the risk of CRC (van der Logt et al., 2004; Martinez et al., 2006; Kury et al., 2008).

Kury et al., and Martinez at al, have also attempted to elucidate the influence of *GSTM3* genetic variants on colorectal cancer risk, however no correlation between these polymorphisms and CRC susceptibility was found (Martinez et al., 2006; Kury et al., 2008). Similarly, no effect of *GSTM3* polymorphism was found in a large study investigating the role of single SNPs within 11 genes of phase I and 15 genes of phase II of xenobiotic metabolism (Landi et al., 2005). Opposite results have been reported for GSTM3*A/GSTM3*B alleles (the latter arising from a 3 bp deletion in intron 6): patients who were carriers of genotypes with at least one GSTM3*B allele (GSTM3 AB and GSTM3 BB combined) had advanced tumour T-stage, increasing Dukes' stage, higher frequency of distant metastases and shorter survival (Holley et al., 2006) Thus, the GSTM3 AA genotype was suggested to be associated with improved prognosis of CRC especially in patients with GSTM1 null genotype (Holley et al., 2006). Analogous results have been reported by Loktionov et al. who found associations between GSTM3*B frequency in patients with distal colorectal cancers particularly when combined with the GSTM1 null genotype (Loktionov et al., 2001).

A very recent study investigated the association between *GSTO2* $N^{142}D$ ($Asn^{142}Asp$) genetic polymorphism and susceptibility to colorectal cancer and reported that ND and DD genotypes were not associated with CRC risk, in comparison with the NN genotype. However subjects with NN genotype and positive family history were at high risk to develop colorectal cancer in comparison with subjects with DD or ND genotypes and negative family history. Thus, GSTO2 NN genotype was suggested to increase the risk of colorectal cancer in persons with positive family history for cancer in the first degree relatives (Masoudi et al., 2010).

The common characteristic of the theta-class GSTs is their high affinity for the organic hydroperoxide species and particularly toward cumene hydroperoxide (GSTT2), underling the importance of GSTT2 activity in protection of cells against toxic ROS and lipid peroxidation products (Tan &Board, 1996), which are a major source of endogenous DNA damage and thus contribute significantly to cancer genesis and progression. In this respect efforts have been done to determine whether *GSTT2* promoter SNPs (-537G>A, -277T>C and -158G>A) are associated with colorectal cancer risk (Jang et al., 2007). Jang at al., reported that -537A allele was associated with colorectal cancer risk, while the -158A allele was protective against colorectal cancer, finally suggesting that SNPs and haplotypes of the *GSTT2* promoter region are associated with colorectal cancer risk in the Korean population (Jang et al., 2007). However, in a Caucasian population there was no such association of GSTT2 polymorphisms with the risk of CRC (Landi et al., 2005)

5. Role of GST-pi in cancer progression

The isoenzyme of class pi, GST-pi, acidic cytosolic protein, possesses unique enzymatic properties: broad substrate specificity (e.g. alkylating antitumor agents such as cisplatin derivatives), glutathione peroxidase activity towards lipid hydroperoxides, and high sensitivity to reactive oxygen species (ROS) (Tsuchida &Sato, 1992; de Bruin et al., 2000; Hoensch et al., 2002). As it was discussed above, GST-pi acts also non-catalytically as intracellular binding protein for a large number of non-substrate molecules of either endogeneous or exogeneous origin, thus contributing to their intracellular transport, sequestration and disposition (Laisney et al., 1984; de Bruin et al., 2000; Hayes et al., 2005). Besides that, GST-pi plays a regulatory role in the MAP kinase pathway that participates in cellular survival and death signals via direct protein:protein interaction with c-Jun-N-terminal Kinase 1 (JNK1) and Apoptosis Signal-regulating Kinase (Ask1) (Adler et al., 1999; Tew &Ronai, 1999; Townsend &Tew, 2003; Hayes et al., 2005; Michael &Doherty, 2005).

Therefore, the increased protein levels and activity of GST-pi found in a variety of neoplastic cancers with different histological origins, including colorectal carcinoma (Moorghen et al., 1991; Ranganathan &Tew, 1991; de Bruin et al., 2000; Dogru-Abbasoglu et al., 2002; Murtagh et al., 2005), are debated as factors responsible, at least partly, for the progression and chemotherapy resistance, observed in many cancers (O'Brien &Tew, 1996; Tew &Ronai, 1999; Townsend &Tew, 2003; Michael &Doherty, 2005).

Earlier we reported our preliminary results concerning the survival of 76 patients with primary CRC according to the level of expression of GST-pi determined by immunohistochemistry (Vlaykova et al., 2005). Further we extended the patient population to 132 and found that the tumors varied according to their GST-pi immune staining: there were tumors negative for GST-pi, others had weak staining and finally tumors exhibiting strong and very strong immune reaction for GST-pi (Figure 2).

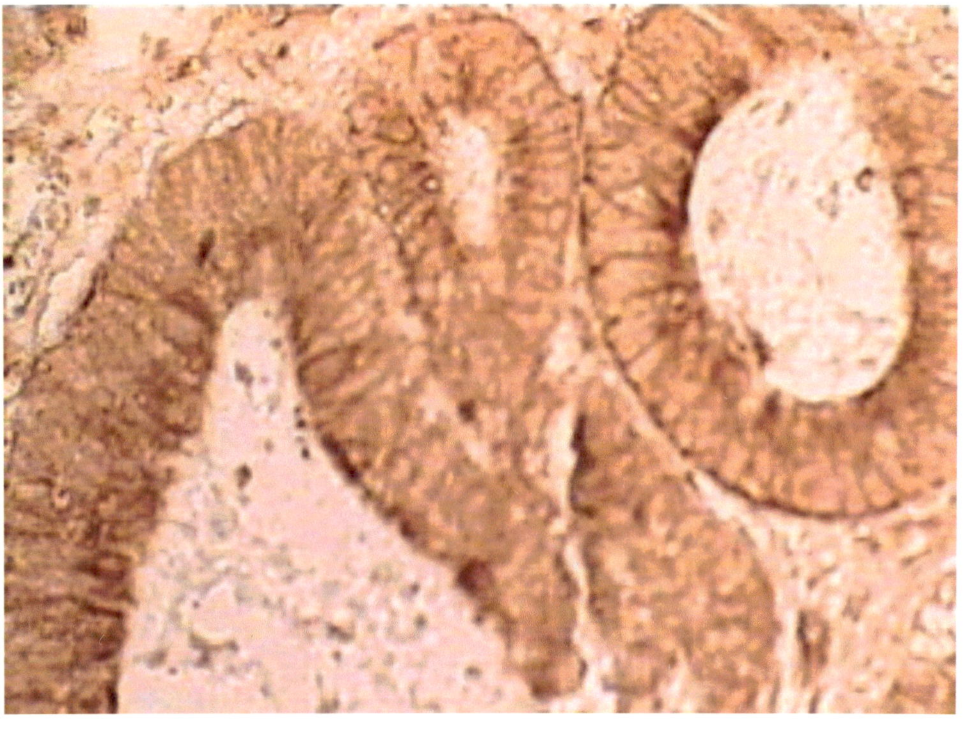

Fig. 2. Intensive cytoplasmic immune reaction for GST-pi in the cells of the tumor glands of a well-differentiated primary colorectal cancer (x 400).

The results concerning survival of the patients with CRC with different level of expression of GST-pi, showed that the higher expression of GST-pi was significantly associated with shorter survival period after surgical therapy (median of 19 months) compared to those negative or with weak GST-pi staining (median of 58 months, p=0.004, Log-rang test) (Figure 3A). This statistically significant association persisted also after stratification for pTNM staging (stage I/II vs. Stage III/IV, p=0.005, Log-rank test) (Figure 3B).
Interestingly, the strong expression of GST-pi retained its impact as unfavorable prognostic factor both for the patients who received an adjuvant chemotherapy (n=63, p=0.008, Log-rank test) (Figure 4A) and for the once without such treatment (n=66, p=0.019, Log-rank test) (Figure 4B). Hence, we suggested that the strong expression of GST-pi may lead to lower effectiveness of the administered anticancer drugs or to inhibiting the apoptosis, thus influencing the survival of the patients.

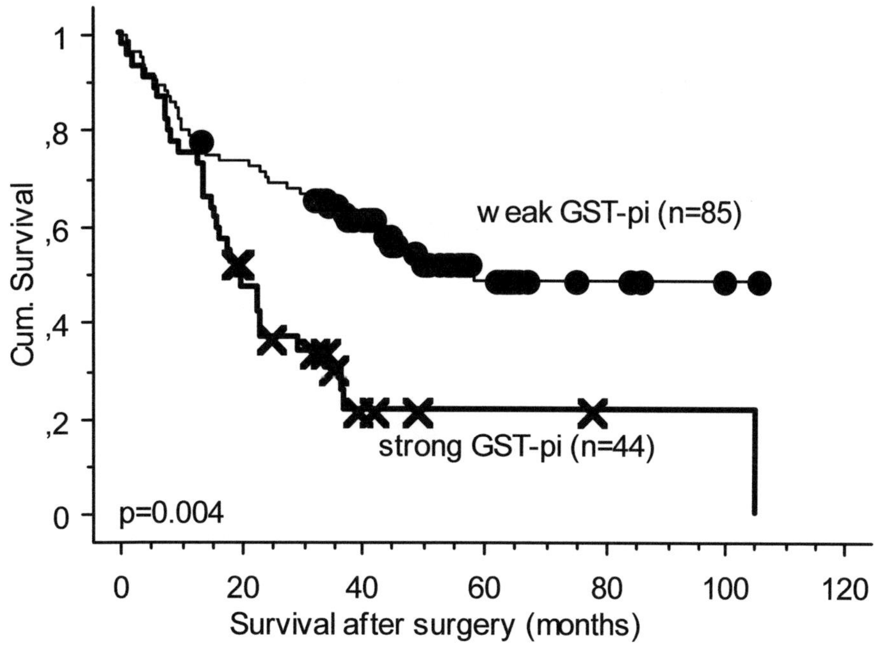

A

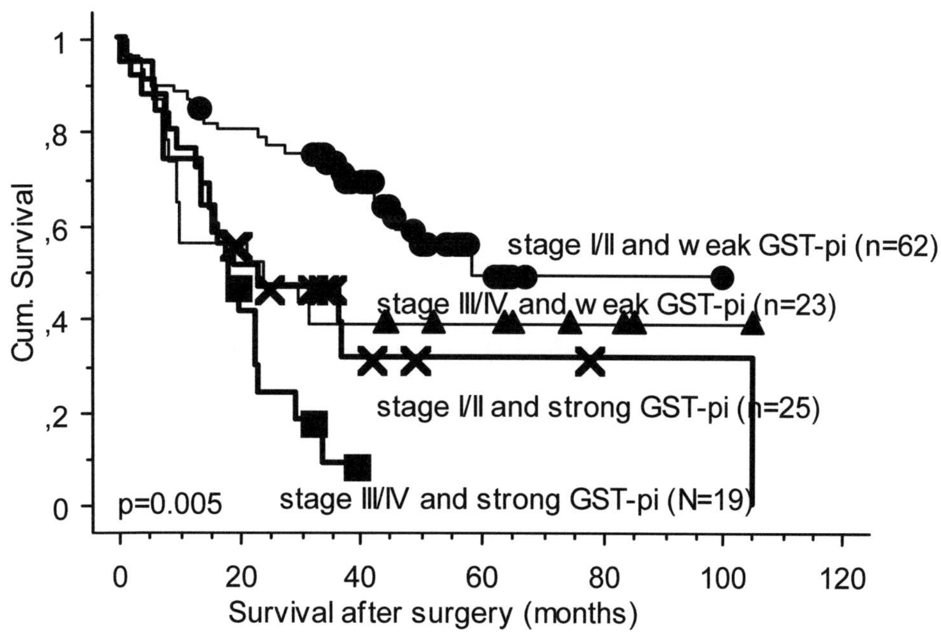

B

Fig. 3. Survival of the whole studied patient population with colorectal carcinoma after surgical treatment according to the level of expression of GST-pi in tumor cells (**A**) and after stratification to pTNM staging (**B**).

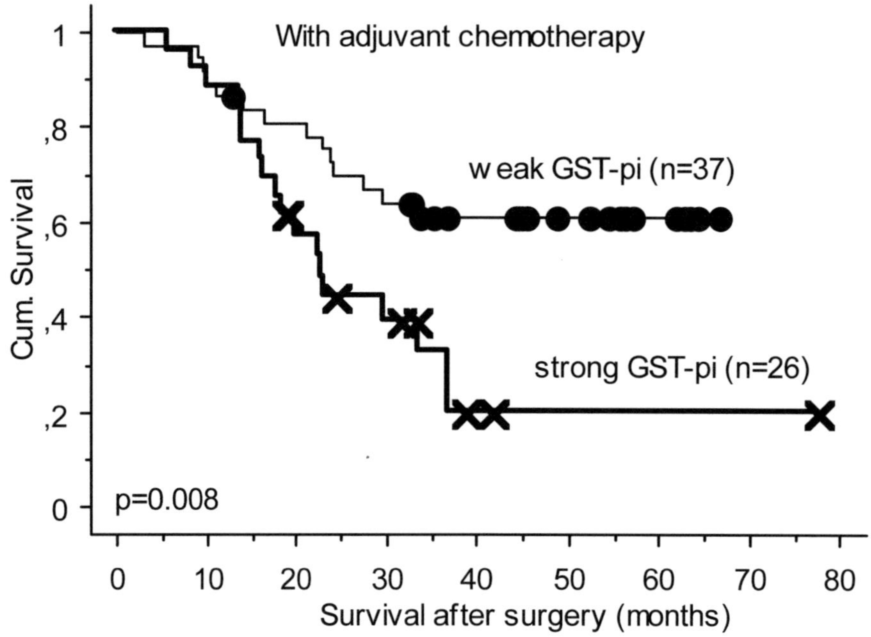

A

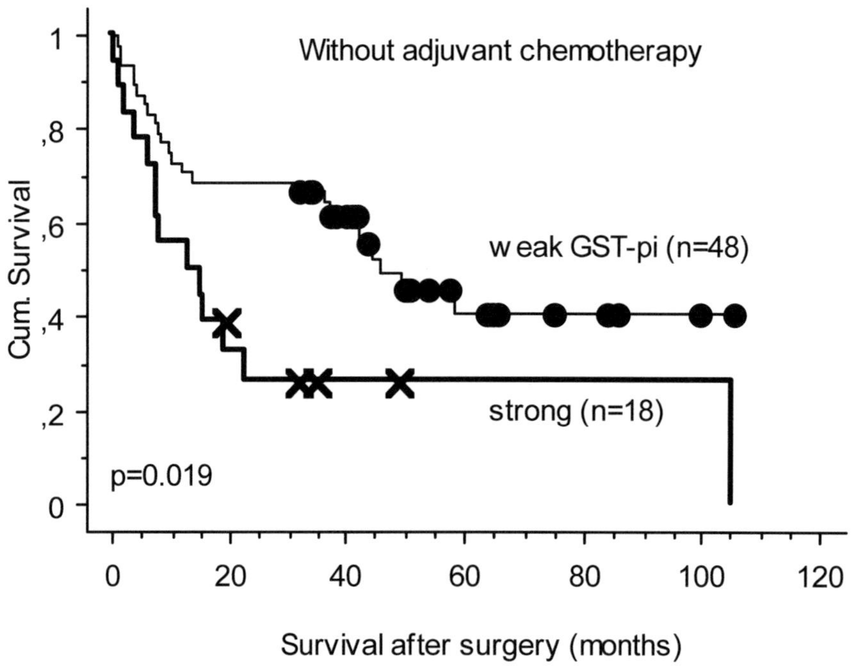

B

Fig. 4. Survival according to the GST-pi expression of patients with CRC subjected to adjuvant chemotherapy **(A)**, Association between the level of expression of GST-pi and survival of patients, who did not receive adjuvant chemotherapy (**B**).

Previously, we also described expression of GST-pi in chromogranin A-positive endocrine cells in colorectal cancers, which also expressed some other antioxidant enzymes, such as SOD1 and SOD2 (Gulubova &Vlaykova, 2010). Moreover, we found that patients having tumors with GST-pi-positive endocrine cells have an unfavorable prognosis. We suggest that not the neuroendocrine differentiation in general, but the presence of endocrine cells with activated antioxidant defense and probably higher metabolic activity might determine a more aggressive type of cancer leading to worse prognosis for patients (Gulubova &Vlaykova, 2010).

The observed heterogeneous expression of GST-pi in tumor glands could be due to different genetic or epigenetic factors. We suppose that the reactive oxygen species, which are generated in high amount during the metabolism of tumor cells could be such factors resulting in overproduction of GST-pi . These ROS are found to induce the expression of the genes of GST-pi and other phase II xenobiotic-biotransformating enzymes (O'Brien &Tew, 1996; Tew &Ronai, 1999; Hoensch et al., 2002). There is a growing evidence that these genes have regulatory sequences recognized by Nrf2 transcription factor, which in turn is regulated by the antioxidant response element (ARE) (O'Brien &Tew, 1996; Tew &Ronai, 1999; Hoensch et al., 2002). Another Zn-dependent mechanism for ROS-induced expression of genes coding GST-pi and other antioxidant enzymes has been proposed (Chung et al., 2005).

Another factor, resulting in overproduction of GST-pi, could be its gene amplification. Such genetic change has been proven for squamous cell carcinoma of head and neck. *GSTP1* amplification has been shown to be a common event and proposed to be associated with cisplatin resistance and poor clinical outcome in head and neck cancer patients treated with cisplatin-based therapy (Wang et al., 1997; Cullen et al., 2003).

On the other hand, the lack of or the low expression of GST-pi could be due to the somatic inactivation by hypermethylation of promoter sequences of GST-pi gene (Yang et al., 2003; Lasabova et al., 2010). Such hypermethylation is the most common event (about 90%) described in prostate adenocarcinoma (Jeronimo et al., 2002).

The results of our studies demonstrated the association between high expression level of GST-pi and unfavorable prognosis for the patients with colorectal carcinoma. This association was valid both for patients who had received adjuvant chemotherapy and for those without such treatment. We suppose that the shorter survival of patients with higher GST-pi could be due to lowering of the effectiveness of administered antineoplastic agents. The high protein level of GST-pi could contribute to this process either via its direct detoxifying effect towards some of the drugs (oxaliplatin) (O'Brien &Tew, 1996; Michael &Doherty, 2005), or via the inhibitory effect of GST-pi on MAP kinase signal pathways of apoptosis, triggered by 5-FU, mitomicin C, camtothecin or other antitumor drugs included in mono- or polychemotherapeutic regiments (Adler et al., 1999; Townsend &Tew, 2003; Hayes et al., 2005; Michael &Doherty, 2005).

The observed association of high GST-pi level with worse prognosis of the patients, who did not received chemotherapy, could also be explained with the ability of this enzyme protein directly to interact with and inhibit proteins involved in regulation of apoptosis (JNK1 and Ask1) (Adler et al., 1999; Townsend &Tew, 2003; Hayes et al., 2005; Michael &Doherty, 2005). In tumors, the high levels of free radicals, which in general are triggering factors and mediators of apoptosis, probably stimulate the expression of GST-pi that can lead to suppression of apoptosis. As a result, the decreased apoptosis can lead to increased tumor burden, which negatively affects patients survival.

6. Conclusions

Colorectal cancer (CRC) is a neoplasm that occurs at high frequency worldwide, including Bulgaria. CRC is a complex and multifactorial disease, since several environmental and endogenous factors, including personal genetic characteristics, are implicated in its etiology, pathogenesis, progression and outcome. The members of the glutathione-S-tranferase (GST) family are important candidates for involvement in susceptibility to carcinogen-associated CRC and for developing of tumor chemotherapy resistance. In this work we presented a short overview of the main cellular functions of some of the GST isoenzymes, their polymorphic nature, and their role as risk factors for development of CRC and of resistance to chemotherapy. We also presented the results of our studies focused on the role of the null *GSTM1* and *GSTT1* polymorphisms, the $Ile^{105}Val$ SNP in *GSTP1* and GST-pi expression as risk and prognostic factors in primary CRC. In conclusion, we suggest that the expression level of GST-pi in primary tumors could be a valuable prognostic factor for patients with colorectal carcinoma both treated with adjuvant chemotherapy and those not subjected to such therapy.

7. References

Adler, V., Yin, Z., Fuchs, S.Y., Benezra, M., Rosario, L., Tew, K.D., Pincus, M.R., Sardana, M., Henderson, C.J., Wolf, C.R., Davis, R.J. & Ronai, Z. (1999). Regulation of JNK signaling by GSTp. *Embo J,* 18, 1321-34.

Agalliu, I., Lin, D.W., Salinas, C.A., Feng, Z. & Stanford, J.L. (2006). Polymorphisms in the glutathione S-transferase M1, T1, and P1 genes and prostate cancer prognosis. *Prostate,* 66, 1535-41.

Alexandrie, A.K., Rannug, A., Juronen, E., Tasa, G. & Warholm, M. (2002). Detection and characterization of a novel functional polymorphism in the GSTT1 gene. *Pharmacogenetics,* 12, 613-9.

Ali-Osman, F., Akande, O., Antoun, G., Mao, J.X. & Buolamwini, J. (1997). Molecular cloning, characterization, and expression in Escherichia coli of full-length cDNAs of three human glutathione S-transferase Pi gene variants. Evidence for differential catalytic activity of the encoded proteins. *J Biol Chem,* 272, 10004-12.

Andonova, I.E., Justenhoven, C., Winter, S., Hamann, U., Baisch, C., Rabstein, S., Spickenheuer, A., Harth, V., Pesch, B., Bruning, T., Ko, Y.D., Ganev, V. & Brauch, H. (2009). No evidence for glutathione S-transferases GSTA2, GSTM2, GSTO1, GSTO2, and GSTZ1 in breast cancer risk. *Breast Cancer Res Treat,* 121, 497-502.

Andonova, I.E., Sarueva, R.B., Horvath, A.D., Simeonov, V.A., Dimitrov, P.S., Petropoulos, E.A. & Ganev, V.S. (2004). Balkan endemic nephropathy and genetic variants of glutathione S-transferases. *J Nephrol,* 17, 390-8.

Ates, N.A., Tamer, L., Ates, C., Ercan, B., Elipek, T., Ocal, K. & Camdeviren, H. (2005). Glutathione S-transferase M1, T1, P1 genotypes and risk for development of colorectal cancer. *Biochem Genet,* 43, 149-63.

Blackburn, A.C., Coggan, M., Tzeng, H.F., Lantum, H., Polekhina, G., Parker, M.W., Anders, M.W. & Board, P.G. (2001). GSTZ1d: a new allele of glutathione transferase zeta and maleylacetoacetate isomerase. *Pharmacogenetics,* 11, 671-8.

Board, P.G. (2011). The omega-class glutathione transferases: structure, function, and genetics. *Drug Metab Rev,* 43, 226-35.

Board, P.G., Coggan, M., Chelvanayagam, G., Easteal, S., Jermiin, L.S., Schulte, G.K., Danley, D.E., Hoth, L.R., Griffor, M.C., Kamath, A.V., Rosner, M.H., Chrunyk, B.A., Perregaux, D.E., Gabel, C.A., Geoghegan, K.F. & Pandit, J. (2000). Identification, characterization, and crystal structure of the Omega class glutathione transferases. *J Biol Chem,* 275, 24798-806.

Bolt, H.M. & Thier, R. (2006). Relevance of the deletion polymorphisms of the glutathione S-transferases GSTT1 and GSTM1 in pharmacology and toxicology. *Curr Drug Metab,* 7, 613-28.

Bostrom, C.E., Gerde, P., Hanberg, A., Jernstrom, B., Johansson, C., Kyrklund, T., Rannug, A., Tornqvist, M., Victorin, K. & Westerholm, R. (2002). Cancer risk assessment, indicators, and guidelines for polycyclic aromatic hydrocarbons in the ambient air. *Environ Health Perspect,* 3, 451-88.

Cantor, K.P., Villanueva, C.M., Silverman, D.T., Figueroa, J.D., Real, F.X., Garcia-Closas, M., Malats, N., Chanock, S., Yeager, M., Tardon, A., Garcia-Closas, R., Serra, C., Carrato, A., Castano-Vinyals, G., Samanic, C., Rothman, N. & Kogevinas, M. (2010). Polymorphisms in GSTT1, GSTZ1, and CYP2E1, disinfection by-products, and risk of bladder cancer in Spain. *Environ Health Perspect,* 118, 1545-50.

Cho, S.G., Lee, Y.H., Park, H.S., Ryoo, K., Kang, K.W., Park, J., Eom, S.J., Kim, M.J., Chang, T.S., Choi, S.Y., Shim, J., Kim, Y., Dong, M.S., Lee, M.J., Kim, S.G., Ichijo, H. & Choi, E.J. (2001). Glutathione S-transferase mu modulates the stress-activated signals by suppressing apoptosis signal-regulating kinase 1. *J Biol Chem,* 276, 12749-55.

Chung, M.J., Walker, P.A., Brown, R.W. & Hogstrand, C. (2005). ZINC-mediated gene expression offers protection against H2O2-induced cytotoxicity. *Toxicol Appl Pharmacol,* 205, 225-36.

Coggan, M., Whitbread, L., Whittington, A. & Board, P. (1998). Structure and organization of the human theta-class glutathione S-transferase and D-dopachrome tautomerase gene complex. *Biochem J,* 334, 617-23.

Coles, B., Nowell, S.A., MacLeod, S.L., Sweeney, C., Lang, N.P. & Kadlubar, F.F. (2001). The role of human glutathione S-transferases (hGSTs) in the detoxification of the food-derived carcinogen metabolite N-acetoxy-PhIP, and the effect of a polymorphism in hGSTA1 on colorectal cancer risk. *Mutat Res,* 482, 3-10.

Coles, B., Yang, M., Lang, N.P. & Kadlubar, F.F. (2000). Expression of hGSTP1 alleles in human lung and catalytic activity of the native protein variants towards 1-chloro-2,4-dinitrobenzene, 4-vinylpyridine and (+)-anti benzo[a]pyrene-7,8-diol-9,10-oxide. *Cancer Lett,* 156, 167-75.

Cotton, S.C., Sharp, L., Little, J. & Brockton, N. (2000). Glutathione S-transferase polymorphisms and colorectal cancer: a HuGE review. *Am J Epidemiol,* 151, 7-32.

Cullen, K.J., Newkirk, K.A., Schumaker, L.M., Aldosari, N., Rone, J.D. & Haddad, B.R. (2003). Glutathione S-transferase pi amplification is associated with cisplatin resistance in head and neck squamous cell carcinoma cell lines and primary tumors. *Cancer Res,* 63, 8097-102.

de Bruin, W.C., Wagenmans, M.J. & Peters, W.H. (2000). Expression of glutathione S-transferase alpha, P1-1 and T1-1 in the human gastrointestinal tract. *Jpn J Cancer Res,* 91, 310-6.

de Jong, M.M., Nolte, I.M., te Meerman, G.J., van der Graaf, W.T., de Vries, E.G., Sijmons, R.H., Hofstra, R.M. & Kleibeuker, J.H. (2002). Low-penetrance genes and their involvement in colorectal cancer susceptibility. *Cancer Epidemiol Biomarkers Prev,* 11, 1332-52.

Di Pietro, G., Magno, L.A. & Rios-Santos, F. (2010). Glutathione S-transferases: an overview in cancer research. *Expert Opin Drug Metab Toxicol,* 6, 153-70.

Dimov, D., Vlaykova, T., Shazie, S. & Ilieva, V. (2008). Investigation of GSTP1, GSTM1 and GSTT1 gene polymorphisms and susceptibility to COPD. . *Trakia J Sci,* 6(4), , 1-8.

Dogru-Abbasoglu, S., Mutlu-Turkoglu, U., Turkoglu, S., Erbil, Y., Barbaros, U., Uysal, M. & Aykac-Toker, G. (2002). Glutathione S-transferase-pi in malignant tissues and plasma of human colorectal and gastric cancers. *J Cancer Res Clin Oncol,* 128, 91-5.

Dorion, S., Lambert, H. & Landry, J. (2002). Activation of the p38 signaling pathway by heat shock involves the dissociation of glutathione S-transferase Mu from Ask1. *J Biol Chem,* 277, 30792-7.

Dulhunty, A., Gage, P., Curtis, S., Chelvanayagam, G. & Board, P. (2001). The glutathione transferase structural family includes a nuclear chloride channel and a ryanodine receptor calcium release channel modulator. *J Biol Chem,* 276, 3319-23.

Eaton, D.L. & Bammler, T.K. (1999). Concise review of the glutathione S-transferases and their significance to toxicology. *Toxicol Sci,* 49, 156-64.

Economopoulos, K.P. & Sergentanis, T.N. (2010). GSTM1, GSTT1, GSTP1, GSTA1 and colorectal cancer risk: a comprehensive meta-analysis. *Eur J Cancer,* 46, 1617-31.

Emin, S., Yordanova, K., Dimov, D., Ilieva, V., Koychev, A., Prakova, G. & Vlaykova, T. (2009). Investigation of the role of null polymorphisms of glutathione-S-transferase genes (GST) for development of COPD and Bronchial asthma. *Eur J Med Res* 14 (Supplement II), 173.

Gao, Y., Cao, Y., Tan, A., Liao, C., Mo, Z. & Gao, F. (2010). Glutathione S-Transferase M1 Polymorphism and Sporadic Colorectal Cancer Risk: An Updating Meta-Analysis and HuGE Review of 36 Case-Control Studies. *Annals of Epidemiology,* 20, 108-121.

Gao, Y., Pan, X., Su, T., Mo, Z., Cao, Y. & Gao, F. (2009). Glutathione S-transferase P1 Ile105Val polymorphism and colorectal cancer risk: A meta-analysis and HuGE review. *European Journal of Cancer,* 45, 3303-3314.

Gsur, A., Haidinger, G., Hinteregger, S., Bernhofer, G., Schatzl, G., Madersbacher, S., Marberger, M., Vutuc, C. & Micksche, M. (2001). Polymorphisms of glutathione-S-transferase genes (GSTP1, GSTM1 and GSTT1) and prostate-cancer risk. *Int J Cancer,* 95, 152-5.

Gulubova, M. & Vlaykova, T. (2010). Expression of the xenobiotic- and reactive oxygen species-detoxifying enzymes, GST-pi, Cu/Zn-SOD, and Mn-SOD in the endocrine cells of colorectal cancer. *Int J Colorectal Dis,* 25, 1397-405.

Guy, C.A., Hoogendoorn, B., Smith, S.K., Coleman, S., O'Donovan, M.C. & Buckland, P.R. (2004). Promoter polymorphisms in glutathione-S-transferase genes affect transcription. *Pharmacogenetics,* 14, 45-51.

Harries, L.W., Stubbins, M.J., Forman, D., Howard, G.C. & Wolf, C.R. (1997). Identification of genetic polymorphisms at the glutathione S-transferase Pi locus and association with susceptibility to bladder, testicular and prostate cancer. *Carcinogenesis,* 18, 641-4.

Hayes, J.D., Flanagan, J.U. & Jowsey, I.R. (2005). Glutathione transferases. *Annu Rev Pharmacol Toxicol,* 45, 51-88.

Hayes, J.D. & Pulford, D.J. (1995). The glutathione S-transferase supergene family: regulation of GST and the contribution of the isoenzymes to cancer chemoprotection and drug resistance. *Crit Rev Biochem Mol Biol,* 30, 445-600.

Hayes, J.D. & Strange, R.C. (1995). Potential contribution of the glutathione S-transferase supergene family to resistance to oxidative stress. *Free Radic Res,* 22, 193-207.

He, J.Q., Connett, J.E., Anthonisen, N.R., Pare, P.D. & Sandford, A.J. (2004). Glutathione S-transferase variants and their interaction with smoking on lung function. *Am J Respir Crit Care Med,* 170, 388-94.

Hoensch, H., Morgenstern, I., Petereit, G., Siepmann, M., Peters, W.H., Roelofs, H.M. & Kirch, W. (2002). Influence of clinical factors, diet, and drugs on the human upper gastrointestinal glutathione system. *Gut,* 50, 235-40.

Holley, S.L., Rajagopal, R., Hoban, P.R., Deakin, M., Fawole, A.S., Elder, J.B., Elder, J., Smith, V., Strange, R.C. & Fryer, A.A. (2006). Polymorphisms in the glutathione S-transferase mu cluster are associated with tumour progression and patient outcome in colorectal cancer. *Int J Oncol,* 28, 231-6.

Inskip, A., Elexperu-Camiruaga, J., Buxton, N., Dias, P.S., MacIntosh, J., Campbell, D., Jones, P.W., Yengi, L., Talbot, J.A., Strange, R.C. & et al. (1995). Identification of polymorphism at the glutathione S-transferase, GSTM3 locus: evidence for linkage with GSTM1*A. *Biochem J,* 312, 713-6.

Ishigaki, S., Abramovitz, M. & Listowsky, I. (1989). Glutathione-S-transferases are major cytosolic thyroid hormone binding proteins. *Arch Biochem Biophys,* 273, 265-72.

Jang, S.G., Kim, I.J., Kang, H.C., Park, H.W., Ahn, S.A., Yoon, H.J., Kim, K., Shin, H.R., Lee, J.S. & Park, J.G. (2007). GSTT2 promoter polymorphisms and colorectal cancer risk. *BMC Cancer,* 7, 16.

Jeronimo, C., Varzim, G., Henrique, R., Oliveira, J., Bento, M.J., Silva, C., Lopes, C. & Sidransky, D. (2002). I105V polymorphism and promoter methylation of the GSTP1 gene in prostate adenocarcinoma. *Cancer Epidemiol Biomarkers Prev,* 11, 445-50.

Johansson, A.S. & Mannervik, B. (2001). Human glutathione transferase A3-3, a highly efficient catalyst of double-bond isomerization in the biosynthetic pathway of steroid hormones. *J Biol Chem,* 276, 33061-5.

Kampranis, S.C., Damianova, R., Atallah, M., Toby, G., Kondi, G., Tsichlis, P.N. & Makris, A.M. (2000). A novel plant glutathione S-transferase/peroxidase suppresses Bax lethality in yeast. *J Biol Chem,* 275, 29207-16.

Katoh, T., Yamano, Y., Tsuji, M. & Watanabe, M. (2008). Genetic polymorphisms of human cytosol glutathione S-transferases and prostate cancer. *Pharmacogenomics,* 9, 93-104.

Kiyohara, C. (2000). Genetic polymorphism of enzymes involved in xenobiotic metabolism and the risk of colorectal cancer. *J Epidemiol,* 10, 349-60.

Kote-Jarai, Z., Easton, D., Edwards, S.M., Jefferies, S., Durocher, F., Jackson, R.A., Singh, R., Ardern-Jones, A., Murkin, A., Dearnaley, D.P., Shearer, R., Kirby, R., Houlston, R. & Eeles, R. (2001). Relationship between glutathione S-transferase M1, P1 and T1 polymorphisms and early onset prostate cancer. *Pharmacogenetics,* 11, 325-30.

Koutros, S., Berndt, S.I., Sinha, R., Ma, X., Chatterjee, N., Alavanja, M.C., Zheng, T., Huang, W.Y., Hayes, R.B. & Cross, A.J. (2009). Xenobiotic metabolizing gene variants, dietary heterocyclic amine intake, and risk of prostate cancer. *Cancer Res,* 69, 1877-84.

Kury, S., Buecher, B., Robiou-du-Pont, S., Scoul, C., Colman, H., Le Neel, T., Le Houerou, C., Faroux, R., Ollivry, J., Lafraise, B., Chupin, L.D., Sebille, V. & Bezieau, S. (2008). Low-penetrance alleles predisposing to sporadic colorectal cancers: a French case-controlled genetic association study. *BMC Cancer,* 8, 326.

Laborde, E. (2010). Glutathione transferases as mediators of signaling pathways involved in cell proliferation and cell death. *Cell Death Differ,* 17, 1373-80.

Laisney, V., Nguyen Van, C., Gross, M.S. & Frezal, J. (1984). Human genes for glutathione S-transferases. *Hum Genet,* 68, 221-7.

Landi, S., Gemignani, F., Moreno, V., Gioia-Patricola, L., Chabrier, A., Guino, E., Navarro, M., de Oca, J., Capella, G. & Canzian, F. (2005). A comprehensive analysis of phase I and phase II metabolism gene polymorphisms and risk of colorectal cancer. *Pharmacogenet Genomics,* 15, 535-46.

Lasabova, Z., Tilandyova, P., Kajo, K., Zubor, P., Burjanivova, T., Danko, J. & Plank, L. (2010). Hypermethylation of the GSTP1 promoter region in breast cancer is associated with prognostic clinicopathological parameters. *Neoplasma,* 57, 35-40.

Liao, L.H., Zhang, H., Lai, M.P., Lau, K.W., Lai, A.K., Zhang, J.H., Wang, Q., Wei, W., Chai, J.H., Lung, M.L., Tai, S.S. & Wu, M. (2007). The association of CYP2C9 gene polymorphisms with colorectal carcinoma in Han Chinese. *Clin Chim Acta,* 380, 191-6.

Litwack, G., Ketterer, B. & Arias, I.M. (1971). Ligandin: a hepatic protein which binds steroids, bilirubin, carcinogens and a number of exogenous organic anions. *Nature,* 234, 466-7.

Liu, X., Campbell, M.R., Pittman, G.S., Faulkner, E.C., Watson, M.A. & Bell, D.A. (2005). Expression-based discovery of variation in the human glutathione S-transferase M3 promoter and functional analysis in a glioma cell line using allele-specific chromatin immunoprecipitation. *Cancer Res,* 65, 99-104.

Lo Bello, M., Nuccetelli, M., Caccuri, A.M., Stella, L., Parker, M.W., Rossjohn, J., McKinstry, W.J., Mozzi, A.F., Federici, G., Polizio, F., Pedersen, J.Z. & Ricci, G. (2001). Human glutathione transferase P1-1 and nitric oxide carriers; a new role for an old enzyme. *J Biol Chem,* 276, 42138-45.

Loktionov, A., Watson, M.A., Gunter, M., Stebbings, W.S., Speakman, C.T. & Bingham, S.A. (2001). Glutathione-S-transferase gene polymorphisms in colorectal cancer patients: interaction between GSTM1 and GSTM3 allele variants as a risk-modulating factor. *Carcinogenesis,* 22, 1053-60.

Manevich, Y., Feinstein, S.I. & Fisher, A.B. (2004). Activation of the antioxidant enzyme 1-CYS peroxiredoxin requires glutathionylation mediated by heterodimerization with pi GST. *Proc Natl Acad Sci U S A,* 101, 3780-5.

Martinez, C., Martin, F., Fernandez, J.M., Garcia-Martin, E., Sastre, J., Diaz-Rubio, M., Agundez, J.A. & Ladero, J.M. (2006). Glutathione S-transferases mu 1, theta 1, pi 1, alpha 1 and mu 3 genetic polymorphisms and the risk of colorectal and gastric cancers in humans. *Pharmacogenomics,* 7, 711-8.

Masoudi, M., Saadat, I., Omidvari, S. & Saadat, M. (2010). Association between N142D genetic polymorphism of GSTO2 and susceptibility to colorectal cancer. *Mol Biol Rep,* 27.

McIlwain, C.C., Townsend, D.M. & Tew, K.D. (2006). Glutathione S-transferase polymorphisms: cancer incidence and therapy. *Oncogene,* 25, 1639-48.

McLellan, R.A., Oscarson, M., Alexandrie, A.K., Seidegard, J., Evans, D.A., Rannug, A. & Ingelman-Sundberg, M. (1997). Characterization of a human glutathione S-transferase mu cluster containing a duplicated GSTM1 gene that causes ultrarapid enzyme activity. *Mol Pharmacol,* 52, 958-65.

Michael, M. & Doherty, M.M. (2005). Tumoral drug metabolism: overview and its implications for cancer therapy. *J Clin Oncol,* 23, 205-29.

Mitrunen, K., Jourenkova, N., Kataja, V., Eskelinen, M., Kosma, V.M., Benhamou, S., Vainio, H., Uusitupa, M. & Hirvonen, A. (2001). Glutathione S-transferase M1, M3, P1, and T1 genetic polymorphisms and susceptibility to breast cancer. *Cancer Epidemiol Biomarkers Prev,* 10, 229-36.

Moorghen, M., Cairns, J., Forrester, L.M., Hayes, J.D., Hall, A., Cattan, A.R., Wolf, C.R. & Harris, A.L. (1991). Enhanced expression of glutathione S-transferases in colorectal carcinoma compared to non-neoplastic mucosa. *Carcinogenesis,* 12, 13-7.

Morgenstern, R., Zhang, J. & Johansson, K. (2011). Microsomal glutathione transferase 1: mechanism and functional roles. *Drug Metab Rev,* 43, 300-6.

Moyer, A.M., Sun, Z., Batzler, A.J., Li, L., Schaid, D.J., Yang, P. & Weinshilboum, R.M. (2010). Glutathione pathway genetic polymorphisms and lung cancer survival after platinum-based chemotherapy. *Cancer Epidemiol Biomarkers Prev,* 19, 811-21.

Murtagh, E., Heaney, L., Gingles, J., Shepherd, R., Kee, F., Patterson, C. & MacMahon, J. (2005). Prevalence of obstructive lung disease in a general population sample: the NICECOPD study. *Eur J Epidemiol,* 20, 443-53.

O'Brien, M.L. & Tew, K.D. (1996). Glutathione and related enzymes in multidrug resistance. *Eur J Cancer,* 6, 967-78.

Pearson, W.R., Vorachek, W.R., Xu, S.J., Berger, R., Hart, I., Vannais, D. & Patterson, D. (1993). Identification of class-mu glutathione transferase genes GSTM1-GSTM5 on human chromosome 1p13. *Am J Hum Genet,* 53, 220-33.

Perera, F.P. (1997). Environment and cancer: who are susceptible? *Science,* 278, 1068-73.

Pistorius, S., Goergens, H., Engel, C., Plaschke, J., Krueger, S., Hoehl, R., Saeger, H.D. & Schackert, H.K. (2007). N-Acetyltransferase (NAT) 2 acetylator status and age of tumour onset in patients with sporadic and familial, microsatellite stable (MSS) colorectal cancer. *Int J Colorectal Dis,* 22, 137-43.

Potter, J.D. (1999). Colorectal cancer: molecules and populations. *J Natl Cancer Inst,* 91, 916-32.

Ranganathan, S. & Tew, K.D. (1991). Immunohistochemical localization of glutathione S-transferases alpha, mu, and pi in normal tissue and carcinomas from human colon. *Carcinogenesis,* 12, 2383-7.

Reszka, E. & Wasowicz, W. (2001). Significance of genetic polymorphisms in glutathione S-transferase multigene family and lung cancer risk. *Int J Occup Med Environ Health,* 14, 99-113.

Reszka, E., Wasowicz, W. & Gromadzinska, J. (2007). Antioxidant defense markers modulated by glutathione S-transferase genetic polymorphism: results of lung cancer case-control study. *Genes Nutr,* 2, 287-94.

Romero, R.Z., Morales, R., Garcia, F., Huarriz, M., Bandres, E., De la Haba, J., Gomez, A., Aranda, E. & Garcia-Foncillas, J. (2006). Potential application of GSTT1-null genotype in predicting toxicity associated to 5-fluouracil irinotecan and leucovorin regimen in advanced stage colorectal cancer patients. *Oncol Rep,* 16, 497-503.

Sau, A., Pellizzari Tregno, F., Valentino, F., Federici, G. & Caccuri, A.M. (2010). Glutathione transferases and development of new principles to overcome drug resistance. *Arch Biochem Biophys,* 500, 116-22.

Sheehan, D., Meade, G., Foley, V.M. & Dowd, C.A. (2001). Structure, function and evolution of glutathione transferases: implications for classification of non-mammalian members of an ancient enzyme superfamily. *Biochem J,* 360, 1-16.

Sorensen, M., Raaschou-Nielsen, O., Brasch-Andersen, C., Tjonneland, A., Overvad, K. & Autrup, H. (2007). Interactions between GSTM1, GSTT1 and GSTP1 polymorphisms and smoking and intake of fruit and vegetables in relation to lung cancer. *Lung Cancer,* 55, 137-44.

Sprenger, R., Schlagenhaufer, R., Kerb, R., Bruhn, C., Brockmoller, J., Roots, I. & Brinkmann, U. (2000). Characterization of the glutathione S-transferase GSTT1 deletion: discrimination of all genotypes by polymerase chain reaction indicates a trimodular genotype-phenotype correlation. *Pharmacogenetics,* 10, 557-65.

Steinhoff, C., Franke, K.H., Golka, K., Thier, R., Romer, H.C., Rotzel, C., Ackermann, R. & Schulz, W.A. (2000). Glutathione transferase isozyme genotypes in patients with prostate and bladder carcinoma. *Arch Toxicol,* 74, 521-6.

Stoehlmacher, J., Park, D.J., Zhang, W., Groshen, S., Tsao-Wei, D.D., Yu, M.C. & Lenz, H.J. (2002). Association between glutathione S-transferase P1, T1, and M1 genetic polymorphism and survival of patients with metastatic colorectal cancer. *J Natl Cancer Inst,* 94, 936-42.

Sundberg, K., Johansson, A.S., Stenberg, G., Widersten, M., Seidel, A., Mannervik, B. & Jernstrom, B. (1998). Differences in the catalytic efficiencies of allelic variants of glutathione transferase P1-1 towards carcinogenic diol epoxides of polycyclic aromatic hydrocarbons. *Carcinogenesis,* 19, 433-6.

Sweeney, C., Coles, B.F., Nowell, S., Lang, N.P. & Kadlubar, F.F. (2002). Novel markers of susceptibility to carcinogens in diet: associations with colorectal cancer. *Toxicology,* 182, 83-7.

Tan, K.L. & Board, P.G. (1996). Purification and characterization of a recombinant human Theta-class glutathione transferase (GSTT2-2). *Biochem J,* 315, 727-32.

Tetlow, N. & Board, P.G. (2004). Functional polymorphism of human glutathione transferase A2. *Pharmacogenetics,* 14, 111-6.

Tetlow, N., Coggan, M., Casarotto, M.G. & Board, P.G. (2004). Functional polymorphism of human glutathione transferase A3: effects on xenobiotic metabolism and steroid biosynthesis. *Pharmacogenetics,* 14, 657-63.

Tetlow, N., Liu, D. & Board, P. (2001). Polymorphism of human Alpha class glutathione transferases. *Pharmacogenetics,* 11, 609-17.

Tew, K.D., Manevich, Y., Grek, C., Xiong, Y., Uys, J. & Townsend, D.M. (2011). The role of glutathione S-transferase P in signaling pathways and S-glutathionylation in cancer. *Free Radic Biol Med,* 51, 299-313.

Tew, K.D. & Ronai, Z. (1999). GST function in drug and stress response. *Drug Resist Updat,* 2, 143-147.

Townsend, D.M., Findlay, V.J., Fazilev, F., Ogle, M., Fraser, J., Saavedra, J.E., Ji, X., Keefer, L.K. & Tew, K.D. (2006). A glutathione S-transferase pi-activated prodrug causes kinase activation concurrent with S-glutathionylation of proteins. *Mol Pharmacol,* 69, 501-8.

Townsend, D.M., Findlay, V.L. & Tew, K.D. (2005). Glutathione S-transferases as regulators of kinase pathways and anticancer drug targets. *Methods Enzymol,* 401, 287-307.

Townsend, D.M., Manevich, Y., He, L., Hutchens, S., Pazoles, C.J. & Tew, K.D. (2009). Novel role for glutathione S-transferase pi. Regulator of protein S-Glutathionylation following oxidative and nitrosative stress. *J Biol Chem,* 284, 436-45.

Townsend, D.M. & Tew, K.D. (2003). The role of glutathione-S-transferase in anti-cancer drug resistance. *Oncogene,* 22, 7369-75.

Tsuchida, S. & Sato, K. (1992). Glutathione transferases and cancer. *Crit Rev Biochem Mol Biol,* 27, 337-84.

van der Logt, E.M., Bergevoet, S.M., Roelofs, H.M., van Hooijdonk, Z., te Morsche, R.H., Wobbes, T., de Kok, J.B., Nagengast, F.M. & Peters, W.H. (2004). Genetic polymorphisms in UDP-glucuronosyltransferases and glutathione S-transferases and colorectal cancer risk. *Carcinogenesis,* 25, 2407-15.

Vasieva, O. (2011). The many faces of glutathione transferase pi. *Curr Mol Med,* 11, 129-39.

Villafania, A., Anwar, K., Amar, S., Chie, L., Way, D., Chung, D.L., Adler, V., Ronai, Z., Brandt-Rauf, P.W., Yamaizumii, Z., Kung, H.F. & Pincus, M.R. (2000). Glutathione-S-Transferase as a selective inhibitor of oncogenic ras-p21-induced mitogenic signaling through blockade of activation of jun by jun-N-terminal kinase. *Ann Clin Lab Sci,* 30, 57-64.

Vlaykova, T., Gulubova, M., Vlaykova, D., Cirovski, G., Yovchev, Y., Dimov, D. & Chilingirov, P. (2009). Possible Influence of GSTM1 and GSTT1 null genotype on the risk for development of sporadic colorectal cancer. *Biotechnol & Biotechnol Equip.,* 23, 1084-1089.

Vlaykova, T., Gulubova, M., Vlaykova, D., Yaneva, K., Cirovski, G., Chilingirov, P. & Stratiev, S. (2005). Expression of GST-pi and its impact on the survival of patients treated with chemotherapy for colorectal cancer. . *Trakia J Sci* 3, 39-44.

Vlaykova, T., Miteva, L., Gulubova, M. & Stanilova, S. (2007). Ile(105)Val GSTP1 polymorphism and susceptibility to colorectal carcinoma in Bulgarian population. *Int J Colorectal Dis,* 22, 1209-15.

Wang, T., Arifoglu, P., Ronai, Z. & Tew, K.D. (2001). Glutathione S-transferase P1-1 (GSTP1-1) inhibits c-Jun N-terminal kinase (JNK1) signaling through interaction with the C terminus. *J Biol Chem,* 276, 20999-1003.

Wang, X., Pavelic, Z.P., Li, Y., Gleich, L., Gartside, P.S., Pavelic, L., Gluckman, J.L. & Stambrook, P.J. (1997). Overexpression and amplification of glutathione S-transferase pi gene in head and neck squamous cell carcinomas. *Clin Cancer Res,* 3, 111-4.

Watson, M.A., Stewart, R.K., Smith, G.B., Massey, T.E. & Bell, D.A. (1998). Human glutathione S-transferase P1 polymorphisms: relationship to lung tissue enzyme activity and population frequency distribution. *Carcinogenesis,* 19, 275-80.

Welfare, M., Monesola Adeokun, A., Bassendine, M.F. & Daly, A.K. (1999). Polymorphisms in GSTP1, GSTM1, and GSTT1 and susceptibility to colorectal cancer. *Cancer Epidemiol Biomarkers Prev,* 8, 289-92.

Whitbread, A.K., Masoumi, A., Tetlow, N., Schmuck, E., Coggan, M. & Board, P.G. (2005). Characterization of the omega class of glutathione transferases. *Methods Enzymol,* 401, 78-99.

Whitbread, A.K., Tetlow, N., Eyre, H.J., Sutherland, G.R. & Board, P.G. (2003). Characterization of the human Omega class glutathione transferase genes and associated polymorphisms. *Pharmacogenetics,* 13, 131-44.

Whyatt, R.M., Perera, F.P., Jedrychowski, W., Santella, R.M., Garte, S. & Bell, D.A. (2000). Association between polycyclic aromatic hydrocarbon-DNA adduct levels in maternal and newborn white blood cells and glutathione S-transferase P1 and CYP1A1 polymorphisms. *Cancer Epidemiol Biomarkers Prev,* 9, 207-12.

Wu, Y., Fan, Y., Xue, B., Luo, L., Shen, J., Zhang, S., Jiang, Y. & Yin, Z. (2006). Human glutathione S-transferase P1-1 interacts with TRAF2 and regulates TRAF2-ASK1 signals. *Oncogene,* 25, 5787-800.

Yang, B., Guo, M., Herman, J.G. & Clark, D.P. (2003). Aberrant promoter methylation profiles of tumor suppressor genes in hepatocellular carcinoma. *Am J Pathol,* 163, 1101-7.

Yu, K.D., Fan, L., Di, G.H., Yuan, W.T., Zheng, Y., Huang, W., Chen, A.X., Yang, C., Wu, J., Shen, Z.Z. & Shao, Z.M. (2009). Genetic variants in GSTM3 gene within GSTM4-GSTM2-GSTM1-GSTM5-GSTM3 cluster influence breast cancer susceptibility depending on GSTM1. *Breast Cancer Res Treat,* 121, 485-96.

Zhao, T., Singhal, S.S., Piper, J.T., Cheng, J., Pandya, U., Clark-Wronski, J., Awasthi, S. & Awasthi, Y.C. (1999). The role of human glutathione S-transferases hGSTA1-1 and hGSTA2-2 in protection against oxidative stress. *Arch Biochem Biophys,* 367, 216-24.

6

Distinct Pathologic Roles for Glycogen Synthase Kinase 3β in Colorectal Cancer Progression

Toshinari Minamoto[1], Masanori Kotake[1,3], Mitsutoshi Nakada[2], Takeo Shimasaki[4], Yoshiharu Motoo[4] and Kazuyuki Kawakami[1]
[1]Division of Translational and Clinical Oncology, Cancer Research Institute,
[2]Department of Neurosurgery, Graduate School of Medical Science,
Kanazawa University, Kanazawa,
[3]Department of Surgery, Ishikawa Prefectural Central Hospital, Kanazawa,
[4]Department of Medical Oncology, Kanazawa Medical University, Uchinada, Ishikawa,
Japan

1. Introduction

Colorectal cancer (CRC) is the third most frequent cancer type and the second leading cause of cancer-related deaths worldwide (Cunningham et al., 2010; Jemal et al., 2010). This is despite the recent trend of stabilizing or declining rates for CRC incidence and mortality in economically developed countries (Center et al., 2009; Edwards et al., 2010; Umar & Greenwald, 2009). Surgical intervention is the initial treatment for most CRC patients. Continuous efforts to optimize surgery for patients with localized CRC has resulted in markedly improved 5-year and 10-year survival rates (Cunningham et al., 2010; Wu & Fazio, 2000). Given the large number of CRC patients who undergo curative surgery, there is now a substantial number who are susceptible to recurrent or metastatic tumors and could therefore benefit from additional systemic therapies. An increasing array of options and protocols for chemotherapies and biologically targeted therapies is now available for use in the adjuvant setting and for the treatment of recurrent and metastatic CRC.
Based on a more detailed knowledge of the molecular characteristics of CRC (Markowitz et al., 2009; Walther et al., 2009), biologically-based therapeutics have been developed for the treatment of advanced stage CRC patients. Currently approved agents for the treatment of advanced and metastatic CRC include therapeutic monoclonal antibodies that target vascular endothelial growth factor (VEGF) and epidermal growth factor receptor (EGFR). Despite a substantial biological rationale for the use of these new classes of therapeutic agents, large-scale clinical trials have observed only incremental clinical benefits for overall patient populations. Clearly, not all patients with recurrent and metastatic CRC benefit from these therapies. This is due to inherent and acquired resistance of tumors to the chemotherapeutic and biologically-based agents. Moreover, there are few reliable markers for predicting the therapeutic and adverse effects of these agents and that would allow patients who benefit from these systemic treatments to be identified. Therefore, new

therapeutic targets are urgently required to further improve the survival of patients with recurrent and metastatic CRC. One such target may be glycogen synthase kinase 3β (GSK3β), a serine/threonine protein kinase that has recently been implicated in various human cancers.

In this Chapter, we briefly summarize the scientific basis and current status of systemic treatments for CRC, including combinations of surgery, chemotherapy and molecular target-directed therapy. Based on our published and ongoing studies, we then focus on GSK3β as an emerging therapeutic target in CRC and other cancer types. We describe the underlying biological mechanism that allows exploration of a novel therapeutic strategy for CRC involving the targeting of aberrant GSK3β.

2. Molecular basis of colorectal cancer

2.1 Multistep and multiple molecular alterations

Colorectal carcinogenesis displays all the major biological hallmarks of cancer (Hanahan & Weinberg, 2011). CRC evolves and develops through orchestrated, multistep genetic and epigenetic alterations in oncogenes, tumor suppressor genes and DNA mismatch repair genes. These include frequent aberrations in certain chromosomes, such as allelic imbalance at several chromosomal loci (e.g., chromosome 5q, 8p, 17p, 18q) and chromosome amplification and translocation. Various combinations of somatic and germ-line alterations in these genes and chromosomes characterize the different genotypes and phenotypes of sporadic and hereditary forms of CRC (Cunningham et al., 2010; Markowitz & Bertagnolli, 2009; Walther et al., 2009). Among the genes involved in the molecular process of CRC development, several genetic markers have been reported to harbor diagnostic and prognostic information and to predict the benefit from or resistance to systemic therapy (Ellis & Hicklin, 2009; Markowitz & Bertagnolli, 2009; Walther et al., 2009).

Recent advances in DNA sequencing technology have allowed sequencing of the entire coding genome of human cancer to become a reality. The high throughput, next-generation sequencing of 18,000 genes in the Reference Sequence data-base of the National Center for Biotechnology Information in the USA has identified cancer-associated somatic mutations in 848 genes. Amongst these, 140 are considered as candidate genes responsible for the development and phenotype of CRC (Sjőblom et al., 2006; Wood et al., 2007).

2.2 Oncogene addiction

The unrestrained survival and proliferation of cancer cells relies on distinct oncogenic signalling pathways in which various oncoproteins, growth factor receptors and their ligands are aberrantly activated, leading to the concept of "oncogene addiction" (Sharma & Settleman, 2007; Weinstein, 2002; Weinstein & Joe, 2006). In theory, acute ablation of oncogene function should lead to the rapid dissipation of its pro-survival signal in cancer cells, thus resulting in apoptotic cell death. This "oncogenic shock" concept underlies the strategy of molecular targeting in cancer therapy (Sharma et al., 2006). The scientific rationale behind the development and application of therapeutic monoclonal antibodies targeting VEGF and EGFR for the treatment of CRC is based on these concepts. Intriguingly, however, the EGFR expression level in primary CRC determined by immunohistochemistry was not observed to correlate with the efficacy of therapeutic anti-EGFR antibodies in clinical trials of metastatic CRC (Hecht et al., 2010; commented by Grothey, 2010).

3. Systemic treatment: An overview

Surgery remains the cornerstone for the cure of localized CRC (Cunningham et al., 2010; Wu & Fazio, 2000). For colon cancer, total resection of the primary tumor with ample surgical margins and regional lymphadenectomy are the requisites for curative surgery. For rectal cancer, curative resection includes total excision of the mesorectum with adequate circumferential and distal surgical margins (R0) and lymphadenectomy along the inferior mesenteric vessels. Laparoscopic surgery has now become prevalent and safe, with long-term oncological outcomes of CRC patients undergoing this surgery reported as comparable to those treated by the open surgical approach (Lacy et al., 2008; The Clinical Outcomes of Surgical Therapy Study Group, 2004). Within 5 years after curative surgical resection, disease relapse (tumor recurrence or metastasis) occurs in 40 to 50% of patients with stage III CRC and in 20% of those with stage II CRC (Midgley & Kerr, 1999). Systemic therapy with

	Chemotherapeutic agents			Therapeutic monoclonal antibodies		
	5-FU Capecitabine	Irinotecan	Oxaliplatin	Bevacizumab	Cetuximab	Panitumumab
Target	TS	Topo-isomerase I	DNA cross-link	VEGF	EGFR	EGFR
Indication	PO adjuvant metastatic	metastatic	PO adjuvant metastatic	metastatic	metastatic	metastatic
Combination						
FOLFOX	+ LV		+	combined	combined	combined
FOLFIRI	+ LV	+		combined	combined	combined
FOLFOXIRI	+ LV	+	+			
Predictive markers	TS, DPD, TP	UGT1A1*	ERCC-1	VEGF? Tumor micro-vessels?	EGFR copy number**, K-ras, B-raf, PI3CA, AREG, EREG	K-ras, B-raf, PI3CA

Table 1. Key agents and their combinations presently used for the treatment of CRC

Abbreviations: AREG, amphyregulin; DPD, dihydropyrimidine dehydrogenase; EGFR, epidermal growth factor receptor; ERCC-1, excision-repair cross-complementing-1; EREG, epiregulin; 5-FU, 5-fluorouracil; FOLFIRI, folinate, 5-FU and irinotecan; FOLFOX, folinate, 5-FU and oxaliplatin; FOLFOXIRI, FOLFOX and irinotecan; LV, leukovorin; PI3KCA, phosphoinositide 3 kinase (PI3K) p110 catalytic subunit gene; PO, postoperative; TP, thymidine phosphorylase; TS, thymidylate synthase; UGT1A1, uridine diphosphate (UDP)-glucuronosyltransferase 1A1; VEGF, vascular endothelial growth factor.

* The number of TA repeats in the TATA element in UGT1A1 gene predicts the drug toxicity and resultant adverse effects.

** EGFR copy number is measured by fluorescence *in-situ* hybridization (FISH).

either chemotherapy and/or targeted therapies have been demonstrated to provide benefit to these CRC patients in both the post-operative adjuvant and advanced disease settings (Inoue et al., 2006; Midgley et al., 2009). Table 1 summarizes the key chemotherapeutic agents and therapeutic monoclonal antibodies targeting VEGF and EGFR and the combinations currently prescribed as adjuvant therapy for relapse-prone CRC patients and patients with metastatic tumors (reviewed in Cunningham et al., 2010; Meyerhardt & Mayer, 2005; Midgley et al., 2009; Wolpin et al., 2007; Wolpin & Mayer, 2008). The putative predictive markers for response to the respective agents are also shown in Table 1 (Walther et al., 2009).

3.1 Adjuvant chemotherapy

The purpose of postoperative adjuvant chemotherapy for stage II or III CRC is to destroy residual tumor cells and/or micrometastatic foci that are latent at the time of curative surgery. The chemotherapeutic mainstay for CRC, 5-fluorouracil (5-FU), exerts its anti-tumor effect by inhibiting thymidylate synthase (TS), a critical enzyme for nucleic acid synthesis. Folinic acid (leucovorin: LV) is frequently used to enhance the anti-tumor effect of 5-FU. The clinical and pharmacological rationale for this combination derives from the biological role of LV in stabilizing the ternary complex between TS and fluoro-deoxyuridine monophosphate (dUMP), an active metabolite of 5-FU, thereby enhancing TS inhibition. Adjuvant treatment regimens consist of oral (capecitabine) or infusional fluoropyrimidine-based chemotherapy as a single agent with LV, or in combination with irinotecan (a topoisomerase I inhibitor), oxaliplatin (a DNA cross-linker) or both (Table 1) (Midgley et al., 2009; Wolpin et al., 2007; Wolpin & Mayer, 2008).

Adjuvant fluoropyrimidine-based chemotherapy reduces the risk of cancer-related mortality by 30% and increases the 5-year survival rate by 5-12% in patients with stage III (node-positive) CRC. Adjuvant chemotherapy for stage II (node-negative) CRC patients is controversial because it increases the 5-year survival rate by just 3-4%. It has been proposed that "high-risk" stage II CRC patients characterized by T4 tumor, luminal stenosis or obstruction, poor histological differentiation, extramural vessel invasion, inadequate lymphadenectomy or surgical margins (R1) should preferentially undergo adjuvant chemotherapy (Cunningham et al., 2010; Midgley et al., 2009). Tumor relapse after curative resection occurs mostly within 3 years, irrespective of adjuvant chemotherapy (Sargent et al., 2007). Several clinical trials have failed to show a survival benefit from combining molecular target-directed agents (e.g., bevacizumab, cetuximab) with adjuvant chemotherapy (reviewed in Cunningham et al., 2010). Improvement in the survival of patients at high risk of tumor relapse therefore depends on intensive surveillance for early diagnosis of metastatic lesions, as well as identification of patients who are susceptible to tumor recurrence and who could thus benefit from more aggressive adjuvant treatment.

3.2 Treatment of metastatic CRC

A series of systemic, fluoropyrimidine-based combinatorial chemotherapies (Table 1) has substantially improved tumor response to treatment and increased the duration of progression-free and overall survival in patients with metastatic CRC. The remarkable advance in treating metastatic CRC in recent years has been due to the emergence and clinical application of molecular targeted therapeutics (Cunningham et al., 2010; Midgley et al., 2009). As stated above, a number of therapeutic monoclonal antibodies that target relevant oncogenic pathways have been tested in clinical trials for CRC. Among them, the most widely used agents are bevacizumab, a recombinant humanized monoclonal antibody against VEGF (Ellis & Hicklin, 2008a; Li & Saif, 2009), cetuximab, a chimeric monoclonal antibody against EGFR (Balko et al, 2010) and panitumumab, a fully humanized monoclonal antibody against EGFR (Davis & Jimeno, 2010). These therapeutic antibodies have been used as monotherapy for the treatment of patients with metastatic CRC, or in combination with systemic chemotherapy (Table 1). Many clinical trials have demonstrated the additive effect of these antibodies on tumor response rate and progression-free survival (reviewed in Cunningham et al., 2010; Midgley et al., 2009). However, the combination of each therapeutic antibody with systemic chemotherapy regimens produced incremental but not always robust benefits to overall survival when compared to chemotherapy alone (Fojo & Parkinson, 2010).

3.3 Obstacles to systemic therapy

3.3.1 Drug resistance and predictive markers

The major obstacles to systemic therapy for CRC include drug resistance (both inherent and acquired) and the lack of reliable biomarkers for predicting response or resistance to drugs in clinical use (Ellis & Hicklin, 2009). This has led to the recent trend of using intensive combinatorial regimens for advanced CRC patients. Surprisingly, some recent clinical trials have shown that combinatorial target-directed therapies resulted in decreased survival, inferior quality of life and unexpected detrimental effects (Douillard et al., 2010; Hecht et al., 2009; Li & Saif, 2009; Tol et al., 2009).

Understanding the molecular mechanisms that underlie drug resistance and identifying predictive markers for drug sensitivity are *one and the same thing*. Pharmacogenomic approaches (Furuta et al., 2009; Walther et al., 2009) have identified a number of factors involved in drug metabolism and secretion, some of which (e.g., *UGT1A1* polymorphism) have been tested in clinical practice (Table 1). Several studies have suggested various biological mechanisms of resistance to VEGF-targeted cancer therapies (Bergers & Hanahan, 2008; Ebos et al., 2008; Ellis & Hicklin, 2008b), but to date there are no clinically useful predictive markers. Mutational activation of oncogenic pathways that lie downstream of EGFR signaling is known to cause intrinsic resistance to therapies that target this receptor. This has led to the identification of predictive markers (e.g., K-*ras*, B-*raf*, *PIK3CA*) that allow better patient selection for such treatments (Banck & Grothey, 2009; Cantwell-Dorris et al., 2011; De Roock et al., 2010a; Sartore-Bianchi et al., 2009). However, the complex pathways involved in tumor progression are often intercalated and therefore single markers cannot accurately predict the efficacy or outcome of CRC patients undergoing molecular targeted therapies (Baldus et al., 2010; De Roock et al., 2010b; Hecht et al., 2010).

Research into the mechanisms of acquired resistance to molecular targeted agents has generated new therapeutic strategies and agents aimed at counteracting the resistance mechanism (Bowles & Jimeno, 2011; Cidón, 2010; Dasari & Messersmith, 2010; Presen et al., 2010). Thus, improving the anti-tumor effects of molecular targeted therapies will depend on the identification of novel molecular pathways, development of new classes of rationally designed biological agents, and identification of predictive markers for response and resistance.

3.3.2 Economic issues

The high cost of developing the biologically-based therapeutic agents shown in Table 1 is a major issue in light of the modest clinical benefits, acquired drug resistance and lack of suitable predictive markers. A recent study reported significantly higher hospital costs for CRC patients with recurrence compared to those without (Macafee et al., 2009). Outside of the United States, the high cost of molecular targeted drugs has restricted their use to patients with sufficient income and/or health insurance. This issue highlights the importance of accurate predictive markers that allow identification of patients who are most likely to benefit from targeted agents, thus improving the cost effectiveness.

4. GSK3β as an emerging therapeutic target

4.1 GSK3β biology

GSK3 was identified as a serine/threonine protein kinase that phosphorylates and inhibits glycogen synthase (GS), a rate-limiting enzyme in the regulation of glucose/glycogen metabolism in response to insulin-mediated signaling (Embi et al., 1980). In contrast to its original name and depending on its substrates and binding partners (Table 2) (Medina & Wandosell, 2011; Xu et al., 2009), GSK3 has been found to participate in many fundamental cellular pathways including proliferation, differentiation, motility, cell cycle and apoptosis (Doble & Woodgett, 2003; Harwood, 2001; Jope & Johnson, 2004; Nakada et al., 2011). The two isoforms of this kinase, GSK3α and GSK3β, are encoded by their respective genes. Their functions do not always overlap (Rayasam et al., 2009) and much recent attention has been directed towards the function of GSK3β.

Unlike most protein kinases, GSK3β is active in normal cells and this activity is controlled by its subcellular localization, differential phosphorylation at serine 9 (S9) and tyrosine 216 (Y216) residues, and different binding partners. A consensus motif and context-based computational analysis of *in vivo* protein phosphorylation sites indicate that GSK3β is one of the kinases with the most substrates (Linding et al., 2007). In normal cells, multiple signaling pathways mediated by phosphoinositide 3 kinase (PI3K)-Akt, Wnt and mitogen-activated protein kinase (MAPK) are known to negatively regulate the activity of GSK3β via S9 phosphorylation (Medina & Wandosell, 2011). The molecular structure and details of the functional and regulatory machinery of GSK3β have been thoroughly described in many excellent reviews cited in this section and are not the focus of this Chapter.

4.2 GSK3β in common chronic diseases

Accumulating evidence suggests pathological roles for GSK3β in glucose intolerance due to inhibition of GS and other signaling cascades involved in the regulation of glucose homeostasis (Frame & Zheleva, 2006; Lee & Kim, 2007) and in neurodegenerative changes through accumulation of the neurotoxic substances amyloid Aβ and tau protein (Annaert & De Strooper, 2002; Bhat & Budd, 2002). Recognition that GSK3β promotes inflammation also implicates this molecule in a broad spectrum of common diseases including type 2 diabetes mellitus and neuropsychiatric disorders involving an inflammatory reaction (Jope et al., 2007). GSK3β has therefore emerged as a therapeutic target in these prevalent diseases (Cohen & Goedert, 2004; Kypta, 2005; Meijer et al., 2004; Phukan et al., 2010). Another line of studies has demonstrated an osteogenic function for the Wnt/β-catenin signaling pathway (Hartman, 2006; Krishnan et al., 2006; Ralston & de Crombrugghe, 2006). This suggests that GSK3β may be a putative therapeutic target for osteoporotic bone disease, since under physiological conditions it is a well established member of a complex that destroys β-catenin

Categories	Substrates
Metabolism	glycogen synthase, ATP citrate lyase, PKA, PDH, acetyl-CoA, carboxylase, PP1, PP2A, PP2A inhibitor, cyclin D1, eIF2B, NGF receptor, axin, APP, Bax, VDAC, hexokinase II, presenilin, LRP5/6
Cell structure	tau, MAP1B, NCAM, neurofilament, CRMP2, dynein, dynein-like protein, maltose binding protein, APC, kinesin light chain
Signaling & Transcription	
Wnt	β-catenin, snail, smad1, Hath1, smad 3
Akt	SRC-3, B-cell lymphoma (BCL)-3, p21
PI3K-Akt	Mcl-1, c-Jun, phosphatase and tensin homologue (PTEN)
Ras-PI3K-Akt	c-Myc, cyclin D1
TNFα	nuclear factor (NF)-κB
Hedgehog	Ci (citrus interruptus), Gli-2
hypoxia	hypoxia inducible factor (HIF)-1α
insulin	glycogen synthase, SREBP
undetermined & others	cyclin E, AP-1, CREB, C/EBP, cdc25A, Notch, p53, $p27^{Kip1}$, NFAT, GR, HSF-1, FGD-1, FGD-3, c-Myb, mCRY2, NACα, MafA, IPF1/PDX1, presenilin 1 C-terminal fragment

Table 2. Known substrates for phosphorylation by GSK3β

Abbreviations: AP-1, activator protein 1; APC, adenomatous polyposis coli; APP, amyloid precursor protein; ATP, adenosine triphosphate; C/EBP, CCAAT (cytidine-cytidine-adenosine-adenosine-thymidine)-enhancer-binding protein; CREB, cyclic adenosine monophosphate (cAMP) response element binding protein; CRMP2, collapsin response mediator protein 2; eIF2B, eukaryotic protein synthesis initiation factor-2B; FGD, FYVE, RhoGEF and PH domain-containing protein; GR, glucocorticoid receptor; HSF-1, heat shock factor protein 1; IPF1, insulin promoter factor 1; LRP5/6, low-density lipoprotein (LDL) receptor-related protein 5/6; MafA, musculoaponeurotic fibrosarcoma oncogene homolog A: MAP1B, microtubule-associated protein 1B; mCRY2, mouse cryptochrome 2; NACα, nascent polypeptide-associated complex α subunit; NCAM, neural cell adhesion molecule; NFAT, nuclear factor of activated T-cells; NGF, nerve growth factor; PDH, pyruvate dehydrogenase; PDX1, pancreatic and duodenal homeobox 1; PKA, protein kinase A; PP, protein phosphatase; SREBP, sterol regulatory element-binding protein; TNFα, tumor necrosis factor α; VDAC, voltage-dependent anion channel.

(Fuchs et al., 2005). In this context, an orally bioavailable GSK3α/β dual inhibitor was generated and tested as a new drug for the treatment of osteoporosis (Kulkarni et al., 2006).

4.3 GSK3β in cancer

An increasing number of cellular structural and functional proteins have been identified as targets for GSK3β phosphorylation-dependent regulation (Table 2). However, this has also generated results that show conflicting roles for the signaling pathways regulated by GSK3β in either suppressing or promoting cancer.

4.3.1 GSK3β suppresses cancer

In physiologically normal cells, many of the substrates for GSK3β-mediated phosphorylation and subsequent ubiquitin-mediated degradation include oncogenic signaling and transcription factors, cell cycle regulators and proto-oncoproteins (Table 2). A previous study showed that GSK3β phosphorylates and stabilizes a major cell cycle regulator, $p27^{Kip1}$ (Surjit & Lal, 2007). Recent studies have shown that inhibition of GSK3β stabilizes snail and induces epithelial-mesenchymal transition (EMT), a morphological and phenotypic change closely associated with tumor cell invasion and metastasis (Bachelder et al., 2005; Zhou et al., 2004; reviewed in Doble & Woodgett, 2007; Schlessinger & Hall, 2004; Zhou & Hung, 2005). These findings are mostly observed in normal but not neoplastic cells and have led to the hypothesis that GSK3β functions as a tumor suppressor (reviewed in Luo, 2009; Manoukian & Woodgett, 2003; Patel & Woodgett, 2008).

Consistent with this hypothesis, a number of studies in breast, lung and non-melanoma skin cancers have shown that GSK3β is inactivated in tumor cells, but that its activation induces apoptosis (reviewed in Luo, 2009; Patel & Woodgett, 2008). It has been reported in several studies that GSK3β renders cancer cells resistant to chemotherapeutic agents (reviewed in Luo, 2009). However, in contrast to the observations described in the next section (**4.3.2**), including our own, none of these studies addressed differences in the expression, activity and biological properties of GSK3β between tumor cells and their normal cell counterparts. Furthermore, these studies did not investigate the direct consequences of GSK3β inhibition for tumor cell survival, proliferation and chemotactic migration and invasion.

4.3.2 Deregulated GSK3β promotes cancer

Wnt signaling plays a crucial role in embryonic development, the regeneration of adult tissues and in many other cellular processes. Aberrant activation of the Wnt pathway due to mutation or deregulated expression of its components mediates the multistep process of colorectal tumorigenesis (Kikuchi, 2007; Klaus & Birchmeier, 2008; Lustig & Behrens, 2003; Willert & Jones, 2006). Over 90% of CRC develops following activation of the Wnt signaling pathway in which β-catenin plays a central role (Fuchs et al., 2005; Giles et al., 2003). GSK3β interrupts activation of the canonical Wnt pathway by phosphorylating β-catenin and recruiting it to ubiquitin-mediated degradation. GSK3β is therefore believed to antagonize tumorigenesis that involves active Wnt signaling (Bienz & Clevers, 2000; Manoukian & Woodgett, 2002; Polakis P, 1999), as represented for example by CRC development. This notion is also supported by the frequent mutational activation of Ras and PI3K-Akt signaling (Markowitz & Bertagnolli, 2009; Parsons et al., 2005), since it is well established that Akt kinase phosphorylates the S9 residue of GSK3β and inhibits its activity (Medina & Wandosell, 2011). However, few studies had focused on the biological properties of GSK3β in cancer until we investigated a putative pathological role for this kinase in CRC, as described below.

Most CRC cell lines and primary CRC tumors in our studies have shown increased expression and activity of GSK3β and deregulation of its activity due to imbalance in the differential phosphorylation of S9 (inactive) and Y216 (active) residues. This is in comparison to non-neoplastic cells (e.g., HEK293) and normal colon mucosa in which GSK3β activity appears to be regulated by the differential phosphorylation. These tumor cell features are unrelated to the activation of β-catenin or Akt (Mai et al., 2009; Shakoori et al., 2005). A non-radioisotopic, *in vitro* kinase assay demonstrated an increased ability of GSK3β derived from most CRC cell lines and primary CRC tumors to phosphorylate its substrate, as compared to non-neoplastic counterparts (Mai et al., 2006, 2009). These observations suggest that, in contrast to having hypothetical tumor suppressor function, GSK3β may actually promote cancer.

A putative pathological role for GSK3β in cancer was demonstrated by subsequent observations that inhibition of GSK3β activity using pharmacological (small-molecule) agents and of its expression by RNA interference reduced the survival and proliferation of CRC cells. Such inhibition also predisposed the cells to apoptosis *in vitro* and in tumor xenografts, suggesting that CRC cells depend on aberrant GSK3β for their survival and proliferation (Mai et al., 2006, 2009; Shakoori et al., 2005, 2007). A series of studies by our group led us to propose that aberrant GSK3β is a novel and potentially important therapeutic target in cancer (Miyashita et al., 2009b; Motoo et al., 2011; Nakada et al., 2011), thus allowing us to apply for domestic and international patents in this field (Minamoto).

Following our studies on the antitumor effects of GSK3β inhibition, similar observations were reported for CRC by other groups (Ghosh & Altieri, 2005; Rottmann et al., 2005; Tan et al., 2005; Tsuchiya et al., 2007) (Table 3). Similar results were also published for other cancer types with underlying biological mechanisms that included GSK3β inhibition of several pathways involved in tumorigenesis (reviewed in Miyashita et al., 2009b; Nakada et al., 2011). A putative role for GSK3β in cancer is still being debated (Luo, 2009; Manoukian & Woodgett, 2003; Patel & Woodgett, 2008) and was discussed in section **4.3.1**. However, the overall results to date indicate that aberrant expression and activity of GSK3β is likely to be a common and fundamental characteristic of a broad spectrum of human cancers.

4.3.3 Oncogene addiction and the effect of GSK3β inhibition against cancer

As stated in section **2.2**, the hypothesis of oncogene addiction has been proposed as a rationale for molecular targeting in cancer treatment. It refers to the observation that a cancer cell, despite its plethora of genetic alterations, seemingly exhibits dependence on a single oncoprotein or oncogenic pathway for its sustained survival and/or proliferation (Sharma & Settleman, 2007; Weinstein, 2002; Weinstein & Joe, 2006). This unique state of dependence by cancer cells is highlighted by the fact that inactivation of the normal counterpart of such proto-oncogene products in non-neoplastic cells is tolerated without obvious consequence. A profound implication of this hypothesis is that acute interruption of the critical oncogenic pathways upon which cancer cells are dependent should have a major detrimental effect (oncogene shock), while sparing normal cells that are not similarly addicted to these pathways (Sharma et al, 2006). In our series of studies, inhibition of GSK3β had little effect on cell survival, growth, apoptosis or senescence in non-neoplastic cells (e.g., HEK293) and on major vital organs in rodents (Mai et al., 2006, 2009; Shakoori et al., 2005, 2007). This concurs with previous reports showing that GSK3β inhibition does not influence the survival or growth of human mammary epithelial cells, embryonic lung fibroblasts (WI38) and mouse embryonic fibroblasts (NIH-3T3) (Kunnimalaiyaan et al., 2007; Ougolkov et al., 2005). With respect to the oncogene addiction hypothesis (Sharma & Settleman, 2007; Weinstein, 2002; Weinstein & Joe, 2006), the selective therapeutic effect of GSK3β inhibition against cancer can be explained by differences in biological properties of GSK3β between neoplastic and non-neoplastic cells (Mai et al., 2006, 2009; Shakoori et al., 2005).

5. GSK3β and the hallmarks of colorectal cancer

Understanding the molecular mechanism behind a pathogenic role for GSK3β in cancer is important for the development of treatment strategies that target this kinase. A current review highlights 8 hallmarks of cancer in which phenotypic properties are progressively

Authors	Study design	Types of GSK3β inhibitors	Pathological roles of GSK3β and underlying mechanism
Shakoori et al, 2005	*in vitro*	AR-A014418, SB-216763, siRNA	Deregulated GSK3β expression and activity are associated with CRC cell survival and proliferation by mechanism independent of activation of Wnt/β-catenin signaling and Akt. GSK3β inhibition attenuates survival and proliferation of colon cancer cells.
Mai et al, 2006	*in vitro*	AR-A014418, SB-216763, siRNA	NRIKA detected higher activity of GSK3β for phosphorylating its substrate (β-catenin) in gastrointestinal cancer cells including CRC cells than non-neoplastic HEK293 cells.
Shakoori et al, 2007	tumor xenograft	AR-A014418, SB-216763	GSK3β inhibition attenuates survival and proliferation of SW480 colon cancer cell xenografts with no detrimental effects on the major vital organs in the rodents.
Mai et al, 2009	*in vitro*, tumor xenograft	AR-A014418, SB-216763, siRNA	GSK3β inhibition attenuates survival and proliferation of colon cancer cells by decreasing hTERT expression and telomerase activity and inducing cell senescence.
Ghosh et al, 2005	*in vitro*	LiCl, TDZD8, SB-216763, siRNA	GSK3β functions against activation of p53-dependent apoptosis in colon cancer cells.
Tan et al, 2005	*in vitro*	LiCl, SB-216763, SB415286, LY2119301	GSK3β functions against activation of p53-dependent apoptosis through a direct Bax-mediated mitochondrial pathway in colon cancer cells.
Rottmann et al, 2005	*in vitro*, tumor xenograft	LiCl, siRNA	GSK3β functions against colon cancer cell apoptosis by inhibiting a TRAIL receptor-dependent synthetic lethal relationship between *Myc* activation and *FBW7* loss of function.
Tsuchiya et al, 2007	*in vitro*	BIO, LiCl, keupaullone	GSK3β inhibits colonocyte differentiation by destabilizing the transcription factor, Hath1.

Table 3. Pathological roles and functions of GSK3β in colorectal cancer

Abbreviations: hTERT, human telomerase reverse transcriptase; NRIKA, non-radioisotopic *in vitro* kinase assay; siRNA, small interfering RNA; TRAIL, tumor necrosis factor (TNF)-related apoptosis-inducing ligand.

acquired during multistep pathogenesis, thus allowing cancer cells to become tumorigenic and ultimately malignant (Hanahan & Weinberg, 2011). These hallmarks are sustained proliferative signaling, evasion of growth suppressors, resistance to cell death, enabling of replicative immortality, induction of angiogenesis, activation of invasion and metastasis, reprogramming of energy metabolism and evasion of immune destruction. The development of each hallmark involves multiple signaling pathways. In this section, we address how GSK3β modulates some of these hallmark characteristics of CRC by referring to the studies shown in Table 3, including our own work.

5.1 Cell proliferation

Unrestrained cell proliferation is the most prominent feature of cancer. Our previous study showed that the effect of GSK3β inhibition against the proliferative capacity of CRC cells was associated with decreased expression of cyclin D1 and cyclin-dependent kinase (CDK) 6 and phosphorylation of the Rb protein (Mai et al., 2009). These observations suggest that Rb function was restored, leading to the binding and inhibition of E2F transcription factor (reviewed in Classon & Harlow, 2002; Knudsen & Knudsen, 2008). This is consistent with a subsequent report that forced expression of exogenous GSK3β promotes the proliferation of ovarian cancer cells by inducing cyclin D1 expression (Cao et al., 2006). Together, the results suggest that suppression of excess cancer cell proliferation via the inhibition of GSK3β is partly due to negative regulation of cell cycling by cyclin D1. In normal or non-neoplastic cells, cyclin D1 is one of the primary targets of GSK3β for phosphorylation and subsequent degradation in the ubiquitin-proteasome system (Diehl et al., 1998) (Table 2). The opposing role of GSK3β in cyclin D1 expression may explain the lack of effect of GSK3β inhibition on cell survival and growth of non-neoplastic cells found in earlier studies (Kunnimalaiyaan et al., 2007; Mai et al., 2009; Ougolkov et al., 2005; Shakoori et al., 2005).

5.2 Resistance to cell death via tumor suppressor pathways

A major mechanism by which cancer cells evade cell death is via the inactivation of tumor suppressor pathways mediated by p53 (Royds & Iacopetta B, 2006; Vousden & Lane, 2007; Zilfou & Lowe, 2009) and Rb (Classon & Harlow, 2002; Knudsen & Knudsen, 2008). The studies listed in Table 3 showed that inhibition of GSK3β induced apoptosis in human CRC cell lines. This effect was associated with increased expression of p53 and of p21 in colon cancer cells with wild-type p53, and decreased Rb phosphorylation in colon cancer cells irrespective of their p53 status (Ghosh & Altieri, 2005; Mai et al., 2009; Tan et al., 2005). Another study showed that GSK3β suppresses the apoptosis of colon cancer cells by inhibiting a tumor necrosis factor (TNF)-related apoptosis-inducing ligand (TRAIL) receptor-dependent synthetic lethal relationship between c-*Myc* activation and *FBW7* (a gene encoding a ubiquitin ligase receptor) loss of function (Rottmann et al., 2005). These studies suggest a putative pathological role for aberrant GSK3β in mediating CRC cell resistance to apoptosis induced by a pathway involving tumor suppressor proteins, TRAIL and c-Myc.

One of the representative pathways for cell survival is mediated by nuclear factor-κB (NF-κB) (Inoue et al., 2007; Karin, 2006, 2009). Based on previous studies showing the potential involvement of GSK3β in NF-κB-mediated cell survival during mouse embryonic development (Hoeflich et al., 2000; Schwabe & Brenner, 2002), it was reported that GSK3β sustains pancreatic cancer cell survival by maintaining transcriptional activity of NF-κB (Ougolkov et al., 2005; Wilson & Baldwin, 2008). While these studies examined the activity of exogenous (transfected) NF-κB, we previously observed no effect of GSK3β inhibition on endogenous NF-κB transcriptional activity in gastrointestinal cancer cells (including CRC) and glioblastoma cells (Mai et al., 2009; Miyashita et al., 2009a). Therefore, a role for GSK3β in regulating NF-κB activity in cancer is controversial.

5.3 Replicative cell immortality

Another critical mechanism used by cancer cells to evade cell death is replicative cell immortality. A close relationship exists in cancer cells between the molecular mechanisms for immortality and escape from replicative senescence (Finkel et al., 2007). Cancer cells acquire constitutive expression and activity of human telomerase reverse transcriptase (hTERT) and telomerase in order to circumvent telomere-dependent pathways of cell mortality (Harley, 2008).

We recently observed a decreased level of hTERT mRNA in colon cancer cells following inhibition of either the activity or expression of GSK3β. Inhibition of GSK3β attenuates telomerase activity and increases the β-galactosidase-positive (senescent) population in colon cancer cells. These effects were associated with increased expression of p53, p21 and c-Jun N-terminal kinase 1 (JNK1) and decreases in CDK6 expression and Rb phosphorylation (Mai et al., 2009). The findings are consistent with the known relationship between these proteins and cell senescence (reviewed in Kiyono, 2007) and with GSK3β activity (Ghosh & Altieri, 2005; Kulikov et al., 2005; Liu et al., 2004; Mai et al., 2009; Qu et al., 2004; Rössig et al., 2002). Consistent with our observation, a recent study found that inhibition of GSK3β suppressed hTERT expression and telomerase activity and shortened the telomere length in various cancer cell lines including HCT116 colon cancer cells, and attenuated cell proliferation and hTERT expression in ovarian cancer xenografts (Bilsland et al., 2009). The putative role for GSK3β in protecting cancer cells from telomere-dependent senescence and mortality is attributed to its effects on hTERT expression and telomerase activity.

5.4 Influence on the cancer microenvironment and tumor invasion

In cancer, various events are orchestrated to produce a distinct tumor microenvironment that dictates the malignant potential. These include depletion of nutrients involved in cell proliferation, tumor cell invasion, tumor neovascularization in response to hypoxic condition, as well as stromal, inflammatory and immune reactions in the host (Joyce, 2005). The promotion of inflammation and immune response by GSK3β (Jope et al, 2007) suggests a broad pathological role for this kinase in the cancer microenvironment.

The pro-invasive phenotype of cancer cells is characterized by EMT, enhanced cell motility and their ability to induce neovascularization. As discussed in section **4.3.1**, inhibition of GSK3β stabilizes snail and induces EMT (Bachelder et al., 2005; Zhou et al., 2004; reviewed in Doble & Woodgett, 2007; Schlessinger & Hall, 2004; Zhou & Hung, 2005). A hypoxic tumor microenvironment induces the expression of hypoxia-inducible factor-1α (HIF-1α), a transcription factor that controls oxygen homeostasis by regulating target genes involved in angiogenesis, glycolysis and cell proliferation (reviewed in Semenza, 2009). A previous study showed that under physiological conditions, GSK3β inhibits angiogenesis by negatively regulating endothelial cell survival and migration in response to PI3K-, MAPK- and protein kinase A (PKA)-dependent signaling pathways (Kim et al., 2002). Another study demonstrated that hypoxia induces a biphasic effect on HIF-1α stabilization in liver cancer cells. Accumulation of HIF-1α occurs in early hypoxia and is dependent on an active PI3K/Akt pathway and inactive GSK3β. In contrast, prolonged hypoxia results in the inactivation of Akt and activation of GSK3β. This negatively regulates HIF-1α activity by inhibiting its accumulation (Mottet et al., 2003). Collectively, it thus appears unlikely that GSK3β participates in cancer cell EMT and in tumor angiogenesis.

Formation of lamellipodia, the characteristic cellular microarchitecture, is responsible not only for cell migration under physiological conditions (e.g., embryonic development, wound healing) but also for cancer cell migration and invasion (Machesky, 2008; Small et al., 2002; Yilmaz & Christofori, 2009). A member of the Rho-GTPase family, Rac1, is known to participate in the formation of lamellipodia and may thus play an important role in cancer progression (Raftpoulou & Hall, 2004; Sahai & Marshall, 2002). It has been reported that GSK3β participates in cell motility by facilitating the formation of lamellipodia (Koivisto et al., 2003) and by activating Rac1 (Farooqui et al., 2006; Kobayashi et al., 2006; Vaidya et al., 2006). Focal adhesion kinase (FAK) is also known to play a key role in regulating cell motility and migration and to be deregulated in cancer (McLean et al., 2005). Earlier studies reported that FAK is one of the downstream effectors in GSK3β-mediated pathways (Kobayashi et al., 2006) and also regulates Rac1 (McLean et al., 2005). Consistent with a recent study for glioblastoma (Nowicki et al., 2008), our preliminary study has shown that inhibition of GSK3β attenuates pancreatic cancer cell migration and invasion by negatively regulating FAK and Rac1 activities (unpublished observation). Therefore, in regard to cancer treatments that target GSK3β, it is important to explore a possible role for GSK3β in CRC cell invasion by investigating its effects on cellular microarchitecture, motility and migration.

5.5 Cancer cell stemness and metabolic traits

Cell stemness and the reprogramming of energy metabolism are primary cell characteristics that share distinct molecular pathways and allow cancer cells to survive, proliferate, invade their host tissues, metastasize and resist treatment. Here, we address future directions in our approach towards ascertaining the potential of GSK3β as a therapeutic target in cancers including CRC.

5.5.1 Cancer cell stemness and GSK3β

Arising from the concept of tissue stem cells, the notion of cancer stem cells has emerged and proposes that cancer initiating cells are a distinct subpopulation within a tumor that have the ability to self-renew and differentiate (Clarke et al., 2006; O'Brien et al., 2010). Similar to other cancer types, a small population of cancer initiating cells has been identified and characterized in CRC (Dalerba et al., 2007; O'Brien et al., 2007; Ricci-Vitiani et al., 2007; reviewed in Yeung & Mortensen, 2009). Current cancer treatments assume that all cancer cells in tumors are homogeneous and have a similar capacity to proliferate, invade and metastasize, as well as having similar susceptibility to chemotherapy and radiation. However, accumulating evidence suggests that cancer stem cells and cancer cells that are undergoing EMT share various biological traits (Polyak & Weinberg, 2009). These cells are also strongly resistant to current forms of therapeutics, thereby identifying this subpopulation of cancer cells as the ultimate target for cancer treatment (Lou & Dean, 2007). Consistent with the physiological roles of GSK3β in Wnt, Hedgehog and Notch signaling (Foltz et al., 2002; Manoukian & Woodgett, 2002; Takenaka et al., 2007), GSK3β inhibition by pharmacological means promotes embryonic stem cell pluripotency (Sato et al., 2004) and hematopoietic stem cell reconstitution (Trowbridge et al., 2006). Conversely, recent studies have demonstrated that GSK3β sustains the respective molecular pathways leading to tumor cell stemness in a specific type of leukemia and in glioblastoma (Korur et al., 2009; Wang et al., 2008). Although the underlying molecular mechanisms are not well understood, these differential roles for GSK3β in normal and cancer stem cells could ultimately benefit cancer treatment strategies by allowing this kinase to be targeted with little harm to patients. As addressed in the next section (**5.5.2**), anaerobic glycolysis and the presence of a distinct niche are thought to be characteristics of cancer stem cells, in addition to their extreme resistance to drug treatment. Therefore, clarification of a putative role for GSK3β in regulating CRC cell stemness is of great interest. This could lead to a new strategy for treatment that targets the biology of cancer cell stemness.

5.5.2 Distinct metabolic traits of cancer cells and GSK3β

Production of excess energy is thought to provide an intrinsic and selective pressure that allows cancer cells to expand clonally and to acquire immortalized and destructive phenotypes. Even under normoxic conditions, most cancer cells depend on increased glucose uptake and aerobic glycolysis to produce their energy source, adenosine triphosphates (ATP) (Kim & Dang, 2006; Vander Heiden & Cantley, 2010). This is known as the Warburg effect and involves truncated oxidative phosphorylation in the tricarboxylic acid (TCA) cycle, thus resulting in mitochondrial uncoupling (Samudio et al., 2009). These properties allow cancer cells to survive and invade host tissues in a microenvironment where the supply of both oxygen and nutrients is deficient, as well as conferring resistance to apoptosis-inducing therapeutic stimuli (Smallbone et al., 2007). Therefore, the glycolytic phenotype of cancer cells is a potential target for cancer diagnosis and treatment (Gatenby & Gillies, 2007; Kroemer & Pouyssegur, 2008). For example, enhanced glucose uptake by cancer cells can be used to visualize cancer by positron emission tomography (PET) using the radioisotope-labeled glucose analogue 2-[^{18}F]-fluoro-2-deoxy-D-glucose (FDG). FDG-PET in combination with computed tomography (PET-CT) enables the detection of metastatic lesions for most cancers with sensitivity and specificity both greater than 90% (Mankoff et al., 2007).

The association between a glycolytic phenotype (*i.e.*, TCA cycle defects) and resistance to apoptosis is attributed to decreased mitochondrial hydrogen peroxide production and cytochrome C release (Samudio et al., 2009; Vander Heiden & Cantley, 2010). Pyruvate dehydrogenase (PDH) plays a crucial role in triggering the TCA cycle by converting pyruvate to citric acid. PDH kinase 1 (PDK1), which phosphorylates and inactivates PDH, is frequently over-activated in cancer cells, resulting in an impaired TCA cycle and mitochondrial hyperpolarization. Thus, inhibition of PDK1 would re-activate PDH and restore mitochondrial membrane polarity, thereby facilitating cancer cell apoptosis in response to chemotherapeutic agents and radiation. Dichloroacetate (DCA), an orally bio-available small molecule, is a well characterized PDK1 inhibitor. The ability of DCA to inhibit lactate production by stimulating PDH and the TCA cycle has long been used to treat lactic acidosis, which is a complication of inherited mitochondrial disorders (Stacpoole, 2003, 2006). A recent study demonstrated that DCA induces cancer cell apoptosis by selectively inhibiting PDK1 in cancer cells, leading to metabolic remodeling from glycolysis to glucose oxidation and the normalization of mitochondrial function (Bonnet et al., 2008). A clinical trial of oral DCA in children with congenital lactic acidosis reported that DCA was well tolerated and safe (Stacpoole, 2006). Thus, orally administered DCA is a promising and selective anticancer agent.

The primary role of GSK3β is to control GS activity (Table 2). It thus acts as a checkpoint at the bifurcation between glycogenesis and glycolysis, the two major pathways of glucose/glycogen metabolism (Lee & Kim, 2007). We recently found that inhibition of GSK3β in colon cancer cells increased GS expression and decreased its S640 phosphorylation (unpublished observation), suggesting that GSK3β inhibition may switch cancer cells from a glycolytic to a glycogenic phenotype. It was previously reported that GSK3β phosphorylates and inactivates PDH (Hoshi et al., 1996) (Table 2), a key enzyme for the TCA cycle in mitochondria. This suggests that deregulated GSK3β contributes to truncation of the TCA cycle and mitochondrial uncoupling in cancer cells, resulting in resistance to chemotherapy and radiation. It has also been reported that the distinct metabolism of cancer cells involves not only anaerobic glycolysis but also other metabolic pathways such as the pentose phosphate pathway, amino acid and nucleic acid synthesis and glutaminolysis (DeBerardinis et al., 2008). GSK3β has a number of key metabolic enzymes as substrates (Table 2), suggesting this molecule could have broad control over various pathological metabolic pathways in cancer cells.

6. Perspectives

Biologically-based therapy of cancer holds great promise, particularly for patients who are refractory to existing forms of therapy. Current paradigms reviewed in the earlier part of this Chapter (**3. Systemic treatment: an overview**) include the targeting of growth factor receptor-type protein tyrosine kinases and angiogenic factors. Such therapies are directed against cancer cell survival, proliferation and tumor angiogenesis; however they are unable to completely eradicate cancer, as demonstrated by most large-scale clinical trials.

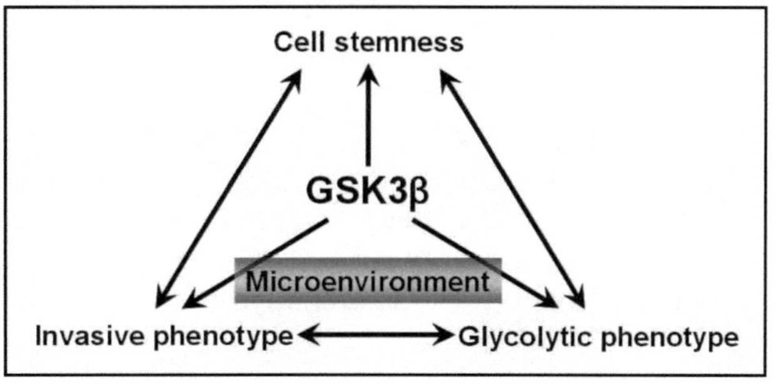

Fig. 1. GSK3β promotes cell stemness, invasive capacity and excess glucose metabolism that interact to produce a distinct cancer microenvironment.

The distinct pathologic properties of GSK3β in cancer described here highlight its potential to be an innovative target for the radical treatment of this disease, including CRC. GSK3β can potentially promote cancer cell stemness, invasive capacity and glucose metabolism, thus creating the selective pressures that allow cancer cells to persist in a distinct microenvironment (Figure 1). Understanding the complex biological mechanisms for the multiple roles of GSK3β in promoting cancer should allow elucidation of novel molecular pathways that lead to cancer development and progression. This will also provide a detailed scientific basis for the development of cancer treatment strategies that target aberrant GSK3β.

Concerns regarding the therapeutic use of GSK3β inhibitors remain because these may activate oncogenic (e.g., Wnt) signaling, thus promoting cell proliferation (Manoukian & Woodgett, 2003). However, this issue has not deterred preclinical studies of GSK3β inhibitors for the treatment of many cancer types (reviewed in Miyashita et al., 2009b) or Phase II clinical trials for the treatment of neurological diseases (Chico et al., 2010). Currently, two clinical trials are being undertaken to test a pharmacological GSK3β inhibitor (LY2090314) for enhancement of the anti-tumor effect of chemotherapeutic agents for advanced solid cancer (phase I: http://clinicaltrials.gov/ct2/show/study/NCT01287520) and leukemia (phase II: http://clinicaltrials.gov/ct2/show/study/NCT01214603). Such trials targeting GSK3β should complement, enhance or substitute the current front line therapies that target growth factor receptors and angiogenic factors in refractory colorectal cancer.

7. Acknowledgments

This study was supported in part by Grants-in-Aid for Scientific Research from the Japanese Ministry of Education, Science, Sports, Technology and Culture (to KK, TM); from the Ministry of Health, Labour and Welfare (to TM); from the Japan Society for the Promotion of Science (to KK, TM); and from the Japan Society for Technology (to KK and TM).

8. References

Annaert, W. & De Strooper, B. (2002). A cell biological perspective on Alzheimer's disease. *Annu Rev Cell Dev Biol.* Vol. 18, pp. 25-51, ISSN: 1081-0706 (Print, Linking), 1530-8995 (Electronic)

Bachelder, R.E., Yoon, S., Franci, C., de Herreros, A.G. & Mercurio, A.M. (2005). Glycogen synthase kinase-3 is an endogenous inhibitor of Snail transcription: implications for the epithelial-mesenchymal transition. *J Cell Biol.* Vol. 168, No. 1, pp. 29-33, ISSN: 0021-9525 (Print, Linking), 1540-8140 (Electronic)

Baldus, S.E., Schaefer, K-L., Engers, R., Hartleb, D., Stoecklein, N.H. & Gabbert, H.E. (2010). Prevalence and heterogeneity of *KRAS*, *BRAF*, and *PIK3CA* mutations in primary colorectal adenocarcinomas and their corresponding metastases. *Clin Cancer Res.* Vol. 16, No. 3, pp. 790-799, ISSN: 1078-0432 (Print, Linking)

Balko, A.L., Black, E.P. & Balko, J.M. (2010). First-line treatment of metastatic cancer: focus on Cetuximab in combination with chemotherapy. *Clin Med Rev Oncol.* Vol. 2, pp. 319-327, ISSN: 1179-2531 (Electronic, Linking)

Banck, M.S. & Grothey, A. (2009). Biomarkers of resistance to epidermal growth factor receptor monoclonal antibodies in patients with metastatic colorectal cancer. *Clin Cancer Res.* Vol. 15, No. 24, pp. 7492-7501, ISSN: 1078-0432 (Print, Linking)

Bergers, G. & Hanahan, D. (2008). Modes of resistance to anti-angiogenic therapy. *Nat Rev Cancer.* Vol. 8, No. 8, pp. 592-603, ISSN: 1474-175X (Print, Linking), 1474-1768 (Electronic)

Bhat, R.V. & Budd, S.L. (2002). GSK3β signalling: casting a wide net in Alzheimer's disease. *Neurosignals.* Vol. 11, No. 5, pp. 251-261, ISSN: 1424-862X (Print, Linking), 1424-8638 (Electronic)

Bienz, M. & Clevers, H. (2000). Linking colorectal cancer to Wnt signaling. *Cell.* Vol. 103, No. 2, pp. 311-320, ISSN: 0092-8674 (Print, Linking), 1097-4172 (Electronic)

Bilsland, A.E., Hoare, S., Stevenson, K., Plumb, J., Gomez-Roman, N., Cairney, C., Burns, S., Lafferty-Whyte, K., Roffey, J., Hammonds, T. & Keith, W.N. (2009). Dynamic telomerase gene suppression via network effects of GSK3 inhibition. *PLoS One.* Vol. 4, No. 7, pp. e6459, ISSN: 1932-6203 (Electronic, Linking)

Bonnet, S., Archer, S.L., Allalunis-Turner, J., Haromy, A., Beaulieu, C., Thompson, R., Lee, C.T., Lopaschuk, G.D., Puttagunta, L., Bonnet, S., Harry, G., Hashimoto, K., Porter, C.J., Andrade, M.A., Thebaud, B. & Michelakis, E.D. (2007). A mitochondria-K^+ channel axis is suppressed in cancer and its normalization promotes apoptosis and inhibits cancer growth. *Cancer Cell.* Vol. 11, No. 1, pp. 37-51, ISSN: 1535-6108 (Print, Linking), 1878-3686 (Electronic)

Bowles, D.W. & Jimeno, A. (2011). New phosphatidylinsitol 3-kinase inhibitors for cancer. *Expert Opin Investig Drugs.* Vol. 20, No. 4, pp. 507-518, ISSN: 1354-3784 (Print, Linking), 1744-7658 (Electronic)

Cantwell-Dorris, E.R., O'Leary, J.J. & Sheils, O.M. (2011). BRAF^{V600E}: implications for carcinogenesis and molecular therapy. *Mol Cancer Ther.* Vol. 10, No. 3, pp. 385-394, ISSN: 1535-7163 (Print, Linking), 1538-8514 (Electronic)

Cao, Q., Lu, X. & Feng, Y. (2006). Glycogen synthase kinase-3β positively regulates the proliferation of human ovarian cancer cells. *Cell Res.* Vol. 16, No. 7, pp. 671-677, ISSN: 1001-0602 (Print, Linking), 1748-7838 (Electronic)

Center, M.M., Jemal, A. & Ward, E. (2009). International trends in colorectal cancer incidence rates. *Cancer Epidemiol Biomarkers Prev.* Vol. 18, No. 6, pp. 1688-1694, ISSN: 1055-9965 (Print, Linking), 1538-7755 (Electronic)

Chico, L.K., Van Eldik, L.J. & Watterson, D.M. (2009). Targeting protein kinases in central nervous system disorders. *Nat Rev Drug Discov.* Vol. 8, No. 11, pp. 892-909, ISSN: 1474-1776 (Print, Linking), 1474-1784 (Electronic)

Cidón, E.U. (2010). The challenge of metastatic colorectal cancer. *Clin Med Insights Oncol.* Vol. 4, pp. 55-60, ISSN: 1179-5549 (Electronic)

Clarke, M.F., Dick, J.E., Dirks, P.B., Eaves, C.J., Jamieson, C.H., Jones, D.L., Visvader, J., Weissman, I.L. & Wahl, G.M. (2006). Cancer stem cells—perspectives on current status and future directions: AACR Workshop on Cancer Stem Cells. *Cancer Res.* Vol., 66, No. 19, pp. 9339-9344, ISSN: 0008-5472 (Print, Linking), 1538-7445 (Electronic)

Classon, M. & Harlow, E. (2002). The retinoblastoma tumor suppressor in development and cancer. *Nat Rev Cancer.* Vol. 2, No. 12, pp. 910-917, ISSN: 1474-175X (Print, Linking), 1474-1768 (Electronic)

Cohen, P. & Goedert, M. (2004). GSK3 inhibitors: development and therapeutic potential. *Nat Rev Drug Discov.* Vol. 3, No. 6, pp. 479-487, ISSN: 1474-1776 (Print, Linking), 1474-1784 (Electronic)

Cunningham, D., Atkin, W., Lenz, H.J., Lynch, H.T., Minsky, B., Nordlinger, B. & Starling, N. (2010). Colorectal cancer. *Lancet.* Vol. 375, No. 9719, pp. 1030-1047, ISSN: 0140-6736 (Print, Linking), 1474-547X (Electronic)

Dalerba, P., Dylla, S.J., Park, I.K., Liu, R., Wang, X., Cho, R.W., Hoey, T., Gurney, A., Huang, E.H., Simeone, D.M., Shelton, A.A., Parmiani, G., Castelli, C. & Clarke, M.F. (2007). Phenotypic characterization of human colorectal cancer stem cells. *Proc Natl Acad Sci U S A.* Vol. 104, No. 24, pp. 10158-10163, ISSN: 0027-8424 (Print, Linking), 1091-6490 (Electronic)

Dasari, A. & Messersmith, W.A. (2010). New strategies in colorectal cancer: biomarkers of response to epidermal growth factor receptor monoclonal antibodies and potential therapeutic targets in phosphoinositide 3-kinase and mitogen-activated protein kinase pathways. *Clin Cancer Res.* Vol. 16, No. 15, pp. 3811-3818, ISSN: 1078-0432 (Print, Linking)

Davis, S.L. & Jimeno, A. (2010). Metastatic colorectal cancer: focus on panitumumab. *Clin Med Rev Oncol.* Vol. 2, pp. 109-121, ISSN: 1179-2531 (Electronic, Linking)

DeBerardinis, R.J., Sayed, N., Ditsworth, D. & Thompson, C.B. (2008). Brick by brick: metabolism and tumor cell growth. *Curr Opin Genet Dev.* Vol. 18, No. 1, pp. 54-61, ISSN: 0959-437X (Print, Linking), 1879-0380 (Electronic)

De Roock, W., Claes, B., Bernasconi, D., De Schutter, J., Biesmans, B., Fountzilas, G., Kalogeras, K.T., Kotoula, V., Papamichael, D., Laurent-Puig, P., Penault-Llorca, F., Rougier, P., Vincenzi, B., Santini, D., Tonini, G., Cappuzzo, F., Frattini, M., Molinari, F., Saletti, P., De Dosso, S., Martini, M., Bardelli, A., Siena, S., Sartore-Bianchi, A., Tabernero, J., Macarulla, T., Di Fiore, F., Gangloff, A.O., Ciardiello, F., Pfeiffer, P., Qvortrup, C., Hansen, T.P., Van Cutsem, E., Piessevaux, H., Lambrechts, D., Delorenzi, M. & Tejpar, S. (2010a). Effects of *KRAS, BRAF, NRAS,* and *PIK3CA* mutations on the efficacy of cetuximab plus chemotherapy in chemotherapy-refractory metastatic colorectal cancer: a retrospective consortium analysis. *Lancet Oncol.* Vol. 11, No. 8, pp. 753-762, ISSN: 1470-2045 (Print, Linking), 1474-5488 (Electronic)

De Roock, W., Jonker, D.J., Di Nicolantonio, F., Sartore-Bianchi, A., Tu, D., Siena, S., Lamba, S., Arena, S., Frattini, M., Piessevaux, H., Van Cutsem, E., O'Callaghan, C.J., Khambata-Ford, S., Zalcberg, J.R., Simes, J., Karapetis, C.S., Bardelli, A. & Tejpar, S. (2010b). Association of KRAS p.G13D mutation with outcome in patients with chemotherapy-refractory metastatic colorectal cancer treated with cetuximab. *JAMA.* Vol. 304, No. 16, pp. 1812-1820, ISSN: 0098-7484 (Print, Linking), 1538-3598 (Electronic)

Diehl, J.A., Cheng, M., Roussel, M.F. & Sherr, C.J. (1998). Glycogen synthase kinase-3β regulates cyclin D1 proteolysis and subcellular localization. *Genes Dev.* Vol. 12, No. 22, pp. 3499-3511, ISSN: 0890-9369 (Print, Linking), 1549-5477 (Electronic)

Doble, B.W. & Woodgett, J.R. (2003). GSK-3: tricks of the trade for a multi-tasking kinase. *J Cell Sci.* Vol. 116, No. Pt7, pp. 1175-1186, ISSN: 0021-9533 (Print, Linking), 1477-9137 (Electronic)

Doble, B.W. & Woodgett, J.R. (2007). Role of glycogen synthase kinase-3 in cell fate and epithelial-mesenchymal transition. *Cells Tissues Organs.* Vol. 185, No. 1-3, pp. 73-84, ISSN: 1422-6405 (Print, Linking), 1422-6421 (Electronic)

Douillard, J.Y., Siena, S., Cassidy, J., Tabernero, J., Burkes, R., Barugel, M., Humblet, Y., Bodoky, G., Cunningham, D., Jassem, J., Rivera, F., Kocákova, I., Ruff, P., Błasińska-Morawiec, M., Šmakal, M., Canon, J.L., Rother, M., Oliner, K.S., Wolf, M. & Gansert, J. (2010). Randomized, phase III trial of panitumumab with infusional fluorouracil, leucovorin, and oxaliplatin (FOLFOX4) versus FOLFOX4 alone as first-line treatment in patients with previously untreated metastatic colorectal cancer: the PRIME study. *J Clin Oncol.* Vol. 28, No. 31, pp. 4697-4705, ISSN: 0732-183X (Print, Linking), 1527-7755 (Electronic)

Ebos, J.M.L., Lee, C.R. & Kerbel, R.S. (2009). Tumor and host-mediated pathways of resistance and disease progression in response to antiangiogenic therapy. *Clin Cancer Res.* Vol. 15, No. 16, pp. 5020-5025, ISSN: 1078-0432 (Print, Linking)

Edwards, B.K., Ward, E., Kohler, B.A., Eheman, C., Zauber, A.G., Anderson, R.N., Jemal, A., Schymura, M.J., Lansdorp-Vogelaar, I., Seeff, L.C., van Ballegooijen, M., Goede, S.L. & Ries, L.A.G. (2010). Annual report to the nation on the status of cancer, 1975-2006, featuring colorectal cancer trends and impact of interventions (risk factors, screening, and treatment) to reduce future rates. *Cancer.* Vol. 116, No. 3, pp. 544-573, ISSN: 0008-543X (Print, Linking), 1097-0142 (Electronic)

Ellis, L.M. & Hicklin, D.J. (2008a). VEGF-targeted therapy: mechanisms of anti-tumor activity. *Nat Rev Cancer.* Vol. 8, No. 8, pp. 579-591, ISSN: 1474-175X (Print, Linking), 1474-1768 (Electronic)

Ellis, L.M. & Hicklin, D.J. (2008b). Pathways mediating resistance to vascular endothelial growth factor–targeted therapy. *Clin Cancer Res.* Vol. 14, No. 20, pp. 6371-6375, ISSN: 1078-0432 (Print, Linking)

Ellis, L.M. & Hicklin, D.J. (2009). Resistance to targeted therapies: refining anticancer therapy in the era of molecular oncology. *Clin Cancer Res.* Vol. 15, No. 24, pp. 7471-7478, ISSN: 1078-0432 (Print, Linking)

Embi, N., Rhylatt, D.B. & Cohen, P. (1980). Glycogen synthase kinase-3 from rabbit skeletal muscle. Separation from cyclic-AMP-dependent protein kinase and phosphorylase kinase. *Eur J Biochem.* Vol. 107, No. 2, pp. 519-527, ISSN: 0014-2956 (Print, Linking), 1432-1033 (Electronic)

Farooqui, R., Zhu, S. & Fenteany, G. (2006). Glycogen synthase kinase-3 acts upstream of ADP-ribosylation factor 6 and Rac1 to regulate epithelial cell migration. *Exp Cell Res.* Vol. 312, No. 9, pp. 1514-1525, ISSN: 0014-4827 (Print, Linking), 1090-2422 (Electronic)

Finkel, T., Serrano, M. & Blasco, M.A. (2007). The common biology of cancer and ageing. *Nature.* Vol. 448, No. 7155, pp. 767-774, ISSN: 0028-0836 (Print, Linking), 1476-4687 (Electronic)

Fojo, T. & Parkinson, D.R. (2010). Biologically targeted cancer therapy and marginal benefits: are we making too much of too little or are we achieving too little by giving too much? *Clin Cancer Res.* Vol. 16, No. 24, pp. 5972-5980, ISSN: 1078-0432 (Print, Linking)

Foltz, D.R., Santiago, M.C., Berechid, B.E. & Nye, J.S. (2002). Glycogen synthase kinase-3β modulates Notch signaling and stability. *Curr Biol.* Vol. 12, No. 12, pp. 1006-1011, ISSN: 0960-9822 (Print, Linking), 1879-0445 (Electronic)

Frame, S. & Zheleva, D. (2006). Targeting glycogen synthase kinase-3 in insulin signalling. *Expert Opin Ther Targets.* Vol. 10, No. 3, pp. 413-428, ISSN: 1472-8222 (Print, Linking), 1744-7631 (Electronic)

Fuchs, S.Y., Ougolkov, A.V., Spiegelman, V.S. & Minamoto, T. (2005). Oncogenic β-catenin signaling networks in colorectal cancer. *Cell Cycle.* Vol. 4, No. 11, pp. 1522-1539, ISSN: 1538-4101 (Print), 1551-4005 (Electronic, Linking)

Furuta, T. (2009). Pharmacogenomics in chemotherapy for GI tract cancer. *J Gastroenterol.* Vol. 44, No. 10, pp. 1016-1025, ISSN: 0944-1174 (Print, Linking), 1435-5922 (Electronic)

Gatenby, R.A. & Gillies, R.J. (2007). Glycolysis in cancer: a potential target for therapy. *Int J Biochem Cell Biol.* Vol. 39, No. 7-8, pp. 1358-1366, ISSN: 1357-2725 (Print, Linking), 1878-5875 (Electronic)

Ghosh, J.C. & Altieri, D.C. (2005). Activation of p53-dependent apoptosis by acute ablation of glycogen synthase kinase-3β in colorectal cancer cells. *Clin Cancer Res.* Vol. 11, No. 12, pp. 4580-4588, ISSN: 1078-0432 (Print, Linking)

Giles, R.H., van Es, J.H. & Clevers, H. (2003). Wnt storm: Wnt signaling in cancer. *Biochim Biophys Acta.* Vol. 1653, No. 1, pp. 1-24, ISSN: 0006-3002 (Print, Linking)

Grothey, A. (2010). EGFR antibodies in colorectal cancer: where do they belong? *J Clin Oncol.* Vol. 28, No. 31, pp. 4668-4670, ISSN: 0732-183X (Print, Linking), 1527-7755 (Electronic)

Hanahan, D. & Weinberg, R.A. (2011). Hallmarks of cancer: the next generation. *Cell.* Vol. 144, No. 5, pp. 646-673, ISSN: 0092-8674 (Print, Linking), 1097-4172 (Electronic)

Harley, C.B. (2008). Telomerase and cancer therapeutics. *Nat Rev Cancer.* Vol. 8, No. 3, pp. 167-179, ISSN: 1474-175X (Print, Linking), 1474-1768 (Electronic)

Hartman, C.A. (2006). A Wnt canon orchestrating osteoblastogenesis. *Trends Cell Biol.* Vol. 16, No. 3, pp. 151-158, ISSN: 0962-8924 (Print, Linking), 1879-3088 (Electronic)

Harwood, A.J. (2001). Regulation of GSK-3: a cellular multiprocessor. *Cell.* Vol. 105, No. 7, pp. 821-824, ISSN: 0092-8674 (Print, Linking), 1097-4172 (Electronic)

Hecht, J. R., Mitchell, E., Chidiac, T., Scroggin, C., Hagenstad, C., Spigel, D., Marshall, J., Cohn, A., McCollum, D., Stella, P., Deeter, R., Shahin, S. & Amado, R.G. (2009). A randomized phase IIIB trial of chemotherapy, bevacizumab, and panitumumab compared with chemotherapy and bevacizumab alone for metastatic colorectal cancer. *J Clin Oncol.* Vol. 27, No. 5, pp. 672-680, ISSN: 0732-183X (Print, Linking), 1527-7755 (Electronic)

Hecht, J.R., Mitchell, E., Neubauer, M.A., Burris, H.A. 3rd, Swanson, P., Lopez, T., Buchanan, G., Reiner, M., Gansert J. & Berlin, J. (2010). Lack of correlation between epidermal growth factor receptor status and response to Panitumumab monotherapy in metastatic colorectal cancer. *Clin Cancer Res.* Vol. 16, No. 7, pp. 2205-2213, ISSN: 1078-0432 (Print, Linking)

Hoeflich, K.P., Luo, J., Rubie, E.A., Tsao, M.S., Jin, O. & Woodgett, J.R. (2000). Requirement for glycogen synthase kinase-3β in cell survival and NF-κB activation. *Nature.* Vol. 406, No. 6791, pp. 86-90, ISSN: 0028-0836 (Print, Linking), 1476-4687 (Electronic)

Hoshi, M., Takashima, A., Noguchi, K., Murayama, M., Sato, M., Kondo, S., Saitoh, Y., Ishiguro, K., Hoshino, T. & Imahori K. (1996). Regulation of mitochondrial pyruvate dehydrogenase activity by tau protein kinase I/glycogen synthase kinase 3β in brain. *Proc Natl Acad Sci U S A.* Vol. 93, No. 7, pp. 2719-2723, ISSN: 0027-8424 (Print, Linking), 1091-6490 (Electronic)

Inoue, Y., Miki, C. & Kusunoki, M. (2006). Current directions in chemotherapy for colorectal cancer. *J Gastroenterol.* Vol. 41, No. 9, pp. 821-831, ISSN: 0944-1174 (Print, Linking), 1435-5922 (Electronic)

Inoue, J-I., Gohda, J., Akiyama, T. & Semba, K. (2007). NF-κB activation in development and progression of cancer. *Cancer Sci.* Vol. 98, No. 3, pp. 268-274, ISSN: 1347-9032 (Print, Linking), 1349-7006 (Electronic)

Jemal, A., Siegel, R., Xu, J. & Ward, E. (2010). Cancer statistics, 2010. *CA Cancer J Clin.* Vol. 60, No. 5, pp. 277-300, ISSN: 0007-9235 (Print, Linking), 1542-4863 (Electronic)

Jope, R.S. & Johnson, G.V. (2004). The glamour and gloom of glycogen synthase kinase-3. *Trends Biochem Sci.* Vol. 29, No. 2, pp. 95-102, ISSN: 0968-0004 (Print, Linking)

Jope, R.S., Yuskaitis, C.J. & Beurel, E. (2007). Glycogen synthase kinase-3 (GSK3): inflammation, diseases, and therapeutics. *Neurochem Res.* Vol. 32, No. 4-5, pp. 577-595, ISSN: 0364-3190 (Print, Linking), 1573-6903 (Electronic)

Joyce, J.A. (2005). Therapeutic targeting of the tumor microenvironment. *Cancer Cell.* Vol. 7, No. 6, pp. 513-520, ISSN: 1535-6108 (Print, Linking), 1878-3686 (Electronic)

Karin, M. (2006). Nuclear factor-κB in cancer development and progression. *Nature.* Vol. 441, No. 7092, pp. 431-436, ISSN: 0028-0836 (Print, Linking), 1476-4687 (Electronic)

Karin, M. (2009). NF-κB as a critical link between inflammation and cancer. *Cold Spring Harb Perspect Biol.* Vol. 1, pp. a000141, ISSN: 1943-0264 (Electronic)

Kikuchi, A. (2007). Tumor formation by genetic mutations in the components of the Wnt signaling pathway. *Cancer Sci.* Vol. 94, No. 3, pp. 225-229, ISSN: 1347-9032 (Print, Linking), 1349-7006 (Electronic)

Kim, H.S., Skurk, C., Thomas, S.R., Bialik, A., Suhara, T., Kureishi, Y., Birnbaum, M., Keaney, J.F. Jr. & Walsh, K. (2002). Regulation of angiogenesis by glycogen synthase kinase-3β. *J Biol Chem.* Vol. 277, No. 44, pp. 41888-41896, ISSN: 0021-9258 (Print, Linking), 1083-351X (Electronic)

Kim, J. & Dang, C.V. (2006). Cancer's molecular sweet tooth and the Warburg effect. *Cancer Res.* Vol. 66, No. 18, pp. 8927-8930, ISSN: 0008-5472 (Print, Linking); 1538-7445 (Electronic)

Korur, S., Huber, R.M., Sivasankaran, B., Petrich, M., Morin, P., Jr., Hemmings, B.A., Merlo, A. & Lino, M.M. (2009). GSK3β regulates differentiation and growth arrest in glioblastoma. *PLoS One.* Vol. 4, No. 10, pp. e7443, ISSN: 1932-6203 (Linking)

Kiyono, T. (2007). Molecular mechanisms of cellular senescence and immortalization of human cells. *Expert Opin Ther Targets.* Vol. 11, No. 12, pp. 1623-1637, ISSN: 1472-8222 (Print, Linking), 1744-7631 (Electronic)

Klaus, A. & Birchmeier, W. (2008). Wnt signalling and its impact on development and cancer. *Nat Rev Cancer.* Vol. 8, No. 5, pp. 387-398, ISSN: 1474-175X (Print, Linking), 1474-1768 (Electronic)

Knudsen, E. & Knudsen, K. (2008). Tailoring to RB: tumour suppressor status and therapeutic response. *Nat Rev Cancer.* Vol. 8, No. 9, pp. 714-724, ISSN: 1474-175X (Print, Linking), 1474-1768 (Electronic)

Kobayashi, T., Hino, S., Oue, N., Asahara, T., Zollo, M., Yasui, W. & Kikuchi, A. (2006). Glycogen synthase kinase 3 and h-prune regulate cell migration by modulating focal adhesions. *Mol Cell Biol.* Vol. 26, No. 3, pp. 898-911, ISSN: 0270-7306 (Print, Linking), 1098-5549 (Electronic)

Koivisto, L., Alavian, K., Hakkinen, L., Pelech, S., McCulloch, C. & Larjava, H. (2003). Glycogen synthase kinase-3 regulates formation of long lamellipodia in human keratinocytes. *J Cell Sci.* Vol. 116, No. Pt 18, pp. 3749-3760, ISSN: 0021-9533 (Print, Linking), 1477-9137 (Electronic)

Krishnan, V., Bryant, H.U. & MacDougald, O.A. (2006). Regulation of bone mass by Wnt signaling. *J Clin Invest.* Vol. 116, No. 5, pp. 1202-1209, ISSN: 0021-9738 (Print, Linking), 1558-8238 (Electronic)

Kroemer, G. & Pouyssegur, J. (2008). Tumor cell metabolism: Cancer's Achilles' heel. *Cancer Cell.* Vol. 13, No. 6, pp. 472-482, ISSN: 1535-6108 (Print, Linking), 1878-3686 (Electronic)

Kulikov, R., Boehme, K.A. & Blattner, C. (2005). Glycogen synthase kinase 3-dependent phosphorylation of Mdm2 regulates p53 abundance. *Mol Cell Biol.* Vol. 25, No. 16, pp. 7170-7180, ISSN: 0270-7306 (Print, Linking), 1098-5549 (Electronic)

Kulkarni, N.H., Onyia, J.E., Zeng, Q., Tian, X., Liu, M., Halladay, D.L., Frolik, C.A., Engler, T., Wei, T., Kriauciunas, A., Martin, T.J., Sato, M., Bryant, H.U. & Ma, Y.L. (2006). Orally bioavailable GSK-3α/β dual inhibitor increases markers of cellular differentiation *in vitro* and bone mass *in vivo*. *J Bone Miner Res.* Vol. 21, No. 6, pp. 910-920, ISSN: 0884-0431 (Print, Linking), 1523-4681 (Electronic)

Kunnimalaiyaan, M., Vaccaro, A.M., Ndiaye, M.A. & Chen, H. (2007). Inactivation of glycogen synthase kinase-3β, a downstream target of the raf-1 pathway, is associated with growth suppression in medullary thyroid cancer cells. *Mol Cancer Ther.* Vol. 6, No. 3, pp. 1151-1158, ISSN: 1535-7163 (Print, Linking), 1538-8514 (Electronic)

Kypta, R.M. (2005). GSK-3 inhibitors and their potential in the treatment of Alzheimer's disease. *Expert Opin Ther Patents.* Vol. 15, No. 10, pp. 1315-1331, ISSN: 1354-3776 (Print, Linking), 1744-7674 (Electronic)

Lacy, A.M., Delgado, S., Castells, A., Prins, H.A., Arroyo, V., Ibarzabal, A. & Pique, J.M. (2008). The long-term results of a randomized clinical trial of laparoscopy-assisted versus open surgery for colon cancer. *Ann Surg.* Vol. 248, No. 1, pp. 1-7, ISSN: 0003-4932 (Print, Linking), 1528-1140 (Electronic)

Lee, J. & Kim, M-S. (2007). The role of GSK3 in glucose homeostasis and the development of insulin resistance. *Diabetes Res Clin Pract.* Vol. 77, No. suppl 1, pp. S49-S57, ISSN: 1572-1671 (Print, Linking)

Li, J. & Saif, M.W. (2009). Current use and potential role of bevacizumab in the treatment of gastrointestinal cancers. *Biologics Targets Ther.* Vol. 3, pp. 429-441, ISSN: 1177-5475 (Print, Linking), 1177-5491 (Electronic)

Linding, R., Jensen, L.J., Ostheimer, G.J., van Vugt, M.A., Jorgensen, C., Miron, I.M., Diella, F., Colwill, K., Taylor, L., Elder, K., Metalnikov, P., Nguyen, V., Pasculescu, A., Jin, J., Park, J.G., Samson, L.D., Woodgett, J.R., Russell, R.B., Bork, P., Yaffe, M.B. & Pawson, T. (2007). Systemic discovery of in vivo phosphorylation networks. *Cell.* Vol. 129, No. 7, pp. 1415-1426, ISSN: 0092-8674 (Print, Linking), 1097-4172 (Electronic)

Liu, S., Yu, S., Hasegawa, Y., LaPushin, R., Xu, H.J., Woodgett, J.R., Mills, G.B. & Fang, X. (2004). Glycogen synthase kinase 3β is a negative regulator of growth factor-induced activation of the c-Jun N-terminal kinase. *J Biol Chem.* Vol. 279, No. 49, pp. 51075-51081, ISSN: 0021-9258 (Print, Linking), 1083-351X (Electronic)

Lou, H. & Dean, M. (2007). Targeted therapy for cancer stem cells: the patched pathway and ABC transporters. *Oncogene.* Vol. 26, No. 9, pp. 1357-1360, ISSN: 0950-9232 (Print, Linking), 1476-5594 (Electronic)

Luo, J. (2009). Glycogen synthase kinase 3β (GSK3β) in tumorigenesis and cancer chemotherapy. *Cancer Lett.* Vol. 273, No. 2, pp. 194-200, ISSN: 0304-3835 (Print, Linking), 1872-7980 (Electronic)

Lustig, B. & Behrens, J. (2003). The Wnt signalling pathway and its role in tumor development. *J Cancer Res Clin Oncol.* Vol. 129, No. 4, pp. 199-221, ISSN: 0171-5216 (Print, Linking), 1432-1335 (Electronic)

Macafee, D.A.L., West, J., Scholefield, J.H. & Whynes, D.K. (2009). Hospital costs of colorectal cancer care. *Clin Med Oncol.* Vol. 3, pp. 27-37, ISSN: 1177-9314 (Electronic, Linking)

Machesky, L.M. (2008). Lamellipodia and filopodia in metastasis and invasion. *FEBS Lett.* Vol. 582, No. 14, pp. 2102-2111, ISSN: 0014-5793 (Print, Linking), 1873-3468 (Electronic)

Mai, W., Miyashita, K., Shakoori, A., Zhang, B., Yu, Z.W., Takahashi, Y., Motoo, Y., Kawakami, K. & Minamoto, T. (2006). Detection of active fraction of GSK3β in cancer cells by non-radioisotopic *in vitro* kinase assay. *Oncology.* Vol. 71, No. 3-4, pp. 297-305, ISSN: 0030-2414 (Print, Linking), 1423-0232 (Electronic)

Mai, W., Kawakami, K., Shakoori, A., Kyo, S., Miyashita, K., Yokoi, K., Jin, M., Shimasaki, T., Motoo, Y. & Minamoto, T. (2009). Deregulated GSK3β sustains gastrointestinal cancer cells survival by modulating human telomerase reverse transcriptase and telomerase. *Clin Cancer Res.* Vol. 15, No. 22, pp. 6810-6819, ISSN: 1078-0432 (Print, Linking)

Mankoff, D.A., Eary, J.F., Link, J.M., Muzi, M., Rajendran, J.G., Spence, A.M. & Krohn, K.A. (2007). Tumor-specific positron emission tomography imaging in patients: [^{18}F] fluorodeoxyglucose and beyond. *Clin Cancer Res.* Vol. 13, No. 12, pp. 3460-3469, ISSN: 1078-0432 (Print, Linking)

Manoukian, S.S. & Woodgett, J. (2002). Role of GSK-3 in cancer: regulation by Wnts and other signaling pathways. *Adv Cancer Res.* Vol. 84, pp. 203-229, ISSN: 0065-230X (Print, Linking)

Markowitz, S.D. & Bertagnolli, M.M. (2009). Molecular basis of colorectal cancer. *N Engl J Med.* Vol. 361, No. 25, pp. 2449-2460, ISSN: 0028-4793 (Print, Linking), 1533-4406 (Electronic)

McLean, G.W., Carragher, N.O., Avizienyte, E., Evans, J., Brunton, V.G. & Frame, M.C. (2005). The role of focal adhesion kinase in cancer - a new therapeutic opportunity. *Nat Rev Cancer.* Vol. 5, No. 7, pp. 505-515, ISSN: 1474-175X (Print, Linking), 1474-1768 (Electronic)

Medina, M. & Wandosell, F. (2011). Deconstructing GSK-3: the fine regulation of its activity. *Int J Alzheimers Dis.* Vol. 2011, Article ID 479249, ISSN: 2090-0252 (Electronic)

Meijer, L., Flajolet, M. & Greengard, P. (2004). Pharmacological inhibitors of glycogen synthase kinase 3. *Trends Pharmacol Sci.* Vol. 25, No. 9, pp. 471-480, ISSN: 0165-6147 (Print, Linking), 1873-3735 (Electronic)

Meyerhardt, J.A. & Mayer, R.J. (2005). Systemic therapy for colorectal cancer. *N Engl J Med.* Vol. 352, No. 5, pp. 476-487, ISSN: 0028-4793 (Print, Linking), 1533-4406 (Electronic)

Midgley, R. & Kerr, D. (1999). Seminar on colorectal cancer. *Lancet.* Vol. 353, No. 9150, pp. 391-399, ISSN: 0140-6736 (Print, Linking), 1474-547X (Electronic)

Midgley, R.S., Yanagisawa, Y. & Kerr, D. (2009). Evolution of nonsurgical therapy for colorectal cancer. *Nat Clin Pract Gastroenterol Hepatol.* Vol. 6, No. 2, pp. 108-120, ISSN: 1743-4378 (Print, Linking), 1743-4386 (Electronic)

Minamoto, T., inventor; National University Corporation Kanazawa University; assignee. Suppression of cancer and method for evaluating anticancer agent based on the effect of inhibiting GSK3β. International patent WO2006/073202. 2006 Jul 13. United States patent US 11/794,716. 2006 Jan 4. European patent EP1845094 2007 Oct 17. Japan patent 2006-550915 2007 Jun 21.

Miyashita, K., Kawakami, K., Mai, W., Shakoori, A., Fujisawa, H., Nakada, M., Hayashi, Y., Hamada, J. & Minamoto, T. (2009a). Potential therapeutic effect of glycogen synthase kinase 3β inhibition against human glioblastoma. *Clin Cancer Res.* Vol. 15, No. 3, pp. 887-897, ISSN: 1078-0432 (Print, Linking)

Miyashita, K., Nakada, M., Shakoori, A., Ishigaki, Y., Shimasaki, T., Motoo, Y., Kawakami, K. & Minamoto, T. (2009b). An emerging strategy for cancer treatment targeting aberrant glycogen synthase kinase 3β. *Anticancer Agents Med Chem.* Vol. 9, No. 10, pp. 1114-1122, ISSN: 1871-5206 (Print, Linking), 1875-5992 (Electronic)

Motoo, Y., Shimasaki, T., Ishigaki, Y., Nakajima, H., Kawakami, K. & Minamoto, T. (2011). Metabolic disorder, inflammation, and deregulated molecular pathways converging in pancreatic cancer development: implications for new therapeutic strategies. *Cancers.* Vol. 3, No. 1, pp. 446-460, ISSN: 2072-6694 (Electronic, Linking)

Mottet, D., Dumont, V., Deccache, Y., Demazy, C., Ninane, N., Raes, M. & Michiels, C. (2003). Regulation of hypoxia-inducible factor-1α protein level during hypoxic conditions by the phosphatidylinositol 3-kinase/Akt/glycogen synthase kinase 3β pathway in HepG2 cells. *J Biol Chem.* Vol. 278, No. 33, pp. 31277-31285, ISSN: 0021-9258 (Print, Linking), 1083-351X (Electronic)

Nakada, M., Minamoto, T., Pyko, I.V., Hayashi, Y. & Hamada, J.I. (2011). The pivotal role of GSK3β in glioma biology, In: *Brain Tumor / Book 2*, Miklos Garami, InTech, ISBN: 978-953-307-587-7, in press

Nowicki, M., Dmitrieva, N., Stein, A.M., Cutter, J.L., Godlewski, J., Saeki, Y., Nita, M., Berens, M.E., Sander, L.M., Newton, H.B., Chiocca, E.A. & Lawler, S. (2008). Lithium inhibits invasion of glioma cells; possible involvement of glycogen synthase kinase-3. *Neuro Oncol.* Vol. 10, No. 5, pp. 690-699, ISSN: 1522-8517 (Print, Linking), 1523-5866 (Electronic)

O'Brien, C.A., Kreso, A. & Jamieson, C.H.M. (2010). Cancer stem cells and self-renewal. *Clin Cancer Res.* Vol. 16, No. 12, pp. 3113-3120, ISSN: 1078-0432 (Print, Linking)

O'Brien, C.A., Pollet, A., Gallinger, S. & Dick, J.E. (2007). A human colon cancer cell capable of initiating tumour growth in immunodeficient mice. *Nature.* Vol. 445, No. 7123, pp. 106-115, ISSN: 0028-0836 (Print, Linking), 1476-4687 (Electronic)

Ougolkov, A.V., Fernandez-Zapico, M.E., Savoy, D.N., Urrutia, R.A. & Billadeau, D.D. (2005). Glycogen synthase kinase-3β participates in nuclear factor κB-mediated gene transcription and cell survival in pancreatic cancer cells. *Cancer Res.* Vol. 65, No. 6, pp. 2076-2081, ISSN: 0008-5472 (Print, Linking), 1538-7445 (Electronic)

Parsons, D.W., Wang, T.L., Samuels, Y., Bardelli, A., Cummins, J.M., DeLong, L., Silliman, N., Ptak, J., Szabo, S., Willson, J.K., Markowitz, S., Kinzler, K.W., Vogelstein, B., Lengauer, C. & Velculescu, V.E. (2005). Colorectal cancer: mutations in a signalling pathway. *Nature.* Vol. 436, No. 7052, pp. 792, ISSN: 0028-0836 (Print, Linking), 1476-4687 (Electronic)

Patel, S. & Woodgett, J. (2008). Glycogen synthase kinase-3 and cancer: good cop, bad cop? *Cancer Cell.* Vol. 14, No. 5, pp. 351-353, ISSN: 1535-6108 (Print, Linking), 1878-3686 (Electronic)

Phukan, S., Babu, V.S., Kannoji, A., Hariharan, R. & Balaji, V.N. (2010). GSK3β: role in therapeutic landscape and development of modulators. *Br J Pharmacol.* Vol. 160, No. 1, pp. 1-19, ISSN: 0007-1188 (Print, Linking), 1476-5381 (Electronic)

Polakis, P. (1999). The oncogenic activation of β-catenin. *Curr Opin Genet Dev.* Vol. 9, No. 1, pp. 15-21, ISSN: 0959-437X (Print, Linking), 1879-0380 (Electronic)

Polyak, K., Weiberg, R.A. (2009). Transitions between epithelial and mesenchymal states: acquisition of malignant and stem cell traits. *Nat Rev Cancer.* Vol. 9, No. 4, pp. 265-273, ISSN: 1474-175X (Print, Linking), 1474-1768 (Electronic)

Prenen, H., Tejpar, S. & Van Cutsem, E. (2010). New strategies for treatment of KRAS mutant metastatic colorectal cancer. *Clin Cancer Res.* Vol. 16, No. 11, pp. 2921-2926, ISSN: 1078-0432 (Print, Linking)

Qu, L., Huang, S., Baltzis, D., Rivas-Estilla, A.M., Pluquet, O., Hatzoglou, M., Koumenis, C., Taya, Y., Yoshimura, A. & Koromilas, A.E. (2004). Endoplasmic reticulum stress induces p53 cytoplasmic localization and prevents p53-dependent apoptosis by a pathway involving glycogen synthase kinase-3β. *Genes Dev*. Vol. 18, No. 3, pp. 261-277, ISSN: 0890-9369 (Print, Linking), 1549-5477 (Electronic)

Raftpoulou, M. & Hall, A. (2004). Cell migration: Rho GTPases lead the way. *Dev Biol.* Vol. 265, No. 1, pp. 23-32, ISSN: 0012-1606 (Print, Linking), 1095-564X (Electronic)

Ralston, S.H. & de Crombrugghe, B. (2006). Genetic regulation of bone mass and susceptibility to osteoporosis. *Genes Dev.* Vol. 20, No. 18, pp. 2492-2506, ISSN: 0890-9369 (Print, Linking), 1549-5477 (Electronic)

Rayasam, G.V., Tulasi, V.K., Sodhi, R., Davis, J.A. & Ray, A. (2009). Glycogen synthase kinase-3: more than a namesake. *Br J Pharmacol.* Vol. 156, No. 6, pp. 885-898, ISSN: 0007-1188 (Print, Linking), 1476-5381 (Electronic)

Ricci-Vitiani, L., Lombardi, D.G., Pilozzi, E., Biffoni, M., Todaro, M., Peschle, C. & De Maria, R. (2007). Identification and expansion of human colon-cancer-initiating cells. *Nature.* Vol. 445, No. 7123, pp. 106-115, ISSN: 0028-0836 (Print, Linking), 1476-4687 (Electronic)

Rössig, L., Badorff, C., Holzmann, Y., Zeiher, A.M. & Dimmeler, S. (2002). Glycogen synthase kinase-3 couples AKT-dependent signaling to the regulation of $p21^{Cip1}$ degradation. *J Biol Chem.* Vol. 277, No. 22, pp. 9684-9689, ISSN: 0021-9258 (Print, Linking), 1083-351X (Electronic)

Rottmann, S., Wang, Y., Nasoff, M., Deveraux, Q.L. & Quon, K.C. (2005). A TRAIL receptor-dependent synthetic lethal relationship between *Myc* activation and GSK3β/FBW7 loss of function. *Proc Natl Acad Sci USA*. Vol. 102, No. 42, pp. 15195-15200, ISSN: 0027-8424 (Print, Linking), 1091-6490 (Electronic)

Royds, J.A. & Iacopetta, B. (2006). p53 and disease: when the guardian angel fails. *Cell Death Diff.* Vol. 13, No. 6, pp. 1017-1026, ISSN: 1350-9047 (Print, Linking), 1476-5403 (Electronic)

Sahai, E. & Marshall, C.J. (2002). Rho-GTPases and cancer. *Nat Rev Cancer.* Vol. 2, No. 2, pp. 133-142, ISSN: 1474-175X (Print, Linking), 1474-1768 (Electronic)

Samudio, I., Fiegl, M. & Andreeff, M. (2009). Mitochondrial uncoupling and the Warburg effect: molecular basis for the reprogrammimg of cancer cell metabolism. *Cancer Res.* Vol. 69, No. 6, pp. 2163-2166, ISSN: 0008-5472 (Print, Linking), 1538-7445 (Electronic)

Sargent, D. J, Patiyil, S., Yothers, G., Haller, D.G., Gray, R., Benedetti, J., Buyse, M., Labianca, R., Seitz, J.F., O'Callaghan, C.J., Francini, G., Grothey, A., O'Connell, M., Catalano, P.J., Kerr, D., Green, E., Wieand, H.S., Goldberg, R.M., de Gramont, A. & ACCENT Group. (2007). End points for colon cancer adjuvant trials: observations and recommendations based on individual patient data from 20,898 patients enrolled onto 18 randomized trials from the ACCENT Group. *J Clin Oncol.* Vol. 25, No. 29, pp. 4569-4574, ISSN: 0732-183X (Print, Linking), 1527-7755 (Electronic)

Sartore-Bianchi, A., Martini, M., Molinari, F., Veronese, S., Nichelatti, M., Artale, S., Di Nicolantonio, F., Saletti, P., De Dosso, S., Mazzucchelli, L., Frattini, M., Siena, S. & Bardelli, A. (2009). PI3CA mutations in colorectal cancer are associated with clinical resistance to EGFR-targeted monoclonal antibodies. *Cancer Res.* Vol. 69, No. 5, pp. 1851-1857, ISSN: 0008-5472 (Print, Linking), 1538-7445 (Electronic)

Sato, N., Meijer, L., Skaltsounis, L., Greengard, P. & Brivanlou, A.H. (2004). Maintenance of pluripotency in human and mouse embryonic stem cells through activation of Wnt signaling by a pharmacological GSK-3-specific inhibitor. *Nat Med.* Vol. 10, No. 1, pp. 55-63, ISSN: 1078-8956 (Print, Linking), 1546-170X (Electronic)

Schlessinger, K. & Hall, A. (2004). GSK-3β sets Snail's pace. *Nat Cell Biol.* Vol. 6, No. 10, pp. 913-915, ISSN: 1465-7392 (Print, Linking), 1476-4679 (Electronic)

Schwabe, R.F. & Brenner, D.A. (2002). Role of glycogen synthase kinase-3 in TNF-α-induced NF-κB activation and apoptosis in hepatocytes. *Am J Physiol Gastrointest Liver Physiol.* Vol. 283, No. 1, pp. G204-211, ISSN: 0193-1857 (Print, Linking), 1522-1547 (Electronic)

Semenza, G.L. (2009). Regulation of oxygen homeostasis by hypoxia-inducible factor 1. *Physiology (Bethesda).* Vol. 24, pp. 97-106, ISSN: 1548-9213 (Print), 1548-9221 (Electronic, Linking)

Shakoori, A., Ougolkov, A., Yu, Z.W., Zhang, B., Modarressi, M.H., Billadeau, D.D., Mai, M., Takahashi, Y. & Minamoto, T. (2005). Deregulated GSK3β activity in colorectal cancer: its association with tumor cell survival and proliferation. *Biochem Biophys Res Commun.* Vol. 334, No. 4, pp. 1365-1373, ISSN: 0006-291X (Print, Linking), 1090-2104 (Electronic)

Shakoori, A., Mai, W., Miyashita, K., Yasumoto, K., Takahashi, Y., Ooi, A., Kawakami, K. & Minamoto, T. (2007). Inhibition of GSK3β attenuates proliferation of human colon cancer cells in rodents. *Cancer Sci.* Vol. 98, No. 9, pp. 1388-1393, ISSN: 1347-9032 (Print, Linking), 1349-7006 (Electronic)

Sharma, S.V., Fischbach, M.A., Haber, D.A. & Settleman, J. (2006). "Oncogenic shock": explaining oncogene addiction through differential signal attenuation. *Clin Cancer Res.* Vol. 12, No. 14 Suppl, pp. 4392s-4395s, ISSN: 1078-0432 (Print, Linking)

Sharma, S.V. & Settleman, J. (2007). Oncogene addiction: setting the stage for molecularly targeted cancer therapy. *Genes Dev.* Vol. 21, No. 24, pp. 3214-3231, ISSN: 0890-9369 (Print, Linking), 1549-5477 (Electronic)

Sjőblom, T., Jones, S., Wood, L.D., Parsons, D.W., Lin, J., Barber, T.D., Mandelker, D., Leary, R.J., Ptak, J., Silliman, N., Szabo, S., Buckhaults, P., Farrell, C., Meeh, P., Markowitz, S.D., Willis, J., Dawson, D., Willson, J.K., Gazdar, A.F., Hartigan, J., Wu, L., Liu, C., Parmigiani, G., Park, B.H., Bachman, K.E., Papadopoulos, N., Vogelstein, B., Kinzler, K.W. & Velculescu, V.E. (2006). The consensus coding sequences of human breast and colorectal cancers. *Science.* Vol. 314, No. 5797, pp. 268-274. ISSN: 0193-4511 (Print, Linking)

Small, J.V., Stradal, T., Vignal, E. & Rottner, K. (2002). The lamellipodium: where motility begins. *Trends Cell Biol.* Vol. 12, No. 3, pp. 112-120, ISSN: 0962-8924 (Print, Linking), 1879-3088 (Electronic)

Smallbone, K., Gatenby, R.A., Gillies, R.J., Maini, P.K. & Gavaghan, D.J. (2007). Metabolic changes during carcinogenesis: potential impact on invasiveness. *J Theor Biol.* Vol. 244, No. 4, pp. 703-713, ISSN: 0022-5193 (Print, Linking), 1095-8541 (Electronic)

Stacpoole, P.W., Nagaraja, N.V. & Hutson, A.D. (2003). Efficacy of dichloroacetate as a lactate-lowering drug. *J Clin Pharmacol.* Vol. 43, No. 7, pp. 683-691, ISSN: 0091-2700 (Print, Linking), 1552-4604 (Electronic)

Stacpoole, P.W., Kerr, D.S., Barnes, C., Bunch, S.T., Carney, P.R., Fennell, E.M., Felitsyn, N.M., Gilmore, R.L., Greer, M., Henderson, G.N., Hutson, A.D., Neiberger, R.E., O'Brien, R.G., Perkins, L.A., Quisling, R.G., Shroads, A.L., Shuster, J.J., Silverstein,

J.H., Theriaque, D.W. & Valenstein, E. (2006). Controlled clinical trial of dichloroacetate for treatment of congenital lactic acidosis in children. *Pediatrics*. Vol. 117, No. 5, pp. 1519-1531, ISSN: 0031-4005 (Print, Linking), 1098-4275 (Electronic)

Surjit, M. & Lal, S.K. (2007). Glycogen synthase kinase-3 phosphorylates and regulates the stability of p27^{kip1} protein. *Cell Cycle*. Vol. 6, No. 5, pp. 580-588, ISSN: 1538-4101 (Print), 1551-4005 (Electronic, Linking)

Takenaka, K., Kise, Y. & Miki, H. (2007). GSK3β positively regulates Hedgehog signaling through Sufu in mammalian cells. *Biochem Biophys Res Commun*. Vol. 353, No. 2, pp. 501-508, ISSN: 0006-291X (Print, Linking), 1090-2104 (Electronic)

Tan, J., Zhuang, L., Leong, H., Iyer, N.G., Liu, E.T. & Yu, Q. (2005). Pharmacologic modulation of glycogen synthase kinase-3β promotes p53-dependent apoptosis through a direct Bax-mediated mitochondrial pathway in colorectal cancer cells. *Cancer Res*. Vol. 65, No. 19, pp. 9012-9020, ISSN: 0008-5472 (Print, Linking), 1538-7445 (Electronic)

The Clinical Outcomes of Surgical Therapy Study Group. (2004). A comparison of laparoscopically assisted and open colectomy for colon cancer. *N Engl J Med*. Vol. 350, No. 20, pp. 2050-2059, ISSN: 0028-4793 (Print, Linking), 1533-4406 (Electronic)

Tol, J., Koopman, M., Cats, A., Rodenburg, C.J., Creemers, G.J., Schrama, J.G., Erdkamp, F.L., Vos, A.H., van Groeningen, C.J., Sinnige, H.A., Richel, D.J., Voest, E.E., Dijkstra, J.R., Vink-Börger, M.E., Antonini, N.F., Mol, L., van Krieken, J.H., Dalesio, O. & Punt, C.J. (2009). Chemotherapy, bevacizumab, and cetuximab in metastatic colorectal cancer. *N Engl J Med*. Vol. 360, No. 6, pp. 563-572, ISSN: 0028-4793 (Print, Linking), 1533-4406 (Electronic)

Trowbridge, J.J., Xenocostas, A., Moon, R.T. & Bhatia, M. (2006). Glycogen synthase kinase-3 is an in vivo regulator of hematopoietic stem cell repopulation. *Nat Med*. Vol. 12, No. 1, pp. 89-98, ISSN: 1078-8956 (Print, Linking), 1546-170X (Electronic)

Tsuchiya, K., Nakamura, T., Okamoto, R., Kanai, T. & Watanabe, M. (2007). Reciprocal targeting of Hath1 and β-catenin by Wnt glycogen synthase kinase 3β in human colon cancer. *Gastroenterology*. Vol. 132, No. 1, pp. 208-220, ISSN: 0016-5085 (Print, Linking), 1528-0012 (Electronic)

Umar, A. & Greenwald, P. (2009). Alarming colorectal cancer incidence trends: a case for early detection and prevention. *Cancer Epidemiol Biomarkers Prev*. Vol. 18, No. 6, pp. 1672-1673, ISSN: 1055-9965 (Print, Linking), 1538-7755 (Electronic)

Vaidya, R.J., Ray, R.M. & Johnson, L.R. (2006). Akt-mediated GSK-3β inhibition prevents migration of polyamine-depleted intestinal epithelial cells via Rac1. *Cell Mol Life Sci*. Vol. 63, No. 23, pp. 2871-2879, ISSN: 1420-682X (Print, Linking), 1420-9071 (Electronic)

Vander Heiden, M.G., Cantley, L.C. & Thompson, C.B. (2010). Understanding the Warburg effect: the metabolic requirements of cell proliferation. *Science*. Vol. 324, No. 5630, pp. 1029-1033, ISSN: 0193-4511 (Print, Linking)

Vousden, K.H. & Lane, D.P. (2007). p53 in health and disease. *Nat Rev Mol Cell Biol*. Vol. 8, No. 4, pp. 275-283, ISSN: 1471-0072 (Print, Linking), 1471-0080 (Electronic)

Walther, A., Johnstone, E., Swanton, C., Midgley, R., Tomlinson, I. & Kerr, D. (2009). Genetic prognostic and predictive markers in colorectal cancer. *Nat Rev Cancer*. Vol. 9, No. 7, pp. 489-499, ISSN: 1474-175X (Print, Linking), 1474-1768 (Electronic)

Wang, Z., Smith, K.S., Murphy, M., Piloto, O., Somervaille, T.C.P. & Cleary, M.L. (2008). Glycogen synthase kinase 3 in *MLL* leukaemia maintenance and targeted therapy.

Nature. Vol. 455, No. 7217, pp. 1205-1209, ISSN: 0028-0836 (Print, Linking), 1476-4687 (Electronic)

Weinstein, I.B. (2002). Cancer: addiction to oncogene—the Achilles' heal of cancer. *Science.* Vol. 297, No. 5578, pp. 63-64, ISSN: 0193-4511 (Print, Linking)

Weinstein, I.B. & Joe, A.K. (2006). Mechanisms of disease: oncogene addiction—a rationale for molecular targeting in cancer therapy. *Nat Clin Pract Oncol.* Vol. 3, No. 8, pp. 448-457, ISSN: 1743-4254 (Print, Linking); 1743-4262 (Electronic)

Willert, K. & Jones, K.A. (2006). Wnt signaling: is the party in the nucleus? *Gene Dev.* Vol. 20, No. 11, pp. 1394-1404, ISSN: 0890-9369 (Print, Linking), 1549-5477 (Electronic)

Wilson, W. 3rd. & Baldwin, A.S. (2008). Maintenance of constitutive IκB kinase activity by glycogen synthase kinase-3α/β in pancreatic cancer. *Cancer Res.* Vol. 68, No. 19, pp. 8156-8163, ISSN: 0008-5472 (Print, Linking), 1538-7445 (Electronic)

Wolpin, B.M., Meyerhardt, J.A., Mamon, H.J. & Mayer, R.J. (2007). Adjuvant treatment of colorectal cancer. *CA Cancer J Clin.* Vol. 57, No. 3, pp. 168-185, ISSN: 0007-9235 (Print, Linking), 1542-4863 (Electronic)

Wolpin, B.M. & Mayer, R.J. (2008). Systemic treatment of colorectal cancer. *Gastroenterology.* Vol. 134, No. 5, pp. 1296-1310, ISSN: 0016-5085 (Print, Linking), 1528-0012 (Electronic)

Wood, L.D., Parsons, D.W., Jones, S., Lin, J., Sjöblom, T., Leary, R.J., Shen, D., Boca, S.M., Barber, T., Ptak, J., Silliman, N., Szabo, S., Dezso, Z., Ustyanksky, V., Nikolskaya, T., Nikolsky, Y., Karchin, R., Wilson, P.A., Kaminker, J.S., Zhang, Z., Croshaw, R., Willis, J., Dawson, D., Shipitsin, M., Willson, J.K., Sukumar, S., Polyak, K., Park, B.H., Pethiyagoda, C.L., Pant, P.V., Ballinger, D.G., Sparks, A.B,, Hartigan, J., Smith, D.R., Suh, E., Papadopoulos, N., Buckhaults, P., Markowitz, S.D., Parmigiani, G., Kinzler, K.W., Velculescu, V.E. & Vogelstein, B. (2007). The genomic landscapes of human breast and colorectal cancers. *Science.* Vol. 318, No. 5853, pp. 1108-1113. ISSN: 0193-4511 (Print, Linking)

Wu, J.S. & Fazio, V.W. (2000). Colon cancer. *Dis Colon Rectum.* Vol. 43, No. 11, pp. 1473-1486, ISSN: 0012-3706 (Print, Linking), 1530-0358 (Electronic)

Xu, C., Kim, N.G. & Gumbiner, B.M. Regulation of protein stability by GSK3 mediated phosphorylation. (2009). *Cell Cycle.* Vol. 8, No. 24, pp. 4032-4039, ISSN: 1538-4101 (Print), 1551-4005 (Electronic, Linking)

Yeung, T.M. & Mortensen, N.J. (2009). Colorectal cancer stem cells. *Dis Colon Rectum.* Vol. 52, No. 10, pp. 1788-1796, ISSN: 0012-3706 (Print, Linking), 1530-0358 (Electronic)

Yilmaz, M. & Christofori, G. (2009). EMT, the cytoskeleton, and cancer cell invasion. *Cancer Metastasis Rev.* Vol. 28, No. 1-2, pp. 15-33, ISSN: 0167-7659 (Print, Linking), 1573-7233 (Electronic)

Zhou, B.P., Deng, J., Xia, W., Xu, J., Li, Y.M., Gunduz, M. & Hung, M.C. (2004). Dual regulation of Snail by GSK-3β-mediated phosphorylation in control of epithelial-mesenchymal transition. *Nat Cell Biol.* Vol. 6, No. 10, pp. 931-940, ISSN: 1465-7392 (Print, Linking), 1476-4679 (Electronic)

Zhou, B.P. & Hung, M.C. (2005). Wnt, hedgehog and β-Trcp in the regulation of metastasis. *Cell Cycle.* Vol. 4, No. 6, pp. 772-776, ISSN: 1538-4101 (Print), 1551-4005 (Electronic, Linking)

Zilfou, J.T. & Lowe, S.W. (2009). Tumor suppressive functions of p53. *Cold Spring Harb Perspect Biol.* Vol. 1, No. 5, pp. a001883, ISSN: 1943-0264 (Electronic)

7

Molecular Traits of the Budding Colorectal Cancer Cells

Boye Schnack Nielsen
Bioneer A/S, Kogle Allé, Hørsholm, Denmark

1. Introduction

The process of cancer cell metastasis is one of the latest steps in cancer progression that involves escape from the primary tumor through the vascular system to local lymph nodes and distant organs, recently reviewed by Chaffer and Weinberg (Chaffer & Weinberg, 2011). For a cancer cell to metastasize, it must escape the primary tumor by obtaining features that allows detachment from neoplastic epithelial structure, invasion through extracellular matrices, intravasation, survival in the blood circulation, extravasation, establishment or *homing* in a novel organ and local *de novo* proliferation. Colorectal cancers (CRC) comprise different subtypes and vary in the degree of differentiation as well as in the local invasion pattern in the tumor periphery. The invasion pattern is partly related to the metastatic ability of the tumor, and the invasion pattern can be fully discerned by microscopy analysis. Molecular characteristics related to the invasion pattern may help in the histopathological diagnosis to provide a prognostic perspective for the patient and potentially identify which patient would benefit from a certain therapy. For CRC, an invasion pattern related to the ability of cancer cells to form buds and focal single cell invasion into the neighboring stroma has obtained much attention. The invasive cancer cells are known as budding cancer cells and the budding phenomenon describes a morphological event, which is becoming better characterized at the molecular level. In this chapter, I will go through some of the molecular characteristics linked to the budding cancer cells and link the observations to the morphologic and molecular changes related to epithelial-to-mesenchymal transition (EMT) often assigned to locally disseminating cancer cells.

1.1 Identification of budding colorectal cancer cells

Two types of metastatic processes can be considered: active and passive. Passive metastasis occurs when cancer cells enter the vascular system, for example by being captured by disrupted vessels in the tumors, and subsequently being trapped in microvessels for example in the liver or lung, where the cancer cells initially proliferate within the vessel and later on disseminate into the parenchyma of the organ. Active metastasis is considered to involve a certain level of EMT in the primary tumor followed by invasion into the vascular system, extravasation by crossing the vascular wall and invasion into the new organ, and then reverting to an epithelial cancer cell capable of *de novo* proliferation and differentiation to form new tumors.

Budding cancer cells likely belong to the category of active metastasis process because their prevalence is directly linked to metastasis and is independent of the TNM classification (Nakamura et al, 2005; Okuyama et al, 2003; Prall et al, 2005; Ueno et al, 2002). Japanese histopathologists have many years tradition for evaluating growth and invasion patterns in CRC including addressing the clinical implications (Fujimori et al, 2009). A clinical significance of budding cancer cells was first described in colon cancers in 1993 by Hase *et al* (Hase et al, 1993). Hase et al (Hase et al, 1993) defined the budding cancer cells as "small clusters of undifferentiated cancer cells located ahead of the invasive front of the lesion".

Hase et al (Hase et al, 1993) evaluated the degree of budding cancer cells in normal hematoxylin and eosin (H&E) stained sections, an approach being widely used by others (Nakamura et al, 2005; Okuyama et al, 2003; Ueno et al, 2002). Because the budding cancer cells are often present in a dense desmoplastic or highly inflamed stroma and because budding cancer cells can acquire morphologically odd shapes (see below), a precise identification of budding cancer cells in H&E stained sections may not always be straight forward (Turner et al, 2007) at least for non-pathologists. Later studies have employed cytokeratin immunohistochemistry whereby budding cancer cells are much easier identified (Prall, 2007; Prall et al, 2005; Turner et al, 2007; Zlobec et al, 2010). The use of cytokeratin immunohistochemistry to detect cancer cell budding versus evaluation in H&E stained sections may lower the proportion of misclassified cases.

The prevalence of tumor cell budding varies strongly from tumor to tumor and Hase et al (Hase et al, 1993) stratified tumors into BD-1 (none or mild) and BD-2 (moderate or severe) based on the H&E stained sections. Prall et al (Prall et al, 2005) stratified tumors into low and high budding based on sections immunohistochemically stained for cytokeratins and counted all cytokeratin-positive cancer cell clusters with less than 5 nuclei. Hase et al (Hase et al, 1993) classified approximately 25% of all CRC analyzed as BD-2 and Prall et al (Prall et al, 2005) classified approximately 30% as high level budding.

Cancer cell budding as it is observed in colon and rectal adenocarcinomas should not be confused with the diffuse growth pattern, which is common in other gastrointestinal cancers and in contrast to tumors with a solid (or expanding) growth pattern. CRC showing a diffuse growth pattern are low differentiated neoplasms and do not show signs of tubular or glandular formations. Therefore quantitative estimation of cancer cell budding even done using cytokeratin immunohistochemistry should be done with some caution.

The degree of cancer cell budding as stratified into groups with none, mild, moderate and strong budding, or less or more than 5 cells in a cluster, indicate that cancer cell budding is not an "all or none" phenomenon, but reflects gradual differences. Nonetheless, both studies (Hase et al, 1993; Prall et al, 2005) showed that tumors with the highest level of budding significantly more often linked to lymph node metastasis than tumors with a low level of budding. The highest level of budding was, not surprisingly, seen in patients with the poorest survival rate, however, cancer biology reflects individual heterogeneity and in fact, some tumors with low budding also show metastatic events (Hase et al, 1993; Prall et al, 2005; Tanaka et al, 2003; Ueno et al, 2002).

1.2 Histo-morphological characterization

One of the morphological features of the budding cancer cells in CRC is their characteristics of dedifferentiation and acquisition of odd shapes as described at the ultra-structural level by Gabbert et al in 1985 (Gabbert et al, 1985). These authors studied DMH-induced colon cancers in rats and found that poorly differentiated tumors, which showed frequency of lymph vessel invasion, also had isolated cancer cells along the invasive front. Gabbert et al (Gabbert et al, 1985) states about the cancer cells located ahead of the invasive front that "Their nuclei are very large and at their cell surface show no signs of differentiation such as formation of microvilli or formation of a basement membrane are discernible." Thus the cellular characteristics of isolated cancer cells suggested general dedifferentiation compared to the cancer cells placed within the adjacent glandular structures. In addition, the isolated cancer cells at the invasive front showed overt cell shape: "The cell shape of more or less isolated tumor cells at the foremost invasion front is extremely variable ... ranging from a round or oval to a sand glass-like." These observations are consistent with the budding cancer cells in human CRC identified both in H&E stained sections as well as cytokeratin immuno-peroxidase stained sections, see for example the studies by Prall and Turner et al (Prall, 2007; Prall et al, 2005; Turner et al, 2007). According to the histological characteristitcs of the budding CRC cells at the invasive front, the stepwise process of budding-directed growth can be divided into the following steps 1) the budding cancer cells detach from the glandular structures, 2) morphologically change cell shape and 3) invade a short distance, say up to 400μm, through the adjacent tumor-associated stroma and 4) settle and 5) found novel glandular structures. Budding CRC cells are rarely seen in the central areas of the tumors, suggesting that the local environment, the stroma constituting the tumor periphery, is dictating the budding process together with the cancer cells. Interestingly, the morphological characteristics of dedifferentiation and dynamic change in cell shape are consistent with characteristics of cells undergoing EMT as described for cultured cells (Kirkland, 2009; Thuault et al, 2006).

Together with the findings that the prevalence of budding cancer cells is linked to more metastatic cancers, strongly suggests that the budding cancer cells also possess cancer stem cell activity. Thus the budding CRC cells possess all canonical requirements for actively metastasizing cancer cells, including the abilities to undergo EMT and the ability of self-renewal. The stepwise process of the budding cancer cell requires significant molecular changes of the cell: for detachment from neoplastic epithelium, dedifferentiation, EMT, cell migration and invasion, and progenitor activity for *de novo* proliferation. Considering that budding CRC cells undergo such a dramatic transient program, probably within a relatively short time frame, the budding CRC cells as an entire cell population constitute a heterogeneous group of cancer cells that possess a strongly modulating molecular profile. In the following I will go through some of the molecular characteristics reported for the budding CRC cells, first cell surface associated proteins and thereafter intracellular molecules. The molecular characteristics involve proteins that participate in regulating differentiation, transcription, translation, cell migration, cell-cell interactions, and adhesion.

2. Laminin-γ2 (Ln-γ2)

The mRNA encoding the Ln-γ2 chain is the first described molecular marker of the budding CRC cells (Pyke et al, 1994). Pyke et al (Pyke et al, 1994) found Ln-γ2 mRNA positive cancer cells in all of 16 colon cancers varying in the presence of positive cells. In a later report, Pyke et al (Pyke et al, 1995) confirmed that the mRNA expression observed in budding colon cancer cells is followed by protein expression in the same cells using a Ln-γ2 specific antibody. Sordat et al (Sordat et al, 1998) reported similar observations in colon cancers using other Ln-γ2 antibody preparations. Laminins are a group of extracellular glycoproteins being important constituents of basement membrane. They are heterotrimers composed of α, β and γ chains of which there are 5, 4 and 3 isoforms, respectively. The currently used systematic nomenclature defines the composition of a laminin heterotrimers (Aumailley et al, 2005), for example laminin-111 is composed of α1, β1 and γ1 chains and has replaced the earlier used name laminin-1, the most predominant laminin in basement membrane.

The Ln-γ2 chain is only present in the laminin-332 variant, previously known as laminin-5 (Guess & Quaranta, 2009). Laminin-332 links the basement membrane via integrins to hemidesmosomes and thereby stabilizes the polarized positioning of epithelial cell to the basement membrane. Laminins are generally secreted from cells as fully composed heterotrimers, Ln-γ2 being the only exception (Guess & Quaranta, 2009). Ln-γ2 can be secreted as monomer or in complex with the Ln-β3 chain (Guess & Quaranta, 2009) and may have an important significance during budding in CRC (Guess et al, 2009). Pyke et al (Pyke et al, 1995) found Ln-γ2 within the cytoplasm of the budding colon cancer cells and only in rare cases observed basement membrane associated Ln-γ2 immunoreactivity. Sordat et al (Sordat et al, 1998) in contrast found prominent Ln-γ2 immunoreactivity both in the cytoplasm of budding CRC cells and in basement membrane along differentiated tumor cell islands. Today, several monoclonal antibodies against Ln-γ2 are commercially available, some recognize both cytoplasmic and basement membrane associated Ln-γ2, and others are specific for the cytoplasmic precursor form (Hansen et al, 2008; Lindberg et al, 2006). Using Ln-γ2 as marker for budding CRC cells, the antibody employed should therefore be chosen with some consideration.

An interesting finding reported by Sordat et al (Sordat et al, 1998), is that budding cancer cells in addition to express Ln-γ2 also express the Ln-β3 chain, but only at a low level express the Ln-α3 chain. These observations suggest that the secreted Ln-γ2 monomer and Ln-β3-γ2 heterodimer may not function by direct integration into the basement membrane. Other functions have in contrast been found for the secreted Ln-γ2 and Ln-β3 chains. Cell surface directed proteolyic activity performed by matrix metalloproteinase (MMP)-2 (Giannelli et al, 1997) and membrane type-1 (MT1)-MMP (Koshikawa et al, 2000) generates fragments of the Ln-γ2 chain constituting epithelial growth factor (EGF)-like domains that stimulates cell motility. In addition, a cleavage product of Ln-β3 chain generated by MT1-MMP promotes cell migration (Udayakumar et al, 2003). The observations taken together suggest that Ln-γ2 and Ln-β3 chains are contributing to the migratory processes of the budding CRC cells.

In clinical studies, the level of tumor budding in CRC correlated with the level of Ln-γ2 positive budding cells (Shinto et al, 2005). Shinto et al (Shinto et al, 2005) also reported that high-grade Ln-γ2 expression was an independent prognostic indicator, and Aoki et al (Aoki et al, 2002) reported a significant association with synchronous liver metastases. Today, Ln-γ2 expression is considered a strong and potentially clinically applicable prognostic marker that reflects the level of cancer cell budding not only in CRC but also in other cancer types including bladder, esophageal and oral cancer (Guess & Quaranta, 2009).

3. Urokinase Plasminogen Activator Receptor (uPAR)

uPAR (CD87) is a 3-domain highly glycosylated, glycolipid anchored protein. uPAR is a specific high affinity binding receptor for (pro-)uPA, but also binds a number of other proteins in the extracellular matrix, in particular vitronectin (Eden et al, 2011; Gardsvoll & Ploug, 2007). The glycosyl-phosphatidylinositol (GPI) moiety of uPAR attaches the protein to the outer lipid layer of the cell membrane and allows uPAR to move laterally on cell surfaces and hence rapidly concentrate at focal sites where it mediates its uPA-directed activity and its interaction with vitronectin to the extracellular matrix. Active plasmin is generated from circulating plasminogen on the cell surfaces by a cascade mechanism involving plasmin-mediated conversion of pro-uPA to active uPA. uPA directed plasminogen activation is strongly enhanced after binding of uPA to uPAR on the cell surface (Ploug, 2003; Romer et al, 2004).

The active plasmin enzymatically cleaves or degrades fibrin and fibronectin deposited in the extracellular matrix (ECM), laminins, including the Ln-β3 chain (Goldfinger et al, 1998), L1CAM described below (Mechtersheimer et al, 2001), and activates other matrix degrading protease including MMPs. Through activation of pro-MMPs, MMP-3 (stromelysin-1), MMP-9 (gelatinase-B), MMP-13 (collagenase-3) and MMP-2 (Hald et al, 2011; Juncker-Jensen & Lund, 2011; Monea et al, 2002; Suzuki et al, 2007), plasmin may also mediate degradation of other ECM components including fibrillar collagens. In addition, plasmin activates growth factors like TGF-β (Odekon et al, 1994). Active TGF-β can transform fibroblasts into myofibroblasts (Ronnov-Jessen & Petersen, 1993) and initiate the EMT process in mammary epithelial cells (Fuxe et al, 2010; Thuault et al, 2006). Thus acceleration of the plasminogen activation cascade pathway may elevate the pericellular proteolytic activity and cause dramatic changes in cellular phenotypes.

uPAR was described in budding CRC cells first time in 1994 identified both at the mRNA and protein level (Pyke et al, 1995). Direct comparison with Ln-γ2 expression indicated a strong overlap with Ln-γ2 mRNA (Pyke et al, 1995). Later studies have shown co-expression of uPAR and Ln-γ2 in double immunofluorescence analyses in budding CRC cells (Illemann et al, 2009). uPAR is highly expressed at the invasive front of most CRC not only in budding cancer cells, but also in the complex stromal environment constituting inflammatory cells and myofibroblasts. Activated macrophages located at the invasive front of CRC express high levels of uPAR on the cell surface, hampering an easy discrimination between uPAR-positive budding cancer cells and macrophages. Therefore, to unambiguously identify uPAR-positive budding CRC cells, combining antibodies against uPAR and the epithelial marker cytokeratin (or Ln-γ2) in a double immunofluorescence analysis, would be necessary (Illemann et al, 2009; Romer et al, 2004). uPA mRNA is also expressed in the budding CRC cells (Illemann et al, 2009) indicating that uPAR may function directly through mediation of uPA-directed activities.

In normal colon tissue, uPAR is expressed in a group of differentiated epithelial cells located at the luminal edge of the villi. It has been suggested that uPAR on these cells serve to promote detachment of terminally differentiated colonocytes to be shedded into the colon lumen (Pyke et al, 1994). One may speculate that detachment of budding CRC cells from the main neoplastic glandular structures may mimic the shedding of terminally differentiated cells. In the case of cancer invasion the cancer cells are shed into the tumor stroma. However, this hypothesis does not corroborate with the fact that budding CRC cells show characteristics of dedifferentiation. Nevertheless, this is an interesting interpretation and the invasion of budding CRC cells remain an abnormal process.

Tissue extracts from colon cancers contain highly elevated levels of uPAR compared to the normal tissue, and the high uPAR levels are associated with adverse outcome. uPAR levels were found to constitute an independent prognostic parameter, importantly being independent of progression stage (Ganesh et al, 1994). A soluble form of uPAR, generated after enzymatic cleavage by uPA or plasmin (Hoyer-Hansen et al, 1997), can be measured in blood, and studies of plasma samples from colon cancer patients substantiate the prognostic significance of uPAR (Stephens et al, 1999; Thurison et al, 2010). As noted above, several different cell types in colon cancers express uPAR, and therefore the prognostic value of uPAR cannot be ascribed solely to the uPAR-positive budding CRC cells. However, in adenocarcinomas, macrophages are by far the predominant uPAR expressing cell type, and therefore most likely account for the elevated levels of uPAR in tumor tissue extracts and in the blood from the cancer patients (Illemann et al, 2009; Romer et al, 2004). uPAR expressing budding cancer cells may nevertheless also contribute to the malignant stage of CRC. uPAR positive cancer cells likely represent a particular malignant cell population since gastric cancer patients with poor prognosis associated with micro-metastatic disease more frequently had uPAR positive cancer cells identified in the bone marrow (Heiss et al, 2002), and uPAR is indeed expressed on invasive cancer cells in gastric cancer (Alpizar-Alpizar et al, 2010).

4. L1 Cell Adhesion Molecule (L1CAM)

L1CAM (L1, CD171) is one of four single-pass trans-membrane proteins forming the group of L1CAM. L1 was first described in 1984 as a neural cell adhesion molecule distinct from the closely related N-CAM group of proteins (Faissner et al, 1984). The other three members of the L1CAM family are NrCAM, CHL1 and neurofascin. All four genes are thoroughly characterized and highly expressed in the nervous system (Chen & Zhou, 2010). The L1CAMs contain 6 immunoglobulin-like motifs and 4 or 5 fibronectin type III repeats. The Cytoplasmic domain allows binding to cytoskeletal ankyrin and ERM proteins (ezrin-radixin-moesin) that associates with actin filaments (Bretscher et al, 2002). L1 is involved in cell-cell adhesion by homophilic interactions, cell-ECM interactions and cell surface interactions by binding integrins and can directly mediate cytoskeletal changes and signal transduction through its cytoplasmic domain (Chen & Zhou, 2010; Kadmon & Altevogt, 1997; Schmid & Maness, 2008). L1 is highly expressed in normal and diseased brain, and plays a critical role for development and organization of neuronal cell groups (Demyanenko et al, 2001; Sakurai et al, 2001). L1 has functions overlapping with NrCAM identified in double-deficient mice that show postnatal lethality in contrast to the corresponding single deficient mice (Sakurai et al, 2001). L1 has been reported to mediate cell adhesion and transendothelial migration also of dendritic cells (Maddaluno et al, 2009).

Expression of L1 in budding CRC cells has been shown both at the protein (Gavert et al, 2005; Kajiwara et al, 2011) and the mRNA level (Kajiwara et al, 2011). Gavert et al (Gavert et al, 2005) found L1 positive budding cancer cells in 68% of 19 colon cancer cases studied. Kajiwara et al (Kajiwara et al, 2011) studied 275 cases of CRC and also found L1 expression at the invasive front. Furthermore the authors showed that the L1 expression increased according to the grade of tumor budding and that L1 expression was correlated with nodal involvement both at the protein and mRNA level. In normal colon mucosa, L1 is expressed on sporadic intramucosal nerve axons and L1 positive enteric nerve axons were found in the deeper layers of the bowel wall (Gavert et al, 2005). In fact, the authors also noted that L1-positive colon cancer cells invaded along L1 positive nerve axons, and suggested that L1-mediated adhesive interactions between the two cell populations may facilitate the invasion of cancer cells. In this connection, it is curious that also uPAR can be found in enteric nerve bundles (Laerum et al, 2008). It is also interesting to note that L1 has been detected in human and murine myeloid and lymphoid cells (Ebeling et al, 1996; Kowitz et al, 1992) and that no L1 immunoreactivity has been reported in tumor stroma of the CRC. Whether the level of L1 in these cells is below the detection limit, is lost by proteolytic shedding, transcriptional or translational downregulation (Hubbe et al, 1993) remains to be clarified.

Proteolytic shedding of the L1 ectodomain has been reported to be performed by the disintegrin and metalloproteinases (ADAM) ADAM10 (Gutwein et al, 2003; Maretzky et al, 2005; Mechtersheimer et al, 2001), ADAM17 (Maretzky et al, 2005), and plasmin (Mechtersheimer et al, 2001). Shedding of the L1 ectodomain will prevent cell-cell interactions and binding interactions with other cell surface proteins and matrix components affecting the biochemical functions of the protein. Cleavage of L1 by ADAM10 releases an approximately 200kDa L1 fragment that can promote cell migration (Gutwein et al, 2003; Maretzky et al, 2005; Mechtersheimer et al, 2001). Similar activity was reported for the plasmin released L1 fragment (Mechtersheimer et al, 2001). In this connection it is important to note that ADAM10 immunoreactivity has been reported to be co-expressed in budding CRC cells (Gavert et al, 2005), and that cleavage can occur to an extent that a soluble L1 fragment can be measured in serum from cancer patients (Fogel et al, 2003). L1 expression in budding CRC cells may therefore be involved in at least 3 different processes during CRC cell budding: detachment from the differentiated neoplastic glandular structures, cell-cell interactions with L1-positive nerve axons or dendritic cells as well as in the contribution to CRC cell migration upon extracellular enzymatic processing.

5. Matrix Metalloproteinase 7 (MMP-7)

A number of other genes have been found to be focally expressed in the budding colon cancer cells. I have already mentioned some of the MMPs in connection with Ln-γ2 processing and plasmin-activated MMPs. MMP-7 (matrilysin-1) belongs to the group of matrix metalloproteinases (MMPs) (Das et al, 2003; Folgueras et al, 2004), which are zinc dependent endopeptidases known for their ability to cleave several ECM proteins. The activity of MMPs is regulated at the level of pro-MMP conversion and blocking by specific tissue inhibitors of metalloproteinases (TIMP) of which 4 are known (Nagase et al, 2006). MMP-7 can digest several ECM proteins including elastin, collagen IV and vitronectin (Ii et al, 2006). In addition, MMP7 has been shown to play important roles in the regulation of a variety of biochemical processes, such as the activation of MMP-2 and MMP-9 and shedding of Fas-ligand, pro-tumor necrosis factor-α, and E-cadherin (Curino et al, 2004; Ii et al, 2006; Nagase et al, 2006). MMP-7 itself is activated by other endoproteinases including plasmin and trypsin. MMP-7 was recently shown to bind and cleave the Ln-β3 chain. The cleaved Ln-β3 fragments was found to mediate cell migration (Remy et al, 2006). MMP-7 immunoreactivity has been reported in budding CRC cancer cells (Kurokawa et al, 2005; Masaki et al, 2001) and was found to co-localize with laminin-5 and Ln-β3 chain in human xenografted colon tumors (Remy et al, 2006). In the relatively small prognostic study by Masaki et al (Masaki et al, 2001), including 38 patients with early CRC, scoring the MMP-7 immunoreactive budding cancer cells was linked to distant metastasis and adverse outcome. However, MMP-7 immunoreactivity was seen in less than half of the cases with moderate to severe budding as determined on H&E stained sections, indicating that MMP-7 is not consistently expressed in budding CRC. In a study of 494 CRC cases, MMP-7 mRNA was found to be an independent risk factor predicting nodal metastasis (Kurokawa et al, 2005). In the context of budding CRC cells, the ability of MMP-7 to shed E-cadherin and cleave the Ln-β3 chain into a motility stimulating fragment suggest that MMP-7 takes part in the early steps involving detachment from the glandular structures and mobilizing cancer cell migration.

6. Membrane Type-1 Matrix Metalloproteinase (MT1-MMP)

MT1-MMP (MMP-14) immunoreactivity has also been demonstrated in budding CRC cells (Hlubek et al, 2004). MT1-MMP belongs to the group of membrane-bound MMPs and is a trans-membrane protein capable of cleaving fibrillar collagen. This MMP is essential for normal development (Holmbeck et al, 1999). MT1-MMP binds extracellular MMP-2 and TIMP-2 into a ternary complex that is important for the regulation of enzymatic activity on the cell surface (Sato & Takino, 2010; Strongin, 2010). The active enzyme can also cleave a number of other membrane-associated proteins including pro-tumor necrosis factor-α and CD44 (Folgueras et al, 2004). Expression of MT1-MMP mRNA is prominent in colon cancer associated stroma (Okada et al, 1995). As also noted above for evaluation of uPAR expression, strong stromal MT1-MMP expression in the invasive front area will prevent unambiguous identification of the protein in budding cancer cells. Expression of MT1-MMP on the surface of budding CRC cells would allow significant surface associated proteolysis either directly or through activation of MMP-2, which together with TIMP-2 would be provided by adjacent stromal cells (Holten-Andersen et al, 2005; Okada et al, 1995; Poulsom et al, 1992). As already mentioned, MT1-MMP can cleave Ln-γ2 alone or in cooperation with MMP-2, which results in a Ln-γ2 fragment with capacity to stimulate migration (Koshikawa et al, 2005; Koshikawa et al, 2004). More immunohistochemical studies are needed to better clarify the expression patterns of MT1-MMP in budding CRC cells.

The activities of the above mentioned proteins Ln-γ2, uPAR, L1, MMP-7 and MT1-MMP are all taking place on the cell surface and pericellular matrix. The following molecules will be related to intracellular acitivities.

7. β-catenin (Wnt pathway)

β-catenin is an important intracellular protein to consider in the characterization of budding CRC cells. Nuclear β-catenin activates transcription of a number of genes including those encoding Ln-γ2, uPAR and MMP-7 (Brabletz et al, 2004; Crawford et al, 1999; Hlubek et al, 2001; Mann et al, 1999). β-catenin is a protein that binds the cytoplasmic domain of E-cadherin and by concomitantly binding actin filaments contributes to maintain the cytoskeleton and the epithelial integrity. The intracellular localization of β-catenin is linked to the status of Wnt activity directed through the trans-membrane receptor Frizzled. Cellular activation by Wnt cause trans-localization of β-catenin to the nuclei, which through binding to transcription factors, affects transcription. β-catenin is expressed both in the differentiated glandular structures and in the budding CRC cells, but the localization changes from cytoplasmic to nuclear. In the case of budding CRC cells, β-catenin is seen in the nuclei (Brabletz et al, 2001; Brabletz et al, 2004; Gavert et al, 2005; Gavert et al, 2011; Hlubek et al, 2001; Jass et al, 2003). Translocation of β-catenin to the nuclei has been used as a reference marker for CRC cell budding to show co-expression of Ln-γ2 (Hlubek et al, 2001), L1 (Gavert et al, 2011), and disruption of E-cadherin (Brabletz et al, 2001). The EMT process and stem cell characteristics has been associated with the activity of β-catenin in cooperation with TGF-β (Brabletz et al, 2005; Fuxe et al, 2010). For a further discussion on signal transduction in budding CRC cells I suggest to consult the review by Prall (Prall, 2007).

8. Hepatocyte growth factor activator inhibitor type 2-Related Small Peptide (H2RSP)

An interesting novel protein identified to be specifically up-regulated in connection with CRC cell budding is hepatocyte growth factor activator inhibitor type 2-related small peptide (H2RSP) (Uchiyama et al, 2007). The H2RSP gene was first described in 2001 by Itoh et al (Itoh et al, 2001), who observed H2RSP expression in tissues obtained from the gastrointestinal tract. H2RSP protein, which is identical to immortalization-upregulated protein (IMUP-1), is a small protein constituting 106 amino acids. Its interaction partner(s) and function(s) remains to be established. An interaction with single stranded G-rich DNA probably via a lysine-rich domain of the protein was discussed to be involved in nuclear translocalization (Uchiyama et al, 2007). Uchiyama et al (Uchiyama et al, 2007) found by immunohistochemistry that H2RSP was located in the cytoplasm of normal un-differentiated epithelial cells in the colon, but found a change in localization to the nuclei in the differentiated epithelial cells. The authors suggested that H2RSP is involved in the transition process from the proliferation phase to terminal differentiation of intestinal epithelium. Looking at colon tumors, they found H2RSP immunoreactivity to be fully lost in the central differentiated tumor areas, but focally upregulated in the invasive front, including in budding CRC cells. In these cells, the H2RSP staining was located in the cytoplasm. The expression of H2RSP coincided with nuclear localization of β-catenin, focal co-expression of p16 and focal loss of proliferation marker Ki67. Thus, H2RSP, as confined to the epithelial cell population, is an interesting marker of budding CRC indicating a stage of dedifferentiation and growth arrest. A potential function in the related hepatocyte growth factor/scatter factor signaling pathway through Met receptor, which is taking place at the cell surface, seems unlikely so far.

9. microRNA-21 (miR-21)

MicroRNAs (miRNA) constitute a group of short, 18-23 base-pair long, non-coding RNAs. MiRNAs are processed from precursor RNA transcripts into mature active forms by a mechanism only partially understood. A generally accepted sequence of steps for the biochemical processing of precursor miRNA to the mature forms is known as the "linear" canonical pathway (Winter et al, 2009). MiRNAs have been found to play particular important roles in cell differentiation by negatively regulating translation (Calin & Croce, 2009; Iorio & Croce, 2009; Lim et al, 2005; Liu & Olson, 2010). miRNAs bind to specific 3'UTR sequences of mRNAs and thereby prevent efficient translation or mediate degradation of target mRNAs. For identification of miRNAs in tissue sections, *in situ* hybridization is an indispensable technique, which different from mRNA *in situ* hybridization cannot be replaced by immunohistochemistry. Specific detection of miRNA *in situ* therefore sets high requirements to the detection probes. Here LNA:DNA chimeric oligo probes have shown to fulfill at least some of the requirement for sufficient specificity and sensitivity (Jorgensen et al, 2010; Kloosterman et al, 2006). In an *in situ* hybridization study of miR-21 expression in stage II CRC, expression of miR-21 was seen in some budding CRC cell located at the invasive front of the tumors (Nielsen et al, 2011). A clear identification and quantitative estimation of the miR-21 positive budding cancer cells was however confounded by high miR-21 signal also in the tumor stroma. Therefore further studies are needed to better address the association of miR-21 to budding CRC cells, including double fluorescence labeling as also discussed above for uPAR. In this case, *in situ* hybridization and immunohistochemistry should be combined as exemplified by Sempere et al (Sempere et al, 2010), who applied this technology in routinely processed clinical paraffin samples.

miR-21 is highly upregulated in CRC compared to normal colon tissue (Nielsen et al, 2011; Schetter et al, 2008) and high expression is linked to adverse outcome in stage II CRC (Nielsen et al, 2011; Schetter et al, 2008). The mechanisms of action of miR-21 in budding cancer cells and in cancer progression in general are unclear. In mice lacking miR-21 (Ma et al, 2011) the number of chemically induced skin tumors was significantly lower than in wild type mice. In keratinocytes from the miR-21 deficient mice, increased expression of SPRY1, PTEN and PDCD4 was found, which is consistent with findings of miR-21 target genes in different human cell lines: *Spry1* in cardiac fibroblasts (Thum et al, 2008), the tumor suppressor *Pten* in hepatocytes and cardiac fibroblasts (Meng et al, 2007; Roy et al, 2009), and the tumor suppressor *Pdcd4* in a variety of cell lines (Asangani et al, 2008; Talotta et al, 2009). In budding CRC cells, miR-21 may suppress the expression level of PTEN and PDCD4 and thereby prevent cell death. miR-21 has also been attributed a central role in TGF-β induced EMT (Zavadil et al, 2007). Whether these regulatory events occur at the invasive front and in budding cancer cells remain to be established.

10. p16, Ki67 and cdx2

In connection with the studies mentioned above a couple of other proteins have been reported to focally change expression pattern in the budding CRC cells. These include p16 (Jass et al, 2003; Uchiyama et al, 2007) and cdx2 (Brabletz et al, 2004). The tumor suppressor p16 plays an important role in regulation of the cell cycle through interaction with p53 and as an inhibitor of cyclin dependent kinase 4 (CDK4). Both Uchiyama et al (Uchiyama et al, 2007) and Jass et al (Jass et al, 2003) noted that p16 was strongly expressed as a cytoplasmic immunoreactivity in the budding CRC cells. The increased expression may block translocation of CDK4 to the nuclei and thereby increase cyclin D1 levels and reduce proliferation (Jass et al, 2003). In fact, the proliferation marker Ki67 is lost in budding CRC cells (Brabletz et al, 2001; Uchiyama et al, 2007). The homeobox *Cdx2* encodes an intestine-specific transcription factor and is considered a tumor suppressor. Cdx2 immunoreactivity was absent in budding CRC cells in contrast to nuclei-related staining in the more differentiated tumor areas (Brabletz et al, 2004). It is intriguing that p16 and Cdx2, as so-called tumor suppressors, present themselves differently with respect to their presence in these highly malignant cells.

Although positive markers of the budding CRC cells provide clues to a mechanistic interpretation, loss of expression or intracellular translocation may provide significant help to characterize the budding process as well. As a final comment, I would like to suggest including the following 3 proteins as reference markers for the dedifferentiated budding CRC cells: Ln-γ2 giving a positive reaction in the cytoplasm, β-catenin giving a positive reaction in the nuclei, and Ki67 being negative (in constrast to the neighboring cancer cells). These markers will complement each other sufficiently as a reference profile and well-characterized antibodies are commercially available and applicable in paraffin embedded specimens.

11. Conclusion

A successful budding CRC cell encounters dramatic challenges during the short local expedition: dedifferentiation and detachment from the established differentiated glandular structure, migration through a foreign stromal tissue rich in inflammatory cells and desmoplastic cells, settlement in the new stromal environment and re-initiation of its own proliferation program. In this chapter I have reviewed current literature in order to compile the molecular traits linked to these cells and put the proteins' function into the budding processes. I propose that budding-initiating factors, such as TGF-β and Wnts, derived from in the stromal environment in the tumor periphery, and that the factors are received by cancer cells with progenitor capacity and which are able to address an activation program involving β-catenin mediated dedifferentiation and migration. From the compiled data, the following sequence of steps could be anticipated: increased levels of ECM degrading proteases, mediated by uPAR/uPA and MT1-MMP/MMP2, and MMP7 taking care of E-cadherin processing. The proliferation program is halted. This could be followed by a discrete EMT program, which transiently changes the morphology of the cells and allows detachment and budding. Upregulation and secretion of Ln-β3 and Ln-γ2 and subsequent extracellular processing will result in strongly motility-inducing fragments that allow migration through the stromal tissue. At the same time L1 is introduced changing the preferred cellular interaction partners to neuronal axons and dendritic cells as well as introducing yet other migration stimulating factors: the ADAM10 and plasmin processed L1 ectodoamins. Budding cancer cells invade as distant as possible into the stroma. One mechanism that could make the invasive cells stop and settle in the stromal environment could be a change in balance between active proteases and protease inhibitors, which may be shifted in favor of the inhibitors. Both PAI-1 and TIMPs are highly expressed in stromal cells at the invasive front (Holten-Andersen et al, 2005; Illemann et al, 2004; Poulsom et al, 1992). Increased protease inhibitor levels would prevent the formation of migration stimulating laminin fragments and also the surface associated proteases needed for invasion through the ECM. After settlement the excess laminins will be deposited and may contribute to form a loose basement membrane for the cancer cell to stick to and polarize, L1 will again be replaced by E-cadherin and proliferation and differentiation programs are reinitiated.

12. References

Alpizar-Alpizar, W., Nielsen, B. S., Sierra, R., Illemann, M., Ramirez, J. A., Arias, A., Duran, S., Skarstein, A., Ovrebo, K., Lund, L. R. & Laerum, O. D. (2010). Urokinase plasminogen activator receptor is expressed in invasive cells in gastric carcinomas from high- and low-risk countries. *Int. J. Cancer*, Vol. 126, No. 2, pp. 405-415.

Aoki, S., Nakanishi, Y., Akimoto, S., Moriya, Y., Yoshimura, K., Kitajima, M., Sakamoto, M. & Hirohashi, S. (2002). Prognostic significance of laminin-5 gamma2 chain expression in colorectal carcinoma: immunohistochemical analysis of 103 cases. *Dis. Colon Rectum*, Vol. 45, No. 11, pp. 1520-1527.

Asangani, I. A., Rasheed, S. A., Nikolova, D. A., Leupold, J. H., Colburn, N. H., Post, S. & Allgayer, H. (2008). MicroRNA-21 (miR-21) post-transcriptionally downregulates tumor suppressor Pdcd4 and stimulates invasion, intravasation and metastasis in colorectal cancer. *Oncogene*, Vol. 27, No. 15, pp. 2128-2136.

Aumailley, M., Bruckner-Tuderman, L., Carter, W. G., Deutzmann, R., Edgar, D., Ekblom, P., Engel, J., Engvall, E., Hohenester, E., Jones, J. C., Kleinman, H. K., Marinkovich, M. P., Martin, G. R., Mayer, U., Meneguzzi, G., Miner, J. H., Miyazaki, K., Patarroyo, M., Paulsson, M., Quaranta, V., Sanes, J. R., Sasaki, T., Sekiguchi, K., Sorokin, L. M., Talts, J. F., Tryggvason, K., Uitto, J., Virtanen, I., von der, M. K., Wewer, U. M., Yamada, Y. & Yurchenco, P. D. (2005). A simplified laminin nomenclature. *Matrix Biol.*, Vol. 24, No. 5, pp. 326-332.

Brabletz, T., Hlubek, F., Spaderna, S., Schmalhofer, O., Hiendlmeyer, E., Jung, A. & Kirchner, T. (2005). Invasion and metastasis in colorectal cancer: epithelial-mesenchymal transition, mesenchymal-epithelial transition, stem cells and beta-catenin. *Cells Tissues. Organs*, Vol. 179, No. 1-2, pp. 56-65.

Brabletz, T., Jung, A., Reu, S., Porzner, M., Hlubek, F., Kunz-Schughart, L. A., Knuechel, R. & Kirchner, T. (2001). Variable beta-catenin expression in colorectal cancers indicates tumor progression driven by the tumor environment. *Proc. Natl. Acad. Sci. U. S. A*, Vol. 98, No. 18, pp. 10356-10361.

Brabletz, T., Spaderna, S., Kolb, J., Hlubek, F., Faller, G., Bruns, C. J., Jung, A., Nentwich, J., Duluc, I., Domon-Dell, C., Kirchner, T. & Freund, J. N. (2004). Down-regulation of the homeodomain factor Cdx2 in colorectal cancer by collagen type I: an active role for the tumor environment in malignant tumor progression. *Cancer Res.*, Vol. 64, No. 19, pp. 6973-6977.

Bretscher, A., Edwards, K. & Fehon, R. G. (2002). ERM proteins and merlin: integrators at the cell cortex. *Nat. Rev. Mol. Cell Biol.*, Vol. 3, No. 8, pp. 586-599.

Calin, G. A. & Croce, C. M. (2009). Chronic lymphocytic leukemia: interplay between noncoding RNAs and protein-coding genes. *Blood*, Vol. 114, No. 23, pp. 4761-4770.

Chaffer, C. L. & Weinberg, R. A. (2011). A perspective on cancer cell metastasis. *Science*, Vol. 331, No. 6024, pp. 1559-1564.

Chen, L. & Zhou, S. (2010). "CRASH"ing with the worm: insights into L1CAM functions and mechanisms. *Dev. Dyn.*, Vol. 239, No. 5, pp. 1490-1501.

Crawford, H. C., Fingleton, B. M., Rudolph-Owen, L. A., Goss, K. J., Rubinfeld, B., Polakis, P. & Matrisian, L. M. (1999). The metalloproteinase matrilysin is a target of beta-catenin transactivation in intestinal tumors. *Oncogene*, Vol. 18, No. 18, pp. 2883-2891.

Curino, A., Patel, V., Nielsen, B. S., Iskander, A. J., Ensley, J. F., Yoo, G. H., Holsinger, F. C., Myers, J. N., El-Nagaar, A., Kellman, R. M., Shillitoe, E. J., Molinolo, A. A., Gutkind, J. S. & Bugge, T. H. (2004). Detection of plasminogen activators in oral cancer by laser capture microdissection combined with zymography. *Oral Oncol.*, Vol. 40, No. 10, pp. 1026-1032.

Das, S., Mandal, M., Chakraborti, T., Mandal, A. & Chakraborti, S. (2003). Structure and evolutionary aspects of matrix metalloproteinases: a brief overview. *Mol. Cell Biochem.*, Vol. 253, No. 1-2, pp. 31-40.

Demyanenko, G. P., Shibata, Y. & Maness, P. F. (2001). Altered distribution of dopaminergic neurons in the brain of L1 null mice. *Brain Res. Dev. Brain Res.*, Vol. 126, No. 1, pp. 21-30.

Ebeling, O., Duczmal, A., Aigner, S., Geiger, C., Schollhammer, S., Kemshead, J. T., Moller, P., Schwartz-Albiez, R. & Altevogt, P. (1996). L1 adhesion molecule on human lymphocytes and monocytes: expression and involvement in binding to alpha v beta 3 integrin. *Eur. J. Immunol.*, Vol. 26, No. 10, pp. 2508-2516.

Eden, G., Archinti, M., Furlan, F., Murphy, R. & Degryse, B. (2011). The Urokinase Receptor Interactome. *Curr. Pharm. Des.* Epub ahead of print.

Faissner, A., Kruse, J., Goridis, C., Bock, E. & Schachner, M. (1984). The neural cell adhesion molecule L1 is distinct from the N-CAM related group of surface antigens BSP-2 and D2. *EMBO J.*, Vol. 3, No. 4, pp. 733-737.

Fogel, M., Gutwein, P., Mechtersheimer, S., Riedle, S., Stoeck, A., Smirnov, A., Edler, L., Ben-Arie, A., Huszar, M. & Altevogt, P. (2003). L1 expression as a predictor of progression and survival in patients with uterine and ovarian carcinomas. *Lancet*, Vol. 362, No. 9387, pp. 869-875.

Folgueras, A. R., Pendas, A. M., Sanchez, L. M. & Lopez-Otin, C. (2004). Matrix metalloproteinases in cancer: from new functions to improved inhibition strategies. *Int. J. Dev. Biol.*, Vol. 48, No. 5-6, pp. 411-424.

Fujimori, T., Fujii, S., Saito, N. & Sugihara, K. (2009). Pathological diagnosis of early colorectal carcinoma and its clinical implications. *Digestion*, Vol. 79 Suppl 1, pp. 40-51.

Fuxe, J., Vincent, T. & Garcia de, H. A. (2010). Transcriptional crosstalk between TGF-beta and stem cell pathways in tumor cell invasion: role of EMT promoting Smad complexes. *Cell Cycle*, Vol. 9, No. 12, pp. 2363-2374.

Gabbert, H., Wagner, R., Moll, R. & Gerharz, C. D. (1985). Tumor dedifferentiation: an important step in tumor invasion. *Clin. Exp. Metastasis*, Vol. 3, No. 4, pp. 257-279.

Ganesh, S., Sier, C. F., Heerding, M. M., Griffioen, G., Lamers, C. B. & Verspaget, H. W. (1994). Urokinase receptor and colorectal cancer survival. *Lancet*, Vol. 344, No. 8919, pp. 401-402.

Gardsvoll, H. & Ploug, M. (2007). Mapping of the vitronectin-binding site on the urokinase receptor: involvement of a coherent receptor interface consisting of residues from both domain I and the flanking interdomain linker region. *J. Biol. Chem.*, Vol. 282, No. 18, pp. 13561-13572.

Gavert, N., Conacci-Sorrell, M., Gast, D., Schneider, A., Altevogt, P., Brabletz, T. & Ben-Ze'ev, A. (2005). L1, a novel target of beta-catenin signaling, transforms cells and is expressed at the invasive front of colon cancers. *J. Cell Biol.*, Vol. 168, No. 4, pp. 633-642.

Gavert, N., Vivanti, A., Hazin, J., Brabletz, T. & Ben-Ze'ev, A. (2011). L1-mediated colon cancer cell metastasis does not require changes in EMT and cancer stem cell markers. *Mol. Cancer Res.*, Vol. 9, No. 1, pp. 14-24.

Giannelli, G., Falk-Marzillier, J., Schiraldi, O., Stetler-Stevenson, W. G. & Quaranta, V. (1997). Induction of cell migration by matrix metalloprotease-2 cleavage of laminin-5. *Science*, Vol. 277, No. 5323, pp. 225-228.

Goldfinger, L. E., Stack, M. S. & Jones, J. C. (1998). Processing of laminin-5 and its functional consequences: role of plasmin and tissue-type plasminogen activator. *J. Cell Biol.*, Vol. 141, No. 1, pp. 255-265.

Guess, C. M., Lafleur, B. J., Weidow, B. L. & Quaranta, V. (2009). A decreased ratio of laminin-332 beta3 to gamma2 subunit mRNA is associated with poor prognosis in colon cancer. *Cancer Epidemiol. Biomarkers Prev.*, Vol. 18, No. 5, pp. 1584-1590.

Guess, C. M. & Quaranta, V. (2009). Defining the role of laminin-332 in carcinoma. *Matrix Biol.*, Vol. 28, No. 8, pp. 445-455.

Gutwein, P., Mechtersheimer, S., Riedle, S., Stoeck, A., Gast, D., Joumaa, S., Zentgraf, H., Fogel, M. & Altevogt, D. P. (2003). ADAM10-mediated cleavage of L1 adhesion molecule at the cell surface and in released membrane vesicles. *FASEB J.*, Vol. 17, No. 2, pp. 292-294.

Hald, A., Rono, B., Melander, M. C., Ding, M., Holck, S. & Lund, L. R. (2011). MMP9 is protective against lethal inflammatory mass lesions in the mouse colon. *Dis. Model. Mech.*, Vol. 4, No. 2, pp. 212-227.

Hansen, L. V., Laerum, O. D., Illemann, M., Nielsen, B. S. & Ploug, M. (2008). Altered expression of the urokinase receptor homologue, C4.4A, in invasive areas of human esophageal squamous cell carcinoma. *Int. J. Cancer*, Vol. 122, No. 4, pp. 734-741.

Hase, K., Shatney, C., Johnson, D., Trollope, M. & Vierra, M. (1993). Prognostic value of tumor "budding" in patients with colorectal cancer. *Dis. Colon Rectum*, Vol. 36, No. 7, pp. 627-635.

Heiss, M. M., Simon, E. H., Beyer, B. C., Gruetzner, K. U., Tarabichi, A., Babic, R., Schildberg, F. W. & Allgayer, H. (2002). Minimal residual disease in gastric cancer: evidence of an independent prognostic relevance of urokinase receptor expression by disseminated tumor cells in the bone marrow. *J. Clin. Oncol.*, Vol. 20, No. 8, pp. 2005-2016.

Hlubek, F., Jung, A., Kotzor, N., Kirchner, T. & Brabletz, T. (2001). Expression of the invasion factor laminin gamma2 in colorectal carcinomas is regulated by beta-catenin. *Cancer Res.*, Vol. 61, No. 22, pp. 8089-8093.

Hlubek, F., Spaderna, S., Jung, A., Kirchner, T. & Brabletz, T. (2004). Beta-catenin activates a coordinated expression of the proinvasive factors laminin-5 gamma2 chain and MT1-MMP in colorectal carcinomas. *Int. J. Cancer*, Vol. 108, No. 2, pp. 321-326.

Holmbeck, K., Bianco, P., Caterina, J., Yamada, S., Kromer, M., Kuznetsov, S. A., Mankani, M., Robey, P. G., Poole, A. R., Pidoux, I., Ward, J. M. & Birkedal-Hansen, H. (1999). MT1-MMP-deficient mice develop dwarfism, osteopenia, arthritis, and connective tissue disease due to inadequate collagen turnover. *Cell*, Vol. 99, No. 1, pp. 81-92.

Holten-Andersen, M. N., Hansen, U., Brunner, N., Nielsen, H. J., Illemann, M. & Nielsen, B. S. (2005). Localization of tissue inhibitor of metalloproteinases 1 (TIMP-1) in human colorectal adenoma and adenocarcinoma. *Int. J. Cancer*, Vol. 113, No. 2, pp. 198-206.

Hoyer-Hansen, G., Ploug, M., Behrendt, N., Ronne, E. & Dano, K. (1997). Cell-surface acceleration of urokinase-catalyzed receptor cleavage. *Eur. J. Biochem.*, Vol. 243, No. 1-2, pp. 21-26.

Hubbe, M., Kowitz, A., Schirrmacher, V., Schachner, M. & Altevogt, P. (1993). L1 adhesion molecule on mouse leukocytes: regulation and involvement in endothelial cell binding. *Eur. J. Immunol.*, Vol. 23, No. 11, pp. 2927-2931.

Ii, M., Yamamoto, H., Adachi, Y., Maruyama, Y. & Shinomura, Y. (2006). Role of matrix metalloproteinase-7 (matrilysin) in human cancer invasion, apoptosis, growth, and angiogenesis. *Exp. Biol. Med. (Maywood.)*, Vol. 231, No. 1, pp. 20-27.

Illemann, M., Bird, N., Majeed, A., Laerum, O. D., Lund, L. R., Dano, K. & Nielsen, B. S. (2009). Two distinct expression patterns of urokinase, urokinase receptor and plasminogen activator inhibitor-1 in colon cancer liver metastases. *Int. J. Cancer*, Vol. 124, No. 8, pp. 1860-1870.

Illemann, M., Hansen, U., Nielsen, H. J., Andreasen, P. A., Hoyer-Hansen, G., Lund, L. R., Dano, K. & Nielsen, B. S. (2004). Leading-edge myofibroblasts in human colon cancer express plasminogen activator inhibitor-1. *Am. J. Clin. Pathol.*, Vol. 122, No. 2, pp. 256-265.

Iorio, M. V. & Croce, C. M. (2009). MicroRNAs in cancer: small molecules with a huge impact. *J. Clin. Oncol.*, Vol. 27, No. 34, pp. 5848-5856.

Itoh, H., Kataoka, H., Yamauchi, M., Naganuma, S., Akiyama, Y., Nuki, Y., Shimomura, T., Miyazawa, K., Kitamura, N. & Koono, M. (2001). Identification of hepatocyte growth factor activator inhibitor type 2 (HAI-2)-related small peptide (H2RSP): its nuclear localization and generation of chimeric mRNA transcribed from both HAI-2 and H2RSP genes. *Biochem. Biophys. Res. Commun.*, Vol. 288, No. 2, pp. 390-399.

Jass, J. R., Barker, M., Fraser, L., Walsh, M. D., Whitehall, V. L., Gabrielli, B., Young, J. & Leggett, B. A. (2003). APC mutation and tumour budding in colorectal cancer. *J. Clin. Pathol.*, Vol. 56, No. 1, pp. 69-73.

Jorgensen, S., Baker, A., Moller, S. & Nielsen, B. S. (2010). Robust one-day in situ hybridization protocol for detection of microRNAs in paraffin samples using LNA probes. *Methods*, Vol. 52, No. 4, pp. 375-381.

Juncker-Jensen, A. & Lund, L. R. (2011). Phenotypic overlap between MMP-13 and the plasminogen activation system during wound healing in mice. *PLoS. One.*, Vol. 6, No. 2, pp. e16954.

Kadmon, G. & Altevogt, P. (1997). The cell adhesion molecule L1: species- and cell-type-dependent multiple binding mechanisms. *Differentiation*, Vol. 61, No. 3, pp. 143-150.

Kajiwara, Y., Ueno, H., Hashiguchi, Y., Shinto, E., Shimazaki, H., Mochizuki, H. & Hase, K. (2011). Expression of l1 cell adhesion molecule and morphologic features at the invasive front of colorectal cancer. *Am. J. Clin. Pathol.*, Vol. 136, No. 1, pp. 138-144.

Kirkland, S. C., (2009). Type I collagen inhibits differentiation and promotes a stem cell-like phenotype in human colorectal carcinoma cells. *Br. J. Cancer*, Vol. 101, No. 2, pp. 320-326.

Kloosterman, W. P., Wienholds, E., de, B. E., Kauppinen, S. & Plasterk, R. H. (2006). In situ detection of miRNAs in animal embryos using LNA-modified oligonucleotide probes. *Nat. Methods*, Vol. 3, No. 1, pp. 27-29.

Koshikawa, N., Giannelli, G., Cirulli, V., Miyazaki, K. & Quaranta, V. (2000). Role of cell surface metalloprotease MT1-MMP in epithelial cell migration over laminin-5. *J. Cell Biol.*, Vol. 148, No. 3, pp. 615-624.

Koshikawa, N., Minegishi, T., Sharabi, A., Quaranta, V. & Seiki, M. (2005). Membrane-type matrix metalloproteinase-1 (MT1-MMP) is a processing enzyme for human laminin gamma 2 chain. *J. Biol. Chem.*, Vol. 280, No. 1, pp. 88-93.

Koshikawa, N., Schenk, S., Moeckel, G., Sharabi, A., Miyazaki, K., Gardner, H., Zent, R. & Quaranta, V. (2004). Proteolytic processing of laminin-5 by MT1-MMP in tissues and its effects on epithelial cell morphology. *FASEB J.*, Vol. 18, No. 2, pp. 364-366.

Kowitz, A., Kadmon, G., Eckert, M., Schirrmacher, V., Schachner, M. & Altevogt, P. (1992). Expression and function of the neural cell adhesion molecule L1 in mouse leukocytes. *Eur. J. Immunol.*, Vol. 22, No. 5, pp. 1199-1205.

Kurokawa, S., Arimura, Y., Yamamoto, H., Adachi, Y., Endo, T., Sato, T., Suga, T., Hosokawa, M., Shinomura, Y. & Imai, K. (2005). Tumour matrilysin expression predicts metastatic potential of stage I (pT1) colon and rectal cancers. *Gut*, Vol. 54, No. 12, pp. 1751-1758.

Laerum, O. D., Illemann, M., Skarstein, A., Helgeland, L., Ovrebo, K., Dano, K. & Nielsen, B. S. (2008). Crohn's disease but not chronic ulcerative colitis induces the expression of PAI-1 in enteric neurons. *Am. J. Gastroenterol.*, Vol. 103, No. 9, pp. 2350-2358.

Lim, L. P., Lau, N. C., Garrett-Engele, P., Grimson, A., Schelter, J. M., Castle, J., Bartel, D. P., Linsley, P. S. & Johnson, J. M. (2005). Microarray analysis shows that some microRNAs downregulate large numbers of target mRNAs. *Nature*, Vol. 433, No. 7027, pp. 769-773.

Lindberg, P., Larsson, A. & Nielsen, B. S. (2006). Expression of plasminogen activator inhibitor-1, urokinase receptor and laminin gamma-2 chain is an early coordinated event in incipient oral squamous cell carcinoma. *Int. J. Cancer*, Vol. 118, No. 12, pp. 2948-2956.

Liu, N. & Olson, E. N. (2010). MicroRNA regulatory networks in cardiovascular development. *Dev. Cell*, Vol. 18, No. 4, pp. 510-525.

Ma, X., Kumar, M., Choudhury, S. N., Becker Buscaglia, L. E., Barker, J. R., Kanakamedala, K., Liu, M. F. & Li, Y. (2011). Loss of the miR-21 allele elevates the expression of its target genes and reduces tumorigenesis. *Proc. Natl. Acad. Sci. U. S. A*, Vol. 108, No. 25, pp. 10144-10149.

Maddaluno, L., Verbrugge, S. E., Martinoli, C., Matteoli, G., Chiavelli, A., Zeng, Y., Williams, E. D., Rescigno, M. & Cavallaro, U. (2009). The adhesion molecule L1 regulates transendothelial migration and trafficking of dendritic cells. *J. Exp. Med.*, Vol. 206, No. 3, pp. 623-635.

Mann, B., Gelos, M., Siedow, A., Hanski, M. L., Gratchev, A., Ilyas, M., Bodmer, W. F., Moyer, M. P., Riecken, E. O., Buhr, H. J. & Hanski, C. (1999). Target genes of beta-catenin-T cell-factor/lymphoid-enhancer-factor signaling in human colorectal carcinomas. *Proc. Natl. Acad. Sci. U. S. A*, Vol. 96, No. 4, pp. 1603-1608.

Maretzky, T., Schulte, M., Ludwig, A., Rose-John, S., Blobel, C., Hartmann, D., Altevogt, P., Saftig, P. & Reiss, K. (2005). L1 is sequentially processed by two differently activated metalloproteases and presenilin/gamma-secretase and regulates neural cell adhesion, cell migration, and neurite outgrowth. *Mol. Cell Biol.*, Vol. 25, No. 20, pp. 9040-9053.

Masaki, T., Matsuoka, H., Sugiyama, M., Abe, N., Goto, A., Sakamoto, A. & Atomi, Y. (2001). Matrilysin (MMP-7) as a significant determinant of malignant potential of early invasive colorectal carcinomas. *Br. J. Cancer*, Vol. 84, No. 10, pp. 1317-1321.

Mechtersheimer, S., Gutwein, P., gmon-Levin, N., Stoeck, A., Oleszewski, M., Riedle, S., Postina, R., Fahrenholz, F., Fogel, M., Lemmon, V. & Altevogt, P. (2001). Ectodomain shedding of L1 adhesion molecule promotes cell migration by autocrine binding to integrins. *J. Cell Biol.*, Vol. 155, No. 4, pp. 661-673.

Meng, F., Henson, R., Wehbe-Janek, H., Ghoshal, K., Jacob, S. T. & Patel, T. (2007). MicroRNA-21 regulates expression of the PTEN tumor suppressor gene in human hepatocellular cancer. *Gastroenterology*, Vol. 133, No. 2, pp. 647-658.

Monea, S., Lehti, K., Keski-Oja, J. & Mignatti, P. (2002). Plasmin activates pro-matrix metalloproteinase-2 with a membrane-type 1 matrix metalloproteinase-dependent mechanism. *J. Cell Physiol*, Vol. 192, No. 2, pp. 160-170.

Nagase, H., Visse, R. & Murphy, G. (2006). Structure and function of matrix metalloproteinases and TIMPs. *Cardiovasc. Res.*, Vol. 69, No. 3, pp. 562-573.

Nakamura, T., Mitomi, H., Kikuchi, S., Ohtani, Y. & Sato, K. (2005). Evaluation of the usefulness of tumor budding on the prediction of metastasis to the lung and liver after curative excision of colorectal cancer. *Hepatogastroenterology*, Vol. 52, No. 65, pp. 1432-1435.

Nielsen, B. S., Jorgensen, S., Fog, J. U., Sokilde, R., Christensen, I. J., Hansen, U., Brunner, N., Baker, A., Moller, S. & Nielsen, H. J. (2011). High levels of microRNA-21 in the stroma of colorectal cancers predict short disease-free survival in stage II colon cancer patients. *Clin. Exp. Metastasis*, Vol. 28, No. 1, pp. 27-38.

Odekon, L. E., Blasi, F. & Rifkin, D. B. (1994). Requirement for receptor-bound urokinase in plasmin-dependent cellular conversion of latent TGF-beta to TGF-beta. *J. Cell Physiol*, Vol. 158, No. 3, pp. 398-407.

Okada, A., Bellocq, J. P., Rouyer, N., Chenard, M. P., Rio, M. C., Chambon, P. & Basset, P. (1995). Membrane-type matrix metalloproteinase (MT-MMP) gene is expressed in stromal cells of human colon, breast, and head and neck carcinomas. *Proc. Natl. Acad. Sci. U. S. A*, Vol. 92, No. 7, pp. 2730-2734.

Okuyama, T., Nakamura, T. & Yamaguchi, M. (2003). Budding is useful to select high-risk patients in stage II well-differentiated or moderately differentiated colon adenocarcinoma. *Dis. Colon Rectum*, Vol. 46, No. 10, pp. 1400-1406.

Ploug, M., (2003). Structure-function relationships in the interaction between the urokinase-type plasminogen activator and its receptor. *Curr. Pharm. Des*, Vol. 9, No. 19, pp. 1499-1528.

Poulsom, R., Pignatelli, M., Stetler-Stevenson, W. G., Liotta, L. A., Wright, P. A., Jeffery, R. E., Longcroft, J. M., Rogers, L. & Stamp, G. W. (1992). Stromal expression of 72 kda type IV collagenase (MMP-2) and TIMP-2 mRNAs in colorectal neoplasia. *Am. J. Pathol.*, Vol. 141, No. 2, pp. 389-396.

Prall, F., (2007). Tumour budding in colorectal carcinoma. *Histopathology*, Vol. 50, No. 1, pp. 151-162.

Prall, F., Nizze, H. & Barten, M. (2005). Tumour budding as prognostic factor in stage I/II colorectal carcinoma. *Histopathology*, Vol. 47, No. 1, pp. 17-24.

Pyke, C., Ralfkiaer, E., Ronne, E., Hoyer-Hansen, G., Kirkeby, L. & Dano, K. (1994). Immunohistochemical detection of the receptor for urokinase plasminogen activator in human colon cancer. *Histopathology*, Vol. 24, No. 2, pp. 131-138.

Pyke, C., Romer, J., Kallunki, P., Lund, L. R., Ralfkiaer, E., Dano, K. & Tryggvason, K. (1994). The gamma 2 chain of kalinin/laminin 5 is preferentially expressed in invading malignant cells in human cancers. *Am. J. Pathol.*, Vol. 145, No. 4, pp. 782-791.

Pyke, C., Salo, S., Ralfkiaer, E., Romer, J., Dano, K. & Tryggvason, K. (1995). Laminin-5 is a marker of invading cancer cells in some human carcinomas and is coexpressed with the receptor for urokinase plasminogen activator in budding cancer cells in colon adenocarcinomas. *Cancer Res.*, Vol. 55, No. 18, pp. 4132-4139.

Remy, L., Trespeuch, C., Bachy, S., Scoazec, J. Y. & Rousselle, P. (2006). Matrilysin 1 influences colon carcinoma cell migration by cleavage of the laminin-5 beta3 chain. *Cancer Res.*, Vol. 66, No. 23, pp. 11228-11237.

Romer, J., Nielsen, B. S. & Ploug, M. (2004). The urokinase receptor as a potential target in cancer therapy. *Curr. Pharm. Des*, Vol. 10, No. 19, pp. 2359-2376.

Ronnov-Jessen, L. & Petersen, O. W. (1993). Induction of alpha-smooth muscle actin by transforming growth factor-beta 1 in quiescent human breast gland fibroblasts. Implications for myofibroblast generation in breast neoplasia. *Lab Invest*, Vol. 68, No. 6, pp. 696-707.

Roy, S., Khanna, S., Hussain, S. R., Biswas, S., Azad, A., Rink, C., Gnyawali, S., Shilo, S., Nuovo, G. J. & Sen, C. K. (2009). MicroRNA expression in response to murine myocardial infarction: miR-21 regulates fibroblast metalloprotease-2 via phosphatase and tensin homologue. *Cardiovasc. Res.*, Vol. 82, No. 1, pp. 21-29.

Sakurai, T., Lustig, M., Babiarz, J., Furley, A. J., Tait, S., Brophy, P. J., Brown, S. A., Brown, L. Y., Mason, C. A. & Grumet, M. (2001). Overlapping functions of the cell adhesion molecules Nr-CAM and L1 in cerebellar granule cell development. *J. Cell Biol.*, Vol. 154, No. 6, pp. 1259-1273.

Sato, H. & Takino, T. (2010). Coordinate action of membrane-type matrix metalloproteinase-1 (MT1-MMP) and MMP-2 enhances pericellular proteolysis and invasion. *Cancer Sci.*, Vol. 101, No. 4, pp. 843-847.

Schetter, A. J., Leung, S. Y., Sohn, J. J., Zanetti, K. A., Bowman, E. D., Yanaihara, N., Yuen, S. T., Chan, T. L., Kwong, D. L., Au, G. K., Liu, C. G., Calin, G. A., Croce, C. M. & Harris, C. C. (2008). MicroRNA expression profiles associated with prognosis and therapeutic outcome in colon adenocarcinoma. *JAMA*, Vol. 299, No. 4, pp. 425-436.

Schmid, R. S. & Maness, P. F. (2008). L1 and NCAM adhesion molecules as signaling coreceptors in neuronal migration and process outgrowth. *Curr. Opin. Neurobiol.*, Vol. 18, No. 3, pp. 245-250.

Sempere, L. F., Preis, M., Yezefski, T., Ouyang, H., Suriawinata, A. A., Silahtaroglu, A., Conejo-Garcia, J. R., Kauppinen, S., Wells, W. & Korc, M. (2010). Fluorescence-based codetection with protein markers reveals distinct cellular compartments for altered MicroRNA expression in solid tumors. *Clin. Cancer Res.*, Vol. 16, No. 16, pp. 4246-4255.

Shinto, E., Tsuda, H., Ueno, H., Hashiguchi, Y., Hase, K., Tamai, S., Mochizuki, H., Inazawa, J. & Matsubara, O. (2005). Prognostic implication of laminin-5 gamma 2 chain expression in the invasive front of colorectal cancers, disclosed by area-specific four-point tissue microarrays. *Lab Invest*, Vol. 85, No. 2, pp. 257-266.

Sordat, I., Bosman, F. T., Dorta, G., Rousselle, P., Aberdam, D., Blum, A. L. & Sordat, B. (1998). Differential expression of laminin-5 subunits and integrin receptors in human colorectal neoplasia. *J. Pathol.*, Vol. 185, No. 1, pp. 44-52.

Stephens, R. W., Nielsen, H. J., Christensen, I. J., Thorlacius-Ussing, O., Sorensen, S., Dano, K. & Brunner, N. (1999). Plasma urokinase receptor levels in patients with colorectal cancer: relationship to prognosis. *J. Natl. Cancer Inst.*, Vol. 91, No. 10, pp. 869-874.

Strongin, A. Y., (2010). Proteolytic and non-proteolytic roles of membrane type-1 matrix metalloproteinase in malignancy. *Biochim. Biophys. Acta*, Vol. 1803, No. 1, pp. 133-141.

Suzuki, Y., Nagai, N., Umemura, K., Collen, D. & Lijnen, H. R. (2007). Stromelysin-1 (MMP-3) is critical for intracranial bleeding after t-PA treatment of stroke in mice. *J. Thromb. Haemost.*, Vol. 5, No. 8, pp. 1732-1739.

Talotta, F., Cimmino, A., Matarazzo, M. R., Casalino, L., De, V. G., D'Esposito, M., Di, L. R. & Verde, P. (2009). An autoregulatory loop mediated by miR-21 and PDCD4 controls the AP-1 activity in RAS transformation. *Oncogene*, Vol. 28, No. 1, pp. 73-84.

Tanaka, M., Hashiguchi, Y., Ueno, H., Hase, K. & Mochizuki, H. (2003). Tumor budding at the invasive margin can predict patients at high risk of recurrence after curative surgery for stage II, T3 colon cancer. *Dis. Colon Rectum*, Vol. 46, No. 8, pp. 1054-1059.

Thuault, S., Valcourt, U., Petersen, M., Manfioletti, G., Heldin, C. H. & Moustakas, A. (2006). Transforming growth factor-beta employs HMGA2 to elicit epithelial-mesenchymal transition. *J. Cell Biol.*, Vol. 174, No. 2, pp. 175-183.

Thum, T., Gross, C., Fiedler, J., Fischer, T., Kissler, S., Bussen, M., Galuppo, P., Just, S., Rottbauer, W., Frantz, S., Castoldi, M., Soutschek, J., Koteliansky, V., Rosenwald, A., Basson, M. A., Licht, J. D., Pena, J. T., Rouhanifard, S. H., Muckenthaler, M. U., Tuschl, T., Martin, G. R., Bauersachs, J. & Engelhardt, S. (2008). MicroRNA-21 contributes to myocardial disease by stimulating MAP kinase signalling in fibroblasts. *Nature*, Vol. 456, No. 7224, pp. 980-984.

Thurison, T., Lomholt, A. F., Rasch, M. G., Lund, I. K., Nielsen, H. J., Christensen, I. J. & Hoyer-Hansen, G. (2010). A new assay for measurement of the liberated domain I of the urokinase receptor in plasma improves the prediction of survival in colorectal cancer. *Clin. Chem.*, Vol. 56, No. 10, pp. 1636-1640.

Turner, R. R., Li, C. & Compton, C. C. (2007). Newer pathologic assessment techniques for colorectal carcinoma. *Clin. Cancer Res.*, Vol. 13, No. 22 Pt 2, pp. 6871s-6876s.

Uchiyama, S., Itoh, H., Naganuma, S., Nagaike, K., Fukushima, T., Tanaka, H., Hamasuna, R., Chijiiwa, K. & Kataoka, H. (2007). Enhanced expression of hepatocyte growth factor activator inhibitor type 2-related small peptide at the invasive front of colon cancers. *Gut*, Vol. 56, No. 2, pp. 215-226.

Udayakumar, T. S., Chen, M. L., Bair, E. L., Von, B., Cress, A. E., Nagle, R. B. & Bowden, G. T. (2003). Membrane type-1-matrix metalloproteinase expressed by prostate carcinoma cells cleaves human laminin-5 beta3 chain and induces cell migration. *Cancer Res.*, Vol. 63, No. 9, pp. 2292-2299.

Ueno, H., Murphy, J., Jass, J. R., Mochizuki, H. & Talbot, I. C. (2002). Tumour 'budding' as an index to estimate the potential of aggressiveness in rectal cancer. *Histopathology*, Vol. 40, No. 2, pp. 127-132.

Winter, J., Jung, S., Keller, S., Gregory, R. I. & Diederichs, S. (2009). Many roads to maturity: microRNA biogenesis pathways and their regulation. *Nat. Cell Biol.*, Vol. 11, No. 3, pp. 228-234.

Zavadil, J., Narasimhan, M., Blumenberg, M. & Schneider, R. J. (2007). Transforming growth factor-beta and microRNA:mRNA regulatory networks in epithelial plasticity. *Cells Tissues. Organs*, Vol. 185, No. 1-3, pp. 157-161.

Zlobec, I., Molinari, F., Martin, V., Mazzucchelli, L., Saletti, P., Trezzi, R., De, D. S., Vlajnic, T., Frattini, M. & Lugli, A. (2010). Tumor budding predicts response to anti-EGFR therapies in metastatic colorectal cancer patients. *World J. Gastroenterol.*, Vol. 16, No. 38, pp. 4823-4831.

8

Lipid Peroxidation in Colorectal Carcinogenesis: Bad and Good News

Stefania Pizzimenti, Cristina Toaldo,
Piergiorgio Pettazzoni, Eric Ciamporcero,
Mario Umberto Dianzani and Giuseppina Barrera
University of Turin,
Italy

1. Introduction

During oxidative stress, membrane lipids are one of the major targets of Reactive Oxygen Species (ROS) that are known to elicit oxidative decomposition of polyunsaturated fatty acids (PUFAs) of membrane phospholipids, a process usually referred to lipid peroxidation (Esterbauer et al., 1991). During this process, a number of carbonylic compounds are generated as final products, including acrolein, malondialdehyde (MDA) and 4-hydroxyalkenals (Esterbauer et al., 1991). Among the 4-hydroxyalkenal class, 4-hydroxynonenal (HNE) is the most abundant aldehyde produced (Dianzani et al., 1999). Over the years, HNE has achieved a status as one of the best recognized and most studied of the cytotoxic products of lipid peroxidation (Poli et al., 2008). In addition to studies on its bioactivity, HNE is commonly used as a biomarker for the occurrence and/or the extent of oxidative stress. It appears to be produced specifically by peroxidation of ω-6 PUFAs, such as linoleic acid, arachidonic acid (AA) and γ-linolenic acid (Esterbauer et al., 1982). HNE has three main functional groups: the aldehyde group, the C=C double bond and the hydroxyl group, which can participate, alone or in sequence, in chemical reactions with other molecules (Esterbauer et al., 1991). HNE is a highly electrophilic molecule, which predisposes it to localize in the cell membranes. It can easily react with low molecular weight compounds, such as glutathione, with proteins, with lipids and, at higher concentration, with DNA (Esterbauer et al., 1991; Uchida, 2003). The double bond, the carbonyl group and the hydroxyl group, all contribute to making HNE highly reactive with nucleophiles with the primary reactivity of the molecule lying at the unsaturated bond of the C-3 atom. HNE has been shown to form Michael adducts via the C-3 atom with the sulfhydryl group of Cys residues, the imidazole group of His residues, and the ε-amino group of Lys residues on a large number of proteins (Esterbauer et al., 1991). Recently, it has been proposed that HNE can also modify Arg residues of proteins (Isom et al., 2004). In addition to Michael adduct formation, Lys residues also form Schiff bases and pentylpyrrole adducts with HNE via the C-1 aldehyde group (Sayre et al., 1993; Petersen & Doorn, 2004; Schaur, 2003)

HNE-modified proteins can be removed by the proteasomal system (Siems & Grune, 2003).

Once formed, HNE is rapidly degraded and its metabolism is dependent upon a set of specific enzymes presenting high affinity toward HNE. In particular HNE metabolism can be divided into glutathione-mediated and oxidative/reductive categories (Siems & Grune, 2003). In the first case, HNE binds the thiol group of GSH resulting in the correspondent emiacetal (Balogh & Atkins, 2011). The reaction with GSH can occur in a spontaneous manner, with low efficiency or through the reaction catalized by Glutathione S Transferases (GSTs). Moreover, although a number of isoforms of GST manifested HNE conjugating activity, it has been widely reported that the isoform GST A4 presents the highest HNE affinity (Balogh & Atkins , 2011). The oxidative/reductive pathway of HNE involves its NAD/NADP-dependent oxidative conversion to 4-hydroxy-2-nonenoic Acid (HNA) catalyzed by aldheyde dehydrogenases (ALDHs) or the reductive conversion to 1,4-dihydroxy-2-nonene (DHN) catalyzed by alchool dehydrogenase (ADH) or aldhehyde reductase (AR) (Hartley et al., 1995; Vander Jagt et al., 1995). However, the majority of HNE is metabolized through forming GS-HNE (Forman et al., 2003). HNE-GSH is then further metabolized and found in urine, mostly, as the mercapturic acid derivative, HNE-MA (Alary, 1995). Indeed, HNE-GSH adduct is further metabolized by γ-glutamyltranspeptidase (γ-GT) and dipeptidases (DP) to the cysteinyl (CYS)-HNE thioether adduct. The cysteinyl thioether adduct is a substrate for acetyltransferases (AT) that catalyze the acetylation of the cysteinyl adduct to generate the acetylcysteinyl (AcCYS), or mercapturic acid, adduct. HNE metabolites also can be found associated with mercapturic acid, such as DHN-MA, HNE-MA and HNA-lactone (Alary et al., 2003). HNE is also partially excreted first with the bile, then with the faeces, under the form of conjugated metabolites. However, biliary metabolites undergo an enterohepatic cycle that limits the final excretion of faecal metabolites (Alary et al., 2003).

HNE, and in general aldehydes formed during membrane lipid peroxidation, are quite long lived, as compared to reactive free radicals and can widely diffuse and react around the site of origin (Esterbauer 1991). As a consequence, HNE and related aldehydes were proposed as putative ultimate toxic messengers, potentially able to mediate stress-related injury at the molecular level (Uchida, 2003). Indeed, HNE has been detected in vivo in several pathological conditions, which entail increased lipid peroxidation, including inflammation, atherosclerosis, chronic degenerative diseases of the nervous system, and chronic liver diseases, reaching a concentration up to about 10 μM (Parola et al., 1999).

However, under physiological conditions, HNE can be found at low concentrations in human tissues and plasma (0.07-2.8 μM) (Esterbauer et al., 1991, Poli et al., 2008) where it participates in the control of biological processes, such as signal transduction, cell proliferation and differentiation. Indeed, HNE, similarly to ROS, plays an important role in controlling the intracellular signal transduction pathways involved in a number of cell responses (Parola et al., 1999; Dianzani et al., 2003; Leonarduzzi et al., 2004).

The contribution of HNE and lipid peroxidation in carcinogenesis is still controversial. Beside pro-tumoral effects, several authors pointed out their protective role. This "two-faced" role has already emerged for ROS (Halliwell, 2007; Wang & Yi, 2008; Pan et al., 2009; Acharya et al., 2010) and increasing evidence is emerging also for a dual role of lipid peroxidation products (Zhi-Hua et al., 2006; Pizzimenti et al., 2010a).

2. HNE and carcinogenesis

2.1 DNA-adducts, mutagenicity and genotoxicity

2.1.1 DNA-adducts

The most substantial evidence of the genotoxic and mutagenic effect of HNE is the formation of HNE-DNA adducts. ROS and HNE seem to share this feature and this has been proposed as the mechanism of tumor induction (Bartsch & Nair, 2005).

One of the most studied HNE-adducts is the propane-type DNA adduct with deoxyguanosine, the 6-(1-hydroxyhexanyl)-8-hydroxy-1, N2-propano-2'deoxyguanine (HNE-dG) (Winter et al., 1986). AA appears to be a major source of HNE-DNA adducts, producing a total of 20.6 µmol of HNE-dG adducts (Chung et al., 2000), by an in vitro assay using 1 mM AA. HNE-dG is also the main lesion produced upon the addition of HNE to DNA (Chung et al., 2000; Wacker et al., 2001); moreover, an increase of HNE-dG adducts was observed in the liver DNA of rats after treatment with CCl4, a well known inducer of lipid peroxidation (Chung et al., 2000). Taken together, these results generate substantial evidence for the endogenous formation of these adducts, thus it has been proposed that lipid peroxidation is a main endogenous pathway leading to propano adduction in DNA (Chung et al., 1999).

In the presence of peroxides and reactive oxygen species, HNE can be further metabolized to an epoxide intermediate that interacts with DNA, forming etheno-type DNA adducts (Chung et al., 1996). However the etheno-type DNA adducts are produced in significantly lower yield, with respect to the HNE-dG adducts, when a pro-oxidant stimulus, such H_2O_2, or HNE is added to cells. Indeed, in these experimental conditions, HNE-dG represent more than 95% of the overall adducts to DNA, suggesting that HNE-dG may represent the best biomarker of the genotoxic effects of HNE (Douki et al., 2004).

All four bases of DNA are the targets for HNE adduct formation (Chung et al., 1996; De Bont et al., 2004), but with different efficiency: G>C>A>T (Kowalczyk et al., 2004).

HNE-DNA adducts have been identified in tissues of untreated rats and humans (Chung et al., 2000), suggesting that the endogenously produced HNE can form adducts with DNA in the physiological condition also.

Removal of these modified bases from DNA plays an important role in the prevention of mutagenesis and carcinogenesis. Each cell has an efficient defence mechanism to repair these types of damage via DNA repair pathways such as base excision repair (BER), nucleotide excision repair (NER), and mismatch repair (MMR) pathways (Min & Eberel, 2009). In human leukocyte treated with 200 µM HNE, DNA damage was repaired after 12 h and returned to the control level at 24 h (Park & Park, 2011).

It has been demonstrated that NER is a major pathway for repairing HNE-dG adducts, since HNE-dG adducts induce a significantly higher level of genotoxicity and mutagenicity in NER-deficient human and E. coli cells than in NER-proficient cells (Feng et al., 2003). Moreover, other authors suggested that HNE can also contribute to carcinogenesis, by inhibiting the nucleotide excision repair (NER) of DNA damage in cancer cells with concentration higher than 50 µM (Feng et al., 2004). In any case, HNE forms adducts with DNA only at higher concentrations, since it can react quickly with amino and sulphydrylic groups of proteins and, primarly, with the sulphydrylic group of GSH. Indeed, it has been calculated that GSH conjugates were 20000 times more numerous than DNA adducts when HNE was exogenously added to the cultured cells (Falletti & Douki, 2008).

2.1.2 Mutagenicity

In this context, it would be important to know whether the HNE-dG adducts are mutagenic. Several authors suggest this possibility, since HNE has been shown to be mutagenic in mammalian cells (Cajelli et al., 1987). HNE was negative in bacterial mutagenicity tests, however its epoxidized form has been tested positive (Chung et al., 1993). HNE was found to be responsible for recombination, base substitutions and frameshift mutations in M13 phage transfected in E.coli (Kowalczyk et al., 2004).

Moreover it has been reported that 50 µM HNE treatment in human cells induces a high frequency of G.C to T.A mutations at the third base of codon 249 (AGG*) of the p53 gene (Hussain et al., 2000), a mutational hot spot in human cancers, particularly in hepatocellular carcinoma (Hsu et al., 1991). Both eheno and propane type HNE-DNA-adduct at codon 249 can be responsible for such transitions (Feng et al., 2003).

The stereochemistry of HNE-dG adducts seems to play an important role in determining mutations. Indeed, two of the HNE-dG adducts, (6R, 8S, 11R) and (6S, 8R, 11S), were significantly more mutagenic than (6R, 8S, 11S) and (6S, 8R, 11R) HNE-dG adducts. Only one of the HNE stereoisomers was able to form interstrand DNA–DNA cross-links. (Fernandes et al., 2003).

2.1.3 Genotoxicity

The genotoxic property of HNE was demonstrated in different cell types, such as on cultured human lymphocytes (Emerit et al., 1991), in primary hepatocytes (Esterbauer et al., 1991) and cerebral microvascular endothelial cells (Eckl, 2003). In these cell lines an increase of micronuclei (a biomarker of chromosome breakage and/or whole chromosome loss), chromosomal aberrations and sister chromatid exchanges was observed after exposure to HNE at relatively low doses, ranging 0.1-10 µM. However these clastrogenic features of low doses of HNE failed to be confirmed in a recent multicentrum study on DNA of normal peripheral blood lymphocytes (Katic et al., 2010).

Currently, the comet assay has been extensively used to measure DNA strand breaks, since it represents a sensitive and rapid assay to detect the mutagenic and genotoxicity of chemicals and xenobiotics (Tice, et al., 1991).

Unfortunately, most HNE-induced DNA lesions are the stable 1,N2-propano adducts and they are not detected by this technique. By using this assay, the genotoxic property of 5-10 µM HNE in the K562 leukemic cell line has been shown; this feature was highly dependent on cellular GSH/GST/AR system (Yadav et al., 2008). The comet test was also used to demonstrate the genotoxicity of 200 µM HNE in human leukocytes (Park & Park, 2011).

2.2 Results in laboratory animals

To date, in contrast with several in vitro experimental results, tumor bioassays in laboratory animals failed to demonstrate the carcinogenic and mutagenic properties of HNE. HNE, in particular its epoxy derivate, has shown that to be a weak tumor-initiating agent, causing the development of renal preneoplastic tubule lesions in new-born mice (Chung et al., 1993). More interestingly, HNE lacks in vivo genotoxicity in lacI transgenic mice, a model for detecting mutagenicity in target organs, even when lethal doses are applied (Nishikawa et al., 2000).

The big gap between the in vitro and the in vivo data can be partially explained by carefully considering the elevated doses frequently used to demonstrated the carcinogenic properties of HNE in vitro. Indeed, several mutagenic assays with HNE have been performed with high doses of HNE (more than 100 μM). It seems rather unlikely that HNE or other aldehydes can reach overall concentrations in the range of 100 μM in cells and organs (Esterbauer et al., 1991). It is conceivable that such levels may be built up locally, near or within peroxidizing membranes for a short time because of their high lipophilicity. It has been calculated, for example, that the concentration of HNE in the lipid bilayer of isolated peroxidizing microsomes is about 4.5 mM (Koster et al., 1986). Nevertheless, a convincing demonstration that this very high concentration can be reached into the cells has remained elusive. On the other hand, when HNE diffuses out from membranes, its concentration is reduced by the surrounding aqueous phase. Moreover, the cytosolic HNE-metabolizing enzymes destroy HNE produced in excess so that the steady-state HNE concentration into the cells, around 1 μM, is reached quickly (Esterbauer et al., 1991; Dianzani et al., 1999).

2.3 Cellular responses and signal transduction

As previously indicated, the adduct formation between HNE and DNA is only one of the several biological effects determined by this aldehyde. Indeed, HNE is considered as a signalling molecule influencing proliferation, differentiation and apoptosis of cancer cells (Dianzani, 2003; Leonarduzzi et al., 2004; Poli et al., 2008; Pizzimenti et al., 2010b). The majority of experimental evidence indicate an antiproliferative role of HNE, when added at low doses (1-10 μM) to cultured cells. The inhibition of proliferation has been observed in leukemic (HL-60, K562, U937, MEL, ML-1) (Barrera et al., 1991; Barrera et al., 1987, Rinaldi et al., 2000; Pizzimenti et al., 2006), neuroblastoma (SK-N-BE) (Laurora et al. 2005), hepatoma (7777, J42) (Muzio et al., 2001; Canuto et al., 1999), osteosarcoma (SaOS2; HOS) (Calonghi et al., 2002; Sunjic et al., 2005), prostate cancer (PC3) (Pettazzoni et al., 2011) cells. This anti-proliferative effect is sustained by the modulation of key genes involved in cell growth control, such as oncogenes (c-myc, c-myb, fos, AP1, cyclins) and anti-oncogenes (pRB, p53, SUFU-1, Mad-1) (Poli et al., 2008; Pizzimenti et al., 2009).

Interestingly, the effect of HNE in normal cell proliferation is more variable if not opposite to that observed in tumor cells. For example, HNE has no effect on normal myeloid stem cells (Hassane et al., 2008) or on human peripheral blood lymphocytes (Semlitsch et al., 2002), while the respective tumour was sensitive to the anti-proliferative effect of aldehyde. On the contrary, in vascular smooth muscle cells 0.1 μM HNE stimulated cell proliferation (Kakishita et al., 2001).

In several cell lines, the inhibition of proliferation was accompanied by apoptosis. The mechanisms of HNE-induced apoptosis through the extrinsic and intrinsic pathways, its self-regulatory role in this process and its interaction with Fas (CD95), p53, and Daxx has been recently reviewed (Awasti et al., 2008).

HNE is also able to induce differentiation, as observed in HL-60, MEL, K562 and SaOS osteosarcoma cells (Barrera et al., 1991; Rinaldi et al., 2000; Calonghi et al., 2002; Cheng et al., 1999; Fazio et al., 1992). Moreover, HNE was shown to induce features of typical differentiated cells, such as chemotaxis (Curzio et al., 1988), phagocytosis and the ability to induce respiratory burst (Barrera et al., 1991) in myeloid cells. HNE also demonstrated the ability to regulate the replicative potential of cells, by inhibiting the telomerase activity. Indeed, in HNE-treated leukemic cells, the expression of the hTERT gene was down-regulated by modulating the expression of transcription factors belonging to the Myc/Mad/Max network (Pizzimenti et al., 2006).

The anti-tumoral properties of HNE are also sustained by the demonstration of anti-angiogenic properties. Stagos and collaborators demonstrated that 5 and 10 μM HNE were able to inhibit the tube formation of human bone marrow endothelial cells (HBMEC) (Stagos et al., 2009). However, conflicting results have been reported, since it has been demonstrated that 1 μM HNE induces an increase of VEGF expression in human retinal pigment epithelial cells (Ayalasomayajula & Kompella, 2002).

The cellular responses to HNE are sustained by affecting cell signalling at multiple levels. Relevant findings in this area have been extensively reviewed (Poli et al., 2008; Leonarduzzi et al., 2004; Dianzani et al., 1999).

In addition to the above cellular responses presented, HNE activates various cytoprotective, stress response pathways, promoting changes in gene expression that facilitate cell survival and recovery from stress (West & Marnett, 2005). For example, HNE activates the transcription factors Nrf2 (Nuclear factor erythroid-derived 2-like 2) and HSF1 (heat shock factor 1), which mediate the antioxidant and heat shock responses, respectively (Jacobs & Marnett, 2007). Nrf2 acts by binding Antioxidant Responsive Elements (ARE) sequences on promoters of certain genes promoting their expression (Thimmulappa et al., 2002). In regard to HNE metabolism, functional ARE sequences have been found on promoter of GST A4 ALDH and ADH (Reddy et al., 2007; Malhotra et al., 2010). Moreover, Nrf2 promotes de novo GSH synthesis by up-regulating expression of the GSH synthesis pathway (Harvey 2009). Nrf2 is controlled by both translational and post-translational mechanisms, in particular the protein Kelch-like ECH-associated protein 1 (KEAP1) mediates Nrf2 ubiquitinaltion followed by proteasomal destruction (Kaspar et al., 2010). In conditions of oxidative stress or in response to many chemicals KEAP1 undergo conformational changes responsible for loss of Nrf2 binding activity. As a consequence Nrf2 can accumulate, translocate in the nucleus and drive expression of the antioxidant program (Reddy et al., 2007).

The heat shock response mediates the induction of a highly conserved set of heat shock proteins (Hsps) (Mosley, 1997). The inducible expression of Hsps is mediated by heat shock transcription factor 1 (HSF1), which translocates to the nucleus upon activation and enhances the expression of genes to form promoters containing heat shoch elements (HSE), such as Hsp70 (Sarge et al., 1993; Baler et al., 1993). A principal function of Hsps is to chaperone other proteins, binding to nascent polypeptide chains as well as to unfolded and damaged proteins. Their function as protein chaperones aids in the recovery of cells from thermal and chemical-induced damage (Hahn & 1982; Howard, 1993). In addition to acting as protein chaperones, Hsps inhibit cell death by directly inhibiting a variety of pro-apoptotic mediators, such as HNE (Jacobs et al., 2007).

It is very likely that the majority of effects observed on cell signalling and cellular responses can be mediated by the reaction of HNE to proteins and peptides. Quantitatively, proteins and, among peptides, the GSH, represent the most important group of HNE-targeted biomolecules. It was estimated that 1–8% of the HNE formed in cells will modify proteins (Siems & Grune, 2003). Most of the identified targets are enzymes, carriers, receptors, ion channels, transport proteins, cytoskeletal, heat shock proteins and others. The biological significance of the HNE-protein adducts identified have been reviewed by several authors (Uchida, 2003; Poli et al., 2008). Some of the protein-adducts identified can explain the anti-tumoral effect exerced by this aldehyde. For example, it was demonstrated that the inhibition of cell proliferation in the human colorectal carcinoma cell line (RKO) and human lung carcinoma cell line (H1299) by HNE was mediated by the direct reaction of HNE with

IκB kinase (IKK), the key enzyme regulating the NF-κB activation (Ji et al., 2001b). Moreover the HNE adducts with alpha-enolase, at the cellular surface of leukemic cells, suggest a new role for HNE in the control of tumour growth and invasion, since HNE causes a dose- and time-dependent reduction of the plasminogen binding to alpha-enolase. As a consequence, HNE reduces adhesion of HL-60 cells to HUVECs (human umbilical vein endothelial cells) (Gentile et al., 2009).

New perspectives of HNE role in cancer-inducing signaling pathways have recently emerged, by recent findings on microRNA (miRNA) (Pizzimenti et al., 2009), a class of conserved non-coding small RNAs, which regulate gene expression by translation repression of coding mRNAs (Bartel, 2004).

2.4 HNE content in human cancers

Several studies on human cancer tissues have analysed the HNE or HNE-protein adduct content, in order to find a possible correlation between this marker of lipid peroxidation and the progression of cancer.

HNE content has been reported to increase along with the progression of breast cancer (Karihtala et al., 2011) and astrocytoma (Zarkovic et al., 2005). In human renal cell carcinoma, immunohistochemistry for HNE-modified proteins showed positive staining in the cytoplasm of tumor cells, with respect to controls, without correlation to the clinical stage (Okamoto et al., 1994).

However other reports have demonstrated the opposite: a low or undetectable lipid peroxidation, as well as HNE content, such as in hepatomas (Dianzani, 1993).

Several studies have shown elevated lipid peroxidation markers in the sera, plasma or urine of breast carcinoma (Hung et al., 1999; Chandramathi et al., 2009), cervical intraepithelial neoplasia and carcinoma of the cervix (Looi et al., 2008), head and neck squamous cell carcinoma (Gupta et al., 2009) and prostate tumor (Kotrikadze et al., 2008), compared to healthy controls. However, these extratumoral measurement are likely, at least partly, to reflect generalized oxidative stress and /or inflammation in the whole body.

3. HNE and colorectal carcinogenesis

3.1 Sources and fate of HNE in colon

Colon cells can be exposed to HNE derived form different sources (Figure 1). It is possible to find HNE directly in the food (Gasc et al., 2007), since it can derived from lipid peroxidation of PUFAs introduced with diet or from endogenous PUFAs presents in cellular membranes. A small amount of HNE can reach the colon also via bile. Following a single intravenous administration of [3H]-HNE, five metabolites were present in the bile, namely GSH–HNE, GSH–DHN, DHN, and HNA-lactone mercapturic acid conjugates (Laurent et al., 1999). Within 4 hr from injection of the radiolabel 3[H]-HNE, 19.5% of the injected radioactivity was found in the bile, whereas only 3% was found in the feces within 48 hr (Laurent et al., 1999). The existence of an enterohepatic circulation for HNE metabolites has been unequivocally demonstrated (Laurent et al., 1999) using a model linking donor rats (injected intravenously with [4-3H]HNE) and recipient rats (to which the bile from donor rats was delivered intraduodenaly). This enterohepatic circulation, approximately 8% of the total dose, may explain the low amount of radioactivity recovered from faeces when rat were dosed intravenously with [4-3H]HNE.

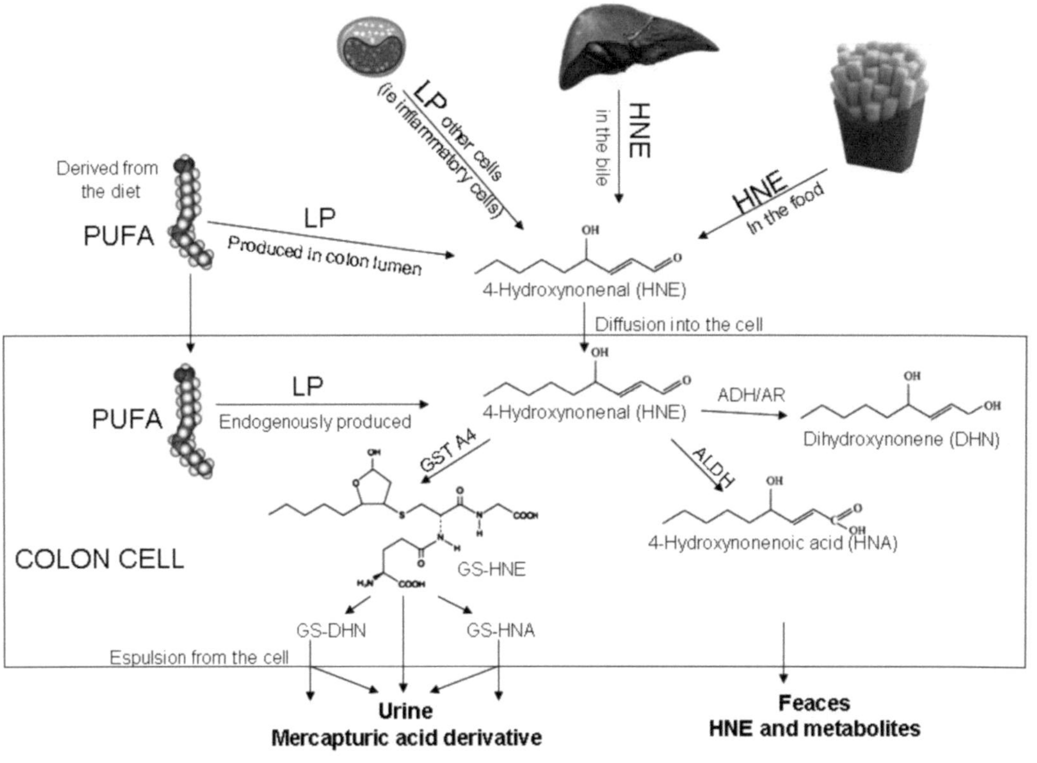

Fig. 1. Sources and fate of HNE in colon

Metabolic transformation of HNE starts in enterocites, where GSH-HNE is the main metabolite produced (Grune et al., 1991). The majority of HNE metabolites are found in the urine. Indeed, following the intravenous administration of [3H]-HNE in rats, 67%, 3%, 0.16%, and 6.5% of the injected radioactive dose was recovered from urine, faeces, liver and remaining tissues, respectively (Alary et al., 2003). The urinary HNE metabolites were separated by HPLC and the resolved peaks were identified as mercapturic acid conjugates of HNA, DHN, HNE and HNA-lactone, where DHN-MA, and to a lesser extent HNA lactone-MA, have been found to be the major urinary metabolites of HNE in rats (Boon et al., 1999). DHN-MA has been confirmed to be the major urinary HNE metabolite also in human urine (Alary et al., 1998).

The microflora of the human intestine can also affect levels of lipid peroxidation, since the antioxidative effect of lactic acid bacteria has been demonstrated (Lin et al., 1999). In particular, the antioxidative activity of Bifidobacterium longum ATCC 15708 and Lactobacillus acidophilus ATCC 4356 was measured based on the inhibition of linoleic acid peroxidation. Both intact cells and intracellular cell-free extracts of B. longum and L. acidophilus demonstrated an antioxidative effect on inhibiting lipid peroxidation. The antioxidative activity ranged from 38 to 48% inhibition of linoleic acid peroxidation. This indicates that B. longum and L. acidophilus have a very strong antioxidative effect on inhibiting lipid peroxidation (Lin et al., 1999).

Low level of HNE and its metabolites can be found also in faecal water (Alary et al., 2003) and numerous studies have emphasized the lipid peroxidation products of faecal water in colon cancer as diet-related factors (Lapre et al., 1992; Glinghammar et al., 1997).

3.2 Pro-tumoral and anti-tumoral role of HNE in colon carcinogenesis

Several authors have reported evidence that sustains the pro-tumoral activity of HNE and other products of lipid peroxidation in colon carcinogenesis. These findings include in vitro (see table 1) and in vivo studies, which demonstrate the genotoxic properties of HNE on coloncarcinoma cell lines, the increase of HNE content along with the progression of colorectal cancer and the increase of HNE-DNA adducts in vivo. However other studies, seem to demonstrate the opposite (see table 1). Consistent with the hypothesis of an anti-tumoral role of HNE are the results showing the inhibition of cell growth, the induction of apoptosis in several colon cancer cell lines, as well as the demonstration that HNE content decreases in biopsies of colon-cancer tissues with respect to normal mucosa. A deeper discussion of these opposite results is here reported.

COLON CANCER CELL LINE	HNE DOSE	OBSERVED EFFECTS	PROTEIN / PATWAY INVOLVED / MAIN RESULTS	REFERENCE
CaCo-2	1 μM	apoptosis, ROS production, enhanced by co-treatement with TGF-β1	HNE activates c-Jun N-terminal kinase (JNK) and Smad4, effects enhanced by co-treatment with TGF-β1	Zanettiet al., 2003; Vizio et al., 2005; Biasi et al., 2006
CaCo-2, HT-29	1 μM	cell growth inhibition, apoptosis	HNE down-regulates telomerase activity and hTERT expression, through modulation of Myc/Mad/Max network	Pizzimenti et al., 2010
CaCo-2	1 μM	cell growth inhibition, apoptosis	HNE induces an increase of c-myc expression and a subsequent down-regulation; HNE increases bax and p-21 expression	Cerbone et al., 2007
RKO	30-75 μM	apoptosis	HNE activates a mitochondrion-dependent pathway, involving cytochrome c release and caspase activation	Ji et al., 2001a
RKO	40 μM	apoptosis	HNE inhibits NF-kB activation by direct interaction with IkB kinase (IKK)	Ji et al., 2001b
RKO	30-60 μM	apoptosis	comparison with other aldehydes producted during lipid peroxidation (HPNE,ONE) and stereoisomers of HNE	West et al., 2004
RKO	5, 20, or 60 μM	5 and 20 μM subcytotoxic, 60 μM apoptosis	by using microarray technology, HNE simultaneously affects multiple stress signaling pathways	West et al., 2005

COLON CANCER CELL LINE	HNE DOSE	OBSERVED EFFECTS	PROTEIN / PATWAY INVOLVED / MAIN RESULTS	REFERENCE
RKO	30-60 µM	apoptosis	beside the activation of pro-apoptotic pathway, HNE activates a protective signal activation through activation of HSF1, Hsp70-1 and Hsp40 and stabilization of Bcl-XL	Jacobs & Marnett, 2007
RKO	45 µM	apoptosis	BAG3, induced by HSF-1, increases cell survival, by stabilizing the level of Bcl-2 family proteins	Jacobs & Marnett, 2009
HCT15	20-80 µM	cell death	AKR1B10-overexpressing cells are resistant to cytotoxicity of HNE	Matsunaga et al., 2011
Apc+/+, Apc+/- colon epithelial cells	10-250 µM	cell death	HNE reduces cellular viability of either Apc+/+ and Apc-/+ cells, with lesser extent in Apc-/+ cells	Pierre et al., 2007
CaCo-2		cell death	HNE increases prostaglandin E2 (PGE2) production and cyclooxygenase (COX)-2 expression; inhibition of AR prevented HNE-induced effects	Tammali et al., 2006
HT-29, HT-29clone19A	100-200 µM	genotoxicity	butyrate reduces DNA damage caused by HNE, through induction of Glutathione S-Transferase	Ebert et al., 2001
primary human colon cells, LT97, HT-29clone19A	100-250 µM	genotoxicity	HNE induces TP53 specific DNA damage	Schaeferhenrich et al., 2003
HT-29	150 µM	genotoxicity	Two fermentation products of wheat bran reduce the genotoxicity of HNE, via up-regulation of the activity of GSTs	Glei et al., 2006
primary human colon cells, LT97	0-250 µM	genotoxicity	HNE induces DNA damage on specific genes (APC,TP53, KRAS)	Glei et al., 2007
HT-29	100-250 µM	genotoxicity	butyrate induces resistance to HNE damage, by inducing GSH syntesis and increasing GSTA4-4 level	Knoll et al., 2005, Scharlau et al., 2009

Table 1. HNE in vitro effects on colon cancer cell lines

3.2.1 HNE-DNA adducts in colon and colon cancer

HNE-dG adducts, were found in normal human colon tissue, as well as DNA adducts with other lipid peroxidation products, such as acrolein and MDA (Chung et al., 2000). The levels of HNE-dG in tissue DNA examined so far are estimated to be in the range of 3-9 adducts per billion bases (3-9 nmol/mol guanine) (Chung et al,. 2000).

The etheno-DNA adducts, inter alia formed from epoxidized HNE, were found at increased level in colonic polyps of familial adenomatous polyposis (FAP) patients. Mean adduct levels in FAP polyps were 65 εdA/109 and 59 εdC/109 parent nucleotides, being 2 to 3 times higher than in unaffected colon tissue (Schmid et al., 2000). Interestingly, the level of etheno-DNA adducts in colon carcinoma tissues were found to be similar to unaffected colon (Schmid et al., 2000), suggesting a possible HNE role in the early events of colon carcinogenesis.

On the contrary, Obtułowicz and collaborators (2010) have found that, in colon cancer patients, the DNA-HNE adducts εdA and εdG, measured both in colon tissues and blood leukocytes, were lower in patients than in controls (Obtułowicz et al., 2010). These authors have measured the two corresponding metabolites also, 1,N6- Ethenoadenine (εAde) and 3,N4-ethenocytosine (εCyt), catalized by BER, the major pathway of etheno adduct elimination from DNA (Obtułowicz et al., 2010). Both excision activities were significantly higher in tumor than in normal colon tissues and this feature could be explained by the increased level of abasic site endonuclease (APE1), belonging to BER system, in coloncancer patients with respect to controls (Obtułowicz et al., 2010).

A possible pro-cancinogenic role of etheno-DNA adducts is also sustained by the finding that in the colon of patients with inflammatory bowel disease εdC, but not εdA, are increased. In particular it has been demonstrated that εdC was 19-fold higher in colonic mucosa of Crohn's disease and 4-fold higher in the colonic mucosa of ulcerative colitis patients, when compared to normal tissues (Nair et al., 2006). Since patients with ulcerative colitis (UC), and Crohn's (CD) have an elevated risk for developing colon cancer (Konner et al., 2003), the authors suggest that the promutagenic etheno-DNA adducts, generated as a consequence of chronic inflammation, can act as a driving force to malignancy in cancer-prone inflammatory diseases (Nair et al., 2006).

HNE can also contribute to induce colon carcinogenesis, by inhibiting the DNA repair mechanism of such adducts. Indeed, Feng and collaborators (2004) demonstrated that 50 μM HNE inhibits NER in the human colon epithelial cell line HCT116. The repair capacity for benzo[a]pyrene diol-epoxide and UV light-induced DNA damage was greatly compromised in cells treated with HNE.

3.2.2 Genotoxicity and mutagenicity of HNE in colon cancer

Comet assay demonstrated that HNE, at concentration higher than 150 μM, displays a genotoxic effect in the colon carcinoma cell line HT-29 (Glei et al., 2006; Ebert et al., 2001; Knoll et al., 2005) and in HT29clone19A, a permanently differentiated sub-clone treated with sodium butyrate (Augeron & Laboisse, 1984). Moreover, such high doses of HNE were able to affect DNA integrity in primary human colon cells (Schaferhenrich et al., 2003; Glei et al., 2007) and in LT97, an established cell line derived from a differentiated microadenoma, representing a model of an early premalignant genotype, carrying adenomatous polyposis coli (APC) and Ki-ras mutated, but normal p53 (Richter et al., 2002), three well-characterized genes involved in coloncancer progression (Fearon et al., 1990).

Genotoxicity of HNE is higly dependent on cellular GSH level. Indeed, GSH depletion leads to and increase of HNE genotoxicity in the HT-29 colon carcinoma cell line (Knoll et al., 2005). Moreover, HNE displayed a higher genotoxicity in LT97 than in HT29clone19A and primary human colon cells. This result can be explained by the lower GST expression found in LT97 compared to HT29clone19A and primary human colon cells (Schaferhenrich et al., 2003).

Recently, by using a refined comet assay (Comet-FISH) (Glei et al., 2009), which combined the classical comet assay with the fluorescence in situ hybridisation, it has been demonstrated that HNE concentrations higher than 150 μM were able to affect DNA integrity on the p53 (Schaferhenrich et al., 2003; Glei et al., 2007), Ki-Ras and APC genes (Glei et al., 2007), in primary human colon cells and the colon adenoma cell LT97. After cell incubation with HNE, the p53 gene, the crucial target gene for the progression of adenoma to carcinoma, migrated more efficiently into the comet tail than the global DNA, indicating a high susceptibility of the p53 gene to HNE (Glei et al., 2007). Moreover, the TP53 gene sensitivity to the DNA damage induced by HNE was significantly higher with respect to APC and KRAS genes. This particular sensitivity is especially apparent in LT97 cells (Glei et al., 2007). This may be due to the fact that LT97 cells normally carry damaged APC and KRAS, but undamaged TP53 (Richter et al., 2002). In normal colonocytes, APC and KRAS were also sensitive to damage (Glei et al., 2007). These findings are highly interesting when considering the sequence of mutational events that occur during human colon carcinogenesis (Vogelstein et al., 1988). APC and KRAS mutations transform normal epithelial (stem) cells into initiated, more rapidly proliferating cells to yield dysplasia and small adenoma. TP53 mutations in adenoma are then crucial alterations leading to further progression and to carcinoma. Based on studies of Glei and collaborators (2007), it is possible to conclude that HNE could potentially contribute to both cancer initiation and progression in the colon, if produced in sufficient amounts. However, as mentioned in the previously chapter, it is unlikely that HNE is reaching such high concentrations (150 μM) in colon in vivo. Moreover it still remains to be studied to what extent the observed genotoxicity of HNE is related to mutagenicity. Consistent with this hypothesis, as previously reported, it has been demonstrated that 50 μM HNE treatment in human TK-6 lymphoblastoid cell line induces a high frequency of G.C to T.A mutations at the third base of codon 249 (AGG*) of the p53 gene (Hussain et al., 2000), a mutational hot spot in human cancers, particularly in hepatocellular carcinoma (Hsu et al., 1991). The adduct of HNE to codon 249 of the p53 gene has been also found by Hu and collaborators (2002). These authors exposed DNA of exons 5, 7 and 8 of human p53 gene, where the large majority of p53 mutations occur, to a very high concentration of HNE (192 mM or more). They identified two main HNE adducts, the first already mentioned at codon 249 (exon 7) and the second at codon 174 (exon 5) (Hu et al., 2002). However, the possible contribution of HNE to p53 mutations, through the formation of DNA adducts remains to demonstrated, since codon 249 and codon 174 of p53 usually are not mutated in colorectal rectal. Indeed, mutations at codon 175, 245, 248, 273, and 282 account for approximately 43% of all p53 mutations in CRC (Soong et al., 2000; Soussi et al., 2000; Soussi & Beroud, 2003).

3.2.3 HNE role in controlling cell proliferation, apoptosis of colon cancer cell

Several findings have been collected through the years related to the anti-proliferative and pro-apoptotic in colon cancer cells. These results, even obtained with very low doses of

HNE, easily reacheable in vivo, cast doubt on the pro-tumoral HNE role. 1 μM HNE is able to inhibit cell proliferation of Caco-2 and HT-29 colon cancer cells (Cerbone et al., 2007; Pizzimenti et al., 2010b; Vizio et al., 2005) and concentrations ranging form 1 to 100 μM are able to induce apoptosis in Caco-2, HT-29, RKO, HCT15 colon cancer cells. (see table I for references). A number of genes or cell signalling pathways have been found to be affected by HNE, and their modulation can explain the biological effects observed.

Results obtained in our laboratories demonstrated that the inhibition of proliferation in Caco-2 and HT-29 colon carcinoma cells by 1 μM HNE is sustained by the down-regulation of telomerase activity and hTERT expression, the catalytic subunit of telomerase (Pizzimenti et al., 2010b). The major mechanism of HNE action seems to be the modulation of expression and activity of transcription factors belonging to the Myc/Mad/Max network (Pizzimenti et al., 2010b).

After HNE treatment, apoptosis of several colon cancer cell lines was investigated by different authors and different pathways were considered to be involved. In Caco-2 human colon adenocarcinoma cell line, 1 μM HNE caused an increase of bax expression (Cerbone et al., 2007) and the apoptosis induction is mediated by JNK activation. Indeed, the HNE-mediated apoptotic cell death was significantly prevented by preincubating the cells with the selective JNK inhibitor SP600125 (Biasi et al., 2006).

Ji and collaborators investigated the mechanism of HNE-induced cell death in human colorectal carcinoma cells and found that HNE-induced apoptosis depends on alteration of mitochondrial function, leading to the release of cytochrome c and subsequent activation of caspase cascade (Ji et al., 2001a). The authors have further demonstrated that HNE inhibited IκB kinase activity by direct interaction with IκB kinase and suggested that HNE is an endogenous inhibitor of NF-κB activation that acts by preventing IκB kinase activation and subsequent IκB degradation (Ji et al., 2001b).

The molecular mechanism of HNE induced apoptosis was investigated in RKO colon cancer cells also. In this cell line, beside the pro-apoptotic stimuli, HNE activates the stress response pathways, that abrogate programmed cell death. Moreover, HNE elicits the nuclear translocation of HSF1 and promotes Hsp40 and Hsp72 expression (Jacobs & Marnett, 2007). The silencing of HSF1 sensitizes the colon cancer cells to HNE-induced apoptosis, through a mechanism involving the control of BCL-XL, BAG3 protein turnover (Jacobs & Marnett, 2007; Jacobs & Marnett, 2009)

3.2.4 HNE content in human colon cancers

Only a few studies have investigated the level of the lipid peroxidation products, in particular HNE, in human colon cancers and results are contradictory. It has been demonstrated that the levels of proteins modified by HNE and MDA in colorectal cancer tissues were significantly increased (Murawaki et al., 2008). By immunohystochemical analysis, Murawaki and collaborators (2008) have demonstrated that the proteins modified by HNE were stained diffusely in the cytoplasm of cancer cells, while they were weakly stained in normal tissues. Similar results have been obtained by Kondo and collaborators (1999). Immunostaining of HNE-histidine adducts was observed in the cytoplasm of colon cancer tissues. Immunoreactivity was also found in the cytosol of infiltrating inflammatory cells. Western blot analysis of HNE-histidine adducts confirmed the results, since larger amounts of modified proteins were detected in carcinomas than in nontumorous epithelial counterparts (Kondo et al., 1999). The authors also demonstrated that HNE content increased along with the progression of colorectal cancer, since tubular adenoma cells revealed a weaker staining, similar to the staining of non-tumorous epithelial cells (Kondo et al., 1999). An increase of HNE content in colon cancer tissues have been found also by Skrzydlewska and collaborators (2005). These authors analyzed the HNE content in homogenates of human colon cancer tissues, by measuring HNE as a fluorimetric derivative. These authors have demonstrated that the level of HNE was significantly increased ($P<0.001$) in cancer tissue compared to control group, with highest in G3-grade adenocarcinoma and mucinous adenocarcinoma and clinical IV stage of colorectal cancer.

In contrast with these results, other scientists demonstrated a decrease of HNE in colon cancer tissues. Indeed, it was demonstrated that HNE was significantly decreased in cancer specimens, with respect to normal tissues, by measuring the HNE content in tissue biopsies from patients with colon adenocarcinoma of different TNM and G stage (Biasi et al., 2002; Zanetti et al., 2003). This result was confirmed later by the same group (Biasi et al., 2006). Moreover, Chiarpotto and collaborators (1997) have demonstrated that the fluorescent adducts with plasma proteins and HNE were significantly lower in the plasma from cancer patients (all stage G3, pT3pN0) than in controls.

3.2.5 HNE metabolism in colon cancer

In colon cells, the enzymes of HNE metabolism are present. Staining with anti GST A4 specific antibodies revealed a significant expression of GST A4 in columnar and crypt epithelial cells of normal colon mucosae (Desmots et al., 2001), as well as in colon cancer cell lines (Scharmach et al., 2009; Knoll et al., 2005). Moreover, both the oxidative and reductive metabolisms of HNE are well represented in colon cells, since both ALDH or ADH have been found to be significantly expressed in colon mucosae (Seitz et al., 1996; Yin et al., 1994). The expression of AR is also enhanced in various forms of cancer, such as hepatoma (Zeindl-Eberhart et al., 1997) and melanoma cancer (Kawamura et al., 1999).

By affecting HNE metabolism enzymes, it is possibly to modulate the HNE concentration inside cells. This could be critical for cancer growth regulation or DNA genotoxicity. Indeed, butyrate, produced during gut fermentation, has a chemoprotective role toward HNE injury, when added at high concentration, such as 100-200 μM in HT-29 colon cancer cells (Knoll et al., 2005). The chemoprotective effect of butyrate seems to be related to the increasing the expression of glutathione S-transferases GSTP1 (Ebert et al., 2001) and hGSTA4-4 (Knoll et al., 2005) able to catalyze the conjugation of HNE with glutathione. Similar results were obtained in HT-29 cells by using two wheat bran-derived arabinoxylans, fermented under anaerobic conditions in human feces. These two fermentation products inhibited growth and reduced the genotoxicity of HNE (100-200 μM) via up-regulation of the activity of GSTs, in absence of a GSTP1 or hGSTA4-4 increase (Glei et al., 2006).

There is a growing interest in targeting aldose reductase (AR), as a novel therapeutic approach in preventing progression of colon cancer (Tammali et al., 2011). AR besides reducing aldo-sugars efficiently reduces toxic lipid aldehydes and their conjugates with glutathione (Tammali et al., 2006). Indeed, inhibition of AR by sorbinil or by antisense ablation, prevented FGF-induced and PDGF-induced proliferation of Caco-2 cells at S-phase (Tammali et al., 2006). Similar results were also obtained in other colon cancer cell lines, by Ramana and collaborators which show that the inhibition of AR prevents epidermal growth factor (EGF)- and basic fibroblast growth factor (bFGF)-induced HT29, and cell proliferation, by accumulating cells at the G1 phase of the cell cycle, through the AKT/Phosphoinositide 3-Kinase/E2F-1 pathway. Analogous results were obtained in SW480 and HCT-116 colon cancer cells (Ramana et al., 2010).

More interestingly, in vivo studies showed that administration of aldose reductase-small interfering RNA (siRNA), or the AR inhibitor fidarest, to nude mice bearing SW480 human colon adenocarcinoma cells, led to a complete arrest of tumor progression. Such evidence suggests a key role for aldose reductase in growth factor-induced proliferation in colon cancer cells and it points to inhibition of aldose reductase as a novel therapeutic approach in preventing progression of colon cancer (Tammali et al., 2006; Ramana et al., 2010).

Recently, the ATP-depent transporter RLIP76 (Ral binding protein1) has been considered for its role in controlling HNE content inside the cells. Indeed, it has been demonstrated that this transporter with multi-specific transport activity towards glutathione-conjugates and chemotherapeutic agents, is also specific for GSH-HNE (Sharma et al., 2002). The expulsion of GS-HNE from cells represents another critical step in HNE detoxification since it avoids the accumulation of adducted GSH and permits the restoration of GSH/GSSG equilibrium. RLIP76 protein is frequently overexpressed in cancer lesions (Vatsyayan et al., 2010), included colon cancers (Singhal et al., 2007), thus there is a growing interest in considering this protein as target in cancer therapy (Vatsyayan et al., 2010). When RLIP76 is inhibited, a rapid increase in HNE-GSH is observed, both in vitro (Awasthi et al., 2003; Cheng et al., 2001; Yang et al., 2003) and in vivo (Vatsyayan et al., 2010). Recent studies show that the inhibition and/or depletion of RLIP76 by antibodies, siRNA, or antisense can lead to a drastic and sustained regression of lung, kidney, melanoma, prostate, and colon cancer xenografts with no observed recurrence of tumors (Vatsyayan et al., 2010). In particular, it has been shown that xenografts of SW480 human colon cancer cells in nude mice can be completely regressed by anti-RalBP1 immunoglubulin G or by suppression of RalBP1 expression using phosphorothioate antisense against it (Singhal et al., 2007).

The super family of aldo-keto reductase (AKR) enzymes seems to be involved in tumor development, and growing evidence is accumulating, suggesting them as a new class of tumor marker. These enzymes are hydroxysteroid dehydrogenases with a broad substrate specificity for other carbonyl compounds including HNE. The isoform AKR1B10 seems to be particulary involved in the transformation of HNE to the oxidized counterpart 4-oxonon-2-enal (4-ONE) (Martin et al., 2009). AKR1B10 is also up-regulated in many types of solid tumors (Fukumoto et al., 2005; Yoshitake et al., 2007; Breton et al., 2008; Satow et al., 2010), and its gene silencing results in growth inhibition of colorectal cancer cells (Yan et al., 2007), as well as in increasing HNE-elicited cell death (Matsunaga et al., 2011).

Recently, some family members of AKR enzymes have been shown to be overexpressed and linked to resistance against anticancer drugs such as anthracyclines, cisplatin, and methotrexate (Veitch et al., 2009; Cheng al., 2008; Selga et al., 2008). As regarding colon cancer, experimental data suggest that the up-regulation of AKR1B10 was related with acquisition of resistance to the anticancer drug mitomycin-c (MMC) in HT-29 colon cancer cells (Matsunaga et al., 2011). The cytotoxic effects of MMC seems to be mediated by the formation of HNE. Thus, the biological significance of the increasing of AKR1B10 in MCC resistant cancer cells would be an ability to better detoxify cytotoxic aldehydes including HNE. (Matsunaga et al., 2011). In the resistant cells, treatment with an AKR1B10 inhibitor decreased their MMC tolerance (Matsunaga et al., 2011), suggesting its use as adjuvant therapy in drug resistant cells, in which AKR1B10 is over-expressed.

Many dietary cancer chemopreventive compounds, such as cruciferous vegetables, could activate the antioxidant responsive element (ARE), a critical regulatory element in the promoter sequence of genes encoding cellular Phase II detoxifying and antioxidant enzymes. Transcriptional activation of ARE is typically mediated by the transcription Nuclear factor-erythroid 2-related factor 2 (Nrf2). Thus, this transcription factor has emerged as a novel target for the prevention of colon cancer (Saw & Kong, 2011). However, stable RNAi-mediated knockdown of Nrf2 in human colon cancer cells suppressed tumor growth in mouse xenograft settings and colon tumor angiogenesis by inhibiting Hypoxia-Induced Activation of HIF-1a (Kim et al., 2011). Thus, the role of Nfr2 in colon carcinogenesis still has to be explored.

3.2.6 HNE and nutrition

It is well accepted that development and progression of colon cancer is generally associated with lifestyle-dependent risk factors, such as dietary choices (Pearson et al., 2009). HNE can be directly found in food (Gasc et al., 2007) or its production can be enhanced by the presence of some nutrients, i.e. ω-6 PUFAs, or some fermentation products of diet, i.e. butyrate, can modulate the metabolism of this aldehyde, thus modifying its concentration. In this context, it is very interesting to explore the connection between HNE, nutrition and colon carcinogenesis.

HNE has been founded in different foods, correlating with the amount of ω-6 (Surh et al., 2010). UsingGC-MS technology, scientists measured 4-hydroxy-alkenaks content in vegetable oils, fish and shellfish, calculating the HNE dietary intake of the Korean population (Surh et al., 2005). Korean daily exposure to 4-hydroxy- 2-alkenals was found to be of 4.3 mg/day and HNE was found to be more represented (2.7 mg). There was an additional exposure to more than 11.8 mg/day 4-hydroxy-2-alkenal from fried foods. The combined exposure would be, therefore, 16.1 mg/day corresponding to 0.3 mg/kg body weight/day for a 60 kg Korean adult. Additionally, the screening of PUFA-fortified foods including infant formulas and baby foods commercially available on the Korean markets were screened, and it was estimated that 3- month to 1-year-old babies sticking exclusively to these products could be exposed to a maximum 20.2 μg/kg BW/ day of 4-hydroxy-2-alkenals (Surh et al., 2007). However, in spite of the biological toxicity of 4-hydroxy-2-alkenals, the risk for humans cannot be quantified due to the lack of a virtually safe dose of the compound (Surh et al., 2005).

A diet high in red and processed meats can increase colon cancer risk by 12–20%. The mechanism of promotion by haem iron is not known, but may be linked to oxidative stress and subsequent events such as lipid pro-oxidation and HNE production (Sesink et al., 1999; Sawa et al., 1998). Indeed, the dietary haem, in the form of either haemoglobin or meat, promotes precancerous lesions, aberrant crypt foci (ACF) and mucin-depleted foci in the colon of rats (Pierre et al., 2003; Pierre et al., 2004). This haem-induced promotion was associated with increased lipid peroxidation in faecal water and strong cytotoxycity activity of faecal water on the cancerous colonic epithelial cell line (Pierre et al., 2003). Further, Pierre and collaborators (2007), have explored the effect of faecal water components of haem-fed rats, on normal APC +/+ or premalignant APC -/+ cells, demonstrating that the toxic effects observed correlated with the presence of HNE in the faeces. Moreover, the premalignat APC -/+ cells were more resistant to apoptosis with respect to normal APC +/+. The authors suggested, thus, that the premalignant mutation confer to cells the resistance to the inhibitory signal, allowing them to undergo further mutations and follow a tumoural pathway (Pierre et al., 2007).

In a randomized human study, the urinary excretion of DHN-MA, the major metabolite of HNE detectable in urine was compared in volunteers consuming different levels of heme iron. The volunteers fed with a low red meat diet (60 g/day) showed a twofold increase of DHN-MA when supplemented with heme iron as blood sausage (70 g/day). Since colon preneoplastic lesions and DHN-MA excretion in the experimental animal were clearly associated with dietary heme iron, urinary DHN-MA was suggested as a promising biomarker of colon carcinogenesis (Pierre et al., 2006).

The role of fat present in the diet in coloncarcinogenesis has been explored by several authors and comprehensive reviews have been published. In particular, diets rich in ω-6 PUFAs, contained in vegetable oils, seem to enhance the development of colon tumors, whereas ω-3 PUFA-containing diets, such as fish oil, reduce colon cancer incidence (Reddy, 2002; Kim & Milner, 2007). Thus, it is possible to suggest a putative HNE role in colon carcinogenesis, since HNE is derived from peroxidation of ω-6. However, the complexity of the issue forces us to be more cautious. Indeed, Eder and collaborators investigated the impact of different fatty-acids composition in the diet on cancer development, measuring the formation of the promutagenic HNE-dG in the mucosa of several organs, such as colon. The correlation between adduct levels and the different fatty acids assumption was not uniform for all organs and they didn't find a clear relationship between fatty acids and adduct levels in the colon (Eder et al., 2008). Moreover, beside lipid peroxidation products it is necessary to consider the eicosanoids, also derived from PUFAs. Indeed, eicosanoids have different properties in cancer cell growth, invasion and angiogenesis when derived from ω-6 or ω-3 fatty acids (Berquim et al., 2008), thus suggesting a role in carcinogenesis.

Epidemiological studies show a reduction in risk for individuals and populations consuming high amounts of vegetables. The protective effect of vegetables may be due to their content of complex carbohydrates such as dietary fiber and starch (Scheppach et al., 1999). A substantial amount of starch escapes digestion in the small intestine (Englyst et al., 1992) and this fraction is called enzyme-resistant starch (RS). Starch and dietary fiber together are the principal substrates controlling the pattern of fermentation in the colon and, thus, the metabolism of compounds, like bile acids, nitrate and enzyme activityes (bacterial and antioxidant enzymes), which have been implicated in carcinogenesis. The effect of enzyme-resistant starch (RS) on the development of colon cancer was reported to include both chemopreventive and tumorigenic activity in humans. Indeed, an inverse association between starch consumption and large bowel cancer incidence has been found in an international comparison in 12 populations worldwide (Cassidy et al., 1994). However, an increased cancer risk with high-starch intake has been also reported (Franceschi et al., 1998; Favero et al., 1999). Wacker and collaborators (2002) have studied the number of 1,N2-propanodeoxyguanosine-30- monophosphate (HNE-dGp) adducts in the colonic mucosa of volunteers fed with starchy foods enriched with a highly resistant amylomaize starch (Hylon VII) and they found an increase of the HNE-dGp adduct, whereas there was no evidence for an increased cell proliferation in the upper crypt.

Finally, as already mentioned, nutrients can modulate the HNE level in the colon, by affecting its metabolism. This is the case of fermented products of diet, such as butyrate (Knoll et al., 2005; Glei et al., 2006) and wheat bran-derived arabinoxylans, that can affect the HNE levels, by upregulating GSTs activities.

4. Conclusion

Lipid peroxidation is a physiological and pathological process that elicits a number of electrophilic compounds able to modulate several cellular processes. Among these, HNE is the most studied aldehyde, due to its high biological activity. Since HNE is a normal constituent of the diet or can be produced in the gut, colon cells can be exposed to this aldehyde.

Low doses of HNE are able to inhibit cell proliferation and induce differentiation of colon cancer cells. Conversely, a high concentration of HNE exhibits genotoxic and mutagenic activity. We believe that the concentration of HNE and other lipid peroxidation products in the colon, represent a steady state level between production and catabolism. The alteration of this equilibrium elicits a stress condition for colon cells and, possibly, could be involved in colon carcinogenesis, although there is no scientific consensus in supporting its pro-tumoral action.

Results on HNE content in human biopsies of coloncancer tissues are contradictory, and the positive correlation between HNE content and cancer progression doesn't allow an assumption whether the HNE increase during the progression of colon cancer may represent a cause or a consequence of this process. However, in colon cancer cells, HNE induces apoptosis and telomerase inhibition. Thus, we can hypothesize that HNE, produced during radiotherapy or chemotherapy, can participate to the control of tumor growth and tumor cell death.

5. References

Acharya, A., Das, I., Chandhok, D. & Saha, T. (2010). Redox regulation in cancer: a double-edged sword with therapeutic potential. Oxidative Medicine and Cellular Longevity, Vol.3, No.1, (January 2010), pp. 23-34, ISSN 1942-0900

Alary, J., Debrauwer, L., Fernandez, Y., Cravedi, J.P., Rao D. & Bories, G. (1998). 1,4-Dihydroxynonene mercapturic acid, the major end metabolite of exogenous 4-hydroxy-2-nonenal, is a physiological component of rat and human urine. Chemical Research in Toxicology, Vol. 11, No.2, (February 1998), pp. 130–135, ISSN 0893-228X

Alary, J., Gueraud, F. & Cravedi, J.P. (2003). Fate of 4-hydroxynonenal in vivo: Disposition and metabolic pathways. Molecular Aspects in Medicine, Vol.24, No.4-5, (August-October 2003), pp. 177–187, ISSN 0098-2997

Augeron, C. & Laboisse C.L. (1984). Emergence of permanently differentiated cell clones in a human colonic cancer cell line in culture after treatment with sodium butyrate. Cancer Research, Vol.44, No.9, (September 1984), pp. 3961–3969, ISSN 0008-5472

Awasthi, S., Singhal, S.S., Singhal, J., Yang, Y., Zimniak, P. & Awasthi, Y.C. (2003). Role of RLIP76 in lung cancer doxorubicin resistance: III. Anti-RLIP76 antibodies trigger apoptosis in lung cancer cells and synergistically increase doxorubicin cytotoxicity. International Journal of Oncology, Vol.22, No.4, (April 2003), pp. 721–732, ISSN 1019-6439

Awasthi, Y.C., Sharma, R., Sharma, A., Yadav, S., Singhal, S.S., Chaudhary, P. & Awasthi, S. (2008). Self-regulatory role of 4-hydroxynonenal in signaling for stress-induced programmed cell death. Free Radical Biology & Medicine, Vol.45, No.2, (July 2008), pp. 111-118, ISSN 0891-5849

Ayalasomayajula, S.P. & Kompella, U.B. (2002), Induction of vascular endothelial growth factor by 4-hydroxynonenal and its prevention by glutathione precursors in retinal pigment epithelial cells. European Journal of Pharmacology, Vol.449, No.3, (August 2002), pp. 213-220, ISSN 0014-2999

Baler, R., Dahl, G., & Voellmy, R. (1993). Activation of human heat shock genes is accompanied by oligomerization, modification, and rapid translocation of heat shock transcription factor HSF. Molecular and Cellular Biology, Vol.13, No.4, (April 1993), pp. 2486–2496, ISSN 0270-7306

Balogh, L.M. & Atkins, W.M. (2011). Interactions of glutathione transferases with 4-hydroxynonenal. Drug Metabolism Review, Vol.43, No.2, (May 2011), pp.165-178, ISSN 0360-2532

Barrera, G., Martinotti, S., Fazio, V., Manzari, V., Paradisi, L., Parola, M., Frati, L. & Dianzani, M.U. (1987). Effect of 4-hydroxynonenal on c-myc expression. Toxicologic Pathology, Vol.15, No.2, (1987), pp. 238-240, ISSN 0192-6233

Barrera, G., Di Mauro, C., Muraca, R., Ferrero, D., Cavalli, G., Fazio, V.M., Paradisi, L. & Dianzani, M.U. (1991). Induction of differentiation in human HL-60 cells by 4-hydroxynonenal.; a product of lipid peroxidation. Experimental Cell Research, Vol.197, No.2, (December 1991), pp. 148-152, ISSN 0014-4827

Bartel, D.P. (2004). MicroRNAs: genomics, biogenesis, mechanism, and function. Cell, Vol.116, No.2, (January 2004), pp. 281–297, ISSN 0092-8674

Bartsch, H. & Nair, J. (2005). Accumulation of lipid peroxidation-derived DNA lesions: potential lead markers for chemoprevention of inflammation-driven malignancies. Mutation Research, Vol.591, No.1-2, (December 2005), pp. 34-44, ISSN 0027-5107

Berquin, I.M., Edwards, I.J. & Chen, Y.Q. (2008). Multi-targeted therapy of cancer by omega-3 fatty acids. Cancer Letters, Vol.269, No.2, (October 2008), pp.363-377, ISSN 0304-3835

Biasi, F., Tessitore, L., Zanetti, D., Cutrin, J.C., Zingaro, B., Chiarpotto, E., Zarkovic, N., Serviddio, G. & Poli G. (2002). Associated changes of lipid peroxidation and transforming growth factor beta1 levels in human colon cancer during tumour progression. Gut, Vol.50, No.3, (March 2002), pp.361-367, ISSN 0017-5749

Biasi, F., Vizio, B., Mascia, C., Gaia, E., Zarkovic, N., Chiarpotto, E., Leonarduzzi, G. & Poli G. (2006). c-Jun N-terminal kinase upregulation as a key event in the proapoptotic interaction between transforming growth factor-beta1 and 4-hydroxynonenal in colon mucosa. Free Radical Biology & Medicine, Vol.41, No.3, (August. 2006), pp.443-54, ISSN 0891-5849

Boon, P.J., Marinho, H.S., Oosting, R. & Mulder, G.J. (1999). Glutathione conjugation of 4-hydroxytrans-2,3-nonenal in the rat in vivo, the isolated perfused liver and erythrocytes. Toxicology and Applied Pharmacology, Vol.159, No.3, (September 1999), pp.214–223, ISSN 0041-008X

Breton, J., Gage, M.C., Hay, A.W., Keen, J.N., Wild, C.P., Donnellan C, Findlay, J.B. & Hardie, L.J. (2008). Proteomic screening of a cell line model of esophageal carcinogenesis identifies cathepsin D and aldo-keto reductase 1C2 and 1B10 dysregulation in Barrett's esophagus and esophageal adenocarcinoma. Journal of Proteome Research, Vol.7, No.5 (May 2008), pp.1953–1962, ISSN 1535-3893

Cajelli, E., Ferraris, A. & Brambilla, G. (1987). Mutagenicity of 4-hydroxynonenal in V79 Chinese hamster cells. Mutation Research, Vol.190, No.2, (February 1987), pp.169-171, ISSN 0027-5107

Calonghi, N., Boga, C., Cappadone, C., Pagnotta, E., Bertucci, C., Fiori, J. & Masotti, L. (2002). Cytotoxic and cytostatic effects induced by 4-hydroxynonenal in human osteosarcoma cells. Biochemical Biophysical Research Communcations, Vol.293, No.5, (May 2002), pp.1502-1507, ISSN 0006-291X

Canuto, R.A., Muzio, G., Ferro, M., Maggiora, M., Federa, R., Bassi, A.M., Lindahl, R. & Dianzani, M.U. (1999). Inhibition of class-3 aldehyde dehydrogenase and cell growth by restored lipid peroxidation in hepatoma cell lines. Free Radical Biology & Medicine, Vol.26, No.3-4, (February 1999), pp. 333-340, ISSN 0891-5849

Cassidy, A., Bingham, S. & Cummings, J. (1994). Starch intake and colorectal cancer risk: an international comparison. British Journal of Cancer, Vol.69, No.5, (May 1994), pp. 937-942, ISSN 0007-0920

Cerbone, A., Toaldo, C., Laurora, S., Briatore, F., Pizzimenti, S., Dianzani, M.U., Ferretti, C. & Barrera G. (2007). 4-Hydroxynonenal and PPARgamma ligands affect proliferation, differentiation, and apoptosis in colon cancer cells. Free Radical Biology & Medicine, Vol. 42, No.11, (June 2007), pp.1661-1670, ISSN 0891-5849

Chandramathi, S., Suresh, K., Anita, Z.B. & Kuppusamy, U.R. (2009). Comparative assessment of urinary oxidative indices in breast and colorectal cancer patients. Journal of Cancer Research and Clinical Oncology, Vol.135, No.2, (February 2009), pp.319–323, ISSN 0171-5216

Chen, J., Adikari, M., Pallai, R., Parekh, H.K. & Simpkins, H. (2008). Dihydrodiol dehydrogenases regulate the generation of reactive oxygen species and the development of cisplatin resistance in human ovarian carcinoma cells. Cancer Chemotherapy and Pharmacology, Vol.61, No.6, (May 2008), pp.979–987, ISSN 0344-5704

Cheng, J.Z., Singhal, S.S., Saini, M., Singhal, J., Piper, J.T., Van Kuijk, F.J., Zimniak, P., Awasthi, Y.C. & Awasthi, S. (1999). Effects of mGST A4 transfection on 4-hydroxynonenal-mediated apoptosis and differentiation of K562 human erythroleukemia cells. Archives of Biochemistry and Biophysics, Vol.372, No.1, (December 1999), pp. 29-36, ISSN 0003-9861

Cheng, J.Z., Sharma, R., Yang, Y., Singhal, S.S., Sharma, A., Saini, M.K., Singh, S.V., Zimniak, P., Awasthi, S. & Awasthi, Y,C. (2001). Accelerated metabolism and exclusion of 4-hydroxy-nonenal through induction of RLIP76 and hGST5.8 is an early adaptive response of cells to heat and oxidative stress. The Journal of Biological Chemistry, Vol.276, No.44, (November 2001), pp.41213–41223, ISSN 0021-9258

Chiarpotto, E., Scavazza, A., Leonarduzzi, G., Camandola, S., Biasi, F., Teggia, P.M., Garavoglia, M., Robecchi, A., Roncari, A. & Poli, G. (1997). Oxidative damage and transforming growth factor beta 1 expression in pretumoral and tumoral lesions of human intestine. Free Radical Biology & Medicine, Vol.22, No.5, (1997), pp.889-894, ISSN 0891-5849

Chung, F.L., Chen, H.J., Guttenplan, J.B., Nishikawa, A. & Hard, G.C. (1993). 2,3-epoxy-4-hydroxynonanal as a potential tumor-initiating agent of lipid peroxidation. Carcinogenesis, Vol.14, No.10, (October 1993), pp. 2073-2077, ISSN 0143-3334

Chung, F.L., Nath, R.G., Nagao, M., Nishikawa, A., Zhou, G.D. & Randerath, K. (1999). Endogenous formation and significance of 1,N2-propanodeoxyguanosine adducts. Mutation Research, Vol. 424, No.1-2, (March 1999), pp.71-78, ISSN 0027-5107

Chung, F.L., Nath, R.G., Ocando, J., Nishikawa, A. & Zhang, L. (2000). Deoxyguanosine adducts of t-4-hydroxy-2-nonenal are endogenous DNA lesions in rodents and humans: detection and potential sources. Cancer Research, Vol.60, No.6, (March 2000), pp.1507-1511, ISSN 0008-5472

Chung, F.L., Chen, H.J. & Nath, R.G. (1996). Lipid peroxidation as a potential endogenous source for the formation of exocyclic DNA adducts. Carcinogenesis, Vol.17, No.10, (October 1996), pp.:2105-2111, ISSN 0143-3334

Curzio M. (1988). Interaction between neutrophils and 4-hydroxyalkenals and consequences on neutrophil motility. Free Radical Research Communications, Vol.5, No.2, (1988), pp.55-66, ISSN 8755-0199

De Bont, R. & van Larebeke, N. (2004). Endogenous DNA damage in humans: a review of quantitative data. Mutagenesis, Vol.19, No.3, (May 2004), pp.169-185, ISSN 0267-8357

Desmots, F., Rissel, M., Loyer, P., Turlin, B. & Guillouzo, A. (2001). Immunohistological analysis of glutathione transferase A4 distribution in several human tissues using a specific polyclonal antibody. Journal of Histochemistry and Cytochemistry, Vol.49, No.12, (December 2001), pp.1573-1580, ISSN 0022-1554

Dianzani, M.U. (1993). Lipid peroxidation and cancer. Critical Reviews in Oncology/Hematology, Vol.15, No.2, (October 1993), pp.125-147, ISSN 1040-8428

Dianzani, M.U., Barrera, G. & Parola, M. (1999). 4-Hydroxy-2,3-nonenal as a signal for cell function and differentiation. Acta Biochimica Polonica, Vol.46, No.1, (1999), pp.61-75, ISSN 0001-527X

Dianzani, M.U. (2003). 4-hydroxynonenal from pathology to physiology. Molecular Aspects in Medicine, Vol.24, No.4-5, (August-October 2003), pp.263-272, ISSN 0098-2997

Douki, T., Odin, F., Caillat, S., Favier, A. & Cadet, J. (2004). Predominance of the 1,N2-propano 20-deoxyguanosine adduct among 4-hydroxy-2-nonenal-induced DNA lesions. Free Radical Biology & Medicine, Vol. 37, No.1, (July 2004), pp.62-70, ISSN 0891-5849

Ebert, M.N., Beyer-Sehlmeyer, G., Liegibel, U.M., Kautenburger, T., Becker, T.W. & Pool-Zobel B.L. (2001). Butyrate induces glutathione S-transferase in human colon cells and protects from genetic damage by 4-hydroxy-2-nonenal. Nutrition and Cancer, Vol.41, No.1-2, (2001), pp.156-164, ISSN 0163-5581

Eckl, P.M. (2003). Genotoxicity of HNE. Molecular Aspects in Medicine, Vol.24, No.4-5, (August-October 2003), pp.161-165, ISSN 0098-2997

Eder, E., Wacker, M., Lutz, U., Nair, J., Fang, X., Bartsch, H., Beland, F.A., Schlatter, J. & Lutz, W.K. (2006). Oxidative stress related DNA adducts in the liver of female rats fed with sunflower-, rapeseed-, olive- or coconut oil supplemented diets. Chemico-Biological Interactions, Vol.159, No.2, (February 2006), pp. 81-89, ISSN 0009-2797

Emerit, I., Khan, S.H. & Esterbauer H. (1991). Hydroxynonenal, a component of clastogenic factors? Free Radical Biology & Medicine, Vol.10, No.6, (1991), pp.371-377. ISSN 0891-5849

Englyst, H.N., Kingman, S.M. & Cummings, J.H. (1992). Classification and measurement of nutritionally important starch fractions. European Journal of Clinical Nutrition, Vol. Suppl 2:S, (October 1992), pp.33-50, ISSN 0954-3007

Esterbauer, H., Cheeseman, K.H., Dianzani, M.U., Poli, G. & Slater, T.F. (1982). Separation and characterization of the aldehydic products of lipid peroxidation stimulated by ADP-Fe2+ in rat liver microsomes. Biochemical Journal, Vol.208, No.1, (October 1982), pp.129-140, ISSN 0264-6021

Esterbauer, H., Schaur, R.J. & Zollner, H. (1991). Chemistry and biochemistry of 4-hydroxynonenal, malonaldehyde and related aldehydes. Free Radical Biology & Medicine, Vol.11, No.1, (1991), pp. 81-128, ISSN 0891-5849

Falletti, O. & Douki, T. (2008). Low glutathione level favors formation of DNA adducts to 4-hydroxy-2(E)-nonenal, a major lipid peroxidation product. Chemical Research in Toxicology, Vol.21, No.11, (November 2008), pp.2097-2105, ISSN 0893-228X

Favero, A., Parpinel, M. & Montella, M. (1999). Energy sources and risk of cancer of the breast and colon-rectum in Italy. Advances in Experimental Medicine and Biology, Vol.472, (1999), pp. 51-55, ISSN 0065-2598

Fazio, V.M., Barrera, G., Martinotti, S., Farace, M.G., Giglioni, B., Frati, L., Manzari, V. & Dianzani, M.U. (1992). 4-Hydroxynonenal, a product of cellular lipid peroxidation, which modulates c-myc and globin gene expression in K562 erythroleukemic cells. Cancer Research, Vol.52, No.18, (September 1992), pp.4866-4871. ISSN 0008-5472

Fearon, E.R. & Vogelstein, B. (1990). A genetic model for colorectal tumorigenesis. Cell, Vol.61, No.5, (June 1990), pp.759-767, ISSN 0092-8674

Feng, Z.H., Hu, W.W., Amin, S. & Tang, M.S. (2003). Mutational spectrum and genotoxicity of the major lipid peroxidation product, trans-4-hydroxy-2-nonenal, induced DNA adducts in nucleotide excision repairproficient and -deficient human cells. Biochemistry, Vol.42, No.25, (July 2003), pp.7848-7854, ISSN 0006-2960

Feng, Z., Hu, W. & Tang, M.S. (2004). Trans-4-hydroxy-2-nonenal inhibits nucleotide excision repair in human cells: a possible mechanism for lipid peroxidation-induced carcinogenesis. Proceedings of the National Academy of Sciences of the United States of America, Vol.101, No.23, (June 2004), pp.8598-8602, ISSN 0027-8424

Fernandes, P.H., Wang, H., Rizzo, C.J. & Lloyd, R.S. (2003). Site-specific mutagenicity of stereochemically defined 1,N-2-deoxyguanosine adducts of trans-4-hydroxynonenal in mammalian cells. Environmental and Molecular Mutagenesis, Vol.42, No.2, (2003), pp.68-74, ISSN 0893-6692

Forman, H.J., Fukuto, J.M., Miller, T., Zhang, H., Rinna, A. & Levy, S. (2008).The chemistry of cell signaling by reactive oxygen and nitrogen species and 4-hydroxynonenal. Archives of Biochemistry and Biophysics, Vol.477, No,2, (September 2008), pp.183-195, ISSN 0003-9861

Franceschi, S., La Vecchia, C., Russo, A., Favero, A., Negri, E., Conti, E., Montella, M., Filiberti, R., Amadori, D. & Decarli, A. (1998). Macronutrient intake and risk of colorectal cancer in Italy. International Journal of Cancer, Vol.76, No.3, (May 1998), pp.321-324, ISSN 0020-7136

Fukumoto, S., Yamauchi, N., Moriguchi, H., Hippo, Y., Watanabe, A., Shibahara, J., Taniguchi, H., Ishikawa, S., Ito, H., Yamamoto, S., Iwanari, H., Hironaka, M.,

Ishikawa, Y., Niki, T., Sohara, Y., Kodama, T., Nishimura, M., Fukayama, M., Dosaka-Akita, H. & Aburatani, H. (2005).

Overexpression of the aldo-keto reductase family protein AKR1B10 is highly correlated with smokers' non-small cell lung carcinomas. Clinical Cancer Research, Vol.11, No.5, (March 2005), pp.1776-1785, ISSN 1078-0432

Gasc, N., Taché, S., Rathahao, E., Bertrand-Michel, J., Roques, V. & Guéraud, F. (2007). 4-hydroxynonenal in foodstuffs: heme concentration, fatty acid composition and freeze-drying are determining factors. Redox Report, Vol.12, No.1, (2007), pp.40-44, ISSN 1351-0002

Gentile, F., Pizzimenti, S., Arcaro, A., Pettazzoni, P., Minelli, R., D'Angelo, D., Mamone, G., Ferranti, P., Toaldo, C., Cetrangolo, G., Formisano, S., Dianzani, M.U., Uchida, K., Dianzani, C. & Barrera, G. (2009). Exposure of HL-60 human leukaemic cells to 4-hydroxynonenal promotes the formation of adduct(s) with alpha-enolase devoid of plasminogen binding activity. Biochemical Journal, Vol.422, No.2, (August 2009), pp.285-294, ISSN 0264-6021

Glei, M., Hofmann, T., Küster, K., Hollmann, J., Lindhauer, M.G. & Pool-Zobel B.L. (2006) Both wheat (Triticum aestivum) bran arabinoxylans and gut flora-mediated fermentation products protect human colon cells from genotoxic activities of 4-hydroxynonenal and hydrogen peroxide. Journal of Agricultural and Food Chemistry, Vol.54, No.6, (March 2006), pp.2088-2095, ISSN 0021-8561

Glei, M., Schaeferhenrich, A., Claussen, U., Kuechler, A., Liehr, T., Weise, A., Marian, B., Sendt, W. & Pool-Zobel B.L. (2007). Comet fluorescence in situ hybridization analysis for oxidative stress-induced DNA damage in colon cancer relevant genes. Toxicological Sciences, Vol.96, No.2 (April 2007), pp. 279-284, ISSN 1096-6080

Glei, M., Hovhannisyan, G. & Pool-Zobel, B.L. (2009) Use of Comet-FISH in the study of DNA damage and repair: review. Mutation Research, Vol.681, No.1, (January-February 2009), pp.33-43, ISSN 0027-5107

Glinghammar, B., Venturi, M., Rowland, I.R. & Rafter, J.J. (1997). Shift from a dairy product-rich to a dairy product-free diet: influence on cytotoxicity and genotoxicity of fecal water—potential risk factors for colon cancer. American Journal of Clinical Nutrition, Vol.66, No.5, (November 1997), pp. 1277-1282, ISSN 0002-9165

Grune, T., Siems, W., Kowalewski, J., Zollner, H. & Esterbauer H. (1991). Identification of metabolic pathways of the lipid peroxidation product 4-hydroxynonenal by enterocytes of rat small intestine. Biochemical International, Vol.25, No.5, (December 1991), pp.963-971, ISSN 0158-5231

Gupta, A., Bhatt, M.L. & Misra, M.K. (2009). Lipid peroxidation and antioxidant status in head and neck squamous cell carcinoma patients. Oxidative Medicine and Cellular Longevity, Vol.2 , No.2, (April-June 2009), pp.68-72, ISSN 1942-0900

Hahn, G.M. & Li, G.C. (1982). Thermotolerance and heat shock proteins in mammalian cells. Radiation Research, Vol.92, No.3, (December 1982), pp.452-457, ISSN 0033-7587

Halliwell, B. (2007). Oxidative stress and cancer: have we moved forward? Biochemical Journal, Vol.401, No.1, (January 2007), pp.1-11, ISSN 0264-6021

Hartley, D.P, Ruth, J.A. & Petersen, D.R. (1995). The hepatocellular metabolism of 4-hydroxynonenal by alcohol dehydrogenase, aldehyde dehydrogenase, and glutathione S-transferas,. Archives of Biochemistry and Biophysics, Vol.316, No.1, (January 1995), pp.197-205, ISSN 0003-9861

Harvey, C.J., Thimmulappa, R.K., Singh, A., Blake, D.J., Ling, G., Wakabayashi, N., Fujii, J., Myers, A. & Biswal, S. (2009). Nrf2-regulated glutathione recycling independent of biosynthesis is critical for cell survival during oxidative stress. Free Radical Biology and Medicine, Vol.46, No.4, (Febraury 2009), pp.443-453, ISSN 0891-5849

Hassane, D.C., Guzman, M.L., Corbett, C., Li, X., Abboud, R., Young, F., Liesveld, J.L.,Carroll, M. & Jordan, C.T. (2008). Discovery of agents that eradicate leukemia stem cells using an in silico screen of public gene expression data. Blood, Vol.111, No.12, (June 2008), pp.5654-5662, ISSN 0006-4971

Howard, M.K., Burke, L.C., Mailhos, C., Pizzey, A., Gilbert, C.S., Lawson, W.D., Collins, M.K., Thomas, N.S. & Latchman, D.S. (1993). Cell cycle arrest of proliferating neuronal cells by serum deprivation can result in either apoptosis or differentiation. Journal of Neurochemistry, Vol.60, No.5, (May 1993), pp.1783-1791, ISSN 0022-3042

Hsu, I.C., Metcalf, R.A., Sun, T., Welsh, J.A., Wang, N.J. & Harris, C.C. (1991). Mutational hotspot in the p53 gene in human hepatocellular carcinomas. Nature, Vol.350, No.6317, (April 1991), pp.427-428, ISSN 0028-0836

Hu, W., Feng, Z., Eveleigh, J., Lyer, G., Pan, J., Amin, S., Chung, F.T. & Tang, M.S. (2002). The major lipid peroxidation product, trans-4-hydroxy-2-nonenal, preferentially forms DNA adducts at codon 249 of human p53 gene, a unique mutational hotspot in hepatocellular carcinoma. Carcinogenesis, Vol.23, No.11, (November 2008), pp.1781-1789, ISSN 0143-3334

Huang, Y.L., Sheu, J.Y. & Lin, T.H. (1999). Association between oxidative stress and changes of trace elements in patients with breast cancer. Clinical Biochemistry, Vol.32, No.2, (March 1999), pp.131-136, ISSN 0009-9120

Hussain, S.P., Raja, K., Amstad, P.A., Sawyer, M., Trudel, L.J., Wogan, G.N., Hofseth, L.J., Shields, P.G., Billiar, T.R., Trautwein, C., Hohler, T., Galle, P.R., Phillips, D.H., Markin, R., Marrogi, A.J. & Harris, C.C. (2000). Increased p53 mutation load in nontumorous human liver of wilson disease and hemochromatosis: oxyradical overload diseases. Proceedings of the National Academy of Sciences of the United States of America, Vol.97, No.23, (November 2000), pp.12770-12775, ISSN 0027-8424

Isom, A.L., Barnes, S., Wilson, L., Kirk, M., Coward, L. & Darley-Usmar, V. (2004). Modification of Cytochrome c by 4-hydroxy- 2-nonenal: evidence for histidine, lysine, and arginine-aldehyde adducts. Journal of The American Society for Mass Spectrometry, Vol.15, No.8, (August 2004), pp.1136-1147, ISSN 1044-0305

Jacobs, A.T. & Marnett, L.J. (2007). Heat shock factor 1 attenuates 4-Hydroxynonenal-mediated apoptosis: critical role for heat shock protein 70 induction and stabilization of Bcl-XL. The Journal of Biological Chemistry, Vol.282, No.46, (November 2007), pp.33412-33420, ISSN 0021-9258

Jacobs, A.T. & Marnett, L.J. (2009). HSF1-mediated BAG3 expression attenuates apoptosis in 4-hydroxynonenal-treated colon cancer cells via stabilization of anti-apoptotic Bcl-2 proteins. The Journal of Biological Chemistry, Vol.284, No.14, (April 2009), pp.9176-9183, ISSN 0021-9258

Ji, C., Amarnath, V., Pietenpol, J.A. & Marnett, L.J. (2001a). 4-hydroxynonenal induces apoptosis via caspase-3 activation and cytochrome c release. Chemical Research in Toxicology, Vol.14, No.8, (August 2001), pp.1090-1096, ISSN 0893-228X

Ji, C., Kozak, K.R. & Marnett, L.J. (2001b). IkappaB kinase, a molecular target for inhibition by 4-hydroxy-2-nonenal. The Journal of Biological Chemistry, Vol.276, No.21, (May 2001), pp.18223-18228, ISSN 0021-9258

Kakishita, H. & Hattori, Y. (2001).Vascular smooth muscle cell activation and growth by 4-hydroxynonenal. Life Sciences, Vol.69, No.6, (June 2001), pp.689-97, ISSN 0024-3205

Karihtala, P., Kauppila, S., Puistola, U. & Jukkola-Vuorinen, A. (2011). Divergent behaviour of oxidative stress markers 8-hydroxydeoxyguanosine (8-OHdG) and 4-hydroxy-2-nonenal (HNE) in breast carcinogenesis. Histopathology, Vol.58, No.6, (May 2011), pp.854-862, ISSN 1365-2559

Kaspar, J.W. & Jaiswal, A.K. (2010).An autoregulatory loop between Nrf2 and Cul3-Rbx1 controlstheir cellular abundance. The Journal of Biological Chemistry, Vol.285, No.28, (July 2010), pp.21349-21358, ISSN 0021-9258

Katic, J., Cemeli, E., Baumgartner, A., Laubenthal, J., Bassano, I., Stølevik, S.B., Granum, B., Namork, E., Nygaard, U.C., Løvik, M., van Leeuwen, D., Vande Loock, K., Anderson, D., Fucić, A. & Decordier, I. (2010). Evaluation of the genotoxicity of 10 selected dietary/environmental compounds with the in vitro micronucleus cytokinesis-block assay in an interlaboratory comparison. Food and Chemical Toxicology, Vol.48, No.10, (June 2010), pp.2612-2623, ISSN 0278-6915

Kawamura, I., Lacey, E., Inami, M., Nishigaki, F., Naoe, Y., Tsujimoto, S., Manda, T. & Goto, T. (1999). Ponalrestat, an aldose reductase inhibitor, inhibits cachexia syndrome in nude mice bearing human melanomas G361 and SEKI. Anticancer Research, Vol.19, No.5B, (September-October 1999), pp.4091-4097, ISSN 0250-7005

Kim, Y.S. & Milner, J.A. (2007). Dietary modulation of colon cancer risk. Journal of Nutrition, Vol.137, No.11 Suppl, (November 2007), pp.2576S-2579S, ISSN 0022-3166

Kim, T.H., Hur, E.G., Kang, S.J., Kim, J.A., Thapa, D., Lee, Y.M., Ku, S.K., Jung, Y. & Kwak, M.K. (2011). NRF2 blockade suppresses colon tumor angiogenesis by inhibiting hypoxia-induced activation of HIF-1α. Cancer Research, Vol.71, No.6, (March 2011), pp.2260-2275, ISSN 0008-5472

Knoll, N., Ruhe, C., Veeriah, S., Sauer, J., Glei, M., Gallagher, E.P. & Pool-Zobel, B.L. (2005). Genotoxicity of 4-hydroxy-2-nonenal in human colon tumor cells is associated with cellular levels of glutathione and the modulation of glutathione S-transferase A4 expression by butyrate. Toxicological Sciences, Vol.86, No.1, (July 2005), pp.27-35, ISSN 1096-6080

Kondo, S., Toyokuni, S., Iwasa, Y., Tanaka, T., Onodera, H., Hiai, H. & Imamura, M. (1999). Persistent oxidative stress in human colorectal carcinoma, but not in adenoma. Free Radical Biology and Medicine, Vol.27, No.3-4, (August 1999), pp.401-410, ISSN 0891-5849

Konner, J., O'Reilly, E. (2002). Pancreatic cancer; epidemiology, genetics, and approaches to screening. Oncology (Williston Park, N.Y.), Vol.16, No.12, (December 2002), pp.1631-1638, ISSN 0890-9091

Koster, J.F., Slee, R.G., Montfoort, A., Lang, J. & Esterbauer, H. (1986). Comparison of the inactivation of microsomal glucose-6-phosphatase by in situ lipid peroxidation-derived 4-hydroxynonenal and exogenous 4-hydroxynonenal. Free radical research communications, Vol.1, No.4, (1986), pp.273-287, ISSN 8755-0199

Kotrikadze, N., Alibegashvili, M., Zibzibadze, M., Abashidze, N., Chigogidze, T., Managadze, L. & Artsivadze, K. (2008). Activity and content of antioxidant enzymes in prostate tumors. Experimental Oncology, Vol.30, No.3, (September 2008), pp.244-247, ISSN 1812-9269

Kowalczyk, P., Ciesla, J.M., Komisarski, M., Kusmierek, J.T. & Tudek, B. (2004). Long-chain adducts of trans-4-hydroxy-2-nonenal to DNA bases cause recombination, base substitutions and frameshift mutations in M13 phage. Mutation Research, Vol.550, No.1-2, (June 2004), pp.33-48, ISSN 1383-5718

Lapre, J.A. & Vandermeer, R. (1992) Diet-induced increase of colonic bile acids stimulates lytic activity of fecal water and proliferation of colonic cells. Carcinogenesis, Vol.13, No.1, (January 1992), pp.41-44, ISSN 0143-3334

Laurent, A., Alary, J., Debrauwer, L. & Cravedi, J.P. (1999). Analysis in the rat of 4-hydroxynonenal metabolites excreted in bile: Evidence of enterohepatic circulation of these byproducts of lipid peroxidation. Chemical Research in Toxicology, Vol.12, No.10, (October 1999), pp.887-894, ISSN 0893-228X

Laurora, S., Tamagno, E., Briatore, F., Bardini, P., Pizzimenti, S., Toaldo, C., Reffo, P., Costelli, P., Dianzani, M.U., Danni, O. & Barrera, G. (2005). 4-Hydroxynonenal modulation of p53 family gene expression in the SK-N-BE neuroblastoma cell line. Free Radical Biology and Medicine, Vol.38, No.2, (January 2005), pp.215-25, ISSN 0891-5849

Leonarduzzi, G., Robbesyn, F. & Poli, G. Signaling kinases modulated by 4-hydroxynonenal. (2004). Free Radical Biology and Medicine, Vol.37, No.11, (December 2004), pp.1694-1702, ISSN 0891-5849

Lin, M.Y. & Yen, C.L. (1999). Antioxidative ability of lactic acid Bacteria. Journal of Agricultural and Food Chemistry, Vol.47, No.4, (April 1999), pp.1460-1466, ISSN 0021-8561

Looi, M.L., Mohd Dali, A.Z., Md Ali, S.A., Wan Ngah, W.Z. & Mohd Yusof, Y.A. (2008). Oxidative damage and antioxidant status in patients with cervical intraepithelial neoplasia and carcinoma of the cervix. European Journal of Cancer Prevention, Vol.17, No.6, (November 2008), pp.555-560, ISSN 0959-8278

Malhotra, D., Portales-Casamar, E., Singh, A., Srivastava, S., Arenillas, D., Happel, C., Shyr, C., Wakabayashi, N., Kensler, T.W., Wasserman, W.W. & Biswal, S. (2010). Global mapping of 22 binding sites for Nrf2 identifies novel targets in cell survival response through ChIP-Seq profiling and network analysis. Nucleic Acids Research, Vol.38, No.17, (September 2010), pp.5718-5734, ISSN 0305-1048

Martin, H.J. & Maser, E. (2009). Role of human aldo-keto-reductase AKR1B10 in the protection against toxic aldehydes. Chemico-Biological Interactions, Vol.178, No.1-3, (March 2009), pp.145-150, ISSN 0009-2797

Matsunaga, T., Yamane, Y., Iida, K., Endo, S., Banno, Y., El-Kabbani, O. & Hara, A. (2011). Involvement of the aldo-keto reductase, AKR1B10, in mitomycin-c resistance through reactive oxygen species-dependent mechanisms. Anti-Cancer Drugs, Vol.22, No.5, (June 2011), pp.402-408, ISSN 1473-5741

Min, K. & Ebeler, S.E. (2009).Quercetin inhibits hydrogen peroxide-induced DNA damage and enhances DNA repair in Caco-2 cells. Food and Chemical Toxicology. Vol.47, No.11, (November 2009), pp.2716-2722, ISSN 0278-6915

Moseley, P.L. (1997). Heat shock proteins and heat adaptation of the whole organism. Journal of Applied Physiology, Vol.83, No.5, (November 1997), pp.1413-1417, ISSN 8750-7587

Murawaki, Y., Tsuchiya, H., Kanbe, T., Harada, K., Yashima, K., Nozaka, K., Tanida, O., Kohno, M., Mukoyama, T., Nishimuki, E., Kojo, H., Matsura, T., Takahashi, K., Osaki, M., Ito, H., Yodoi, J., Murawaki, Y. & Shiota, G. (2008). Aberrant expression of selenoproteins in the progression of colorectal cancer. Cancer Letters, Vol.259, No.2, (Febraury 2008), pp.218-230, ISSN 0304-3835

Muzio, G., Canuto, R.A., Trombetta, A. & Maggiora, M. (2001). Inhibition of cytosolic class 3 aldehyde dehydrogenase by antisense oligonucleotides in rat hepatoma cells. Chemico-Biological Interactions, Vol.130-132, No.1-3, (January 2001), pp.219-225, ISSN 0009-2797

Nair, J., Gansauge, F., Beger, H., Dolara, P., Winde, G. & Bartsch, H. (2006). Increased etheno-DNA adducts in affected tissues of patients suffering from Crohn's disease, ulcerative colitis, and chronic pancreatitis. Antioxidants & Redox Signaling, Vol.8, No.5-6, (May-June 2006), pp.1003-1010, ISSN 1523-0864

Nishikawa, A., Furukawa, F., Kasahara, K., Ikezaki, S., Itoh, T., Suzuki, T., Uchida, K., Kurihara, M., Hayashi, M., Miyata, N. & Hirose, M. (2000). Trans-4-hydroxy-2-nonenal, an aldehydic lipid peroxidation product, lacks genotoxicity in lacI transgenic mice. Cancer Letters, Vol.148, No.1, (January 2000), pp.81-86, ISSN 0304-3835

Obtułowicz, T., Winczura, A., Speina, E., Swoboda, M., Janik, J., Janowska, B., Cieśla, J.M., Kowalczyk, P., Jawien, A., Gackowski, D., Banaszkiewicz, Z., Krasnodebski, I., Chaber, A., Olinski, R., Nair, J., Bartsch, H., Douki, T., Cadet, J. & Tudek, B. (2010). Aberrant repair of etheno-DNA adducts in leukocytes and colon tissue of colon cancer patients. Free Radical Biology and Medicine, Vol.49, No.6, (September 2010), pp.1064-1071, ISSN 0891-5849

Okamoto, K., Toyokuni, S., Uchida, K., Ogawa, O., Takenawa, J., Kakehi, Y., Kinoshita, H., Hattori-Nakakuki, Y., Hiai, H. & Yoshida, O. (1994). Formation of 8-hydroxy-2′-deoxyguanosine and 4-hydroxy-2-nonenal-modified proteins in human renal-cell carcinoma. International Journal of Cancer, Vol.58, No.6, (September 1994), pp.825-829, ISSN 1097-0215

Pan, J.S., Hong, M.Z. & Ren, J.L. (2009). Reactive oxygen species: a double-edged sword in oncogenesis. World Journal of Gastroenterology, Vol.15, No.14, (April 2009), pp.1702-1707, ISSN 1007-9327

Park, J.H. & Park, E. (2011). Influence of iron-overload on DNA damage and its repair in human leukocytes in vitro. Mutation Research, Vol.718, No.1-2, (January 2011), pp.56-61, ISSN 1383-5718

Parola, M., Bellomo, G., Robino, G., Barrera, G. & Dianzani, M.U. (1999). 4-Hydroxynonenal as a biological signal: molecular basis and pathophysiological implications.

Antioxidants & Redox Signaling, Vol.3, No.1, (Fall 1999), pp.255-284, ISSN 1523-0864

Pearson, J.R., Gill, C.I. & Rowland, I.R. (2004). Diet, fecal water, and colon cancer--development of a biomarker. Nutrition Reviews, Vol.67, No.9, (September 2009), pp.509-526, ISSN 0029-6643

Petersen, D.R. & Doorn, J.A. (2004). Reactions of 4-hydroxynonenal with proteins and cellular targets. Free Radical Biology and Medicine, Vol.37, No.7, (October 2004), pp.937-945, ISSN 0891-5849

Pettazzoni, P., Pizzimenti, S., Toaldo, C., Sotomayor, P., Tagliavacca, L., Liu, S., Wang, D., Minelli, R., Ellis, L., Atadja, P., Ciamporcero, E., Dianzani, M.U., Barrera, G. & Pili, R. (2011). Induction of cell cycle arrest and DNA damage by the HDAC inhibitor panobinostat (LBH589) and the lipid peroxidation end product 4-hydroxynonenal in prostate cancer cells. Free Radical Biology and Medicine, Vol.50, No.2, (January 2011), pp.313-322, ISSN 0891-5849

Pierre, F., Tache, S., Petit, C.R., Van der Meer, R. & Corpet, D.E. (2003) Meat and cancer: haemoglobin and haemin in a low-calcium diet promote colorectal carcinogenesis at the aberrant crypt stage in rats. Carcinogenesis, Vol.24, No.10, (October 2003), pp.1683-1690, ISSN 0143-3334

Pierre, F., Freeman, A., Tache, S., Van der Meer, R. & Corpet, D.E. (2004). Beef meat and blood sausage promote the formation of azoxymethaneinduced mucin-depleted foci and aberrant crypt foci in rat colons. Journal of Nutrition, Vol.134, No.10, (October 2004), pp.2711-2716, ISSN 0022-3166

Pierre, F., Peiro, G., Tache, S., Cross, A.J., Bingham, S.A., Gasc, N., Gottardi, G., Corpet, D.E. & Guéraud, F. (2006). Newmarker of colon cancer risk associated with heme intake: 1,4-dihydroxynonane mercapturic acid. Cancer Epidemiology, Biomarkers & Prevention, Vol.15, No.11, (November 2006), pp.2274-2279, ISSN 1538-7755

Pierre, F., Tache, S., Guéraud, F., Rerole, A.L., Jourdan, M.L. & Petit, C. (2007). Apc mutation induces resistance of colonic cells to lipoperoxide-triggered apoptosis induced by faecal water from haem-fed rats. Carcinogenesis, Vol.28, No.2, (February 2007), pp.321-327, ISSN 0143-3334

Pizzimenti, S., Briatore, F., Laurora, S., Toaldo, C., Maggio, M., De Grandi, M., Meaglia, L., Menegatti, E., Giglioni, B., Dianzani, M.U. & Barrera, G. (2006). 4-Hydroxynonenal inhibits telomerase activity and hTERT expression in human leukemic cell lines. Free Radical Biology and Medicine, Vol.40, No.9, (May 2006), pp.1578-1591, ISSN 0891-5849

Pizzimenti, S., Ferracin, M., Sabbioni, S., Toaldo, C., Pettazzoni, P., Dianzani, M.U., Negrini, M. & Barrera, G. (2009). MicroRNA expression changes during human leukemic HL-60 cell differentiation induced by 4-hydroxynonenal, a product of lipid peroxidation. Free Radical Biology and Medicine, Vol.46, No.2, (January 2009), pp.282-288, ISSN 0891-5849

Pizzimenti, S., Toaldo, C., Pettazzoni, P., Dianzani, M.U. & Barrera, G. (2010a). The "Two-Faced" Effects of Reactive Oxygen Species and the Lipid Peroxidation Product 4-Hydroxynonenal in the Hallmarks of Cancer. Cancers, Vol.2, No.2, (March 2010), pp.338-363, ISSN 1097-0142

Pizzimenti, S., Menegatti, E., Berardi, D., Toaldo, C., Pettazzoni, P., Minelli, R., Giglioni, B., Cerbone, A., Dianzani, M.U., Ferretti, C. & Barrera, G. (2010b). 4-hydroxynonenal, a lipid peroxidation product of dietary polyunsaturated fatty acids, has anticarcinogenic properties in colon carcinoma cell lines through the inhibition of telomerase activity. The Journal of Nutritional Biochemistry, Vol.21, No.9, (September 2010), pp.818-826, ISSN 0955-2863

Poli, G., Schaur, R.J., Siems, W.G. & Leonarduzzi, G. (2008). 4-hydroxynonenal: a membrane lipid oxidation product of medicinal interest. Medicinal Research Reviews, Vol.28, No.4, (July 2008), pp.569-631, ISSN 0198-6325

Poljak-Blazi, M., Kralj, M., Hadzija, M.P., Zarković, N., Zarković, K. & Waeg, G. (2000). Involvement of lipid peroxidation, oncogene expression and induction of apoptosis in the antitumorous activity of ferric-sorbitol-citrate. Cancer Biotherapy and Radiopharmaceuticals, Vol.15, No.3, (June 2000), pp.285-293, ISSN 1084-9785

Ramana, K.V., Tammali, R. & Srivastava, S.K. (2010). Inhibition of aldose reductase prevents growth factor-induced G1-S phase transition through the AKT/phosphoinositide 3-kinase/E2F-1 pathway in human colon cancer cells. Molecular Cancer Therapeutics, Vol.9, No.4, (April 2010), pp.813-824, ISSN 1535-7163

Reddy, B.S. (2002). Types and amount of dietary fat and colon cancer risk: Prevention by omega-3 fatty acid-rich diets. Environmental Health and Preventive Medicine, Vol.7, No.3, (July 2002), pp.95-102, ISSN 1342-078X

Reddy, N.M., Kleeberger, S.R., Yamamoto, M., Kensler, T.W., Scollick, C., Biswal, S. & Reddy, S.P. (2007). Genetic dissection of the Nrf2-dependent redox signaling-regulated transcriptional programs of cell proliferation and cytoprotection. Physiological Genomics, Vol.32, No.1, (December 2007), pp. 74-81, ISSN 1094-8341

Richter, M., Jurek, D., Wrba, F., Kaserer, K., Wurzer, G., Karner-Hanusch, J. & Marian B. (2002). Cells obtained from colorectal microadenomas mirror early premalignant growth patterns in vitro. European Journal of Cancer, Vol.38, No.14, (September 2002), pp. 1937–1945. ISSN 0959-8049

Rinaldi, M., Barrera, G., Aquino, A., Spinsanti, P., Pizzimenti, S., Farace, M.G., Dianzani, M.U. & Fazio, V.M. (2000). 4-Hydroxynonenal-induced MEL cell differentiation involves PKC activity translocation. Biochemical and Biophysical Research Communications, Vol.272, No.1, (May 2000), pp. 75-80, ISSN 0006-291X

Sarge, K.D., Murphy, S.P., & Morimoto, R.I. (1993). Activation of heat shock gene transcription by heat shock factor 1 involves oligomerization, acquisition of DNA-binding activity, and nuclear localization and can occur in the absence of stress. Molecular and Cellular Biology, Vol.13, No.3, (March 1993), pp. 1392–1407, ISSN 0270-7306

Satow, R., Shitashige, M., Kanai, Y., Takeshita, F., Ojima, H., Jigami, T., Honda, K., Kosuge, T., Ochiya, T., Hirohashi, S. & Yamada T. (2010). Combined functional genome survey of therapeutic targets for hepatocellular carcinoma. Clinical Cancer Research, Vol.16, No.9, (May 2010), pp. 2518–2528, ISSN 1078-0432

Saw, C.L. & Kong, A.N. (2011). Nuclear factor-erythroid 2-related factor 2 as a chemopreventive target in colorectal cancer. Expert Opinion on Therapeutic Targets, Vol.15, No.3, (March 2011), pp. 281-295, ISSN 1472-8222

Sawa,T., Akaike,T., Kida, K., Fukushima,Y., Takagi, K., & Maeda, H. (1998). Lipid peroxyl radicals from oxidized oils and heme-iron: implication of a high-fat diet in colon carcinogenesis. Cancer Epidemiology, Biomarkers & Prevention, Vol.7, No.11, (November 1998), pp. 1007–1012, ISSN 1055-9965

Sayre, L.M., Arora, P.K., Iyer, R.S. & Salomon, R.G. (1993). Pyrrole formation from 4-hydroxynonenal and primary amines. Chemical Research in Toxicology , Vol.6, No.1, (January-February 1993), pp. 19-22, ISSN 0893-228X

Schaeferhenrich, A., Beyer-Sehlmeyer, G., Festag, G., Kuechler, A., Haag, N., Weise, A., Liehr, T., Claussen, U., Marian, B., Sendt, W., Scheele, J. & Pool-Zobel B.L. (2003). Human adenoma cells are highly susceptible to the genotoxic action of 4-hydroxy-2-nonenal. Mutation Research - Fundamental and Molecular Mechanisms of Mutagenesis, Vol.526, No.1-2, (May 2003), pp. 19-32, ISSN: 0027-5107

Scharlau, D., Borowicki, A., Habermann, N., Hofmann, T., Klenow, S., Miene, C., Munjal, U., Stein, K. & Glei M. (2009). Mechanisms of primary cancer prevention by butyrate and other products formed during gut flora-mediated fermentation of dietary fibre. Mutatation Research - Reviews, Vol.682, No.1, (July-August 2009), pp. 39-53, ISSN 1383-5742

Scharmach, E., Hessel, S., Niemann, B. & Lampen, A. (2009). Glutathione S-transferase expression and isoenzyme composition during cell differentiation of Caco-2 cells. Toxicology, Vol.265, No.3, (November 2009), pp. 122-126, ISSN 0300-483X

Schaur, R.J. (2003). Basic aspects of the biochemical reactivity of 4-hydroxynonenal. Molecular Aspects of Medicine, Vol.24, No. 4-5, (August-October 2003), pp. 149-59, ISSN: 0098-2997

Scheppach, W., Bingham, S., Boutron-Ruault, M., Verdier, M. G. D., Moreno, V., Nagengast, F., Reifen, R., Riboli, E., Seitz, H. &Wahrendorf, J. (1999). WHO consensus statement on the role of nutrition in colorectal cancer. European Journal of Cancer Prevention, Vol.8, No.1, (February 1999), pp. 57–62, ISSN 0959-8278

Schmid, K., Nair, J., Winde, G., Velic, I., & Bartsch, H. (2000). Increased levels of promutagenic etheno-DNA adducts in colonic polyps of FAP patients. International Journal of Cancer , Vol.87, No.1, (July 2000), pp. 1-4, ISSN 0020-7136

Seitz, H.K., Egerer, G., Oneta, C., Krämer, S., Sieg, A., Klee, F. & Simanowski, U.A. (1996). Alcohol dehydrogenase in the human colon and rectum. Digestion, Vol.57, No.2, pp. 105-108, ISSN 0012-2823

Selga, E., Noé, V., & Ciudad, C.J. (2008). Transcriptional regulation of aldo-keto reductase 1C1 in HT29 human colon cancer cells resistant to methotrexate: role in the cell cycle and apoptosis. Biochemical Pharmacology,. Vol.75, No.2, (January 2008), pp. 414–426, ISSN 0006-2952

Semlitsch, T., Tillian, H.M., Zarkovic, N., Borovic, S., Purtscher, M., Hohenwarter, O., & Schaur, R.J. (2002). Differential influence of the lipid peroxidation product 4-hydroxynonenal on the growth of human lymphatic leukaemia cells and human peripheral blood lymphocytes. Anticancer Research, Vol.22, No.3, (May-June 2002), pp. 1689-1697, ISSN 0250-7005

Sesink, A.L.A., Termont, D.S.M.L., Kleibeuker, J.H. & Vandermeer, R. (1999). Red meat and colon cancer: the cytotoxic and hyperproliferative effects of dietary heme. Cancer Research, Vol.59, No.22, (November 1999), pp. 5704–5709, ISSN 0008-5472

Sharma, R., Sharma, A., Yang, Y., Awasthi, S., Singhal, S.S., Zimniak, P. & Awasthi, Y.C. (2002). Functional reconstitution of Ral-binding GTPase activating protein, RLIP76, in proteoliposomes catalyzing ATP-dependent transport of glutathione conjugate of 4-hydroxynonenal. Acta Biochimica Polonica, Vol.49, No.3, pp. 693-701, ISSN 0001-527X

Siems, W. & Grune, T. (2003). Intracellular metabolism of 4-hydroxynonenal. Molecular Aspects of Medicine, Vol.24, No.4-5, (August-October 2003), pp. 167- 175, ISSN: 0098-2997

Singhal, S.S., Singhal, J., Yadav, S., Dwivedi, S., Boor, P.J., Awasthi, Y.C., & Awasthi, S. (2007). Regression of lung and colon cancer xenografts by depleting or inhibiting RLIP76 (Ral-binding protein 1). Cancer Research, Vol.67, No. 9, (May 2007), pp. 4382-4389, ISSN 0008-5472

Skrzydlewska, E., Sulkowski, S., Koda, M., Zalewski, B., Kanczuga-Koda, L. & Sulkowska, M. (2005). Lipid peroxidation and antioxidant status in colorectal cancer. World Journal of Gastroenterology, Vol.11, No.3, pp. 403-406, ISSN 1007-9327

Soong, R., Powell, B., Elsaleh, H., Gnanasampanthan, G., Smith, D.R., Goh, H.S., Joseph, D. & Iacopetta, B. (2000). Prognostic significance of TP53 gene mutation in 995 cases of colorectal carcinoma. Influence of tumour site, stage, adjuvant chemotherapy and type of mutation. European Journal of Cancer, Vol. 36, No.16, (October 2000), pp. 2053–2060, ISSN 0959-8049

Soussi, T., Dehouche, K. & Beroud, C. (2000). p53 website and analysis of p53 gene mutations in human cancer: forging a link between epidemiology and carcinogenesis. Human Mutation, Vol.15, No.1, pp. 105–113, ISSN: 1059-7794

Soussi, T. & Beroud, C. (2003). Significance of p53 mutations in human cancer: a critical analysis of mutations at CpG dinucleotides. Human Mutation, Vol.21, No3, pp. 192–200, ISSN: 1059-7794

Stagos, D., Zhou, H., Ross, D. & Vasiliou, V. (2009). 4-HNE inhibits tube formation and up-regulates chondromodulin-I in human endothelial cells. Biochemical and Biophysical Research Communications, Vol.379, No.3, (February 2009), pp. 654-658, ISSN 0006-291X

Sunjic, S.B., Cipak, A., Rabuzin, F., Wildburger, R. & Zarkovic, N. (2005). The influence of 4-hydroxy-2-nonenal on proliferation, differentiation and apoptosis of human osteosarcoma cells. Biofactors, Vol. 24, No.1-4, pp. 141-148, ISSN 1872-8081

Surh, J., & Kwon, H. (2005). Estimation of daily exposure to 4-hydroxy-2-alkenals in Korean foods containing n-3 and n-6 polyunsaturated fatty acids. Food Additives & Contaminants., Vol.22, No.8, (August 2005), pp. 701–708, ISSN 1944-0049

Surh, J., Lee, S. & Kwon, H. (2007). 4-Hydroxy-2-alkenals in polyunsaturated fatty acids-fortified infant formulas and other commercial food products. Food Additives & Contaminants, Vol. 24, No.11, (November 2007), pp. 1209-1218, ISSN 1944-0049

Surh, J., Lee, B.Y. & Kwon, H. (2010). Influence of Fatty Acids Compositions and Manufacturing Type on the Formation of 4-Hydroxy-2-alkenals in Food Lipids. Food Science and Biotechnology, Vol.19, No.2, (April 2010), pp.297-303, ISSN 1226-7708

Tammali, R., Ramana, K.V., Singhal, S.S., Awasthi, S., & Srivastava, S.K. (2006). Aldose reductase regulates growth factor-induced cyclooxygenase-2 expression and prostaglandin E2 production in human colon cancer cells. Cancer Research, Vol.66, No.19, (October 2006), pp. 9705-9713, ISSN 0008-5472

Tammali, R., Srivastava, S.K. & Ramana, K.V. (2011). Targeting aldose reductase for the treatment of cancer. Current Cancer Drug Targets, Vol.11, No.5, (June 2011), pp. 560-571, ISSN 1568-0096

Thimmulappa, R.K., Mai, K.H., Srisuma, S., Kensler, T.W., Yamamoto, M. & Biswal, S. (2002). Identification of Nrf2-regulated genes induced by the chemopreventive agent sulforaphane by oligonucleotide microarray. Cancer Research, Vol.62, No.18, (September 2002), pp. 5196-5203, ISSN 0008-5472

Tice, R.P., Andrews, P.W., Hirai, O. & Singh, N.P. (1991). The single cell gel (SCG) assay: an electrophoretic technique for the detection of DNA damage in individual cells. Advances in Experimental Medicine and Biology, Vol. 283, pp. 157–164, ISSN 0065-2598

Uchida, K. (2003). 4-Hydroxy-2-nonenal: a product and mediator of oxidative stress. Progress in lipid research, Vol.42, No.4, (July 2003), pp. 318-343, ISSN 0163-7827

Vander Jagt, D.L., Kolb, N.S., Vander Jagt, T.J., Chino, J., Martinez, F.J., Hunsaker, L.A. & Royer, R.E. (1995). Substrate specificity of human aldose reductase: Identification of 4-hydroxynonenal as an endogenous substrate. Biochimica et Biophysica Acta, Vol.1249, No.2, (June 1995), pp. 117–126, ISSN 0006-3002

Vatsyayan, R., Lelsani, P.C., Awasthi, S., & Singhal, S.S. (2010). RLIP76: a versatile transporter and an emerging target for cancer therapy. Biochemical Pharmacology, Vol.79, No.12, (June 2010), pp. 1699-1705, ISSN 0006-2952

Veitch, Z.W., Guo, B., Hembruff, S.L., Bewick, A.J., Heibein, A.D., Eng, J., Cull, S., Maclean, D.A., & Parissenti, A.M. (2009). Induction of 1C aldoketoreductases and other drug dose-dependent genes upon acquisition of anthracycline resistance. Pharmacogenetics and Genomics, Vol.19, No.6, (June 2009), pp. 477–488, ISSN 1744-6872

Vizio, B., Poli, G., Chiarpotto, E. & Biasi, F. (2005). 4-hydroxynonenal and TGF-beta1 concur in inducing antiproliferative effects on the CaCo-2 human colon adenocarcinoma cell line. Biofactors., Vol.24, No.1-4, pp. 237-246, ISSN 1872-8081

Vogelstein, B., Fearon, E.R., Hamilton, S.R., Kern, S.E., Preisinger, A.C., Leppert, M., Nakamura, Y., White, R., Smits, A.M. & Bos, J.L. (1988). Genetic alterations during colorectal tumor development. The New England Journal of Medicine, Vol.319, No.9, (September 1988), pp. 525–532, ISSN 0028-4793

Wacker, M., Wanek, P., Eder, E., Hylla, S., Gostner, A. & Scheppach, W. (2002). Effect of enzyme-resistant starch on formation of 1,N(2)-propanodeoxyguanosine adducts of trans-4-hydroxy-2-nonenal and cell proliferation in the colonic mucosa of healthy volunteers. Cancer Epidemiology, Biomarkers & Prevention, Vol.11, No.9, (September 2002), pp. 915-920, ISSN 1055-9965

Wacker, M., Wanek, P. & Eder, E. (2001). Detection of 1,N2-propanodeoxyguanosine adducts of trans-4-hydroxy-2-nonenal after gavage of trans-4-hydroxy-2-nonenal or induction of lipid peroxidation with carbon tetrachloride in F344 rats. Chemico-Biological Interactions, Vol.137, No.3, (September 2001), pp. 269–283, ISSN 0009-2797

Wang, J. & Yi, J. (2008). Cancer cell killing via ROS: to increase or decrease, that is the question. Cancer Biology and Therapy, Vol.7, No.12, (December 2008), pp. 1875-1884, ISSN 1538-4047

West, J.D., Ji, C., Duncan, S.T., Amarnath, V., Schneider, C., Rizzo, C.J., Brash, A.R. & Marnett L.J. (2004). Induction of apoptosis in colorectal carcinoma cells treated with 4-hydroxy-2-nonenal and structurally related aldehydic products of lipid peroxidation. Chemical Research in Toxicology, Vol. 17, No. 4, (April 2004), pp. 453-462, ISSN 0893-228X

West, J.D. & Marnett, L.J. (2005). Alterations in gene expression induced by the lipid peroxidation product, 4-hydroxy-2-nonenal. Chemical Research in Toxicology, Vol.18, No.11, (November 2001), pp. 1642-1653, ISSN 0893-228X

Winter, C.K., Segall. H.J. & Haddon.W.F. (1986). Formation of cyclic adducts of deoxyguanosine with the aldehydes trans-4-hydroxy-2-hexenal and trans-4-hydroxy-2-nonenal in vitro. Cancer Research, Vol.46, No.11, (November 1986), pp. 5682-5686, ISSN 0008-5472

Yadav, U.C., Ramana, K.V., Awasthi, Y.C. & Srivastava, S.K. (2008). Glutathione level regulates HNE-induced genotoxicity in human erythroleukemia cells. Toxicology and Applied Pharmacology, Vol.227, No.2, (March 2008), pp. 257-264, ISSN 0041-008X

Yan, R., Zu, X., Ma, J., Liu, Z., Adeyanju, M. & Cao, D. (2007). Aldo-keto reductase family 1B10 gene silencing results in growth inhibition of colorectal cancer cells: implication for cancer intervention. International Journal of Cancer, Vol.121, No.10, (November 2007), pp. 2301–2306, ISSN 0020-7136

Yang, Y., Sharma, A., Sharma, R., Patrick, B., Singhal, S.S., Zimniak, P., Awasthi, S. & Awasthi, Y.C. (2003). Cells preconditioned with mild, transient UVA irradiation acquire resistance to oxidative stress and UVA-induced apoptosis: role of 4-hydroxynonenal in UVA mediated signalling for apoptosis. The Journal of Biological Chemistry, Vol.278, No.42, (October 2003), pp. 41380–41388, ISSN 0021-9258

Yin, S.J., Liao, C.S., Lee, Y.C., Wu, C.W. & Jao, S.W. (1994).Genetic polymorphism and activities of human colon alcohol and aldehyde dehydrogenases: no gender and age differences. Alcoholism, clinical and experimental research, Vol.18, No.5, (October1994), pp. 1256-1260, ISSN 1530-0277

Yoshitake, H., Takahashi, M., Ishikawa, H., Nojima, M., Iwanari, H., Watanabe, A., Aburatani, H., Yoshida, K., Ishi, K., Takamori, K., Ogawa, H., Hamakubo, T., Kodama, T. & Araki, Y. (2007). Aldo-keto reductase family 1, member B10 in uterine carcinomas: a potential risk factor of recurrence after surgical therapy in cervical cancer. International Journal of Gynecological Cancer. Vol.17, No.6, (November-December 2007), pp. 1300–1306, ISSN 1048-891X

Zanetti, D., Poli, G., Vizio, B., Zingaro, B., Chiarpotto, E. & Biasi, F. (2003). 4-hydroxynonenal and transforming growth factor-beta1 expression in colon cancer. Molecular Aspects of Medicine, Vol.24, No.4-5, (August-October 2003), pp. 273-280, ISSN 0098-2997

Zarkovic, K., Juric, G., Waeg, G., Kolenc, D. & Zarkovic, N. (2005). Immunohistochemical appearance of HNE-protein conjugates in human astrocytomas. Biofactors, Vol.24, No.1-4, pp. 33-40, ISSN 1872-8081

Zeindl-Eberhart, E., Jungblut, P.R., Otto, A., Kerler, R., Rabes, H.M. (1997). Further characterization of a rat hepatomaderived aldose-reductase-like protein-organ distribution and modulation in vitro. European Journal of Biochemistry, Vol.247, No.3, (August 1997), pp. 792–800, ISSN 0014-2956

Zhi-Hua, C. & Etsuo, N. (2006). 4-Hydroxynonenal (4-HNE) has been widely accepted as an inducer of oxidative stress. Is this the whole truth about it or can 4-HNE also exert protective effects? IUBMB Life, Vol.58, No.5-6, (May-june 2006), pp. 372–373, ISSN 1521-6543

9

Growth Factors and the Redox State as New Therapeutic Targets for Colorectal Cancer

Teodoro Palomares, Marta Caramés,
Ignacio García-Alonso and Ana Alonso-Varona
University of the Basque Country,
Spain

1. Introduction

Colorectal cancer (CRC) is an important health problem in many western countries due to its significant morbidity/mortality. Despite advances in its diagnosis and treatment, survival associated with this cancer when it has extended to adjacent organs, lymphatic nodules or distal organs is drastically reduced. The liver is the most common site of CRC metastasis, since it represents a unique microenvironment for the formation of metastases, not only due to its sinusoidal endothelium (Barberá-Guillén et al., 1989), but also due to its abundant expression of growth factors (GFs) (Stoeltzing et al., 2003).

At present, curative treatment of localized metastases is possible via partial liver resection. However, this surgical procedure is only potentially curative, since 65% of patients subjected to resection of liver metastases experience relapse within 5 years (Sun & Tang, 2003; Allendorf et al., 2004). In the light of this frequent recurrence, it is essential to develop new preventive therapeutic strategies, which require a detailed knowledge of the biological events that occur following hepatectomy. In this sense, we have previously demonstrated the tumor-enhancing effect associated with liver resection in a mouse tumor model; in addition, we showed that hepatectomized rat serum increased cell proliferation *in vitro*, when compared with laparotomized rat serum or fetal calf serum (García-Alonso et al., 2003; García-Alonso et al., 2008a, 2008b). These findings indicated that GFs produced by the liver promote the development of metastases.

At present, CRC treatment includes various active drugs, either as individual agents or in combination: 5-fluorouracil (5-FU), capecitabine, irinotecan and oxaliplatin, among others. Despite this wide array of anti-tumor agents, relapse often occurs in CRC patients, due in large part to the resistance of the tumor cells to these anti-neoplastic agents. Various different mechanisms have been reported as being responsible for the development of chemoresistance and, though each may be important in itself, they take on an even greater significance if we consider how they may be interrelated.

One of these mechanisms of resistance to anti-neoplastic agents is the presence of GFs, which may be able to protect certain tumor cells against cytotoxic cell death. For this reason, one of the most promising cell targets nowadays are these GFs and their receptors. Thus, since 2004, three new agents have been approved which in combination with cytotoxic agents are administered in cases of advanced and metastatic CRC: bevacizumab, a monoclonal antibody to vascular endothelial growth factor (VEGF) (Hurwitz et al., 2004), and cetuximab and panitumumab, which are monoclonal antibodies to the epidermal growth factor receptor (EGFR) (Cunningham et al., 2004; Odom et al., 2011).

An increasing amount of evidence indicates that the intracellular redox state plays an essential role in the mechanisms underlying the actions of GFs. In particular, GFs have been reported to generate reactive oxygen species (ROS) which can function as second messengers, mediating important cellular functions, such as proliferation and programmed cell death. Intracellular redox homeostasis is sustained primarily by glutathione (GSH), which has long been known to be an important factor in cancer chemoresistance.

In the present chapter, we analyze three important concerns in relation to CRC chemoresistance:

- The influence of GFs in CRC biology and in the response to current cytotoxic therapies.
- The involvement of the redox state in the mechanisms of action of GFs in CRC cells.
- The exogenous modulation of the redox state as a new pharmacological strategy to improve the response to chemotherapeutic agents.

2. Growth factors and colorectal cancer

GFs play a fundamental role in CRC biology, mediating critical functions in cancerous cells, such as proliferation, angiogenesis and the inhibition of cell death. The recurrence of cancer after excision surgery is still a major clinical problem. Accumulating clinical and experimental evidence has indicated that specific factors involved in liver regeneration may influence the growth patterns of residual or dormant micrometastases after resection, suggesting that the process of hepatic regeneration has a significant proliferative effect on tumor cells. In this regard, GFs appear to be involved in tumor recurrence and in metastasis formation. Thus, after partial resection of liver metastases, various types of GFs, which are responsible for liver regeneration, are locally released. However, these may also stimulate the proliferation of undetected tumor cells in the remaining liver, i.e. highly metastatic colon cancer cells can respond to liver regeneration associated mitogens, whose expression is induced after hepatectomy. GFs such as hepatocyte growth factor (HGF), epidermal growth factor (EGF), transforming growth factor alpha (TGF-α), transforming growth factor beta (TGF-β), basic-fibroblastic growth factor (b-FGF), insulin growth factor–I (IGFI) and vascular endothelial growth factor (VEGF) have been reported to be associated with tumor progression and metastasis (Christophi et al., 2008).

Hepatocyte Growth Factor (HGF) is essential for the process of hepatic regeneration. It is a potent mitogenic agent produced by stellate, endothelial and Kupffer sinusoidal cells, which binds to a receptor of the tyrosine kinase (TK) family. This family of genes is encoded by the proto-oncogene c-Met which is expressed in hepatocytes, as well as in other cell types, including tumor cells (Di Renzo et al., 1991). It has a pro-angiogenic effect and stimulates cell motility as well as the secretion of matrix metalloproteinases (MMPs) by pericytes, suggesting an important role in tumor invasion. In the case of CRC, the co-expression of HGF and its receptor is correlated with tumor pathogenesis and with the metastatic phenotype, and for this reason, it has been proposed as a possible molecular marker to be incorporated into CRC staging procedures (Kammula et al., 2007). Moreover, it is known that epithelial tumor metastases undergo an epithelial to mesenchymal transition (EMT) before becoming invasive. The stimuli which promote this transition include HGF and other

GFs such as b-FGF, EGF, TGF-β, as well as extracellular matrix (ECM) constituents including MMPs (Kalluri & Zeisberg, 2006; Christophi et al., 2008). For these reasons, HGF is considered to be a potentially valuable new therapeutic target for different tumors. Studies using NK4, a HGF antagonist, have shown an inhibitory effect on proliferation, invasion and angiogenesis in cell lines of gastric and pancreatic carcinoma, and of CRC (Hirao et al., 2002; Wen et al., 2007). In addition, anti-HGF monoclonal antibodies have been developed, thereby blocking binding to its receptor (Cao et al., 2001). Other developments include anti c-Met antibodies (Jin et al., 2008), and strategies aimed at silencing the expression of c-Met or HGF via antisense oligonucleotides (Stabile et al., 2004), o iRNA (Shinomiya et al., 2004).

Epidermal Growth Factor Receptor (EGFR) ligands, the most physiologically relevant of which include EGF, TGF-α, and Amphiregulin (AR). All of these bind to the extracellular domain of EGFR, which is a member of the ErbB transmembrane TK receptor family (Hynes & Lane, 2005). Binding of these ligands to the receptor activates the Ras/Raf/MAPK and PI3K-AKT signaling pathways which are involved in tumor cell proliferation, inhibition of apoptosis, invasion, migration and angiogenesis (Le Golvan & Resnick, 2010; Wanebo & Berz, 2010). Abnormal expression of these ligands has been demonstrated in many advanced tumors, including breast cancers, gliomas, and lung cancer. In the case of CRC, EGFR overexpression has been detected in 60-80% of cases (Le Golvan & Resnick, 2010) and a correlation has been reported with early tumor recurrence and extra-hepatic metastasis (Christophi et al., 2008). However, its exact role in the CRC metastatic cascade has not yet been characterized due to controversial results obtained with anti-EGFR antibody therapy. In this regard, the therapeutic use of two monoclonal antibody agents (cetuximab and panitumumab) has been authorized in patients with metastatic CRC; although they have a modest effect when used as single agents, they have been found to be beneficial in some patients when used in combination with conventional chemotherapeutic agents (Wanebo & Berz, 2010; Tol & Punt, 2010). In fact, it has been shown that the response to this therapy is independent of EGFR expression in tumor tissue (Chung et al., 2005). Thus, some studies suggest that EGFR expression in the primary tumor does not necessarily correspond with the same level of expression in metastatic tissue, while other studies have reported 78-100% concordance in EGFR expression in both tissue compartments (Tol & Punt, 2010). These discrepancies may partially be due to differences in the detection techniques employed. Nevertheless, recent studies have demonstrated that the therapeutic efficacy of the anti-EGFR antibody is limited to patients in whom the K-Ras oncogene is not mutated, since mutation of this oncogene can induce constitutive activation of the Ras/Raf/MAPK signaling pathway, which is independent of the activation of EGFR via ligand binding (Benvenuti et al., 2007; Tol & Punt, 2010).

Transforming Growth Factor β (TGF-β) acts as a tumor suppressor due to its inhibition of growth and its activation of apoptosis. However, in CRC, this suppressor activity is lost due to the existence of mutations in the genes which encode TGF-β, the type II receptor (TGFR β 2), or SMAD proteins, in such a way that the antiproliferative signal associated with this factor is interrupted (Markowitz & Bertagnolli, 2009). On the other hand, TGF-β has a pro-tumor effect due to its effect on the stroma, promoting angiogenesis, and on the tumor cells themselves, stimulating their motility and their invasive capacity (Blobe & Gordon, 2000). Thus, TGF-β, whose serum values are correlated with a poor CRC prognosis, acts as a tumor promoter, inducing the development of hepatic metastasis (Shim et al., 1999).

Insulin Growth Factor I (IGF-I) and its TK receptor are implicated in the development and progression of CRC due to their induction of proliferation. A correlation has been found between serum levels of IGF-I, high levels of IGF-IR expression in tumor cells and the development of hepatic metastasis. This pro-tumor effect is due to the fact that the signal induced by the binding of IGF-I to its receptor promotes the migration of endothelial cells, invasion and the formation of new blood vessels following the stimulation of VEGF production by endothelial cells (Wu et al., 2002), suggesting that IGF-I is an important contributor to tumor growth and hepatic metastatic development after hepatectomy (Christophi et al., 2008).

Vascular Endothelial Growth Factor (VEGF) is an endothelial cell mitogen which induces cell migration, proliferation, invasion and increased vascular permeability and has a potent pro-angiogenic activity. It has been shown that a large percentage of tumors which produce high levels of VEGF are associated with a high density of vessels in the tumor, metastasis, chemoresistance and poor prognosis (Sullivan & Brekken, 2010).

The VEGF family is made up of six growth factors. These exert their effects via binding to one of the three VEGFRs which belong to the tyrosine kinase receptor (TKR) family. These are localized predominantly on endothelial cells and angioblasts (Tol & Punt, 2010). In addition, in solid tumors, it is postulated that the production of VEGF is increased following liberation of hypoxia-inducible factor 1α (HIF-1α) (Kaur et al., 2005), EGF (Niu et al., 2002) and HGF (Dong et al., 2001). In turn, VEGF induces the synthesis of other factors related to tumor development, such as stroma-derived factor 1 (SDF-1) which induces an increase in the population of cancer-associated fibroblasts (CAFs) (Kalluri & Zeisberg, 2006, Christophi et al., 2008).

The risk of developing hepatic metastasis associated with CRC may be related to the expression of different VEGF isoforms which bind to the different VEGFRs. Thus, it has been shown that in 50% of CRCs, VEGFR-2 is expressed on the surface of the tumor cells (Duff et al., 2006). This extensive expression, which reflects the dependence of some solid tumors on neoangiogenesis, has led to the proposal that VEGF and VEGFR may be therapeutic targets in the treatment of CRC. Bevacizumab is a humanized monoclonal antibody which binds to VEGFA blocking the binding of this GF to VEGFR, thereby avoiding the corresponding intracellular signal transduction. Although parameters which allow a prediction of the efficacy of this monoclonal antibody have not been reported, bevacizumab has been approved as a first and second-line therapy for the treatment of metastatic CRC, enhancing survival, stabilizing the disease and achieving partial regression when used with chemotherapy. Two recent and complete reviews by Tol & Punt (2010) and Wanebo & Berz, (2010) analyze randomized and non-randomized trials of neo-adjuvant therapy using bevacizumab in metastatic CRC.

3. The role of the redox state in the mechanism of action of growth factors

The redox state is a key characteristic which influences important cell biological processes including enzymatic reactions, cell signaling, cell proliferation and apoptosis. The term redox signaling refers to a regulatory process in which the signal is transmitted through redox reactions. The intra- and extracellular redox levels allow the carrying out of different extra and intracellular signaling (intra-cytoplasmic and nuclear), which subsequently give rise to the cascade of effector signals that regulate diverse cellular activities such as cell proliferation.

GF signals are transmitted from the cell surface by means of the activation of TK-type transmembrane receptors and the induction of the corresponding intracellular effects.

Among these signal transduction pathways, protein phosphorylation plays a fundamental role. This process is reversible and dynamic, being controlled by the opposing actions of protein tyrosine kinases (PTKs) and protein tyrosine phosphatases (PTPs). As a consequence of the binding of GF to its specific receptor, dimerization occurs followed by the autophosphorylation of tyrosine residues in the intracellular domain of the receptor (Cadena & Gill, 1992). These residues are key sites of interaction with cytoplasmic proteins which contain SH2 (*Src homology type 2*) domains; these mediate the signal transduction of GFs, such as PLC- γ, GAP-ras (*GTP-ase-activating protein of ras*), PIK3 and Grb2 (Johnson & Vaillancourt, 1994). The action of all these proteins, via different mechanisms, converges to activate the Ras protein, which in its turn, activates the Raf tyrosine. Subsequently, a phosphorylation cascade is produced in such a manner that Raf phosphorylates another kinase, the MAPK kinase which phosphorylates members of a family of serine/threonine kinases, the MAP kinases. Finally, MAP kinases phosphorylate the transcription factors which promote the transcription of genes necessary for the final cellular response (Davis, 1993).

Many studies have demonstrated that the cellular redox status plays a key role in GF-mediated signaling systems (Thannickal & Fanburg, 2000). Although there is evidence that GFs generate ROS, it is not yet clear how ROS activate these cell signaling pathways. One plausible mechanism is that ROS could act as second messengers which participate in phosphorylation/dephosphorylation processes (Storz, 2005). ROS, such as hydrogen peroxidase (H_2O_2), induce the phosphorylation and activation of some PTKs, such as the kinases implicated in the MAP kinase cascade (Rao, 1996). In contrast, PTPs have a cysteine residue in their catalytic domain, which must be in its reduced form for total activity of the receptor. It has been shown that in cell signaling phenomena, ROS may induce the inactivation of PTPs (Rhee et al., 2000). Interestingly, ROS play a crucial role in vascular angiogenesis, not only due to their induction of VEGF (Sen et al., 2002), but also to their implication in the VEGF signaling pathway. Thus, VEGF stimulates ROS production via the activation of nicotinamide adenine dinucleotide phosphate (NADPH) oxidase, which is essential for the satisfactory propagation of the angiogenic signal (Roy et al., 2008); in fact, NADPH oxidase has been proposed as a target for anticancer therapy (Ushio-Fukai & Nakamura, 2008).

Similarly, it has been demonstrated that EGF stimulates ROS production in cells and that inhibition of this production leads to a weakening of the signaling system of the corresponding factor (Mills et al., 1998). A ROS mediated signaling cascade has also been reported to be activated following stimulation of the c-Met/HGF system; this cascade has been found to be associated with the crucial role of the receptor in the development of metastasis (Ferraro et al., 2006).

All of these biological effects occur at low to moderate concentrations of ROS. For this reason, redox regulation is essential for the maintenance of an optimal level of oxidation which permits precise signal transduction and the appropriate cellular response.

4. Glutathione metabolism in colorectal cancer

Cells are exposed to oxidative stress which is generated by normal metabolism and also by exogenous factors, such as ionizing radiation, some chemotherapeutic drugs and xenobiotics. The oxidative modification of cell components via ROS is one of the most potentially damaging processes for normal cellular activity (Halliwell, 1991). However, ROS are well recognized for playing a dual role. Thus, a number of studies have provided convincing evidence that, depending on the level of oxidative stress, ROS can function as pro-life signals in certain contexts (as mentioned above, low or mild increases in ROS play a pivotal role in many physiological reactions, such as the regulation of transcription factors and cellular signaling pathways) (Maellaro et al., 2000) and pro-death signals in others (high concentrations of ROS can induce apoptosis) (Le Bras et al., 2005). Consequently, the maintenance of the redox status is a key factor for cell survival, in the case of both normal and cancer cells.

In order to maintain redox balance and also to protect themselves from oxidative stress, cells possess powerful redox regulation systems, known as the *"redox buffer"*, including GSH and thioredoxin (TRX), as well as antioxidant enzymes, such as superoxide dismutase (SOD), catalase, GSH peroxidase (GPx) and thioredoxin reductase (TrxR). In addition, cells also have available other non-enzymatic antioxidants which are obtained via the diet, among which are ascorbic acid (vitamin C), α-tocopherol (vitamin E), flavonoids, carotenoids and selenium.

Intracellular redox homeostasis is sustained primarily by GSH, the most prevalent intracellular non-protein thiol. In fact, the ratio between its reduced and oxidized states (GSH/GSSG) is considered to be an indicator of the redox status of the cell. GSH is intracellularly synthesized from the three amino acids glutamic acid, cysteine and glycine; it possesses an unusual γ peptide bond between glutamic acid and cysteine, and has a thiol group on the latter aminoacid. The biosynthesis and degradation of GSH occurs within the γ-glutamyl cycle, in which GSH is transported to the extracellular space and γ-glutamyl-aminoacids are transported to the intracellular space. GSH is synthesized from glutamate by two consecutive reactions which are catalyzed by the γ-glutamylcysteine synthetase (γ-GCS) and GSH synthetase enzymes. GSH can be exported outside the cell, although its constituent aminoacids can be reincorporated into the cell, thanks to a transpeptidation reaction catalyzed by the γ-glutamyl transpeptidase (γ-GT) enzyme, which is a glycoprotein localized on the outer surface of the plasma membrane. Transpeptidation occurs in the presence of aminoacids, giving rise to γ-glutamyl-aminoacids and cysteinylglycine (Cys-Gly). The γ-glutamyl-aminoacids are transported into the cell, whereas in the case of cysteinylglycine, bond breakage by means of a dipeptidase is first required. This dipeptidase is present on the outer surface of the plasma membrane, thereby allowing the incorporation of the peptides into the cell. The γ-glutamyl-aminoacids are the substrate of the γ-glutamyl cyclotransferase enzyme, which transforms the glutamyl residue into 5-oxoproline, liberating the remaining aminoacids. Next, by means of the 5-oxo-L-prolinase (5-OPase) enzyme, 5-oxoproline is transformed into glutamate and this reaction involves the consumption of ATP. The cycle is completed with the action again of γ-GCS and GSH synthetase (Fig. 1) (Meister & Anderson, 1983).

Due to its structural characteristics, GSH participates in numerous processes which are essential for cell physiology. GSH and its related enzymes are involved in cell proliferation and participate in the cell cycle, in the synthesis of proteins and in DNA synthesis and repair (Higuchi, 2004). In addition, its capacity as a reducing and antioxidant agent renders GSH an essential component for the maintenance of the integrity of the protein and lipid components of the cell, as well as a substrate for antioxidant GSH peroxidase enzymes, a selenium-dependent system. As indicated previously, another of its important functions consists in the protection of the cell from free radicals, endogenous and exogenous toxic substances, and carcinogens. GSH also defends the cell against the effects produced by radiation and some chemotherapeutic drugs, such as alkylating agents. The formation of GSH S-conjugated products generated during intracellular detoxification may occur due to the non-enzymatic reaction of exogenous electrophilic compounds or to the action of GSH S-transferase (GST) enzymes. GST conjugates can then be eliminated via an ATP-dependent GS-X pump.

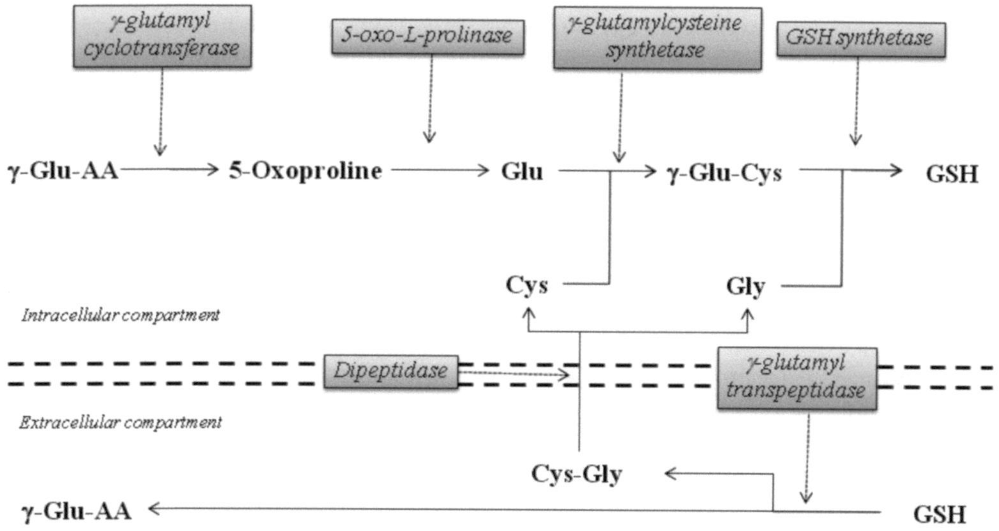

Fig. 1. The γ-glutamyl cycle. Abbreviations: γ-glu-AA, γ-glutamyl-aminoacids; Glu, glutamic acid; Cys, cysteine; Gly, glycine.

In addition to its essential role in normal growth, GSH is also involved in cell differentiation. Thus, it has been reported that as the cell progresses from proliferation to differentiation, cellular GSH content decreases. For example, it has been observed that butyrate-induced differentiation of the HT-29 human colon cell line is associated with reduced levels of cellular GSH (Bernard & Balasubramanian, 1997). These findings led to the notion that thiol status may be dependent on cellular energy metabolism. In this regard, the tumor cells have a very high cellular metabolism and, consequently, they generate high levels of ROS. Here, we should underline the importance of regulation of redox balance for the survival of malignant cells; the activation of redox regulatory systems, in which GSH plays an important role, could be considered to be the first line of adaptation of cancerous cells to oxidative stress. In fact it has been reported that non-differentiated and highly metastatic melanoma cells have a significantly higher GSH content than non-tumorigenic melanocytes (Thrall et al., 1991). Moreover, it has been demonstrated that whereas elevation of intracellular GSH is associated with mitogenic stimulation (Palomares et al., 1997), GSH depletion decreases the rate of cell proliferation and inhibits cancer growth (Del Olmo et al., 2000).

Increased levels of ROS in cancerous cells may have profound consequences, including enhanced cell proliferation, increased incidence of mutations and genetic instability, and reduced sensitivity of cells to anticancer agents, leading to resistance. In the case of CRC, intense oxidative stress and significant oxidative DNA adducts have been found during all stages of colorectal carcinogenesis (Schmid, et al., 2000). In fact, these DNA adducts, as well as GST polymorphisms, have been suggested as molecular biomarkers for the detection of early CRC and the prediction of the clinical effectiveness of chemopreventive drugs (Garcea et al., 2003). Elevated GST expression (Naidu et al., 2003) and a significant increase in GSH levels (Balendiran et al., 2004) have been found in CRC; these are often associated with an increased resistance to cancer chemotherapy drugs via GSH conjugation. Elevated GSH levels may also be related to γ-GCS, another GSH-related enzyme whose levels have also been found to be elevated in CRC (Tatebe et al., 2002). Finally, it should be remembered that GSH and its related enzymes is only one of the redox regulation systems which are implicated in CRC, since an increased expression of TRX-1 in human CRC has been found to be associated with reduced survival times of patients (Raffel et al., 2003).

In summary, the GSH system involves complex and dynamic processes in which several related enzymes participate. Although it may be difficult to know *a priori* what type of GSH metabolism a given CRC may have, the fact that some CRC cells contain high levels of GSH has led to the suggestion that it may be an important factor in limiting the therapeutic efficiency of conventional cancer treatment.

5. The influence of glutathione metabolism in the response to chemotherapy

A common cause of treatment failure in CRC is chemoresistance. This resistance to current cytotoxic therapies limits their success in the majority of advanced cancer patients. This is particularly true in the case of liver metastases.

GSH is able to modulate cell susceptibility to chemotherapy. In particular, GSH plays an important role in the protection against cell injury caused by various anticancer agents (see Balendiran et al., 2004 for review), and elevated GSH levels render tumor cells resistant to chemotherapeutic drugs. In the particular case of CRC, there is also evidence that the GSH status of colon cancer cells is a critical determinant of cell damage by various agents. Indeed, it has been proposed that elevated intracellular GSH levels may be a cause of acquired resistance to 5-FU, platinum agents and camptothecins. In this regard, it has been suggested that the increased levels of antioxidant enzymes in response to the generation of ROS by 5-FU, a standard drug for the treatment of this disease, may underlie the acquired resistance to this anti-tumor agent (Hwang et al., 2007). In *in vitro* studies, we have shown that treatment with 5-FU produced the greatest antiproliferative effect after 24 hours of incubation and that later, once drug treatment had been stopped, the growth of tumor cells rebounded (Palomares et al., 2009). This finding may be due to the recovery of GSH levels after the initial 5-FU-induced reduction, which has also been suggested by other authors (Chen et al., 1995).

It has also been reported that GSH may modulate the cytotoxicity of platinum agents (Sadowitz et al., 2002). However, intracellular GSH levels do not appear to influence the cell growth-inhibiting activity of these compounds in cells not previously exposed to platinum complexes (Boubakari et al., 2004), suggesting that GSH may be more relevant in acquired resistance. Furthermore, several authors have reported the influence of GSH on sensitivity to camptothecins (Yoshida et al., 2006).

In order to decrease the resistance of tumor cells to chemotherapeutic drugs, many GSH-based therapeutic strategies have focused on lowering GSH levels, principally via the use of agents which reduce this tripeptide or inhibit its synthesis. The agent which is most frequently used to reduce the levels of this thiol, not only in basic research but also in clinical assays, is L-buthionine-[S,R]-sulfoximine (BSO) (Fig. 2). We found that this potent inhibitor of γ-GCS enhances the sensitivity of tumor cells to treatment with ionizing radiation and cytostatic drugs, such as alkylating agents (Palomares et al., 1999). We have also found that the reduction in GSH content (around 52%) produced by BSO significantly inhibits the proliferation of colon cancer WiDr cells (Palomares et al., 2009).

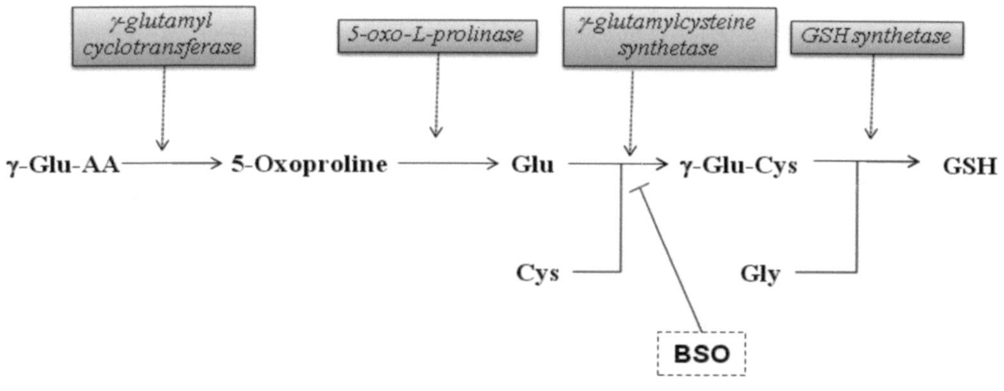

Fig. 2. Inhibition of γ-glutamylcysteine synthetase by L-buthionine-[S,R]-sulfoximine (BSO).

However, the anti-tumor efficacy of BSO is accompanied by increased toxicity, due to the fact that BSO exerts its effects in a non-selective manner. In fact, it reduces GSH levels in both tumor and normal cells and thus sensitizes both cell populations to the toxic effect of anticancer agents. This finding has been reported in clinical studies, such as that of Bailey et al. (1998), who upon combining BSO and melphalan, found an important increase in medullar toxicity with respect to that produced by the administration of the alkylating agent alone. Thus, BSO treatment produces toxicity at the level of the immune, gastrointestinal, urinary and central nervous systems. This toxicity limits, *de facto*, the therapeutic potential of BSO and of other non-selective GSH reducing agents.

One of the principal reasons for the limited effects of chemotherapy is the insufficient therapeutic index of available drugs. This index could be increased by regimes which protect healthy tissues against toxicity and at the same time enhance the sensitivity of tumor tissue to anticancer drugs. Since GSH is highly relevant in protecting both normal and tumor cells, one way of achieving this objective would be to selectively modulate GSH levels. An increase in GSH levels or in the capacity of normal cells to synthesize GSH, would enhance their resistance, leading to a protector effect. In contrast, a reduction in GSH content or in the capacity of tumor cells to synthesize this tripeptide would enhance sensitivity to the effects of anti-tumor agents. In this regard, it was suggested many years ago that agents which induce a selective modulation in GSH levels could be beneficially added to conventional treatments in order to enhance the anti-tumor efficacy of radiotherapy and/or chemotherapy (Russo et al., 1986).

Selective modulation of GSH as a therapeutic strategy requires an in-depth knowledge of the physiological differences in GSH synthesis and metabolism between healthy and tumor cells, as well as of the level of expression of GSH-related enzymes. In this regard, lower expression of the 5-OPase enzyme has been found in some tumor cell lines in comparison to healthy cells, leading to the suggestion that this enzyme may be a key player in obtaining the required selective modulation of GSH (Chen & Batist, 1998).

Within the γ-glutamyl cycle, 5-OPase catalyses the hydrolysis of 5-oxo-L-proline to L-glutamate, one of the three aminoacids which participate in GSH synthesis, joining in this way the reactions of GSH synthesis and metabolism in this cycle (see Fig. 1). It has also been observed that L-2-oxothiazolidine-4-carboxylate (OTZ) –an analog of 5-oxo-proline– also acts as a substrate of 5-OPase, thereby converting this cysteine prodrug into S-carboxycysteine, hydrolyzing it subsequently to cysteine and CO2 (Fig. 3).
Some studies have found that in contrast to BSO, OTZ treatment is selective, increasing GSH levels in healthy tissue and reducing it paradoxically in tumor tissue (Chen & Batist, 1998). These authors have suggested that OTZ, by competing with 5-oxo-L-proline for 5-OPase, could exert two different effects on GSH levels, depending on the level of expression of the 5-OPase enzyme and on the quantity of aminoacids necessary for the synthesis of the said tripeptide. In this way, OTZ would increase intracellular levels of GSH in healthy cells by means of increasing the contribution of cysteine - in normal conditions, the limiting aminoacid in GSH synthesis in these cells - (Meister A, 1983), but would reduce GSH content in tumor cells by means of the inhibition of glutamate synthesis from 5-oxo-L-proline. In fact, it has been observed that in tumor cells and in other cells under conditions of oxidative stress, glutama`te is the limiting factor in GSH synthesis (Kang, 1993)

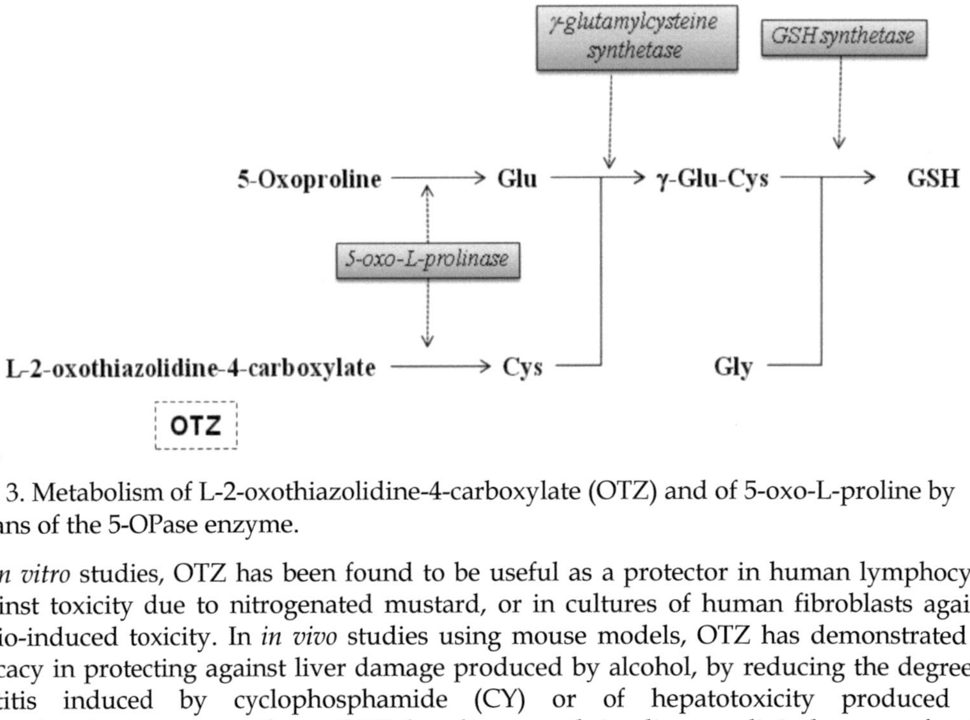

Fig. 3. Metabolism of L-2-oxothiazolidine-4-carboxylate (OTZ) and of 5-oxo-L-proline by means of the 5-OPase enzyme.

In *in vitro* studies, OTZ has been found to be useful as a protector in human lymphocytes against toxicity due to nitrogenated mustard, or in cultures of human fibroblasts against radio-induced toxicity. In *in vivo* studies using mouse models, OTZ has demonstrated its efficacy in protecting against liver damage produced by alcohol, by reducing the degree of cystitis induced by cyclophosphamide (CY) or of hepatotoxicity produced by acetaminophen, among others. OTZ has been used in diverse clinical assays for the treatment of a variety of pathologies associated with ROS generation and with reduced GSH levels. Diseases in which OTZ treatment has been successfully employed include acute respiratory distress syndrome (Morris et al., 2008), amyotrophic lateral sclerosis (Cudkowicz et al., 1999) and atherosclerosis (Vita et al., 1998). Patients subjected to peritoneal dialysis (Moberly et al., 1998) and patients infected with the AIDS virus (Barditch-Crovo et al., 1998) have also benefited from this treatment.

Paradoxically, in contrast to the effect produced in healthy tissue, OTZ reduces GSH levels in some human tumor cell lines including breast adenocarcinoma and ovary adenocarcinoma (Chen & Batist, 1998). In the same way, we have also demonstrated the selective character of GSH modulation by OTZ, *in vitro* as well as *in vivo*. Thus, OTZ was found to reduce the intracellular content of GSH in melanoma cells, producing reduced proliferation and increased chemosensitivity, whereas it increased GSH levels in peripheral blood mononuclear cells, exhibiting a corresponding cytoprotector effect (Del Olmo et al., 2000, 2006; Bilbao et al., 2002).

Several authors have pointed to the usefulness of GSH modulating agents as an adjuvant in chemotherapy treatments for CRC. Regarding 5-FU, a number of studies support the therapeutic use of antioxidant compounds in combination with this drug. Thus, therapy with high doses of antioxidants such as pyrrolidine dithiocarbamate (PDTC) and N-acetylcysteine (NAC) seem to enhance the therapeutic efficacy of 5-FU (Bach et al., 2001).

NAC is a prodrug of cysteine, which is an essential element for GSH synthesis. It was developed to avoid the important toxicity produced as a consequence of the direct administration of this aminoacid. The mechanisms of protection of this thiol against mutagenesis and carcinogenesis are related to a large number of biological effects, including antioxidant activity, involvement in DNA repair mechanisms, modulation of gene expression and of signal transduction, immunological activity, regulation of cell survival and of apoptosis, inhibition of cell transformation, of invasion and metastasis and of angiogenic activity, among others (Morini et al., 1999). However, some authors have reported contradictory effects of NAC in its anticancer action. Moreover, it has been demonstrated that antioxidant protection therapy in cancer patients should be used with caution, since it can give rise to counterproductive effects (Brizel & Overgaard, 2003). The reduction in the concentration of free radicals due to the excessive administration of antioxidants can stimulate the survival of damaged cells, enhancing the neoplastic stage, thereby promoting carcinogenesis more than inhibiting it. Furthermore, we and others have demonstrated that the increase in GSH levels induced by NAC is not specific to normal cells; rather, this can also occur in tumor cells, such as melanoma, increasing its proliferative capacity and protecting it against the cytotoxic effects of acrolein, one of the active metabolites of CY (Del Olmo et al., 2000).

It has also been found that the reduced levels of GSH induced by BSO and OTZ, lead to an increased cytotoxic effect of 5-FU in different human CRC cells (Meurette et al., 2005; Palomares et al., 2009). It has also been observed that BSO enhances the activity of SN-38 (an active metabolite of the anticancer drug irinotecan) in WiDr colon cancer cells (Caramés et al., 2010), and in cell lines of ovary cancer resistant to cisplatin, as well as of breast cancer. BSO is also capable of reverting resistance to SN-38 in leukemia cells with increased GSH levels (Yoshida et al., 2006). This increased anti-tumor effect of SN-38 may be related to the reduced activity of the transcription factor NF-κB, which is dependent on the intracellular redox status and thus sensitive to a reduced content of intracellular GSH. In fact, SN-38 is known to activate NF-κB and so the pharmacological inhibition of this NF-κB signaling pathway can enhance the anti-tumor activity of SN-38 in colon cancer cells *in vitro* and of irinotecan *in vivo* (Lagadec et al., 2008).

Regarding platinum compounds, various authors have demonstrated that GSH participates in the detoxification of these agents and that reduced GSH levels sensitize cancer cells to the cytotoxic effects of these anti-tumor agents (Jansen et al., 2002). We have found that both BSO and OTZ increase the efficacy of oxaliplatin in the WiDr human colon cancer cell line

(Caramés et al., 2010). Thus, reduced GSH levels mediated by BSO or OTZ lead to an increase in cytotoxicity induced by drugs which are more frequently used nowadays for CRC therapy, with an additive effect being observed in the antiproliferative effects of these combinations.

6. The influence of growth factors in the sensitivity of tumor cells to chemotherapy

Research on the phenomenon of chemotherapy resistance has traditionally focused on the tumor cells themselves. However, it has become apparent that the tumor microenvironment may also influence chemoresistance in an important way. In this regard, it is necessary to underline the fundamental role of GFs in cancer biology and in the formation of metastasis, since they control critical functions in cancer cells, such as proliferation, angiogenesis and the inhibition of apoptosis. Thus, GFs, due to their capacity to modulate the sensitivity of tumor cells to cytotoxic drugs, have become important targets for the development of new anti-cancer therapies, either as individual agents or in combination with conventional chemotherapy, with the aim of enhancing the efficacy of anti-cancer drugs.

It has been demonstrated that the presence of GFs significantly reduces the cytotoxic activity of a number of commonly used drugs. In this regard, some authors have pointed out that HGF protects tumor cells against the cytotoxicity and apoptosis induced by DNA-damaging agents, such as ionizing radiation or adriamycin (Shen et al., 2007), and that it may contribute to the resistance of RMS cells to conventional treatment (Jankowski et al., 2003). Similarly, it has been suggested that this factor could induce resistance to cisplatin in lung cancer cells (Chen et al., 2008). Nevertheless, in contrast to expectations, it has also been observed that HGF sensitizes ovary cancer cells to the drugs paclitaxel and cisplatin (Bardella et al., 2007). These findings indicate that HGF effects depend on the targeted tumor type. Indeed, various other studies have reported the effect of VEGF in reducing the efficacy of endocrine therapy in breast cancer (Qu et al., 2008). It has also been found that VEGF diminishes the response to drugs in myeloid leukemia (De Jonge et al., 2008) and that doxorubicin exerts a milder inhibitory effect in the presence of VEGF overexpression in soft-tissue sarcoma (Zhang et al., 2006). Regarding EGF, it has been widely demonstrated that this GF reduces the response of tumors, such as human breast carcinoma, to cytotoxic compounds and to radiotherapy (Schmidt & Lichtner, 2002).

In the case of CRC, we (Palomares et al., 2009) and others (Sun & Tang, 2003; Allendorf et al., 2004) have demonstrated that HGF, EGF and VEGF significantly reduce the efficacy of drugs currently used in CRC. In particular, the increased expression of HGF and VEGF results in fluoropyrimidine-based adjuvant chemotherapy being less effective, increasing the risk of recurrence. In relation to EGF, it has been shown that its receptor, EGFR, increases resistance to 5-FU. Moreover, 5-FU itself induces the activation of EGFR, which protect colon cancer cells against chemotherapy (Hiro et al., 2008). Moreover, it has been reported that SN-38, through a mechanism involving ROS, induces the activation of EGF and EGFR, and this could contribute to resistance to irinotecan (Kishida et al., 2005). These data suggest that inhibition of the EGFR signaling pathway could revert resistance to treatment with the fluoropyrimidines and irinotecan. On the basis of this hypothesis, some authors have carried out assays using tyrosine kinase inhibitors of EGFR, such as gefitinib (Stebbing et al., 2008), as well as inhibitors of the Src tyrosine kinase (Ischenko et al., 2008).

The molecular mechanisms underlying GF-mediated resistance continue to be largely unknown. On the one hand, GFs induce cell proliferation and the activation of anti-apoptotic signaling pathways, via proteins such as Bcl-XL, thereby contributing to the resistance to apoptosis in CRC cells following treatment with 5-FU, oxaliplatin and irinotecan (Schulze-Bergkamen et al., 2008). In addition, it has also been suggested that GFs may also induce an increase in the repair of damaged DNA (Hiro et al., 2008). On the other hand, it has been observed that the EGFR-Src-STAT3 oncogenic signaling pathway plays an important role in CRC, contributing to proliferation, cell survival and treatment resistance (Hbibi et al., 2008). In fact, it has been demonstrated that this pathway is activated in response to treatment with topoisomerase I inhibitors, such as camptothecins, reducing DNA damage and enhancing cell survival (Vigneron et al, 2008).

Moreover, as we have recently shown, GFs give rise to an increase in GSH levels which, as mentioned earlier, is an important mechanism of cell defense against oxidative stress and against the effects produced by radiation and by some chemotherapeutic agents; this increase in GSH levels has been correlated with diminished 5-FU anti-tumor activity in colon cancer cells (Palomares et al., 2009). In this regard, it has been reported that the combination of an EGFR inhibitor with doxorubicin leads to enhanced cytotoxic effects via the generation of oxidative stress, due to ROS induction and reduced GSH content in rat hepatoma cells (Ortiz et al., 2008).

Additionally, it has been suggested that GF-induced increases in intracellular GSH levels and the activation of the redox-sensitive transcription factor NF-κB could play a major role in inducible chemoresistance. This cell survival transcription factor, which is subject to regulation by GSH (Lou & Kaplowitz, 2007), has been shown to be constitutively activated in many colon cancer cells. NF-κB has been shown to be associated with the proliferation of tumor cells, with invasion, angiogenesis and the production of metastasis (Bours et al., 1994). It has been demonstrated that HGF, via the PI3K/Akt signaling pathway, leads to the activation of NF-κB, by means of which cells are protected against adriamycin and irinotecan (Fan et al., 2005). In the same way, the transmission of the proliferative signal induced by EGF is also mediated by the activation of NF-κB (Sethi et al., 2007), which plays an important role in the regulation of EGFR ligands via a ROS-mediated mechanism (Murillo et al., 2007). Moreover, NF-κB activation in response to exposure to anti-cancer drugs has been shown to be one of the mechanisms of tumor resistance to chemotherapy, as has been reported in the cases of 5-FU and irinotecan (Ahn et al., 2008). In contrast, inhibition of NF-κB has been shown to enhance the sensitivity of colon cancer tumor cells to HT-29 and 5-FU (Voboril et al., 2004).

Overall, these data indicate that GFs play a critical role in the resistance of colon cancer cells to chemotherapeutic agents. In consequence, these factors are potential therapeutic targets for increasing the anti-tumor activity of cytotoxic drugs.

7. New therapeutic strategies to enhance the response of CRC to chemotherapy by reversion of the growth factor pro-tumour effects

Based on the aforementioned data, GFs have been identified as important targets to be considered in the development of new anticancer drugs and, consequently, many experimental studies have been carried out to evaluate the effects of blocking GF effects on tumor cells. These attempts could be classified into three categories, according to the mechanism chosen to avoid the GF stimulation of these cells. The first approach was to administer monoclonal antibodies (MoAb) against one or several GFs, and the results have been quite exciting. Another idea was to produce MoAb against the membrane receptors for different GFs, and again the results have been very promising. In fact, several of these MoAb have already entered the armamentarium for cancer therapy and others are currently at different stages of clinical trials. The third exciting arm of these GF-based therapies consists of the so-called "small molecules" which block the activation of the intracellular part of GF receptors.

The combination of conventional cytotoxic drugs with new agents that specifically interfere with GF signaling pathways presents the advantage of avoiding crossed resistance, since these approaches are directed against different cell targets and have different underlying mechanisms of action. In this regard, many studies have indicated that inhibitors of GFs or of their receptors enhance the efficacy of conventional cytotoxic agents (Wanebo & Berz, 2010). The GF inhibitors bevacizumab and cetuximab are particularly noteworthy. Currently, bevacizumab is used in combination with regimes which contain 5-FU (FOLFOX or FOLFIRI) as a first line therapy in advanced or metastatic CRC (Giantonio et al., 2007; Tol & Punt, 2010). On the other hand, combined therapy consisting of irinotecan and cetuximab is indicated after progression in patients who have previously received 5-FU based therapy (Cunningham et al., 2004).

Other agents, such as gefitinib, have been found in preclinical studies to exhibit synergistic inhibitory effects when administered in combination with different cytotoxic drugs. For example, some authors have observed that gefitinib and irinotecan act synergistically in WiDr cells, as a result of the inhibition of the survival signal induced by irinotecan via the phosphorylation of EGFR (Koizumi et al., 2004). Similarly, *in vitro* studies have shown that the combination of gefitinib and oxaliplatin has a synergistic effect in colon cancer cells due, at least in part, to the fact that the EGFR inhibitor reduces the activity of γ-GT. This enzyme, which participates in the γ-glutamyl cycle, helps to salvage extracellular GSH and contributes to redox control by providing a substrate for GSH synthesis during oxidative stress, thereby preventing apoptosis, as we have showed previously (Castro et al., 2002). Reduced γ-GT activity thereby leads to increased cellular oxaliplatin accumulation and platinum-DNA adducts (Xu et al., 2003).

However, these anti-tumor agents also have their inconveniences. They induce diverse side effects which complicates their clinical use (Mulder et al., 2011). Also, as happens with other chemotherapeutic agents, the development of resistance to these GF-based agents has already been reported (Giaccone & Wang, 2011). For these reasons, it is important to continue the search for new therapeutic strategies which could be used in combination in order to enhance the efficacy of GF-related targeted agents. In this sense, the therapeutic biomodulation of GSH metabolism may hold promise for the improvement of the efficacy of anticancer treatments. Many lines of evidence indicate that this may be an effective approach to treating cancer: i) the fact that tumor cells are under high levels of oxidative stress may represent a great opportunity given that it means they are particularly vulnerable to further increases in ROS levels; ii) colon cancer cells contain particularly high levels of GSH; iii) GF-induced signal transduction pathways are redox sensitive, and accordingly, alterations in cellular GSH content may affect the growth of GF-sensitive cells; and iv) the fact that NF-κB is involved in GF-dependent proliferation and that the activity of this transcription factor might also be subject to regulation by GSH suggests that depletion of cellular GSH could interrupt NF-κB activity and consequently lead to growth inhibition.

In this regard, we have recently demonstrated that GSH-induced depletion by BSO or OTZ abrogated the growth-promoting effects of GFs in WiDr colon cancer cells (Palomares et al., 2009). Similarly, other authors have demonstrated that BSO inhibits GSH upregulation induced by HGF, thereby blocking its mitogenic effect (Yang et al., 2008) and the protection against apoptosis afforded by this factor. It has likewise been reported that BSO interferes with EGF-induced proliferation and that extended exposure (for 48 h or more) of cells to BSO induces cell death, probably via a necrotic mechanism (Carmona-Cuenca et al., 2006). Regarding VEGF, it has also been reported that BSO treatment reverts increased GSH activity induced by this factor and, in this way, its vasculoprotective function (Kuzuya et al., 2001). In contrast, decreased GSH levels produced by BSO have been shown to promote the autocrine secretion of VEGF (Sreekumar et al., 2006).

Thus, the two effects derived from the biomodulation of GSH intracellular content with BSO or OTZ, i.e. i) the reversion of the pro-tumor effect of GFs and ii) the enhanced efficacy of chemotherapy, may contribute to enhancing the therapeutic benefit of chemotherapy treatment. In fact, we have shown that, in the presence of GFs, the combination of either of the GSH modulators with chemotherapeutic drugs produced greater anti-tumor activity than the cytotoxic drugs alone. Thus, we found that both BSO and OTZ completely reverted the resistance (due to the presence of GFs) of WiDr colon cancer cells to 5-FU, a finding which holds promise for more successful anticancer treatment, particularly after surgical resection of hepatic metastases (Palomares et al., 2009). Indeed, 5-FU activity was enhanced by 40% following the addition of GSH modulators. The activity of oxaliplatin was also found to be significantly enhanced (by nearly 25%). Moreover, combined therapy with SN-38 was found to produce the optimal chemotherapeutic combination; thus, OTZ pretreatment combined with SN-38 resulted in an increase of almost 70% in the cytotoxic activity of SN-38 (Caramés et al., 2010). To this benefit, we must also add the advantage of OTZ with respect to BSO, i.e. the selective reduction of GSH levels in tumor cells, protecting healthy cells, as mentioned above.

Other interesting approaches to the GF problem in cancer therapy have been developed. Thus, as cell proliferation and differentiation are deregulated in tumor cells, the induction of cell differentiation with retinoids could help to neutralize the pro-tumor effect of GFs. The mechanisms of action which underlie the effects of retinoids include the activation of nuclear retinoic acid receptors (RAR), but also, curiously, the induction of enhanced ROS levels (Palomares et al. , 2006) and a direct interaction of retinoids with the GSH-dependent protein kinase C, a key regulatory enzyme in signal transduction (Radominska-Pandya et al., 2000). In this sense, we have analyzed the effect of all-trans-retinoic acid (ATRA), a well known pro-differentiating agent, on the growth-promoting effect of GFs in two tumor models. This drug was found to reduce the proliferative rate of RMS (García-Alonso et al., 2005) and CRC cells (Martínez-Astorquiza et al., 2008), and hindered or completely abolished the stimulus produced by serum obtained from hepatectomized rats, and by a wide variety of GFs (HGF, VEGF, PDGF, EGF, bFGF). Furthermore, we also found that cells cultured in medium containing ATRA do not develop resistance to the drug, and these ATRA-preexposed cells responded to subsequent ATRA treatments in the same manner as non-treated cells. However, we observed that the antiproliferative effect of ATRA *in vitro* is not permanent: forty eight hours after removing the drug from the culture medium the cells recovered their normal proliferative rate (Díaz et al., 2009). Nevertheless, in *in vitro* studies, we found that ATRA did not interfere with the antiproliferative effect of chemotherapeutics drugs, such as 5-FU; moreover, when both drugs were administered together, an additive effect was observed (García-Alonso et al., 2010).

In order to corroborate these findings *in vivo*, we designed an experimental model in which daily intraperitoneal doses of ATRA were administered for two weeks, starting three days before a partial hepatectomy was performed in animals bearing liver metastases. These *in vivo* experiments confirmed the efficacy of ATRA in reducing the proliferative rate of tumor cells. In rats bearing RMS S4MH liver metastases, the mean number of liver metastases, as well as their mean size, were significantly reduced and significantly longer survival was achieved. Using this tumor model, we also analyzed the synergistic effect of ATRA with commonly used chemotherapeutic agents such as CY. Once again, animals treated with ATRA+CY presented a significant reduction in the mean number of liver metastases and also an increase in survival compared to animals treated with CY alone. Similar experiments were carried out with the murine CC-531 colon cancer cell line, and similar, albeit not so dramatic, results were found (unpublished data). Thus, the mean number of liver metastases was unmodified by ATRA, but the mean size of the liver foci was significantly reduced, suggesting that tumor progression had been retarded. However, survival remained unaltered. Regarding drug tolerance, ATRA was well tolerated by the animals, with no repercussion on hematological cell counts, serum enzymes or weight gain. These findings point to the need to enhance ATRA effects via other mechanisms. In this regard, it has recently been shown that the selective COX-2 inhibitor celecoxib, increased the expression of RARbeta in human colon cancer cells, as well as sensitivity to ATRA through COX-2-independent mechanisms (Liu et al., 2010).

Novel synthetic derivatives of ATRA have been developed recently and examined in clinical trials (Sogno et al, 2010). However, these trials involve administration of the drug as a conventional chemotherapeutic agent (Kummar et al, 2011). In the light of the above, it is apparent that retinoids (or pro-differentiating agents in general) should be tested as a complementary treatment, and administered as part of a combined therapy during the early postoperative period, when their action would be most effective. Otherwise, it is unlikely that significant improvements will be found in patients treated with these agents in monotherapy.

Overall, and in the light of the important role of GFs in tumor recurrence following surgical resection of hepatic metastases, the use of GSH modulators and pro-differentiating agents seems to hold promise as a novel therapeutic strategy for metastatic CRC, by reversing GF pro-tumor effects and improving the efficacy of chemotherapy.

8. Conclusion

Growth factors play a pivotal role in the regulation of CRC progression and metastasis. They are involved not only in promoting tumor growth, but also in reducing the responsiveness of tumor cells to cytotoxic compounds. The mechanisms of action underlying GF effects include the redox state of the tumor, in particular GSH metabolism, and the level of expression of related enzymes. The biomodulation of GSH metabolism via agents such as BSO or OTZ, could reverse the growth-promoting effects of GFs and enhance the therapeutic benefit of chemotherapeutic drugs. The use of pro-differentiating agents may also represent a promising anti-tumor strategy to block the pro-tumor effects of GFs. The development of more effective retinoids, used either alone or preferably in combination with other dugs, may also provide more effective anti-tumor benefits. These new types of strategies to neutralize the pro-tumor effects of GFs may well be crucial in the treatment of metastatic disease and the prevention of the recurrence of liver metastases arising from CRC.

9. Acknowledgments

This work was supported by research grants from the University of the Basque Country (Project GIU 10/16) and Gangoiti Barrera Foundation.

10. References

Ahn KS, Sethi G & Aggarwal BB. (2008). Reversal of chemoresistance and enhancement of apoptosis by statins through down-regulation of the NF-kappaB pathway. *Biochem Pharmacol*, Vol.75, No4 (2008 Feb 15), pp 907-13. Epub 2007 Oct 16. ISSN: 0006-2952.

Allendorf J, Ippagunta N & Emond J. (2004). Management of liver metastases: new horizons for biologically based therapy. *J Surg Res*, Vol.117, No.1 (March 2004), pp.144-153, **ISSN:** 0022-4804.

Bach SP, Williamson SE, Marshman E, Kumar S, O`Dwyer ST, Potten CS & Watson AJ. (2001). The antioxidant N-acetylcysteine increases 5-fluorouracil activity against colorectal cancer xenografts in nude mice. *J Gastrointest Surg*, Vol.5, No.1 (January-February 2001), pp. 91-97, ISSN: 1091-255X.

Bailey HH. (1998). L-S,R-buthionine sulfoximine: historical development and clinical issues. *Chem Biol Interact*, Vol.112, (April 1998), pp.239-254, ISSN: 0009-2797.

Balendiran GK, Dabur R & Fraser D. (2004). The role of glutathione in cancer. *Cell Biochem Funct*, Vol.22, No.6 (November-December 2004), pp.343–352, ISSN: 0263-6484.

Barberá-Guillem E, Alonso-Varona A & Vidal-Vanaclocha F. (1989). Selective implantation and growth in rats and mice of experimental liver metastasis in acinar zone one. *Cancer Res*, Vol.49, No.14 (July 1989), pp.4003-4010, ISSN: 0008-5472.

Bardella C, Dettori D, Olivero M, Coltella N, Mazzone M & Di Renzo MF. (2007). The therapeutic potential of hepatocyte growth factor to sensitize ovarian cancer cells to cisplatin and paclitaxel *in vivo.Clin Cancer Res*, Vol.13, No.7 (April 2007), pp.2191-2198, ISSN: 1078-0432.

Barditch-Crovo P, Noe D, Skowron G, Lederman M, Kalayjian RC, Borum P, Buier R, Rowe WB, Goldberg D & Lietman P. (1998). A phase I/II evaluation of oral L-2-oxothiazolidine-4-carboxylic acid in asymptomatic patients infected with human immunodeficiency virus. *J Clin Pharmacol, Vol.*38, No.4 (April 1998), pp.357-363, ISSN: 0091-2700.

Benvenuti S, Sartore-Bianchi A, Di Nicolantonio F, Zanon C, Moroni M, Veronese S, Siena S & Bardelli A. (2007). Oncogenic activation of the RAS/RAF signaling pathway impairs the response of metastatic colorectal cancers to anti-epidermal growth factor receptor antibody therapies. *Cancer Research,* Vol.67, No.6 (March 2007), pp.2643-2648, ISSN: **0008**-5472.

Bernard O & Balasubramanian KA. (1997). Modulation of glutathione level during butyrate-induced differentiation in human colon derived HT-29 cells. *Mol Cell Biochem,* Vol.170, No.1-2 (May 1997), pp.109-114, ISSN: 0300-8177.

Bilbao P, Del Olmo M, Alonso-Varona A, Castro B, Bilbao J & Palomares T. (2002). L-2-Oxothiazolidine-4-Carboxylate reverses the tumour growth-promoting effect of interleukin-2 and improves the anti-tumour efficacy of biochemotherapy in mice bearing B16 melanoma liver metastases. *Melanoma Res,* Vol.12, No.1 (February 2002), pp.17-26, ISSN: 0960-8931.

Blobe GC & Gordon KJ. (2000). Role of transforming growth factor beta in human disease.*Bioch et Bioph Acta Molec Basis of Disease,* Vol.1782, No.4 (April 2008), pp.1350-1358, ISSN: 0925-4439.

Boubakari, Bracht K, Neumann C, Grunert R & Bednarski PJ. (2004). No correlation between GSH levels in human cancer cell lines and the cell growth inhibitory activities of platinum diamine complexes. *Arch Pharm,* Vol.337, No.12 (December 2004), pp.668-671, ISSN: 0365-6233.

Bours V, Dejardin E, Goujon-Letawe F, Merville MP & Castronovo V. (1994). The NF-kappa B transcription factor and cancer: high expression of NF-kappa B- and I kappa B-related proteins in tumor cell lines. *Biochem Pharmacol,* Vol.47, No.1 (January 1994), pp.145-149, ISSN: 0006-2952.

Brizel DM & Overgaard J (2003). Does amifostine have a role in chemoradiation treatment? *Lancet Oncol.* Vol.4, No.6 (2003 Jun), pp.378-381. ISSN: 1470-2045.

Cadena DL & Gill GN. (1992). Receptor tyrosine kinases. *FASEB J,* Vol.6, No.6 (March 1992), pp.2332-2337, ISSN: 0892-6638.

Cao B, Su Y, Oskarsson M, Zhao P, Kort EJ, Fisher RJ, Wang LM & Vande Woude GF.(2001). Neutralizing monoclonal antibodies to hepatocyte growth factor/scatter factor (HGF/SF) display antitumor activity in animal models. *Proc Natl Acad Sci U S A,* Vol.98, No.13 (June 2001), pp.7443-7448, ISSN: 0027-8424.

Caramés, M, Alonso-Varona A, García-Alonso I & Palomares T. (2010). Glutathione modulators reverse the pro-tumour effect of growth factors enhancing WiDr cell response to chemotherapeutic agents. *Anticancer Res,* Vol.30, No.4 (April 2010), pp.1223-1231, ISSN: 0250-7005.

Carmona-Cuenca I, Herrera B, Ventura JJ, Roncero C, Fernández M & Fabregat I. (2006). EGF blocks NADPH oxidase activation by TGF-beta in fetal rat hepatocytes, impairing oxidative stress, and cell death. *J Cell Physiol,* Vol.207, No.2 (May 2006), pp.322-330, ISSN: 0021-9541.

Castro B, Alonso-Varona A, del Olmo M, Bilbao P & Palomares T. (2002). Role of gamma-glutamyltranspeptidase on the response of poorly and moderately differentieted rhabdomyosarcoma cell lines to buthionine sulfoximine-induced inhibition of glutathione synthesis. *Anti-Cancer Drugs,* Vol.13, No.3 (March 2002), pp.281-291, ISSN: 0959-4973.

Chen JT, Huang CY, Chiang YY, Chen WH, Chiou SH, Chen CY & Chow KC. (2008). HGF increases cisplatin resistance via down-regulation of AIF in lung cancer cells. *Am J Respir Cell Mol Biol.* Vol. 38, No.5 (2008 May), pp.559-65. Epub 2007 Dec 20. ISSN: 1044-1549.

Chen MF, Chen LT & Bouce HW Jr. (1995). 5-Fluorouracil cytotoxicity in human colon HT-29 cells with moderately increased or decreased cellular gluthatione level. *Anticancer Res*, Vol.15, No.1 (January-February 1995), pp.163-167, ISSN: 0250-7005.

Chen X & Batist G. (1998). Sensitization effect of L-2-oxothiazolidine-4-carboxylate on tumor cells to melpahalan and the role of 5-oxo-L-prolinase in glutathione modulation in tumor cells. *Biochem Pharmacol*, Vol.56, No.6 (September 1998), pp.743-749, ISSN: 0006-2952.

Christophi C, Harun N & Fifis T. (2008). Liver regeneration and tumor stimulation-A review of Cytokine and angiogenic factors. *Journal of Gastrointestinal Surgery*, Vol.12, No.5 (May 2008), pp.966-980, ISSN: 1091-255X.

Chung KY, Shia J, Kemeny NE, Shah M, Schwartz GK, Tse A, Hamilton A, Pan D, Schrag D, Schwartz L, Klimstra DS, Fridman D, Kelsen DP & Saltz LB. (2005). Cetuximab shows activity in colorectal cancer patients with tumors that do not express the epidermal growth factor receptor by immunohistochemistry. *Journal of Clinical Oncology*, Vol.23, No.9 (March 2005), pp.1803-1810, ISSN: 0732-183X.

Cudkowicz ME, Sexton PM, Ellis T, Hayden DL, Gwilt PR, Whalen J & Brown RH Jr. (1999). The pharmacokinetics and pharmaco-dynamics of procysteine in amyotrophic lateral sclerosis. *Neurology*, Vol.52, No.7 (April 1999), pp.1492-1494, ISSN: 0028-3878.

Cunningham D, Humblet Y, Siena S, Khayat D, Bleiberg H, Santero A, Bets D, Mueser M, Harstrick A, Verslype C, Chau I & Van Cutsem E. (2004). Cetuximab monotherapy and cetuximab plus irinotecan in irinotecan-refractory metastatic colorectal cancer. *N Engl J Med*, Vol.351, No.4 (July 2004), pp.337-345, ISSN: 0028-4793.

Davis RJ. (1993). The mitogen-activated protein kinase signal transduction pathway. *J Biol Chem*, Vol.268, No.20 (July 1993), pp.14553-14556, ISSN: 0021-9258.

De Jonge HJ, Weidenaar AC, Ter Elst A, Boezen HM, Scherpen FJ, Bouma-Ter Steege JC, Kaspers GJ, Goemans BF, Creutzig U, Zimmermann M, Kamps WA & de Bont ES. (2008). Endogenous vascular endothelial growth factor-C expression is associated with decreased drug responsiveness in childhood acute myeloid leukemia. *Clin Cancer Res*, Vol.14, No.3 (February 2008), pp.924-930, ISSN: 1078-0432.

Del Olmo M, Alonso-Varona A, Castro B, Calle Y, Bilbao P & Palomares T. (2000). Effects of L-2-oxothiazolidine-4-carboxylate on the cytotoxic activity and toxicity of cyclophosphamide in mice bearing B16F10 melanoma liver metastases. *Melanoma Res*, Vol.10, No.2 (April 2000), pp.103-112, ISSN: 0960-8931.

Del Olmo M, Alonso-Varona A, Castro B, Bilbao P, & Palomares T. (2006). Cytomodulation of interleukin-2-effect by L-2-oxothiazolidine-4-carboxylate on human malignant melanoma. *Cancer Immunol Immunother*, Vol.55, No.8 (August 2006), pp.948-957, ISSN: 0340-7004.

Di Renzo MF, Narsimhan RP, Olivero M, Bretti S, Giordano S, Medico E, Gaglia P, Zara P & Comoglio PM. (1991). Expression of the Met/HGF receptor in normal and neoplastic human tissues. *Oncogene*, Vol.6, No.11 (November 1991), pp.1997-2003, ISSN: 0950-9232.

Díaz I, Palomares T, Marín H, Alonso-Varona A, Herrero B & García-Alonso I. (2009). ATRA blockage of cancer cells' proliferation *in vitro* depends on the continuous presence of the drug. *Br J Surg,* Vol.96, No.S5 (May2009), pp.42, ISSN: 1365-2168.

Dong G, Chen Z, Li ZY, Yeh NT, Bancroft CC & Van Waes C. (2001). Hepatocyte growth factor/scatter factor-induced activation of MEK and PI3K signal pathways contributes to expression of proangiogenic cytokines interleukin-8 and vascular endothelial growth factor in head and neck squamous cell carcinoma. *Cancer Res,* Vol.61, No.15 (August 2001), pp.5911-5918, ISSN: 0008-5472.

Duff SE, Jeziorska M, Rosa DD, Kumar S, Haboubi N, Sherlock D, O'Dwyer ST & Jayson GC. (2006) Vascular endothelial growth factors and receptors in colorectal cancer: implications for anti-angiogenic therapy. *European Journal of Cancer,* Vol.42, No.1 (January 2006), pp.112-117, ISSN: 0959-8049.

Fan S, Gao M, Meng Q, Laterra JJ, Symons MH, Coniglio S, Pestell RG, Goldberg ID & Rosen EM. (2005). Role of NF-kappaB signaling in hepatocyte growth factor/scatter factor-mediated cell protection. *Oncogene,* Vol.24, No.10 (March 2005), pp.1749-1766, ISSN: 0950-9232.

Ferraro D, Corso S, Fasano E, Panieri E, Santangelo R, Borrello S, Giordano S, Pani G & Galeotti T. (2006). Pro-metastatic signaling by c-Met through RAC-1 and reactive oxygen species (ROS). *Oncogene,* Vol.25, No.26 (June 2006), pp.3689-3698, ISSN: 0950-9232.

Garcea G, Sharma RA, Dennison A, Steward WP, Gescher A & Berry DP. (2003). Molecular biomarkers of colorectal carcinogenesis and their role in surveillance and early intervention. *Eur J Cancer,* Vol.39, No.8 (May 2003), pp.1041–1052, ISSN: 0959-8049.

García-Alonso I, Palomares T, Alonso A, Portugal V, Castro B, Caramés J & Méndez J. (2003). Effect of hepatic resection on development of liver metastasis. *Rev Esp Enferm Dig,* Vol.95, No.11 (November 2003), pp.771-776, ISSN: 1130-0108.

García-Alonso I, Palomares T, Alonso-Varona A, Castro B, Del Olmo M, Portugal V & Méndez J (2005). Effects of all-trans retinoic acid on tumor recurrence and metastasis. *Rev Esp Enferm Di, Vol.97, No.4 (*2005 Apr), pp.240-248, ISSN: 1130-0108.

García-Alonso I, Díaz-Sanz I, Palomares T, San Cristóbal J, Martínez-Astorquiza T, Marín H. (2008a) Effect of hepatic growth factors on CC-531 adenocarcinoma cancer cells. *Br J Surg,* Vol.95, No.S6 (May 2008), pp.19-20, ISSN: 1365-2168.

García-Alonso I, Palomares T, Alonso A, Echenique-Elizondo M, Caramés J, Castro B & Méndez J. (2008b). Effect of liver resection on the progression and growth of rhabdomyosarcoma metastases in a rat model. *J Surg Res,* Vol.148, No.2 (August 2008), pp.185-190, ISSN: 0022-4804.

García-Alonso I, Palomares T, Alonso-Varona A, Díaz-Sanz I, Miró B, Méndez J. (2010) All-Trans Retinoic Acid blocks the proliferative effect of growth factors on rat colocarcinoma cells. *Br J Surg,* Vol.97, No.S4 (June 2010), pp.15, ISSN: 1365-2168.

Giantonio BJ, Catalano PJ, Meropol NJ, O´Dwyer PJ, Mitchell EP, Alberts SR, Schawartz MA & Benson AB 3rd. (2007). Bevacizumab in combination with oxaliplatin, fluorouracil, and leucovorin (FOLFOX4) for previously treated metastatic colorectal cancer: results from the Eastern Cooperative Oncology Group Study E3200. *J Clin Oncol*, Vol.25, No.12 (April 2007), pp.1539-1544, ISSN: 0732-183X.

Giaccone G & Wang Y. (2011) Strategies for overcoming resistance to EGFR family tyrosine kinase inhibitors. *Cancer treatment reviews*, (February 2011), DOI: 10.1016/j.ctrv.2011.01.003, ISSN: 0305-7372.

Halliwell B. (1991). Reactive oxygen species in living systems: source, biochemistry, and role in human disease. *Am J Med, (suppl. 3C)*, Vol.91, (September 1991), pp.S14-S22, ISSN: 0002-9343.

Hbibi AT, Lagorce C, Wind P, Spano JP, Des Guetz G, Milano G, Benamouzig R, Rixe O, Morere JF, Breau JL, Martin A & Fagard R. (2008). Identification of a functional EGF-R/p60c-src/STAT3 pathway in colorectal carcinoma: analysis of its long-term prognostic value. *Cancer Biomark*, Vol.4, No.2 (June 2008), pp.83-91, ISSN: 1574-0153.

Higuchi Y. (2004). Glutathione depletion-induced chromosomal DNA fragmentation associated with apoptosis and necrosis. *J Cell Mol Med*, Vol.8, No.4 (October-December 2004), pp.455-464, ISSN: 1582-1838.

Hirao S, Yamada Y, Koyama F, Fujimoto H, Takahama Y, Ueno M, Kamada K, Mizuno T, Maemondo M, Nukiwa T, Matsumoto K, Nakamura T & Nakajima Y. (2002). Tumor suppression effect using NK4, a molecule acting as an antagonist of HGF, on human gastric carcinomas. *Cancer Gene Ther*, Vol.9, No.8 (August 2002), pp.700-707, ISSN: 0929-1903.

Hiro J, Inoue Y, Toiyama Y, Miki C & Kusunoki M. (2008). Mechanism of resistance to chemoradiation in p53 mutant human colon cancer. *Int J Oncol*, Vol.32, No.6 (June 2008), pp.1305-1310, ISSN: 1019-6439.

Hurwitz H, Fehrenbacher L, Novotny W, Cartwright T, Hainsworth J, Heim W, Berlin J, Baron A, Griffing S, Holmgren E, Ferrara N, Fyfe G, Rogers B, Ross R & Kabbinavar F. (2004). Bevacizumab plus irinotecan, fluorouracil, and leucovorin for metastatic colorectal cancer. *New England Journal of Medicine*, Vol.350, No.23 (June 2004), pp.2335-2342, ISSN: 0028-4793.

Hwang IT, Chung YM, Kim JJ, Chung JS, Kim BS, Kim HJ. Kim JS & Yoo YD. (2007). Drug resistance to 5-FU linked to reactive oxygen species modulator 1. *Biochem Biophys Res Commun*, Vol.359, No.2 (July 2007), pp.304-310, ISSN: 0006-291X.

Hynes NE & Lane HA. (2005). ERBB receptors and cancer: the complexity of targeted inhibitors. *Nat Rev Cancer*, Vol.5, No.7 (July 2005), pp.341-354, ISSN: 1474-175X.

Ischenko I, Camaj P, Seeliger H, Kleespies A, Guba M, De Toni EN, Schwarz B, Graeb C, Eichhorn ME, Jauch KW & Bruns JC. (2008). Inhibition of Src tyrosine kinase reverts chemoresistance toward 5-fluorouracil in human pancreatic carcinoma cells: an involvement of epidermal growth factor receptor signaling. *Oncogene*, Vol.27, No.57 (December 2008), pp.7212-7222, ISSN: 0950-9232.

Jankowski K, Kucia M, Wyscoczynski M, Reca R, Zhao DL, Trzyna E, Trent J, Peiper S, Zembala M, Ratajczak J, Houghton P, Janowska-Wieczorek A & Ratajczak MZ (2003). Both hepatocyte growth factor (HGF) and stromal-derived factor-1 regulate metastatic behaviour of human rhabdomyosarcoma cells, but only HGF enhances their resistance to radiochemotherapy. *Cancer Res*, Vol.63, No.22 (November 2003), pp.7926-7935, ISSN: 0008-5472.

Jansen BA, Brouwer J & Reedijk J. (2002). Glutathione induces cellular resistance against cationic dinuclear platinum anticancer drugs. *J Inorg Biochem*,Vol.89, No.3-4 (April 2002), pp.197-202, ISSN: 0162-0134.

Jin H, Yang R, Zheng Z, Romero M, Ross J, Bou-Reslan H, Carano RA, Kasman I, Mai E, Young J, Zha J, Zhang Z, Ross S, Schwall R, Colbern G & Merchant M. (2008). MetMAb, the one-armed 5D5 anti-c-Met antibody, inhibits orthotopic pancreatic tumor growth and improves survival. *Cancer Res*, Vol.68, No.11 (June 2008), pp.4360-4368, ISSN: 0008-5472.

Johnson GL & Vaillancourt RR. (1994). Sequential protein kinase reactions controlling cell growth and differentiation. *Curr Opin Cell Biol*, Vol.6, No.2 (April 1994), pp.230-238, ISSN: 0955-0674.

Kalluri R & Zeisberg M. (2006). Fibroblasts in cancer. *Nature Reviews in Cancer*, Vol.6, No.5 (May 2006), pp.392-401, ISSN: 1474-175X.

Kammula US, Kuntz EJ, Francone TD, Zeng Z, Shia J, Landmann RG, Paty PB & Weiser MR. (2007). Molecular co-expression of the c-Met oncogene and hepatocyte growth factor in primary colon cancer predicts tumor stage and clinical outcome. *Cancer Lett*, Vol.248, No.2 (April 2007), pp.219-228, ISSN: 0304-3835.

Kang YJ. (1993). Buthionine sulfoximine spares intracellular glutamate: a possible mechanism for cell growth stimulation. *Cell Mol Biol Res*, Vol.39, No.7 (May 1993), pp.675-684, ISSN: 0968-8773.

Kaur B, Khwaja FW, Severson EA, Matheny SL, Brat DJ & Van Meir EG. (2005). Hypoxia and the hipoxya-inducible factor pathway in glioma growth and angiogenesis. *Neuro-oncol*, Vol.7, No.2 (April 2005), pp.134-153, ISSN: 1522-8517.

Kishida O, Miyazaki Y, Murayama Y, Ogasa M, Miyazaki T, Yamamoto T, Watabe K, Tsutsui S, Kiyohara T, Shimomura I & Shinomura Y. (2005). Gefitinib ("Iressa", ZD1839) inhibits SN-38-triggered EGF signals and IL-8 production in gastric cancer cells. *Cancer Chemother Pharmacol*, Vol.55, No.4 (April 2005), pp.393-403, ISSN: 0344-5704.

Koizumi F, Kanzawa F, Ueda Y, Koh Y, Tsukiyama S, Taguchi F, Tamura T, Saijo N & Nishio K. (2004). Synergistic interaction between the EGFR tyrosine kinase inhibitor gefitinib ("Iressa") and the DNA topoisomerase I inhibitor CPT-11 (irinotecan) in human colorectal cancer cells. *Int J Cancer.*, Vol.108, No.3 (January 2004), pp.464-472, ISSN: 0020-7136.

Kummar S, Gutierrez ME, Maurer BJ, Reynolds CP, Kang M, Singh H, Crandon S, Murgo AJ & Doroshow JH. (2011). Phase I trial of fenretinide lym-x-sorb oral powder in adults with solid tumors and lymphomas. *Anticancer Res*, Vol.31, No.3 (2011 Mar), pp.961-966, ISSN: 0250-7005.

Kuzuya M, Ramos MA, Kanda S, Koike T, Asai T, Maeda K, Shitara K, Shibuya M & Iguchi A. (2001). VEGF protects against oxidized LDL toxicity to endothelial cells by an intracellular glutathione-dependent mechanism through the KDR receptor. *Arterioscler Thromb Vasc Biol*, Vol.21, No.5 (May 2001), pp.765-770, ISSN: 1079-5642.

Lagadec P, Griessinger E, Nawrot MP, Fenouille N, Colosetti P, Imbert V, Mari M, Hofman P, Czerucka D, Rousseau D, Berard E, Dreano M & Peyron JF. (2008). Pharmacological targeting of NF-kappaB potentiates the effect of the topoisomerase inhibitor CPT-11 on colon cancer cells. *Br J Cancer,* Vol.98, No.2 (January 2008), pp.335-344, ISSN: 0007-0920.

Le Bras M, Clément MV, Pervaiz S & Brenner C. (2005). Reactive oxygen species and the mitochondrial signalling pathway of cell death. *Histol Histopathol,* Vol.20, No.1 (January 2005), pp.205-219, ISSN: 0213-3911.

LeGolvan MP & Resnick M. (2010). Pathobiology of colorectal cancer hepatic metastases with an emphasis on prognostic factors. *Journal of Surgical Oncology,* Vol.102, No.8 (December 2010), pp.898-908, ISSN: 0022-4790.

Liu JP, Wei HB, Zheng ZH, Guo WP & Fang JF. (2010). Celecoxib increases retinoid sensitivity in human colon cancer cell lines. *Cell Mol Biol Lett,* Vol.15, No.3 (2010 Sep), pp.440-450, ISSN: 1425-8153.

Lou H & Kaplowitz N (2007). Glutathione depletion down-regulates tumor necrosis factor alpha-induced NF-kappaB activity via IkappaB kinase-dependent and -independent mechanisms. *J Biol Chem,* Vol.282, No.40 (October 2007), pp.29470-29481, ISSN: 0021-9258.

Maellaro E, Dominici S, Del Bello B, Valentini MA, Pieri L, Perego P, Supino R, Zunino F, Lorenzini E, Paolicchi A, Comporti M & Pompella A. (2000). Membrane gamma-glutamyltranspeptidase activity of melanoma cells: effects on cellular H_2O_2 production, cell surface protein thiol oxidation and NF-κB activation status. *J Cell Sci,* Vol.113, No.15 (August 2000), pp.2671-2678, ISSN: 0021-9533.

Markowitz SD & Bertagnolli MM. (2009). Molecular origins of cancer: Molecular basis of colorectal cancer. *New England Journal of Medicine,* Vol.361, No.25 (December 2009), pp.2449-2460, ISSN: 0028-4793.

Martínez-Astorquiza T, Palomares T, San Cristóbal J, Marín H, Quintana A & García-Alonso I. (2008) Effect of all-trans retinoic acid on the development of colon carcinoma liver metastases following partial hepatectomy in rats. *Br J Surg,* Vol.95, No.S6, (May 2008), pp.34, ISSN: 1365-2168.

Meister A & Anderson ME. (1983). Glutathione. *Annu Rev Biochem,* Vol.52, (November 1983), pp.711-760, ISSN: 0066-4154.

Meurette O, Lefeuvre-Orfila L, Rebillard A, Lagadic-Gossmann D & Dimanche-Boitrel MT. (2005). Role of intracellular glutathione in cell sensitivity to the apoptosis induced by tumor necrosis factor {alpha}-related apoptosis-inducing ligand/anticancer drug combinations. *Clin Cancer Res,* Vol.11, No.8 (April 2005), pp.3075-3083, ISSN: 1078-0432.

Mills EM, Takeda K, Yu ZX, Ferrans V, Katagiri Y, Jiang H, Lavigne MC,Leto TL & Guroff G. (1998). Nerve growth factor treatment prevents the increase in superoxide produced by epidermal growth factor in PC12 cells. *J Biol Chem,* Vol.273, No.35 (August 1998), pp.22165-22168, ISSN: 0021-9258.

Moberly JB, Logan J, Borum PR, Story KO, Webb LE, Jassal SV, Mupas L, Rodela H, Alghamdi GA, Moran JE, Wolfson M, Martis L & Oeropoulos DG. (1998). Elevation of whole-blood glutathione in peritoneal dialysis patients by L-2-oxothiazolidine-4-carboxylate, a cysteine prodrug (Procysteine (R)). *J Am Soc Nephrol,* Vol.9, No.6 (June 1998), pp.1093-1099, ISSN: 1046-6673.

Morini M, Cai T, Aluigi MG, Noonan DM, Masiello L, De Flora S, D´Agostini F, Albini A & Fassina G. (1999). The role of the thiol N-acetylcysteine in the prevention of tumor invasion and angiogenesis. *Int. J. Biol. Markers,* Vol.14, No.4 (October-December 1999), pp.268-271, ISSN: 0393-6155.

Morris PE, Papadakos P, Russell JA, Wunderink R, Schuster DP, Truwit JD, Vincent JL & Bernard GR. (2008). A double-blind placebo-controlled study to evaluate the safety and efficacy of L-2-oxothiazolidine-4-carboxylic acid in the treatment of patients with acute respiratory distress syndrome. *Crit Care Med,* Vol.36, No.3 (March 2008), pp.782-788, ISSN: 0090-3493.

Mulder K, Scarfe A, Chua N, Spratlin J. (2011) The role of bevacizumab in colorectal cancer: understanding its benefits and limitations. *Expert Opinion on Biological Therapy,* Vol.11, No.3 (March 2011), pp.405-413, ISSN: 1471-2598.

Murillo MM, Carmona-Cuenca I, Del Castillo G, Ortiz C, Roncero C, Sánchez A, Fernández M & Fabregat I. (2007). Activation of NADPH oxidase by transforming growth factor-beta in hepatocytes mediates up-regulation of epidermal growth factor receptor ligands through a nuclear factor-kappaB-dependent mechanism. *Biochem J,* Vol.405 (part 2), No.? (July 2007), pp.251-259, ISSN: 0264-6021.

Naidu KA, Nasir A, Pinkas H, Kaiser HE, Brady P & Coppola D. (2003). Glutathione-S-transferase pi expression and activity is increased in colonic neoplasia. *In Vivo,* Vol.17, No.5 (September-October 2003), pp.479–482, ISSN: 0258-851X.

Niu G, Wright KL, Huang M, Song LX, Haura E, Turkson J, Zhang SM, Wang TH, Sinibaldi D, Coppola D, Heller R, Ellis LM, Karras J, Bromberg J, Pardoll D, Jove R & Yu H. (2002). Constitutive Stat3 activity up-regulates VEGF expression and tumor angiogenesis. *Oncogene,* Vol.21, No.13 (March 2002), pp.2000-2008, ISSN: 0950-9232.

Odom D, Barber B, Bennett L, Peeters M, Zhao Z, Kaye J, Wolf M, Wiezorek J. (2011) Health-related quality of life and colorectal cancer-specific symptoms in patients with chemotherapy-refractory metastatic disease treated with panitumumab. *Int J Colorectal Dis,* Vol.26, No.2 (February 2011), pp.173-181, ISSN 0179-1958.

Ortiz C, Caja L, Sancho P, Bertran E & Fabregat I. (2008). Inhibition of the EGF receptor blocks autocrine growth and increases the cytotoxic effects of doxorubicin in rat hepatoma cells: role of reactive oxygen species production and glutathione depletion. *Biochem Pharmacol,* Vol.75, No.10 (May 2008), pp.1935-1945, ISSN: 0006-2952.

Palomares T, Alonso-Varona A, Alvarez A, Castro B, Calle Y & Bilbao P. (1997). Interleukin-2 increases intracellular glutathione levels and reverses the growth inhibiting effects of cyclophosphamide on B16 melanoma cells. *Clin Exp Metastasis,* Vol.15, No.3 (May 1997), pp.329-337, ISSN: 0262-0898.

Palomares T, Bilbao P, del Olmo M, Castro B, Calle Y & Alonso-Varona A. (1999). *In vitro* and *in vivo* comparison between the effects of treatment with adenosine triphosphate and treatment with buthionine sulfoximine on chemosensitization and tumour growth of B16 melanoma. *Melanoma Res,* Vol.9, No.3 (June 1999), pp.233-242, ISSN: 0960-8931.

Palomares T, Caramés M, García-Alonso I & Alonso-Varona A. (2009). Glutathione modulation reverses the growth-promoting effect of growth factors, improving the

5-fluorouracil anti-tumour response in WiDr human colon cancer cell line. *Anti-Cancer Res*, Vol.29, No.10 (October 2009), pp.3957-3965, ISSN: 0250-7005.

Qu Z, Van Ginkel S, Roy AM, Westbrook L, Nasrin M, Maxuitenko Y, Frost AR, Carey D, Wang W, Li R, Grizzle WE, Thottassery JV & Kern FG. (2008). Vascular endothelial growth factor reduces tamoxifen efficacy and promotes metastatic colonization and desmoplasia in breast tumors. *Cancer Res,* Vol.68, No.15 (August 2008), pp.6232-6240, ISSN: 0008-5472.

Radominska-Pandya A, Chen G, Czernik PJ, Little JM, Samokyszyn VM, Carter CA, et al. (2000). Direct interaction of all-trans-retinoic acid with protein kinase C (PKC). J Biol Chem, Vol.275, No.29 (July 2000), pp.22324-22330, ISSN: 0021- 9258.

Raffel J, Bhattacharyya AK, Gallegos A, Cui HY, Einspahr JG, Alberts DS & Powis G. (2003). Increased expression of thioredoxin-1 in human colorectal cancer is associated with decreased patient survival. *J Lab Clin Med,* Vol.142, No.1 (July 2003), pp.46–51, ISSN: 0022-2143.

Rao GN. (1996). Hydrogen peroxide induces complex formation of SHC-Grb2-SOS with receptor tyrosine kinase and activates Ras and extracellular signal-regulated protein kinases group of mitogen-activated protein kinases. *Oncogene,* Vol.13, No.4 (August 1996), pp.713-719, ISSN: 0950-9232.

Rhee SG, Bae YS, Lee C, Yang KS, Lee SR & Kwon J. (2000). Hydrogen peroxide in peptide growth factor signaling. Faseb Journal, Vol.14, No.8 (May 2000), pp.A1505-A1505, ISSN: 0892-6638.

Roy S, Khanna S & Sen CK. (2008). Redox regulation of the VEGF signaling path and tissue vascularization: Hydrogen peroxide, the common link between physical exercise and cutaneous wound healing. *Free Radic Biol Medic,* Vol.44, No.2 (January 2008), pp.180-192, ISSN: 0891-5849.

Russo A, DeGraff W, Friedman N & Mitchell JB. (1986). Selective modulation of glutathione levels in human normal versus tumor cells and subsequent differential response to chemotherapy drugs. *Cancer Res,* Vol.46, No.6 (June 1986), pp.2845-2848, ISSN: 0008-5472.

Sadowitz PD, Hubbard BA, Dabrowiak JC, Goodisman J, Tacka KA, Aktas MK, Cunningham MJ, Dubowy RL & Souid AK. (2002). Kinetics of cisplatin binding to cellular DNA and modulations by thiol-blocking agents and thiol drugs. *Drug Metabol Dispos,* Vol.30, No.2 (February 2002), pp.183-190, ISSN: 0090-9556.

Schmid K, Nair J, Winde G, Velic I & Bartcsh H. (2000). Increased levels of DNA adducts in colonic polyps of Fap patients. *Int J Cancer,* Vol.87, No.1 (July 2000), pp.1–4, ISSN: 0020-7136.

Schmidt M & Lichtner RB. (2002). EGF receptor targeting in therapy-resistant human tumors. *Drug Resist Updat,* Vol.5, No.1 (February 2002), pp.11-18, ISSN: 1368-7646.

Schulze-Bergkamen H, Ehrenberg R, Hickmann L, Vick B, Urbanik T, Schimanski CC, Berger MR, Schad A, Weber A, Heeger S, Galle PR & Moehler M. (2008). Bcl-x(L) and Myeloid cell leukaemia-1 contribute to apoptosis resistance of colorectal cancer cells. *World J Gastroenterol,* Vol.14, No.24 (June 2008), pp.3829-3840, ISSN: 1007-9327.

Sen CK, Khanna S, Babior BM, Hunt TK, Ellison EC & Roy S. (2002). Oxidant-induced vascular endothelial growth factor expression in human keratinocytes and cutaneous wound healing. *J Biol Chem,* Vol.277, No.36 (September 2002), pp.33284-33290, ISSN: 0021-9258.

Sethi G, Ahn KS, Chaturvedi MM & Aggarwal BB. (2007). Epidermal growth factor (EGF) activates nuclear factor-kappaB through I kappa B alpha kinase-independent but EGF receptor-kinase dependent tyrosine 42 phosphorylation of I kappa B alpha. *Oncogene,* Vol.26, No.52 (November 2007), pp.7324-7232, ISSN: 0950-9232.

Shen JG, Cheong JH, Noh SH & Wang LB. (2007). Effects of hepatocyte growth factor gene transfection on adriamycin-induced apoptosis of gastric cancer cells *in vitro.* *Zhonghua Zhong Liu Za Zhi,* Vol.29, No.5 (May 2007), pp.338-341, ISSN: 0253-3766.

Shim KS, Kim KH, Han WS & Park EB. (1999). Elevated serum levels of transforming growth factor-beta 1 in patients with colorectal carcinoma: Its association with tumor progression and its significant decrease after curative surgical resection. *Cancer,* Vol.85, No.3 (February 1999), pp.554-561, ISSN: 0008-543X.

Shinomiya N, Gao CF, Xie Q, Gustafson M, Waters DJ, Zhang YW & Woude GF. (2004). RNA interference reveals that ligand-independent met activity is required for tumor cell signaling and survival. *Cancer Res,* Vol.64, No.21 (November 2004), pp.7962-7970, ISSN: 0008-5472.

Sogno I, Venè R, Ferrari N, De Censi A, Imperatori A, Noonan DM, Tosetti F & Albini A. (2010). Angioprevention with fenretinide: targeting angiogenesis in prevention and therapeutic strategies. *Crit Rev Oncol Hematol,* Vol.75, No.1 (July 2010), pp.2-14, ISSN: 1040-8428.

Sreekumar PG, Kannan R, de Silva AT, Burton R, Ryan SJ & Hinton DR. (2006). Thiol regulation of vascular endothelial growth factor-A and its receptors in human retinal pigment epithelial cells. *Biochem Biophys Res Commun,* Vol.346, No.4 (August 2006), pp.1200-1206, ISSN: 0006-291X.

Stabile LP, Lyker JS, Huang L & Siegfried JM. (2004). Inhibition of human non-small cell lung tumors by a c-Met antisense/U6 expression plasmid strategy. *Gene Ther,* Vol.11, No.3 (February 2004), pp.325-335, ISSN: 0969-7128.

Stebbing J, Harrison M, Glynne-Jones R, Bridgewater J & Propper D. (2008). A phase II study to determine the ability of gefitinib to reverse fluoropyrimidine resistance in metastatic colorectal cancer (the INFORM study). *Br J Cancer,* Vol.98, No.4 (February 2008), pp.716-719, ISSN: 0007-0920.

Stoeltzing O, Liu W, Reinmuth N, Parikh A, Ahmad SA, Jung YD, Fan F & Ellis LM. (2003). Angiogenesis and antiangiogenic therapy of colon cancer liver metastasis. *Ann Surg Oncol,* Vol.10, No.7 (August 2003), pp.722-733, ISSN: 1068-9265.

Storz P. (2005). Reactive oxygen species in tumor progression. *Front Biosci,* Vol.10, (May 2005), pp.1881-1896, ISSN: 1093-9946.

Sullivan LA & Brekken RA. (2010). The VEGF family in cancer and antibody-based strategies for their inhibition. *Mabs,* Vol.2, No.2 (March 2010), pp.165-175, ISSN: 19420862.

Sun HC & Tang ZY (2003). Preventive treatments for recurrence after curative resection of hepatocellular carcinoma. A literature review of randomised control trials. *World J Gastroenterol,* Vol.9, No.4 (April 2003), pp.635-640, ISSN: 1007-9327.

Tatebe S, Unate H, Sinicrope FA, Sakatini T, Sugumura K, Makino M, Ito H, Savaraj N, Kaibara N & Kuo MT. (2002). Expression of heavy subunit of gamma-glutamylcysteine synthetase (gamma-GCSh) in human colorectal carcinoma. *Int J Cancer,* Vol.97, No.1 (January 2002), pp.21–27, ISSN: 0020-7136.

Thannickal VJ & Fanburg BL. (2000). Reactive oxygen species in cell signaling. *Am J Physiol Lung Cell Mol Physiol,* Vol.279, No.6 (December 2000), pp.L1005-L1028, ISSN: 1040-0605.

Thrall BD, Raha GA, Springer DL & Meadows GG. (1991). Differential sensitivities of murine melanocytes and melanoma cells to buthionine sulfoximine and anticancer drugs. *Pigment Cell Res,* Vol.4, No.5-6 (December 1991), pp.234-239, ISSN: 0893-5785.

Tol J & Punt CJA. (2010). Monoclonal antibodies in the treatment of metastatic colorectal cancer: a review. *Clinical Therapeutics,* Vol.32, No.3 (March 2010), pp.437-453, ISSN: 0149-2918.

Ushio-Fukai M & Nakamura Y. (2008). Reactive oxygen species and angiogenesis: NADPH oxidase as target for cancer therapy. *Cancer lett,* Vol.266, No.1 (July 2008), pp.37-52, ISSN: 0304-3835.

Vigneron A, Gamelin E & Coqueret O. (2008). The EGFR-STAT3 oncogenic pathway up-regulates the Eme1 endonuclease to reduce DNA damage after topoisomerase I inhibition. *Cancer Res,* Vol.68, No.3 (February 2008), pp.815-825, ISSN: 0008-5472.

Vita JA, Frei B, Holbrook M, Gokce N, Leaf C & Keany JF Jr. (1998). L-2-oxothiazolidine-4-carboxylic acid reverses endothelial dysfunction in patients with coronary artery disease. *J Clin Invest,* Vol.101, No.6 (March 1998), pp.1408-1414, ISSN: 0021-9738.

Voboril R, Hochwald SN, Li J, Brank A, Weberova J, Wessels F, Moldawer LL, Camp ER & MacKay SL. (2004). Inhibition of NF-kappa B augments sensitivity to 5-fluorouracil/folinic acid in colon cancer. *J Surg Res,* Vol.120, No.2 (August 2004), pp.178-188, ISSN: 0022-4804.

Wanebo HJ & Berz D. (2010). The neoadjuvant therapy of colorectal hepatic metastases and the role of biologic sensitizing and resistance factors. *Journal of Surgical Oncology,* Vol.102, No.8 (December 2010), pp.891-897, ISSN: 0022-4790.

Wen JH, Matsumoto K, Taniura N, Tomioka D & Nakamura T. (2007). Inhibition of colon cancer growth and metastasis by NK4 gene repetitive delivery in mice. *Biochem Biophys Res Commun,* Vol.358, No.1 (June 2007), pp.117-123, ISSN: 0006-291X.

Wu YP, Yakar S, Zhao L, Hennighausen L & Le Roith D. (2002). Circulating insulin-like growth factor-I levels regulate colon cancer growth and metastasis. *Cancer Res,* Vol.62, No.4 (February 2002), pp.1030-1035, ISSN: 0008-5472.

Xu JM, Azzariti A, Colucci G & Paradiso A. (2003). The effect of gefitinib (Iressa, ZD1839) in combination with oxaliplatin is schedule-dependent in colon cancer cell lines. *Cancer Chemother Pharmacol,* Vol.52, No.6 (December 2003), pp.442-448, ISSN: 0344-5704.

Yang H, Magilnick N, Xia M & Lu SC. (2008). Effects of hepatocyte growth factor on glutathione synthesis, growth, and apoptosis is cell density-dependent. *Exp Cell Res,* Vol.314, No.2 (January 2008), pp.398-412, ISSN: 0014-4827.

Yoshida A, Takemura H, Inoue H, Miyashita T & Ueda T. (2006). Inhibition of glutathione synthesis overcomes Bcl-2-mediated topoisomerase inhibitor resistance and induces nonapoptotic cell death via mitochondrial-independent pathway. *Cancer Res*, Vol.66, No.11 (June 2006), pp.5772-5780, ISSN: 0008-5472.

Zhang L, Hannay JA, Liu J, Das P, Zhan M, Nguyen T, Hicklin DJ, Yu D, Pollock RE & Lev D. (2006). Vascular endothelial growth factor overexpression by soft tissue sarcoma cells: implications for tumor growth, metastasis, and chemoresistance. *Cancer Res*, Vol.66, No.17 (September 2006), pp.8770-8778, ISSN: 0008-5472.

10

Human Tip60 (NuA4) Complex and Cancer

Hiroshi Y. Yamada
University of Oklahoma Health Sciences Center (OUHSC), USA

1. Introduction

Recent publications implicate human Tip60 (NuA4) complex in colorectal and other cancers. Our lab and others discovered deregulations in the components of human Tip60 (NuA4) complex in advanced colon cancers, and the functional significance and the potential as a therapeutic target, has been investigated. Human Tip60 (NuA4) complex likely represents a fusion form of yeast NuA4 and SWR1 complexes, and the functions seem to be evolutionarily preserved. This notion has greatly contributed in understanding functions of human Tip60 (NuA4) complex. The Tip60 (NuA4) complex is a multiprotein complex with at least 16 subunits. It is thought to function in at least two ways; (a) as a chromatin remodeling factor, it controls chromatin structure and transcription through its Histone Acetyl Transferase (HAT) activity, and (b) it controls activities of other non-histone proteins, such as metabolic enzymes, through protein acetylation. Through the enzymatic activity and other interactions, Tip60 (NuA4) complex is involved in wide variety of cellular functions, including transcriptional activation, DNA repair, cell cycle progression, chromosome stability, stem cell maintenance and differentiation, and cell migration and invasion. This review will discuss functions of Tip60 (NuA4) complex, consequences of the defect in the subunit, its connection to human cancer, and its potential as a therapeutic target in clinic.

2. A chromatin remodeling factor with Histone Acetyl Transferase (HAT) activity, Tip60 (NuA4) complex

Readout of genomic information is regulated through multiple mechanisms. A major part of the regulatory role is played by chromatin remodeling factors; enzyme complexes that modify DNA or chromatin proteins. The modifications change local chromatin structure, thus change accessibility of transcription factors and availability of genomic information (Kouzarides 2007). In the case of Histones and major chromatin proteins, protein modifications occur in a variety of ways, including phosphorylation, acetylation, methylation, ubiquitylation, and ADP-ribosylation. These different types of modifications may functionally influence each other, creating possibilities of multiple layers of regulations, which have been referred as the "Histone code". Although the possibility has been pointed out, the multiple layers of regulations (the "Histone code") have not fully been deciphered yet.

Among the modifications, acetylation has a defined role: To change surface charge distribution of the target protein and change accessibility to DNA and/or to other proteins.

The histones are acetylated and deacetylated on lysine residues in the N-terminal tail. These acetylation/deacetylation reactions are catalyzed by two groups of enzymes, Histone Acetyl Transferase (HAT) and Histone DeACetylase (HDAC), respectively. Histones are not the only target for these enzymes. HATs and HDACs can acetylate/deacetylate non-histone proteins as well.

In this review, we will focus on a human multisubunit and multifunctional HAT complex, Tip60 (NuA4) (Nucleosomal Acetyltransferase of H4) complex. We will describe the complex and known functions from the standpoint of each subunit and discuss new insights relevant to cancer, especially in colon cancer. We will also discuss the possibility of targeting Tip60 (NuA4) subunits for therapeutic purposes.

3. Human Tip60 (NuA4) complex; Its components and functions

Human Tip60 (NuA4) complex is a multiprotein complex with at least 16 subunits, and it has HAT activity (Cai et al., 2003, Doyon et al., 2004). The subunit composition suggests that Human Tip60 (NuA4) complex is a fusion form of two yeast HAT complexes, NuA4 and SWR (Allard et al, 1999) (Table 1). As seen in Table1, these two yeast HAT complexes share four components (Eaf2, Arp4, Act1 and Yaf9), together they correspond to all human subunits. Supporting the fusion theory, the expression of a chimeric Eaf1-Swr1 protein provides a scaffold for the complex assembly and recreates a single human-like complex in yeast cells (Auger et al, 2008).

Historically speaking, yeast has been a superior model system to investigate functions of molecular and cellular machineries with its genetical tractability, its ease of experimental manipulations, feasibility for biochemistry and its short life cycle and time span for experiments. Several cellular functions of NuA4 and SWR complex were identified directly with yeast studies and later confirmed in human cultured cells. The known acetylation targets of yeast NuA4 *in vivo* are histone H4 (Mitchell et al., 2008) and the histone H2A variant Htz1 (Babiarz et al., 2006, Keogh et al., 2006, Mizuguchi et al., 2004). Yeast NuA4 complex also targets non-histone proteins, which are equally important to evaluate cellular functions of NuA4 complex. With yeast protein array, Lin et al. (2009) screened the target proteins. Among 5800 proteins screened for *in vitro* acetylation with NuA4 complex, 91 candidates were identified, 20 were selected for validation, and 13 were validated. The functions of validated proteins encompass metabolism, transcription, cell cycle, RNA processing, and stress response. The authors focused on Pck1, a key metabolic enzyme that regulates gluconeogenesis, and showed that Pck1 activity and glucose secretion is regulated through NuA4-mediated acetylation in yeast and in human hepatocellular carcinoma cells HepG2. Thus NuA4 is implicated in metabolism and energy generation through its non-histone targets.

The human TIP60 complex has at least three interrelated enzymatic activities: histone H4/H2A acetyltransferase, ATP-dependent H2AZ-H2B histone dimer exchange, and DNA helicase (Auger et al., 2008). Only a limited number of non-histone targets, including human Pck1, has been identified so far (Liu et al., 2009).

Knockdown and/or mutational studies have been performed to identify functions of the subunits of human Tip60 (NuA4) complex. The studies implicate following biological events to Tip60 (NuA4) complex, directly or indirectly.

- DNA repair
- Transcriptional regulation
- Chromatin structure alteration
- Interaction and/or regulation with factors relevant to tumorigenesis (e.g. c-myc, E1A, E2F1, p53, STAT3, NF-kappaB)
- Cell migration and invasion
- Mitosis
- Genomic instability
- Stem cell maintenance and differentiation

In addition, RNAi-based screening with nematode *C. elegans* implicated Tip60 (NuA4) complex in attenuation of *ras*-signaling involving development of vulva in the model. The *C. elegans* MLL (Mixed Lineage Leukaemia (MLL)) complex-like complex cooperates with the TIP60 (NuA4) complex to regulate the expression of a novel *ras*-signaling attenuator, AJM-1 (Fischer et al., 2010).

4. Functions of each subunit

In the following section we will discuss each of the subunits.

4.1 TRRAP/Tra1/*

(human protein/yeast protein in NuA4 complex/ yeast protein in Swr complex. Asterisk * if not applicable)

Human TRRAP (transformation/transcription domain-associated protein) has a FATC (FRAP, ATM, TRRAP C-terminal) domain and a kinase domain, and belongs to ATM/PI3K family. However, TRRAP does not appear to possess kinase activity, because the kinase domain in TRRAP lacks the conserved amino acids required for ATP binding and catalytic activity for phosphate transfer. For that reason, it is speculated that TRRAP has evolved as a specialized PIKK member to serve as an adaptor/scaffold for protein–protein interaction and multiprotein assemblies or as a platform for recruitment of different regulatory factors and complexes to chromatin (Murr et al 2007). The FATC domain in the C-terminus likely affects the protein stability in an oxidation/redox-dependent manner (Dames et al., 2005).

TRRAP is a common component of many HAT complexes (e.g. SAGA, PCAF and Tip60 (NuA4) complex). As such, targeting TRRAP will influence a broader range of biological events and pathways than targeting more specialized components in Tip60 (NuA4) complex.

TRRAP is one of the frequently mutated genes in melanoma. TRRAP harbored a recurrent mutation that clustered in one position (p. Ser722Phe) in 6 out of 167 affected individuals (~4%), although the effects of the mutation on the protein function is unclear (Wei et al., 2011). Expression profiling revealed that TRRAP is frequently both amplified and overexpressed in Pancreatic Ductal AdenoCarcinoma (PDAC), and the overexpression is associated with poor prognosis (Bashyam et al., 2005, Loukopoulos et al,2007). In brain tumor-initiating cell, knockdown of TRRAP significantly increased differentiation and decreased cell cycle progression, leading to overall inhibition of tumor formation. The result indicates a critical role for TRRAP in maintaining a tumorigenic, stem cell-like state (Wurdak et al., 2010). TRRAP is shown to regulate a major player in colon cancer, beta-catenin. TRRAP interacts with Skp1/SCF and mediates its recruitment to beta-catenin target promoter in chromatin. TRRAP deletion leads to a reduced level of beta-catenin

Human Tip60 (NuA4) complex subunits	Yeast NuA4 complex subunits	Yeast SWR1 complex subunits	Protein domain(s)	Yeast null phenotype	Inhibition (e.g. siRNA) in cultured cells	Knockout in mouse	Relationship to cancer (See text)
TRRAP (transformation/transcription domain-associated protein)	Tra1		ATM/PI3K family kinase, FATC domain	inviable	Mitotic defect with Mad1 and Mad2 misregulation	Embryonic lethal	High expression in mouse leukemogenic cell lines; co-factor for c-myc oncogenic transformation
hDomino p400/EP400	Eaf1 (HAS/SANT)	Swr1 (HAS/SWI2)	SWI2/SNF2 related, ATPase, Trico Peptide Repeat (TPR) domain	Viable; decreased growth, genome instability		Embryonic lethal	
Brd8 (Bromodomain 8)		Bdf1	Bromodomain	Viable; decreased growth, multidrug sensitivity, enhanced salt sensitivity by mitochondrial dysfunction	Enhanced spindle poison sensitivity	ND	Protein accumulated in rat colon cancer and human colon cancer cell lines
EPC1/EPC-like (Enhancer of Polycomb homolog)	Epl1			inviable			Locates in chromosomal breaking point in ATLL
Tip60 (TAT interactive protein)	Esa1			inviable		Embryonic lethal	Prostate cancer promotion; tumor suppressor candidate/ expression reduced in cancers
DMAP1 (DNA methyltransferase 1-associated protein 1)	Eaf2/swc4	Eaf2/swc4	a SWI3-ADA2-N-CoR-TF IIIB (SANT) domain	Inviable; G2/M arrest		lethal during preimplantation	Binds to DNA methyltransferase 1 (DNMT1), which is progressively upregulated in colon adenoma-carcinoma sequence
ING3 (Inhibitor of Growth Protein 3)	Yng2		PHD finger	Viable			Tumor suppressor candidate; Overexpression inhibits cell growth and promote apoptosis; allelic loss detected in head and neck cancers
YL-1 (Vacuolar protein sorting-associated protein 72 homolog)		Vps72		Viable; decreased fitness			
RuvBL1		Rvb1/Tip49A		inviable			Binds to beta-catenin
RuvBL2		Rvb2/Tip49B		inviable			
BAF53a	Arp4	Arp4	Actin-related	inviable			
Actin	Act1	Act1	actin	inviable			
MRG15	Eaf3			Viable; increased lifespan			
GAS41	Yaf9	Yaf9		Viable; Enhanced spindle poison sensitivity, multidrug sensitivity, decreased chromosome maintenance			
?	Eaf5			Viable			
MRGBP	Eaf7			Viable; decreased fitness			Overexpressed in human colon cancer
hEaf6	Eaf6			Viable			

Table 1. Subunits of Human Tip60 (NuA4); (columns from left) subunits of the yeast counterpart complexes NuA4 and SWR1; notable protein domains; yeast mutant phenotypes that implicate functions; inhibition in cultured cells and mice; and information relevant to cancer. ND: Not Determined. The order listed is following the size of the protein. Larger subunit is shown on top.

ubiquitination, lower degradation rate and accumulation of beta-catenin protein. Furthermore, recruitment of Skp1 to chromatin and ubiquitination of chromatin-bound beta-catenin are abolished upon TRRAP knock-down, leading to an abnormal retention of beta-catenin at the chromatin and concomitant hyperactivation of the canonical Wnt pathway (Finkbeiner et al., 2008). TRRAP is also involved in DNA damage repair. TRRAP depletion impairs both DNA-damage-induced histone H4 hyperacetylation and accumulation of repair molecules at sites of Double Strand Breaks (DSBs), resulting in defective homologous recombination (HR) repair, albeit with the presence of a functional ATM-dependent DNA-damage signaling cascade (Murr et al., 2006). TRRAP regulates expressions of many cancer-relevant genes, including mitotic checkpoint proteins Mad1 and Mad2 (Li et al., 2004) and mdm2 (Ard et al., 2002).

Consistent with the loss of mitotic checkpoint proteins essential for cellular survival, null mutation of Trrap (mouse homolog of human TRRAP) results in peri-implantation lethality due to a blocked proliferation of blastocysts. Loss of Trrap blocks cell proliferation because of an aberrant mitotic exit accompanied by cytokinesis failure and endoreduplication. Trrap-deficient cells failed to sustain mitotic arrest despite chromosome missegregation and disrupted spindles, and display compromised cdk1 activity. Thus, Trrap is essential for early development and required for the mitotic checkpoint, presumably through expression control of mad1 and mad2, and normal cell cycle progression (Herceg et al., 2001).

In yeast, deletion of TRRAP homolog Tra1 is also lethal. Tra1 is identified as a component of multiple yeast transcription regulator complexes, Ada-Spt, SAGA and NuA4 (Saleh et al., 1998; Grant et al., 1998; Allard et al., 1999). Tra1 directly interacts with the acidic transcriptional activators Gcn4, Hap4, and Gal4 (Brown et al., 2001). Tra1 is required for both the acetylation of Histone H4 surrounding the promoters and the transcription of Gcn4-dependent genes, suggesting that Tra1 may mediate the recruitment of NuA4 to certain promoters.

4.2 hDomino p400/Eaf1/Swr1

hDomino (also known as p400, EP400, E1A binding protein p400) is a DEXH-box class of RNA-dependent ATPase subunit in Tip60 (NuA4) complex, and can destabilize histone-DNA interactions in reconstituted nucleosomes in an ATP-dependent manner. hDomino also contains a highly conserved SANT (SWI3–ADA2–NcoR–TFIIIB) domain, a histone tail-binding module (Boyer et al. 2004). The protein is related to yeast Swi2/Snf2 (SWItch 2/Sucrose NonFermentable 2) and to Domino in fruit fly *Drosophila*. *Drosophila* Domino was isolated in search of immune system mutants devoid of circulating larval hemocytes from P-element insertion-based mutant library. Because of the very striking lymph gland phenotype that results in mutant larvae with two black dots visible on the anterior half, the authors named the mutation *domino* (Braun et al., 1997).

Through the Swi2/Snf2 domain, hDomino binds to adenovirus oncoprotein E1A. Mutational loss of E1A binding results in the loss of transformation, indicating that the binding plays a critical role in cellular transformation. hDomino also binds to c-myc with different protein components (Fuchs et al., 2001). In most human colorectal carcinoma, the ratio between Tip60 and p400 mRNAs is affected. Reversing the p400/Tip60 imbalance by Tip60 overexpression or the use of siRNAs resulted in increased apoptosis and decreased proliferation of colon-cancer-derived cells, suggesting that this ratio defect is important for cancer progression (Mattera et al., 2009).

In mice, p400 knockout results in embryonic lethality. Homozygous knockout mice died on embryonic day 11.5 (E11.5), and displayed an anemic appearance and slight deformity of the neural tube. Their results suggest that p400/mDomino plays a critical role in embryonic hematopoiesis by regulating the expression of developmentally essential genes such as those in the Hox gene cluster (Ueda et al., 2007). Tip60-p400 is necessary to maintain characteristic features of Embryonic Stem Cells (ESCs) (Fazzio et al., 2008). Through an RNAi screen in mouse ESCs of 1008 loci encoding chromatin protein, the authors identified 68 proteins that exhibit diverse phenotypes upon knockdown, including seven subunits of the Tip60-p400 complex, Trrap, Tip60, p400, DMAP1, RuvBL1, RuvBL2 and GAS41. Phenotypic analyses revealed that p400 localization to the promoters of both silent and active genes is dependent upon histone H3 lysine 4 trimethylation (H3K4me3). The Tip60-p400 knockdown gene expression profile is enriched for developmental regulators and significantly overlaps with that of the transcription factor Nanog. Depletion of Nanog reduces p400 binding to target promoters without affecting H3K4me3 levels. Together, these data indicate that Tip60-p400 integrates signals from Nanog and H3K4me3 to regulate gene expression in ESCs (Fazzio et al., 2008).

Yeast p400 homolog Eaf1 (Esa1-associated Factor 1, VID21) is the only subunit exclusively found in the NuA4 complex in biochemical preparation. Eaf1 is the platform on which four different functional modules of the other subunits are assembled into the native complex (Auger et al., 2008). Although eaf1 deletion strain is viable, the cells show genome instability and high incidences of sporulation defects and aneuploidy. The mutant is also highly sensitive to DNA damage-inducing stress such as X-ray (Auger et al., 2008; Hughes et al., 2000; Krogan et al., 2004).

4.3 Brd8/*/Bdf1

Human Brd8 was functionally identified as a Thyroid hormone receptor coactivator p120 (Monden et al., 1997; Yuan et al., 1998). Later, its role as a transcriptional coactivator with RXR/PPAR-gamma was also reported, establishing the role as a nuclear receptor coactivator (Monden et al., 1999). Human Brd8 has one or two Bromodomain(s), depending on the isoform. The Bromodomain is a domain that can bind to acetylated lysine, typically observed in histones, suggesting its role in regulating protein-protein interactions in histone-directed chromatin remodeling and gene transcription. (Zeng and Zhou, 2002; Mujtaba et al., 2007).

Brd8 was isolated through a HeLa cell-based expression cloning for genes that influence sensitivity to a microtubule inhibitor (Yamada and Gorbsky, 2006). Ectopic expression of Brd8 provides partial resistance to microtubule inhibitors and proteasome inhibitor, and knockdown sensitized cells to the drugs, suggesting Brd8 influences sensitivity to microtubule inhibitors and proteasome inhibitor (Yamada and Rao, 2008). Human Brd8 protein is overexpressed in human metastatic colorectal cancer cell lines. Brd8 is also overexpressed in advanced colon adenocarcinoma in rats induced with Dextran sulfate and azoxymethane (an inflammatory colon cancer model system). SiRNA-mediated Brd8 knockdown resulted in cell death in HCT116 and growth delay in DLD1, both are colorectal cancer cells (Yamada and Rao, 2008). With shRNA, an independent lab showed that inhibition of Brd8 resulted in growth inhibition (Yamaguchi et al., 2010), thus Brd8 is suspected to provide survival fitness and growth advantage. In our lab, transcriptome analysis showed little difference in the amount of Brd8 transcripts in colonic normal-looking epithelial and cancer cells, yet the protein accumulates in cancer cells. The protein accumulation is enhanced with an addition of proteasome inhibitor in cultured human colon cancer cells, suggesting that a post translational, proteasome-dependent pathway is involved in the regulation (unpublished results).

Yeast homolog Bdf1p (Bromo Domain Factor 1) contains two bromodomains and is thought to correspond to a missing piece of TFIID (Matangkasombut et al., 2000). Bdf1 deletion in yeast is viable, but affects general transcription including small nuclear RNA, sporulation, mitochondrial function and stress-induced cell death (Lygerou et al., 1994; Liu et al, 2009). Overexpression of Bdf1 can suppress phenotypes and defects of yaf9 (human GAS41 homolog) deletion, indicating functional overlap between Bdf1 and Yaf9 (Bianchi et al., 2004).

4.4 Epc1/Epl1/*

In *Drosophila,* EPC1 (Enhancer of PolyComb 1) mutation was isolated as a mutation that enhances the effect of homeotic proteins Polycomb. Although homozygotic mutations of Epc1 in *Drosophila* are lethal in the embryo, heterozygous mutations do not by themselves result in a zygotic homeotic phenotype (Stankunas et al, 1998). Epc1 protein is a chromatin protein with no known enzymatic activity by itself.

EPC1 deregulation is observed in Adult T-cell leukemia/lymphoma (ATLL), a malignant tumor caused by latent human T-lymphotropic virus 1 (HTLV-1) infection. In acute-type ATLL, there is a common breakpoint cluster region at 10p11.2. The chromosomal breakpoints are localized within the enhancer of polycomb 1 (EPC1) gene locus (Nakahata et al., 2009).

In mice development, Epc1 is involved in skeletal muscle differentiation. The expression of *Epc1* mRNA is gradually decreased with aging from embryonic day 11.5 to postnatal week 8. Epc1 is highly expressed in skeletal muscles and heart ventricle in week 8 mice (Kee et al., 2007). Epc1 knockdown caused a decrease in the acetylation of histones associated with serum response element (SRE) of the skeletal alpha-actin promoter. The Epc1.SRF (Serum Response Factor) complex bound to the SRE, and the knockdown of Epc1 resulted in a decrease in SRF binding to the skeletal alpha-actin promoter. Epc1 recruited histone acetyltransferase activity, which was potentiated by cotransfection with p300 but abolished by siRNA-mediated p300 inhibition. Epc1 directly bound to p300 in myoblast cells. Epc1 heterozygous mice showed distortion of skeletal alpha-actin, and the isolated myoblasts from the mice had impaired muscle differentiation. These results suggest that Epc1 is required for skeletal muscle differentiation by recruiting both SRF and p300 to the SRE of muscle-specific gene promoters (Kim et al., 2009).

Deletion of Yeast homolog Epl1 (Enhancer of Polycomb Like 1) is inviable, causes cells to accumulate in G2/M and global loss of acetylated histones H4 and H2A (Boudreault et al., 2003).

4.5 Tip60/Esa1/*

TIP60 in humans and Esa1 in yeast are the catalytic (acetyltransferase) subunit of the NuA4 complex (Ikura et al., 2000; Smith et al., 1998) and play a central role in Tip60 (NuA4) complex function. MYC associates with TIP60 and recruits it to chromatin *in vivo* with four other components of the TIP60 complex: TRRAP, p400, RuvBL1 and RuvBL2 (Frank et al., 2003)

The Tip60 histone acetyltransferase has been recently shown to be underexpressed in many human cancers from various origins (Lleonart et al., 2006; Gorrini et al., 2007). Moreover, in a model of tumor induction mice, it has been shown to function as a haploinsufficient tumor suppressor, providing a causal link between Tip60 underexpression and tumorigenesis (Gorrini et al., 2007).

A down-regulation of the TIP60 gene was observed in 28 out of 46 (61%) specimens of primary gastric cancer (Sakuraba et al, 2011). As mentioned in p400, in colon cancer expression ratio of Tip60-p400 is altered, and it may be involved in tumor growth (Mattera et al., 2009).

In yeast the catalytic subunit Esa1 is the only HAT protein essential for viability and is responsible for the bulk of histone H4 and H2A acetylation in vivo (Doyon and Cote, 2004). *esa1* temperature sensitive (ts) mutants provoke a *RAD9*-dependent G2/M delay (Megee et al., 1995; Clarke et al., 1999). Yeast Esa1 mutation is inviable, and *esa1* conditional mutation serve to dissolve whole complex (Allard et al., 1999).

4.6 DMAP1/Eaf2/Eaf2

Human DMAP1 and its yeast homolog Eaf2 contain a highly conserved SANT (SWI3–ADA2–NcoR–TFIIIB) domain, a histone tail-binding module (Boyer et al. 2004). DMAP1 (DNA methyltransferase (DNMT)-1 associated protein 1) is a subunit of the TIP60-p400 complex that maintains embryonic stem (ES) cell pluripotency (Fazzio et al., 2008) and also a subunit of a complex containing the somatic form of DNA methyltransferase 1 (DNMT1s). The lack of DNMT1 in the purified TIP60-p400 complex indicates that DMAP1 interacts with DNMT1 in a distinct complex, thus DMAP1 functions in two distinct manner, as a Tip60 (NuA4) complex and with DNMT1 (Cai et al. 2003, Doyon et al., 2004). The non-catalytic amino terminus of DNMT1 binds to HDAC2 and can mediate transcriptional repression (Rountree et al, 2000). DNMT1 is essential for epidermal progenitor cell function and replenishing the tissue (Sen et al., 2010).

DMAP1 associated proteins (DNMT1,3A and 3B) were progressively upregulated in colorectal adenoma-carcinoma sequence (Schmidt et al., 2007). Since counteracting demethylase MBD2 amount remained unchanged, the authors suggested that epigenetic regulation in the adenoma-carcinoma sequence may be driven by increased methylating activity by DNMTs rather than suppressed demethylation.

In mice, DMAP1 homozygous knockout resulted in lethality during preimplantation (Mohan et al., 2010). Reduction of the expression of DMAP1 caused a loss of characteristic ES cell morphology and activation of genes associated with cell differentiation (Fazzio et al., 2008), and it is a likely cause of the embryonic lethal phenotype. Dmap1 knockdown in mouse embryonic fibroblasts (MEFs) lead to spontaneous double-strand breaks (DSBs), resulting in growth arrest because of p53-dependent cell cycle checkpoint activation (Negishi et al., 2009).

Yeast homolog Eaf2 (also known as SWC4) is a shared component of NuA4 and SWR1 complexes. Mutant yeasts are highly sensitive to DNA breaks induced by DNA-damaging agents, suggesting an essential role for these two proteins in DNA repair (Auger et al., 2008).

4.7 Ing3/Yng2/*

Human ING1 (Inhibitor of Growth 1) was identified as a tumor suppressor candidate, and subsequently the "Ing family" proteins (ING1-ING5) were investigated. Human Ing3 is a

47kd protein with a C-terminal plant homeodomain (PHD)-finger motif, common in proteins involved in chromatin remodeling and is a sequence-specific histone recognition protein module (Gunduz et al., 2002; Nagashima et al., 2003; Sanchez and Zhou, 2011). p47ING3 activates p53-transactivated promoters, including promoters of p21/waf1 and bax. Thus p47ING3 modulates p53-mediated transcription, cell cycle control, and apoptosis. Later, ING family proteins are identified as components of chromatin remodeling complexes; ING1 in mSin3A HDAC, ING2 in an HDAC complex similar to ING1, ING3 in Tip60 (NuA4) HAT complex, ING4 in HBO1 HAT, and ING5 fractionates with two distinct complexes containing HBO1 or nucleosomal H3-specific MOZ/MORF HATs. (Doyon et al., 2006).

Consistent with the proposed function as a tumor suppressor, a decrease of ING3 expression or LOH are observed in tumors. Decreased or no expression of ING3 mRNA was observed in 50% of primary head and neck squamous cell carcinomas (HNSCC) as compared with that of matched normal samples. About 63% of tongue and larynx tumors showed the decrease, and a tendency of higher mortality was observed in cases with decreased ING3 expression. It suggests that the ING3 gene functions as a tumor suppressor in a subset of HNSCC (Gunduz et al., 2002). Expression of ING3 is correlated with poor prognosis in HNSCC (Gunduz et al., 2008). Distorted ING3 expression has been found in several lymphoma-derived cell lines (Fadlelmola et al., 2008). Nuclear ING3 expression was reduced in melanomas in a Skp2-ubiquitin/proteasome pathway-dependent manner (Chen et al., 2010). This reduction was correlated with a poorer patient survival (Wang et al., 2007). Decreased ING3 expression is associated with melanoma progression and poor prognosis.

The yeast Saccharomyces cerevisiae has three homologs of ING family proteins. Homolog of human ING3 is Yng2 (Loewith et al., 2000). Yng2 is a plant homeodomain (PHD)-finger protein and a NuA4 complex subunit. Deletion of YNG2 results in several phenotypes, including an abnormal multibudded morphology, an inability to utilize nonfermentable carbon sources, heat shock sensitivity, slow growth, temperature sensitivity, and sensitivity to caffeine (Loeweth et al., 2000). Also notable was its requirement for normal progression through mitosis and meiosis. Some of the phenotypes were suppressed by HDAC inhibitor Tricostatin A, demonstrating that the phenotypes are based on defects in acetylation cycle (Choy et al., 2001). Yng2p is stabilized by the proteasome inhibitor MG-132, and is likely regulated through an ubiquitin-proteasome pathway (Lin et al., 2008).

4.8 YL-1/*/Vps72

Human YL-1 is a nuclear protein with an acidic region and a proline-rich region (Horikawa et al., 1995), and was identified as a component of Tip60 (NuA4) complex with biochemical purification and mass spectrometry. YL-1 is also a part of human counterpart of yeast SWR1 complex (Cai et al., 2005). Notably, mammalian SRCAP and *Drosophila* Tip60 complexes are associated with histone H2AZ or its fly counterpart H2AvD. These similarities suggest that YL-1 may serve as a binding module for histone H2AZ in metazoans, as does Swc2 in yeast (Wu et al., 2005).

In the Kirsten sarcoma virus–transformed NIH3T3 cells highly expressing the exogenous human YL-1 protein, the anchorage-independent growth (colony-forming ability in soft agar medium) was markedly suppressed. However, in contrast to the suppression of anchorage-independent growth, the forced expression of YL-1 did not affect the transformed phenotypes in adherent culture and tumorigenicity in nude mice. The data suggest that YL-

1 is involved in the transformation process, and once cells are transformed, additional YL-1 expression does not play additional role in tumor growth (Horikawa et al., 1995).
Yeast homolog VPS72 (Vascular Protein Sorting 72, also known as SWC2) is a histone variant H2AZ (Htz1p)-binding component of the SWR1 complex, which exchanges Htz1p for chromatin-bound histone H2A (Wu et al., 2005).

4.9 RuvBL1/*/Rvb1(Tip49A) and 4.10 RuvBL2/*/Rvb2(Tip49B)

RuvBL1 and RuvBL2 belong to the family of AAA+ ATPases (ATPases Associated with various cellular Activities). Ruvbl1 is also called Pontin, NMP238, ECP54, TAP54α, TIH1 or Tip49, while Ruvbl2 is also called Reptin, ECP51, TAP54α, TIH2 or Tip48. RuvBL1 and RuvBL2 bind each other and function as a hexameric helicase (Ikura et al., 2000; Shen et al., 2000). The names come from their homology with the bacterial RuvB helicase, which is involved in DNA recombination and repair. In bacteria, the ruvA-ruvB complex in the presence of ATP renatures cruciform structure in supercoiled DNA with palindromic sequence, indicating that it may promote strand exchange reactions in homologous recombination. RuvAB is a helicase that mediates the Holliday junction migration by localized denaturation and reannealing.
Human RuvBL1 and RuvBL2 are components of multiple multiprotein complexes, INO80, SRCAP, URI-1, R2TP and Tip60 (NuA4) complex. RuvBL1 and RuvBL2 were co-immunoprecipitated or affinity-purified with at least 48 proteins (Grigoletto et al., 2011).
Human RuvBL1 and RuvBL2 are overexpressed in a variety of cancers inculding colorectal (Carlson et al., 2003). Regulation of COX-2 transcription in a colon cancer cell line by Pontin52/TIP49a, (Lauscher et al.; 2007; Ki et al., 2007), gastric (Li et al., 2010), bladder (Sanchez-Carbayo et al., 2006), mesothelioma (Zhan et al., 2007), non-small cell lung cancer (Dehan et al., 2007), as well as in several types of acute (Andersson et al., 2007) or chronic leukemias (Haslinger et al., 2004), in multiple myeloma (Zhan et al., 2007) and high-grade lymphoma (Nishiu et al., 2002). In ovarian cancer cell lines, microcell-mediated chromosome transfer and expression microarray analysis identified nine genes associated with functional suppression of tumorogenicity; AIFM2, AKTIP, AXIN2, CASP5, FILIP1L, RBBP8, RGC32, RUVBL1 and STAG3. Two SNPs in RUVBL1 were associated with increased risk of serous ovarian cancer (Notaridou et al., 2011). The expression of an ATPase-deficient mutant form of RuvBL1/TIP49 substantially inhibited β-catenin-mediated neoplastic transformation of immortalized rat epithelial cells and anchorage-independent growth of human colon cancer cells with deregulated β-catenin (Feng et al., 2003).
Disruption of the yeast RuvBL1 (Kanemaki et al., 1999; Lim et al., 2000) or RuvBL2 genes (Lim et al., 2000) is lethal.

4.11 BAF53a (ACTL6a)/Arp4/Arp4

Human BAF53a (BRG1-associated factor 53a) is also known as ACTL6a (Actin-like 6a). As the name implies, the protein has a 36% identity and 50% similarity with the human beta-actin. BAF53 is a part of Tip60 (NuA4) complex (Cai et al., 2003, Doyon et al., 2004, 2006). In addition, BAF53a is also a part of other multiple multiprotein complexes, including INO80, SWI/SNF, and myc-containing nuclear cofactor complex (Park et al., 2002; Sung et al., 2001). For SWI/SNF-like protein complex, beta-actin and BAF53 are required for maximal ATPase activity of BRG1 and are also required with BRG1 for association of the complex with chromatin/matrix (Zhao et al., 1998). Baf53 protein was also identified as a major binding target for HIV Tat protein through affinity chromatography coupled with mass spectrometry. The result suggests that Baf53 and Tip60 (NuA4) complex is a major target for HIV-1 proviral gene silencing and activation (Gautier et al., 2009).

In yeast, Arp4/Act3 was identified as a component of NuA4 complex with affinity-purification followed by mass spectrometry (Galarneau et al., 2000). *ARP4* gene is essential for growth in yeast (Harata et al., 1994). In temperature-sensitive *arp4* mutants, NuA4 complex disintegrated and lost its activity in restrictive temperature, demonstrating the critical role of Arp4 in the NuA4 complex (Galarneau et al., 2000). Upon DNA damage, Arp4 recognizes and interacts with histone H2A phosphorylated at serine 129. This action recruits NuA4 to regions of DNA double-strand breaks where histone H4 acetylation is required for DNA double-strand break repair (Bird et al., 2002; Downs et al., 2004).

4.12 Actin/Act1/Act1

A major cytoskeletal protein beta-actin is also a subunit of Tip60 (NuA4) complex (Cai et al., 2003; Doyon et al., 2004, 2006). As in BAF53a, Actin is also a subunit of other multiprotein complex. Inhibition of Actin with the Actin monomer sequestering natural product Latrunculin B blocks chromatin-dependent ATPase activation of the BAF complex, indicating that Actin is a functionally critical component of SWI/SNF complex (Zhao et al., 1998). As a major cytoskeletal component, beta-actin (Actb) gene is an essential gene, and its hypomorph is embryonic lethal in mice (Tondeleir et al., 2009).

In yeast, in addition to cytoskeletal roles, Act1 is shown to be a component of distinctive chromatin remodeling complexes including INO80, SWR and NuA4 (Shen et al., 2000; Krogan et al., 2003; Galarneau et al., 2000). Act1 deletion is lethal.

4.13 MRG15/Eaf3/*

MRG 15 (Morf-related genes (Mrg) on chromosomes 15 (Mrg15)) belongs to Morf family proteins. From cellular senescent study to identify single chromosomes from normal human cells that can inhibit growth of immortal human cells, an intronless transcription factor-like protein, mortality factor on chromosome 4 (*MORF4*) was identified. From structural homology, other family proteins including MRG15 and MRGX were identified and investigated. MRG15 has helix-loop-helix and leucine zipper domains, which are typically found in transcriptional regulators, and a chromodomain thought to be involved in protein-protein interaction in chromatin remodeling factors. MRG15 and -MRGX are expressed ubiquitously in all cells and tissues. Currently, MRG proteins, which have pro-growth activity, are hypothesized to antagonize growth inhibition activity by Morf4.

Mrg15 knockout mice are embryonic lethal, and mouse embryonic fibroblasts derived from Mrg15 null embryos proliferate poorly, enter senescence rapidly, and have impaired DNA repair compared to wild type mice (Tominaga et al., 2005). Mrg15 null embryonic neural stem and progenitor cells also have a decreased capacity for proliferation and differentiation (Garcia et al., 2007). Expression of the cyclin-dependent kinase inhibitor p21 is specifically up-regulated in Mrg15 deficient neural stem/progenitor cells (NSCs). Mrg15 deficient NSCs exhibit severe defects in DNA damage response following ionizing radiation (Chen et al., 2011).

So far, cancer association of Mrg15 has been poorly shown. No alterations or mutations were identified for MRG15/MORF4L1 in unclassified FA patients and Breast Cancer (BrCa) familial cases. No significant associations between common MORF4L1 variants and BrCa risk for BRCA1 or BRCA2 mutation carriers were identified (Martrat et al., 2011).

Yeast Eaf3 is a shared component of the NuA4 complex and Rpd3 histone deacetylase complex. The loss of Eaf3 greatly alters the genomic profile of histone acetylation (Reid et al., 2004).

4.14 GAS41/Yaf9/Yaf9

GAS41 (Glioma Amplified Sequence 41) is a nuclear protein containing a C-terminal alpha-acidic activation domain and an N-terminal YEATS domain (Fischer et al., 1997). The YEATS domain family of proteins is well conserved from yeast to human, and functions as transcriptional regulators as a part of multiprotein complexes. GAS41 is associated with TFIIF via its YEATS domain. GAS41 is also a subunit of the human TIP60 and SCRAP complexes (Doyon et al., 2004; Cai et al., 2005). In addition, GAS41 physically interacts with transforming acidic coiled-coil 1(TACC1) protein, microtubule-associated colonic and hepatic tumor overexpressed (ch-TOG) protein and nuclear matrix (NuMA) protein (Lauffart et al., 2002; Harborth et al., 2000).

Yeast homolog Yaf9 encodes a protein of 226 residues, containing an N-terminal YEATS domain and a C-terminal predicted coiled-coil sequence (Le Masson et al., 2003). Deletion of Yaf9 shows pleiotropic effect, including sensitivity to a variety of drugs such as cadmium, cecium chrolide, cycloheximide, and microtubule inhibitor benomyl. The phenotype is associated with a change in transcriptome. The transcriptomic change can be suppressed by Bdf1 multicopy expression, suggesting functional overlapping between these two components (Bianchi et al., 2004). Since human Brd8 (Bdf1) was isolated from a screen that influenced sensitivity to microtubule inhibitors, it is tempting to speculate that Brd8-GAS41 (Bdf1-yaf9) may be an interface module to genes involved in sensitivity to microtubule inhibitors.

4.15 */Eaf5/*

Yeast Eaf5 (Esa1p-associated factor 5) is a component of yeast NuA4 complex (Nourani et al., 2001). Its direct human counterpart is unclear. Eaf5 protein forms subcomplex with Eaf7, and Eaf5 interacts with NuA4 complex (Mitchell et al., 2008). Eaf5 deletion strain is viable, and shows resistance to chemicals such as acetic acid and lactic acid (Kawahata et al., 2006). Deletion strains of *eaf5* and *eaf7* display similarity in microarray transcriptional profiles (Krogan et al., 2006).

4.16 MRGBP/Eaf7/*

MRGBP (MRG Binding Protein) was identified as a NuA4 component with biochemical purification (Cai et al., 2003). MRGBP is also a component of the human INO80 complex (Jin et al., 2005). Crystal structure determination of the MRG domain indicated that MRGBP has structural similarity to DNA binding domains of the tyrosine site-specific recombinases XerD, lambda integrase, and Cre (Bowman et al., 2006).

In human colon cancer, MRGBP was upregulated in the majority of the cancers. Inhibition of MRGBP with shRNA in vitro resulted in an inhibition of cell growth (Yamaguchi et al., 2010). High levels of MRGBP expression were observed more frequently in human colonic carcinomas (45%) than adenomas (5%), linking its role to malignant properties of colorectal tumors (Yamaguchi et al., 2011).

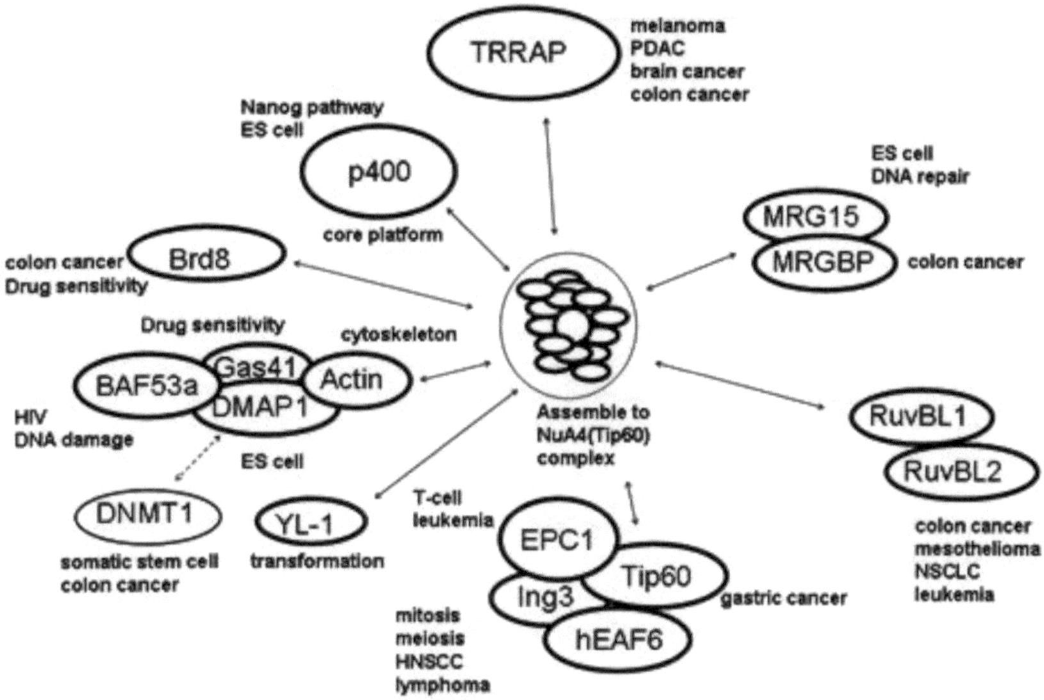

Fig. 1. Tip60 (NuA4) complex is assembled by combining subcomplexes and subunits. Each subunit of Tip60 (NuA4) complex is linked to different biological events, presumably because each subunit represents an interface to the proteins involved in the particular events. Inhibition of a subunit results in different phenotypes, which may provide intervention opportunities for cancer prevention and/or therapeutic purpose. Abbreviations: PDAC (Pancreatic Ductal Adeno Carcinoma); ES cell (Embryonic Stem cell); NSCLC (Non Small Cell Lung Cancer); HNSCC (Head and Neck Small Cell Carcinoma).

4.17 hEaf6/Eaf6/*

Human Eaf6 was isolated as a component of Tip60 (NuA4) complex (Doyon et al., 2004). hEaf6 is also a component of HBO and/or MOZ/MORF HAT complex (Ullah et al., 2008; Saksouk et al., 2009).

5. Relevance to colon cancer

Among multiple subunits, Brd8, MRGBP, RuvBL1 and RuvBL2 show particularly strong connections to colon cancer. These subunits are overexpressed in colon cancer (Yamada and Rao, 2009; Yamaguchi et al.,2010, 2011; Carlson et al., 2003; Lauscher et al., 2007; Graudens et al., 2006; Ki et al., 2007). Brd8 plays a role in survival and/or drug resistance of cultured colon cancer cells. MRGBP also plays a role in survival of cultured colon cancer cells. RuvBL1 is an important cofactor in beta-catenin/TCF gene regulation, and expression of its dominant-negative form inhibited β-catenin-mediated neoplastic transformation of

immortalized rat epithelial cells and anchorage-independent growth of human colon cancer cells with deregulated β-catenin (Feng et al., 2003).
In addition, DMAP1 associated proteins (DNMT1,3A and 3B) were progressively upregulated in colorectal adenoma-carcinoma sequence (Schmidt et al., 2007). DNMT1 may play a role in colon cancer progression directly or indirectly.

6. Subunit-specific targeting strategy

As in above, deregulations in subunits of human Tip60 (NuA4) complex are common in various cancers, and the complex is gaining attention as a potential target for cancer therapy. However, concerns for targeting whole Tip60 (NuA4) complex are raised because the complex plays essential roles for cellular survival and targeting the core components of the complex would impair the essential functions, which may lead to general toxicity to both normal and cancer cells. Although many successful drugs in existence do target essential and ubiquitous cellular components (e.g. Taxol for microtubule, Velcade for proteasome), the concern needs to be addressed.
As a rebuttal, targeting of each component has been proposed. Although the Tip60 (NuA4) complex is thought to function as a complex, targeting each subunit does not necessarily show the same biological effect and phenotype empirically, suggesting unique roles of each subunit. This fact may be exploited for developing therapeutic strategy. Further investigation of the unique roles of each subunit would allow us to develop subunit-specific targeting strategies for therapeutic purpose.
Extrapolating from yeast and mice results, the following subunits of Tip60 (NuA4) complex are essential for cellular survival; TRRAP, p400, EPC1, Tip60, DMAP1, RuvBL1, RuvBL2, BAF53a and Actin. Inhibiting these subunits may require caution. Components whose inhibition may not directly or immediately kill cells are; Brd8, ING3, YL-1, MRG15, GAS41, MRGBP and hEaf6. Inhibition of these components may prove valuable as an adjuvant approach to improve other therapies such as chemo- and radio-therapies.
In some subunits and associating factors (Brd8, MRGBP, DNMT1), overexpression is correlated to stage advancement of colon cancer, thus drug-mediated inhibition seems intuitively appropriate. GAS41 and Brd8 may have a more prominent effect on cellular sensitivity to anti-microtubule drugs. It is possible that chemoresistance of colon cancer is at least in part provided by deregulation of these subunits, and drug-mediated inhibition of these subunits results in enhancement of the effect of these drugs.

7. Conclusion

Accumulating evidence supports that the Tip60 (NuA4) complex plays a role in various cancers including that in colon, and possibly in drug sensitivity/resistance of cells. Targeting the components may prove successful in preventing cancer and/or in killing or chemosensitizing cancer cells. Since the major hindrance to a colon cancer cure is its chemoresistance, chemosensitizing through modulation of the Tip60 (NuA4) complex component seems to be a novel and attractive strategy. However, thus far validation of Tip60 (NuA4) complex, or the subunit(s), as a therapeutic target is yet to be performed. Continuing investigation is required to translate current knowledge to clinical or translational studies. Strategies for targeting (e.g. siRNA, small molecule) should be explored.

8. Acknowledgements

Dr. Chinthalapally V. Rao (OUHSC) for support. Dr. Kiyoshi Yamaguchi for sharing manuscript prior to publication. A part of this work is supported by Kerley-Cade chair Research endowment (OUHSC).

9. References

Allard, S.; Utley, R.T.; Savard, J.; Clarke, A.; Grant, P.; Brandl, C. J.; Pillus, L.; Workman, J.L.; Côté, J. (1999). NuA4, an essential transcription adaptor/histone H4 acetyltransferase complex containing Esa1p and the ATM-related cofactor Tra1p. *EMBO J* Vol. 18(18), pp. 5108-5119.

Andersson, A.; Ritz, C.; Lindgren, D.; Eden, P.; Lassen, C.; Heldrup, J.; et al. (2007). Microarray-based classification of a consecutive series of 121 childhood acute leukemias: prediction of leukemic and genetic subtype as well as of minimal residual disease status. *Leukemia* Vol. 21, pp. 1198–1203.

Ard, P.G.; Chatterjee, C.; Kunjibettu, S.; Adside, L.R.; Gralinski, L.E.; McMahon, S.B. (2002). Transcriptional regulation of the mdm2 oncogene by p53 requires TRRAP acetyltransferase complexes. *Mol Cell Biol* Vol. 22(16), pp.5650-5661.

Auger, A.; Galarneau, L.; Altaf, M.; Nourani, A.; Doyon, Y.; Utley, R. T.; Cronier, D.; Allard, S.; Côté, J.(2008). Eaf1 is the platform for NuA4 molecular assembly that evolutionarily links chromatin acetylation to ATP-dependent exchange of histone H2A variants. *Mol Cell Biol* Vol. 28 (7), pp.2257-2270.

Babiarz, J. E.; Halley, J. E. ; Rine, J. (2006). Telomeric heterochromatin boundaries require NuA4-dependent acetylation of histone variant H2A.Z in Saccharomyces cerevisiae. Genes Dev Vol. 20, pp. 700-710.

Basso, K.; Margolin, A.A.; Stolovitzky, G.; Klein, U.; Dalla-Favera, R.; Califano, A. (2005). Reverse engineering of regulatory networks in human B cells. *Nat. Genet* Vol. 37, pp. 382–390.

Bianchi, M.M.; Costanzo, G.; Chelstowska, A.; Grabowska, D.; Mazzoni, C.; Piccinni, E.; Cavalli, A.; Ciceroni, F.; Rytka, J.; Slonimski, P.P.; Frontali, L.; Negri, R. (2004). The bromodomain-containing protein Bdf1p acts as a phenotypic and transcriptional multicopy suppressor of YAF9 deletion in yeast. *Mol Microbiol* Vol. 53(3), pp. 953-968.

Bird, A. W.; Yu, D. Y.; Pray-Grant, M. G.; Qiu, Q.; Harmon, K. E.; Megee, P. C.; Grant, P. A.; Smith, M. M.; Christman, M. F. (2002). Acetylation of histone H4 by Esa1 is required for DNA double-strand break repair. *Nature* Vol. 419, pp. 411-415

Boudreault, A.A.; Cronier, D.; Selleck, W.; Lacoste, N.; Utley, R.T.; Allard, S.; Savard, J.; Lane, W.S.; Tan, S.; Côté, J. (2003). Yeast enhancer of polycomb defines global Esa1-dependent acetylation of chromatin. *Genes Dev* Vol. 17(11), pp. 1415-1428.

Bowman, B.R.; Moure, C.M.; Kirtane, B.M.; Welschhans, R.L.; Tominaga, K.; Pereira-Smith, O.M.; Quiocho, F.A. (2006). Multipurpose MRG domain involved in cell senescence and proliferation exhibits structural homology to a DNA-interacting domain. *Structure* Vol.14(1), pp.151-158.

Boyer, L.A.; Latek, R.R.; Peterson, C.L. (2004) The SANT domain: a unique histone-tail-binding module? Nat. Rev. *Mol Cell Biol* Vol. 5, pp. 158–163.

Braun, A.; Lemaitre, B.; Lanot, R.; Zachary, D.; Meister, M. (1997) Drosophila immunity: analysis of larval hemocytes by P-element-mediated enhancer trap. *Genetics* Vol. 147 (2), pp. 623-634.

Brown, C. E.; L. Howe; K. Sousa, S. C.; Alley, M. J.; Carrozza, S.; Tan, and J. L. Workman. (2001). Recruitment of HAT complexes by direct activator interactions with the ATM-related Tra1 subunit. *Science* Vol. 292, pp. 2333-2337.

Cai, Y.; Jin, J.; Tomomori-Sato, C.; Sato, S.; Sorokina, I.; Parmely, T. J.; Conaway, R. C.; Conaway, J. W. (2003) Identification of new subunits of the multiprotein mammalian TRRAP/TIP60-containing histone acetyltransferase complex. *J Biol Chem* Vol. 278 (44), pp. 42733-42736.

Cai, Y.; Jin, J.; Florens, L.; Swanson, S.K.; Kusch, T.; Li, B.; Workman, J.L.; Washburn, M.P.; Conaway, R.C.; Conaway, J.W. (2005). The mammalian YL1 protein is a shared subunit of the TRRAP/TIP60 histone acetyltransferase and SRCAP complexes. *J Biol Chem* Vol. 280(14), pp. 13665-13670.

Carlson, M.L.; Wilson, E.T.; Prescott, S.M. (2003). Regulation of COX-2 transcription in a colon cancer cell line by Pontin52/TIP49a. *Mol Cancer* Vol. 2, pp. 42.

Chen, M.; Pereira-Smith, O.M.; Tominaga, K. (2011). Loss of the chromatin regulator MRG15 limits neural stem/progenitor cell proliferation via increased expression of the p21 Cdk inhibitor. *Stem Cell Res* Vol. 7(1), pp. 75-88.

Choy, J.S.; Tobe, B.T.; Huh, J.H.; Kron, S.J. (2001). Yng2p-dependent NuA4 histone H4 acetylation activity is required for mitotic and meiotic progression. *J Biol Chem* Vol. 276(47), pp. 43653-43662.

Chua, P.; Roeder, G.S. (1995). Bdf1, a yeast chromosomal protein required for sporulation. *Mol Cell Biol* Vol. 15(7), pp. 3685-3696.

Couture, J.F.; Trievel, R.C. (2006). Histone-modifying enzymes: encrypting an enigmatic epigenetic code. *Curr Opin Struct Biol* Vol. 16(6), pp.753-760.

Dames, S.A.; Mulet, J.M.; Rathgeb-Szabo, K.; Hall, M.N.; Grzesiek, S. (2005).The solution structure of the FATC domain of the protein kinase target of rapamycin suggests a role for redox-dependent structural and cellular stability. *J Biol Chem* Vol. 280 (21), pp. 20558-20564.

Dehan, E.; Ben-Dor, A.; Liao, W.; Lipson, D.; Frimer, H.; Rienstein, S.; Simansky, D.; Krupsky, M.; Yaron, P.; Friedman, E.; Rechavi, G.; Perlman, M, et al. (2007). Chromosomal aberrations and gene expression profiles in non-small cell lung cancer. *Lung Cancer* Vol. 56, pp. 175–184.

Downs, J. A.; Allard, S.; Jobin-Robitaille, A.; Javaheri, A.; Auger, N.; Bouchard, S.; Kron, S. J.; Jackson, S. P.; Cote, J. (2004). Binding of chromatin-modifying activities to phosphorylated histone H2A at DNA damage sites. *Mol Cell* Vol. 16, pp.979-990.

Doyon, Y.; Selleck, W.; Lane, W. S.; Tan, S.; Côté, J. (2004) Structural and functional conservation of the NuA4 histone acetyltransferase complex from yeast to humans. *Mol cell biol* Vol. 5, pp.1884-1896.

Doyon, Y.; Cayrou, C.; Ullah, M.; Landry, A.J.; Côté, V.; Selleck, W.; Lane, W.S.; Tan, S.; Yang, X.J.; Côté, J. (2006). ING tumor suppressor proteins are critical regulators of chromatin acetylation required for genome expression and perpetuation. *Mol Cell* Vol. 21(1), pp. 51-64.

Fadlelmola, F.M.; Zhou, M.; de Leeuw, R.J.; Dosanjh, N. S.; Harmer, K.; Huntsman, D. et al. (2008). Sub-megabase resolution tiling (SMRT) array-based comparative genomic hybridization profiling reveals novel gains and losses of chromosomal regions in Hodgkin lymphoma and anaplastic large cell lymphoma cell lines. *Mol Cancer* Vol. 7, pp. 2.

Fazzio, T.G.; Huff, J.T.; Panning, B. (2008). An RNAi screen of chromatin proteins identifies Tip60-p400 as a regulator of embryonic stem cell identity. *Cell* Vol. 134(1), pp. 162-174.

Feng, Y.; Lee, N.; Fearon, E.R. (2003) .TIP49 regulates beta-catenin-mediated neoplastic transformation and T-cell factor target gene induction via effects on chromatin remodeling. *Cancer Res* Vol. 63(24), pp.8726-8734.

Fischer, U.; Heckel, D.; Michel, A.; Janka, M.; Hulsebos, T.; Meese, E. (1997). Cloning of a novel transcription factor-like gene amplified in human glioma including astrocytoma grade I. *Hum Mol Genet* Vol. 6, pp. 1817-1822.

Fuchs, M.; Gerber, J.; Drapkin, R.; Sif, S.; Ikura, T.; Ogryzko, V.; Lane, W.S.; Nakatani, Y.; Livingston, D.M. (2001). The p400 complex is an essential E1A transformation target. *Cell* Vol. 106(3), pp. 297-307.

Galarneau, L.; Nourani, A.; Boudreault, A.A.; Zhang, Y.; Héliot, L.; Allard, S.; Savard, J.; Lane, W.S.; Stillman ,D.J.; Côté, J. (2000). Multiple links between the NuA4 histone acetyltransferase complex and epigenetic control of transcription. *Mol Cell* Vol. 5(6), pp. 927-937.

Garcia, S.N.; Kirtane, B.M.; Podlutsky, A.J.; Pereira-Smith, O.M.; Tominaga, K. (2007). Mrg15 null and heterozygous mouse embryonic fibroblasts exhibit DNA-repair defects post exposure to gamma ionizing radiation. *FEBS Lett* Vol. 581(27), pp. 5275-5281.

Gautier, V.W.; Gu, L.; O'Donoghue, N.; Pennington, S.; Sheehy, N.; Hall, W.W. (2009). In vitro nuclear interactome of the HIV-1 Tat protein. *Retrovirology* Vol. 6, pp. 47.

Grant, P.A.; Schieltz, D.; Pray-Grant, M.G.; Yates, J.R. 3rd.; Workman, J.L.(1998). The ATM-related cofactor Tra1 is a component of the purified SAGA complex. *Mol Cell* Vol. 2(6), pp. 863-867.

Grigoletto, A.; Lestienne, P.; Rosenbaum, J. (2011). The multifaceted proteins Reptin and Pontin as major players in cancer. *Biochim Biophys Acta* Vol. 1815(2), pp. 147-157.

Gunduz, M.; Ouchida, M.; Fukushima, K.; Ito, S.; Jitsumori, Y.; Nakashima, T.; Nagai, N.; Nishizaki, K.; Shimizu, K. (2002). Allelic loss and reduced expression of the ING3, a candidate tumor suppressor gene at 7q31, in human head and neck cancers. *Oncogene* Vol. 21(28), pp. 4462-4470.

Gunduz, M.; Beder, L.B.; Gunduz, E.; Nagatsuka, H.; Fukushima, K.; Pehlivan, D.; Cetin, E.; Yamanaka, N.; Nishizaki, K.; Shimizu K.; Nagai, N. (2008). Downregulation of

ING3 mRNA expression predicts poor prognosis in head and neck cancer. *Cancer Sci* Vol. 99(3), pp. 531-538.

Harata, M.; Karwan, A.; Wintersberger, U. (1994). An essential gene of Saccharomyces cerevisiae coding for an actin-related protein. *Proc. Natl. Acad. Sci. USA* Vol. 91, pp. 8258–8262.

Harborth, J.; Weber, K.; Osborn, M. (2000). GAS41, a highly conserved protein in eukaryotic nuclei, binds to NuMA. *J Biol Chem* Vol. 275(41), pp.31979-31985.

Haslinger, C.; Schweifer, N.; Stilgenbauer, S.; Dohner, H.; Lichter, P.; Kraut, N.; Stratowa, C.; Abseher, R. (2004). Microarray gene expression profiling of B-cell chronic lymphocytic leukemia subgroups defined by genomic aberrations and VH mutation status. *J Clin Oncol* Vol. 22, pp. 3937–3949.

Herceg, Z.; Hulla, W.; Gell, D.; Cuenin, C.; Lleonart, M.; Jackson, S.; Wang, Z. Q. (2001). Disruption of Trrap causes early embryonic lethality and defects in cell cycle progression. *Nat Genet* Vol. 29(2), pp. 206-211.

Horikawa, I.; Tanaka, H.; Yuasa, Y.; Suzuki, M.; Oshimura, M. (1995a). Molecular cloning of a novel human cDNA on chromosome 1q21 and its mouse homolog encoding a nuclear protein with DNA-binding ability. *Biochem Biophys Res Commun* Vol. 208(3), pp. 999-1007.

Horikawa, I.; Tanaka, H.; Yuasa, Y.; Suzuki, M.; Shimizu, M.; Oshimura, M. (1995b). Forced expression of YL-1 protein suppresses the anchorage-independent growth of Kirsten sarcoma virus-transformed NIH3T3 cells. *Exp Cell Res* Vol. 220(1), pp. 11-17.

Hughes, T. R.; C. J. Roberts, H.; Dai, A. R.; Jones, M. R.; Meyer, D.; Slade, J.; Burchard, S.; Dow, T. R.; Ward, M. J.; Kidd, et al. (2000). Widespread aneuploidy revealed by DNA microarray expression profiling. *Nat Genet* Vol. 25, pp. 333-337.

Ikura, T.; Ogryzko, V.V.; Grigoriev, M.; Groisman, R.; Wang, J.; Horikoshi, M.; Scully, R.; Qin, J.; Nakatani Y. (2000). Involvement of the TIP60 histone acetylase complex in DNA repair and apoptosis. *Cell* Vol.102(4), pp.463-473.

Imbeaud, S. (2006). Deciphering cellular states of innate tumor drug responses. *Genome Biol* Vol. 7, pp. R19.

Jin, J.; Cai, Y.; Yao, T.; Gottschalk, A.J.; Florens, L.; Swanson, S.K.; Gutiérrez, J.L.; Coleman, M.K.; Workman, J.L.; Mushegian, A.; Washburn, M.P.; Conaway, R.C.; Conaway, J.W. (2005) A mammalian chromatin remodeling complex with similarities to the yeast INO80 complex. *J Biol Chem* Vol. 280(50), pp. 41207-41212.

Kanemaki, M.; Kurokawa, Y.; Matsu-ura, T.; Makino, Y. Masani, A.; Okazaki, K.; Morishita, T.; Tamura, T.A. (1999). TIP49b, a new RuvB-like DNA helicase, is included in a complex together with another RuvB-like DNA helicase, TIP49a, *J Biol Chem* Vol, 274 , pp. 22437–22444.

Kawahata, M. Masaki, K.; Fujii, T.; Iefuji, H. (2006). Yeast genes involved in response to lactic acid and acetic acid: acidic conditions caused by the organic acids in Saccharomyces cerevisiae cultures induce expression of intracellular metal metabolism genes regulated by Aft1p. *FEMS Yeast Res* Vol. 6(6), pp. 924-936.

Keogh, M. C.; Mennella, T. A.; Sawa, C.; Berthelet, S.; Krogan, N. J.; Wolek, A.; Podolny, V.; Carpenter, L. R.; Greenblatt, J. F.; Baetz, K.; Buratowski, S. (2006). The

Saccharomyces cerevisiae histone H2A variant Htz1 is acetylated by NuA4. *Genes Dev* Vol. 20, pp. 660-665.

Ki, D.H.; Jeung, H.C.; Park, C.H.; Kang, S.H.; Lee, G.Y.; Lee, W.S.; Kim, N.K.; Chung, H.C.; Rha, S.Y. (2007). Whole genome analysis for liver metastasis gene signatures in colorectal cancer. *Int J Cancer* Vol. 121, pp. 2005–2012.

Kim, J.R.; Kee, H.J.; Kim, J.Y.; Joung, H.; Nam, K.I.; Eom, G.H.; Choe, N.; Kim, H.S.; Kim, J.C.; Kook, H.; Seo, S.B.; Kook, H. (2009). Enhancer of polycomb1 acts on serum response factor to regulate skeletal muscle differentiation. *J Biol Chem* Vol. 284(24), pp. 16308-16316.

Kouzarides, T. (2007). Chromatin modifications and their function. *Cell* Vol. 128, pp. 693–705.

Krogan, N.J.; Keogh, M.C.; Datta, N.; Sawa, C.; Ryan, O.W.; Ding, H.; et al. (2003) A Snf2 family ATPase complex required for recruitment of the histone H2A variant Htz1. *Mol Cell* Vol. 12(6), pp. 1565-1576.

Krogan, N. J.; Baetz, K.; Keogh, M.C.; Datta, N.; Sawa, C.; Kwok, T. C.; Thompson, N. J.; Davey, M. G.; Pootoolal, J.; Hughes, T. R.; Emili, A.; Buratowski, S.; Hieter, P.; Greenblatt, J. F. (2004). Regulation of chromosome stability by the histone H2A variant Htz1, the Swr1 chromatin remodeling complex, and the histone acetyltransferase NuA4. *Proc Natl Acad Sci U S A* Vol. 101(37), pp.13513-13518.

Krogan, N.J.; Cagney, G.; Yu, H.; Zhong, G.; Guo, X.; Ignatchenko, A.; et al. (2006). Global landscape of protein complexes in the yeast Saccharomyces cerevisiae. *Nature* Vol. 440(7084), pp. 637-43.

Lauffart, B.; Howell, S.J.; Tasch, J.E.; Cowell, J.K.; Still, I.H. (2002). Interaction of the transforming acidic coiled-coil 1 (TACC1) protein with ch-TOG and GAS41/NuBI1 suggests multiple TACC1-containing protein complexes in human cells. *Biochem J* Vol. 363(Pt 1), pp.195-200.

Lauscher, J.C.; Loddenkemper, C.; Kosel, L.; Grone, J.; Buhr, H.J.; Huber, O. (2007). Increased pontin expression in human colorectal cancer tissue. *Hum Pathol* Vol. 38, pp. 978–985.

Le Masson, I.; Yu, D.Y.; Jensen, K.; Chevalier, A.; Courbeyrette, R.; Boulard, Y.; Smith, M.M.; Mann, C. (2003). Yaf9, a novel NuA4 histone acetyltransferase subunit, is required for the cellular response to spindle stress in yeast. *Mol Cell Biol* Vol. 23(17), pp. 6086-6102.

Li, H.; Cuenin, C.; Murr, R, Wang, Z.Q.; Herceg, Z. (2004). HAT cofactor Trrap regulates the mitotic checkpoint by modulation of Mad1 and Mad2 expression. *EMBO J* Vol. 23(24), pp. 4824-4834.

Li, W.; Zeng, J.; Li, Q.; Zhao, L.; Liu, T.; Bjorkholm, M.; Jia, J.; Xu, D. (2010). Reptin is required for the transcription of telomerase reverse transcriptase and over-expressed in gastric cancer. *Mol Cancer* Vol. 9, pp. 132

Lim, C.R.; Kimata, Y.; Ohdate, H.; Kokubo, T.; Kikuchi, N.; Horigome, T.; Kohno K. (2000). The Saccharomyces cerevisiae RuvB-like protein, Tih2p, is required for cell cycle progression and RNA polymerase II-directed transcription, *J Biol Chem* Vol. 275 (2000), pp. 22409–22417.

Lin, Y.Y.; Lu, J.Y.; Zhang, J.; Walter, W.; Dang, W.; Wan, J.; Tao, S. C.; Qian, J.; Zhao, Y.; Boeke, J.D.; Berger, S.L.; Zhu, H. (2009). Protein acetylation microarray reveals that NuA4 controls key metabolic target regulating gluconeogenesis. *Cell* Vol. 136 (6), pp.1073-1084.

Lin, Y.Y.; Qi, Y.; Lu, J.Y.; Pan, X.; Yuan, D.S.; Zhao, Y.; Bader, J.S.; Boeke, J.D. (2008). A comprehensive synthetic genetic interaction network governing yeast histone acetylation and deacetylation. *Genes Dev* Vol. 22(15), pp.2062-2074.

Liu, X.; Yang, H.; Zhang, X.; Liu, L.; Lei, M.; Zhang, Z.; Bao, X. (2009). Bdf1p deletion affects mitochondrial function and causes apoptotic cell death under salt stress. *FEMS Yeast Res* Vol. 9(2), pp. 240-246.

Loewith, R.; Meijer, M.; Lees-Miller, S.P.; Riabowol, K.; Young, D. (2000). Three yeast proteins related to the human candidate tumor suppressor p33(ING1) are associated with histone acetyltransferase activities. *Mol Cell Biol* 20(11), pp. 3807-3816.

Loukopoulos, P.; Shibata, T.; Katoh, H.; Kokubu, A.; Sakamoto, M.; Yamazaki, K.; Kosuge, T, Kanai, Y.; Hosoda, F.; Imoto, I.; Ohki, M.; Inazawa, J.; Hirohashi, S. (2007). Genome-wide array-based comparative genomic hybridization analysis of pancreatic adenocarcinoma: identification of genetic indicators that predict patient outcome. *Cancer Sci* Vol.; 98(3), pp. 392-400.

Lygerou, Z.; Conesa, C.; Lesage, P.; Swanson, R.N.; Ruet, A.; Carlson, M.; Sentenac, A.; Séraphin, B. (1994). The yeast BDF1 gene encodes a transcription factor involved in the expression of a broad class of genes including snRNAs. *Nucleic Acids Res* Vol. 22(24), pp. 5332-5340.

Martrat, G.; Maxwell, C.A.; Tominaga, E.; Porta-de-la-Riva, M.; Bonifaci, N.; Gómez-Baldó, L.; et al. (2011). Exploring the link between MORF4L1 and risk of breast cancer.*Breast Cancer Res* Vol. 13(2), pp.R40.

Matangkasombut, O.; Buratowski, R.M.; Swilling, N.W.; Buratowski, S. (2000). Bromodomain factor 1 corresponds to a missing piece of yeast TFIID. *Genes Dev* Vol. 14(8), pp.951-962.

Mattera, L.; Escaffit, F.; Pillaire, M.J.; Selves, J.; Tyteca, S, Hoffmann, J.S.; Gourraud, P.A.; Chevillard-Briet, M.; Cazaux, C.; Trouche, D. (2009). The p400/Tip60 ratio is critical for colorectal cancer cell proliferation through DNA damage response pathways. *Oncogene* Vol. 28(12), pp. 1506-1517.

Mitchell, L.; Lambert, J.P.; Gerdes, M.; Al-Madhoun, A.S.; Skerjanc, I.S.; Figeys, D.; Baetz, K. (2008). Functional dissection of the NuA4 histone acetyltransferase reveals its role as a genetic hub and that Eaf1 is essential for complex integrity. *Mol Cell Biol* Vol. 28(7), pp. 2244-2256.

Mizuguchi, G.; Shen, X.; Landry, J.; Wu, W. H. ; Sen, S.; Wu, C.. (2004). ATP-driven exchange of histone H2AZ variant catalyzed by SWR1 chromatin remodeling complex. Science Vol. 303, pp. 343-348.

Mohan, K.N.; Ding, F.; Chaillet, J.R. (2011). Distinct Roles of DMAP1 in Mouse Development. *Mol Cell Biol* Vol. 31(9), pp. 1861-1869.

Monden, T.; Wondisford, F.E.; Hollenberg, A. N. (1997). Isolation and characterization of a novel ligand-dependent thyroid hormone receptor-coactivating protein. *J Biol Chem* Vol. 272(47), pp. 29834-29841.

Monden, T.; Kishi, M.; Hosoya, T.; Satoh, T.; Wondisford, F.E.; Hollenberg, A.N.; Yamada, M.; Mori, M. (1999). p120 acts as a specific coactivator for 9-cis-retinoic acid receptor (RXR) on peroxisome proliferator-activated receptor-gamma/RXR heterodimers. *Mol Endocrinol* Vol. 13(10), pp. 1695-1703.

Mujtaba, S.; Zeng, L.; Zhou, M.M. (2007). Structure and acetyl-lysine recognition of the bromodomain. *Oncogene* Vol.;26(37), pp. 5521-5527.

Murr, R.; Loizou, J.I.; Yang, Y.G.; Cuenin, C.; Li, H.; Wang, Z.Q.; Herceg, Z. (2006). Histone acetylation by Trrap-Tip60 modulates loading of repair proteins and repair of DNA double-strand breaks. *Nat Cell Biol* Vol. 8(1), pp. 91-99.

Murr, R.; Vaissière, T.; Sawan, C.; Shukla, V.; Herceg, Z. (2007) Orchestration of chromatin-based processes: mind the TRRAP. *Oncogene* Vol. 26(37), pp. 5358-5372.

Nagashima, M.; Shiseki, M.; Pedeux, R.M.; Okamura, S.; Kitahama-Shiseki, M.; Miura, K.; Yokota, J.; Harris, C.C. (2003). A novel PHD-finger motif protein, p47ING3, modulates p53-mediated transcription, cell cycle control, and apoptosis. *Oncogene* Vol. 22(3), pp. 343-350.

Nakahata, S.; Saito, Y.; Hamasaki, M.; Hidaka, T.; Arai, Y.; Taki, T.; Taniwaki, M.; Morishita, K. (2009). Alteration of enhancer of polycomb 1 at 10p11.2 is one of the genetic events leading to development of adult T-cell leukemia/lymphoma. *Genes Chromosomes Cancer* Vol. 48(9), pp. 768-776.

Negishi, M.; Chiba, T.; Saraya, A.; Miyagi, S.; Iwama, A. (2009). Dmap1 plays an essential role in the maintenance of genome integrity through the DNA repair process. *Genes Cells* Vol. 14(11), pp.1347-1357.

Nishiu, M.; Yanagawa, R.; Nakatsuka, S.; Yao, M.; Tsunoda, T.; Nakamura, Y. Aozasa, K. (2002). Microarray analysis of gene-expression profiles in diffuse large B-cell lymphoma: identification of genes related to disease progression, Jpn J. *Cancer Res* Vol. 93, pp. 894–901.

Notaridou, M.; Quaye, L.; Dafou, D.; Jones, C.; Song, H.; Høgdall, E.; Kjaer, S.K.; Christensen, L.; Høgdall, C.; Blaakaer, J.; McGuire, V.; Wu, A.H.; et al. (2011). Common alleles in candidate susceptibility genes associated with risk and development of epithelial ovarian cancer. *Int J Cancer* Vol. 128(9), pp. 2063-2074.

Park, J.; Wood, M.A.; Cole, M.D. (2002). BAF53 forms distinct nuclear complexes and functions as a critical c-Myc-interacting nuclear cofactor for oncogenic transformation. *Mol Cell Biol* Vol. 22(5), pp.1307-1316.

Reid, J.L.; Moqtaderi, Z.; Struhl, K. (2004). Eaf3 regulates the global pattern of histone acetylation in Saccharomyces cerevisiae. *Mol Cell Biol* Vol. 24(2), pp.757-764.

Rountree, M.R.; Bachman, K.E.; Baylin, S.B. (2000). DNMT1 binds HDAC2 and a new co-repressor, DMAP1, to form a complex at replication foci. *Nat Genet* Vol. 25(3), pp. 269-277.

Saksouk, N.; Avvakumov, N.; Champagne, K.S.; Hung, T.; Doyon, Y.; Cayrou, C.; Paquet, E.; Ullah, M.; Landry, A.J.; Côté, V.; Yang, X.J.; Gozani, O.; Kutateladze, T.G.; Côté, J.

(2009). HBO HAT complexes target chromatin throughout gene coding regions via multiple PHD finger interactions with histone H3 tail. *Mol Cell* Vol. 33(2), pp. 257-265.

Saleh, A.; Schieltz, D.; Ting, N.; McMahon, S.B.; Litchfield, D.W.; Yates, J.R. 3rd; Lees-Miller, S.P.; Cole, M.D.; Brandl, C. J.(1998). Tra1p is a component of the yeast Ada.Spt transcriptional regulatory complexes. *J Biol Chem* Vol. 273(41), pp. 26559-26565.

Sanchez, R.; Zhou, M.M. (2011). The PHD finger: a versatile epigenome reader. *Trends Biochem Sci* [Epub ahead of print]

Sanchez-Carbayo, M.; Socci, N.D.; Lozano, J.; Saint, F. Cordon-Cardo, C. (2006). Defining molecular profiles of poor outcome in patients with invasive bladder cancer using oligonucleotide microarrays. *J Clin Oncol* Vol. 24, pp. 778–789.

Sardiu, M.E.; Cai, Y.; Jin, J.; Swanson, S.K.; Conaway, R.C.; Conaway, J.W.; Florens, L.; Washburn, M.P. (2008). Probabilistic assembly of human protein interaction networks from label-free quantitative proteomics. *Proc Natl Acad Sci U S A* Vol.105(5), pp.1454-1459.

Sen, G.L.; Reuter, J.A.;, Webster, D.E.; Zhu, L.; Khavari, P.A. (2010). DNMT1 maintains progenitor function in self-renewing somatic tissue. *Nature* 2010 Vol.; 463(7280), pp. 563-567.

Shen, X. Mizuguchi, G.; Hamiche, A.; Wu, C. (2000). A chromatin remodelling complex involved in transcription and DNA processing. *Nature* Vol. 406(6795), pp. 541-544

Stankunas, K.; Berger, J.; Ruse, C.; Sinclair, D.A.; Randazzo, F.; Brock, H.W. (1998). The enhancer of polycomb gene of Drosophila encodes a chromatin protein conserved in yeast and mammals. *Development* Vol. 125(20), pp. 4055-4066.

Sung, Y.H.; Choi, E.Y.; Kwon, H. (2001). Identification of a nuclear protein ArpN as a component of human SWI/SNF complex and its selective association with a subset of active genes. *Mol Cells* Vol. 11(1), pp. 75-81.

Tominaga, K.; Kirtane, B.; Jackson, J.G.; Ikeno, Y.; Ikeda, T.; Hawks, C.; Smith, J.R.; Matzuk, M.M.; Pereira-Smith, O.M. (2005). MRG15 regulates embryonic development and cell proliferation. *Mol Cell Biol* Vol. 25(8), pp. 2924-2937.

Tondeleir, D.; Vandamme, D.; Vandekerckhove, J.; Ampe, C.; Lambrechts, A. (2009). Actin isoform expression patterns during mammalian development and in pathology: insights from mouse models. *Cell Motil Cytoskeleton* Vol. 66(10), pp.798-815

Ueda, T.; Watanabe-Fukunaga, R.; Ogawa, H.; Fukuyama, H.; Higashi, Y.; Nagata, S.; Fukunaga, R. (2007). Critical role of the p400/mDomino chromatin-remodeling ATPase in embryonic hematopoiesis. *Genes Cells* Vol. 12(5), pp. 581-592.

Ullah, M.; Pelletier, N.; Xiao, L.; Zhao, S.P.; Wang, K.; Degerny, C.; Tahmasebi, S.; Cayrou, C.; Doyon, Y.; Goh, S.L.; Champagne, N.; Côté, J.; Yang, X.J. (2008). Molecular architecture of quartet MOZ/MORF histone acetyltransferase complexes. *Mol Cell Biol* Vol. 28(22), pp.6828-6843.

Wang, Y.; Dai, D.L.; Martinka, M.; Li, G. (2007). Prognostic significance of nuclear ING3 expression in human cutaneous melanoma. *Clin Cancer Res* Vol. 13(14), pp. 4111-4116.

Wei, X.; Walia, V.; Lin, J.C.; Teer, J.K.; Prickett, T.D.; Gartner, J.; Davis, S.; NISC Comparative Sequencing Program; Stemke-Hale, K.; Davies, M.A.; Gershenwald, J. E.; Robinson, W.; Robinson, S.; Rosenberg, S.A.; Samuels, Y. (2011). Exome sequencing identifies GRIN2A as frequently mutated in melanoma. *Nat Genet* Vol. 43(5), pp. 442-446.

Wu, W.H.; Alami, S.; Luk, E.; Wu, C.H.; Sen, S.; Mizuguchi, G.; Wei, D.; Wu, C. (2005). Swc2 is a widely conserved H2AZ-binding module essential for ATP-dependent histone exchange. *Nat Struct Mol Biol* Vol. 12(12), pp. 1064-1071.

Wurdak, H.; Zhu, S.; Romero, A.; Lorger, M.; Watson, J.; Chiang, C.Y.; Zhang, J.; Natu, V.S.; Lairson, L.L.; Walker, J.R.; Trussell, C.M.; Harsh, G.R.; Vogel, H.; Felding-Habermann, B.; Orth, A.P.; Miraglia, L.J.; Rines, D.R.; Skirboll, S.L.; Schultz, P.G. (2010). An RNAi screen identifies TRRAP as a regulator of brain tumor-initiating cell differentiation. *Cell Stem Cell* Vol. 6(1), pp. 37-47.

Yamada, H.Y.; Gorbsky, G.J. (2006) Cell-based expression cloning for identification of polypeptides that hypersensitize mammalian cells to mitotic arrest. *Biol Proced Online*. Vol. 8, pp.36-43.

Yamada, H.Y.; Rao, C.V. (2009). BRD8 is a potential chemosensitizing target for spindle poisons in colorectal cancer therapy. *Int J Oncol* Vol. 35(5), pp.1101-1109.

Yamaguchi, K.; Sakai, M.; Shimokawa, T.; Yamada, Y.; Nakamura, Y.; Furukawa, Y. (2010). C20orf20 (MRG-binding protein) as a potential therapeutic target for colorectal cancer.*Br J Cancer* Vol. 102(2), pp.325-31.

Yamaguchi, K.; Sakai, M.; Kim, J.; Tsunesumi, S.; Fujii, T.; Ikenoue, T.; Yamada, Y.; Akiyama, Y.; Muto, Y.; Yamaguchi, R.; Miyano, S.; Nakamura, Y.; Furukawa, Y. (2011). MRG-binding protein contributes to colorectal cancer development. *Cancer Sci* Vol. 102(8), pp.1486-1492.

Yuan, C.X.; Ito, M.; Fondell, J.D.; Fu, Z.Y.; Roeder, R.G. (1998). The TRAP220 component of a thyroid hormone receptor- associated protein (TRAP) coactivator complex interacts directly with nuclear receptors in a ligand-dependent fashion. *Proc Natl Acad Sci U S A* Vol. 95(14), pp. 7939-7944

Zeng L.; Zhou, M.M. (2002). Bromodomain: an acetyl-lysine binding domain. *FEBS Lett* Vol. 513(1), pp. 124-128.

Zhan, F.; Barlogie, B.; Arzoumanian, V.; Huang, Y.; Williams, D.R.; Hollmig, K.; Pineda-Roman, M.; Tricot, G.; van Rhee, F.; Zangari, M.; Dhodapkar, M. Shaughnessy Jr., J.D. (2007). Gene-expression signature of benign monoclonal gammopathy evident in multiple myeloma is linked to good prognosis. *Blood* Vol. 109, pp. 1692–1700.

Zhang, H.; Richardson, D.O.; Roberts, D.N.; Utley, R.; Erdjument-Bromage, H.; Tempst, P.; Côté, J, Cairns, B.R. (2004). The Yaf9 component of the SWR1 and NuA4 complexes is required for proper gene expression, histone H4 acetylation, and Htz1 replacement near telomeres. *Mol Cell Biol* Vol. 24(21), pp. 9424-9436.

Zhao, K.; Wang, W.; Rando, O.J.; Xue, Y.; Swiderek, K.; Kuo, A.; Crabtree, G.R. (1998). Rapid and phosphoinositol-dependent binding of the SWI/SNF-like BAF complex to chromatin after T lymphocyte receptor signaling. *Cell* Vol. 95(5), pp. 625-636.

11

Characterization of the Cell Membrane During Cancer Transformation

Barbara Szachowicz-Petelska[1], Izabela Dobrzyńska[1], Stanisław Sulkowski[2] and Zbigniew A. Figaszewski[1,3]

[1]Institute of Chemistry, University in Bialystok,
[2]Department of General Pathomorphology, Medical University of Bialystok,
[3]Faculty of Chemistry, University of Warsaw,
Poland

1. Introduction

Colorectal cancer is one of the most common cancers diagnosed worldwide. The development of colorectal cancer, like many types of cancer is a multistage process that involves many different pathways. In particular, deregulation of cell-cell communication plays an important role. Moreover, cell-cell comunication is indispensable for the maintenance of homeostasis in a multicellular organism. *Gap*-type junctions are one of the most common and perhaps most interesting, mediators of intercellular communications. Digestive tract gap junctions are also important and are flanked by various cell types within each layer of the wall. The composition and organisation of gap junction channel subunits plays a critical role in determining the properties of these channels, including conductance properties and pH sensitivity. Structurally, gap junctions are composed of transmembrane proteins which form structures called connexons, with a single connexon consistings of six peripherally arranged subunits of integral membrane proteins known as connexins. Correspondingly, normal human epithelial cells in the colon have been found to express the connexins, Cx32 and Cx43. Moreover, in our previous studies Cx26 expression was detected in normal colon epithelium as well as in colorectal cancer tissues (Contreras et al., 2002, Cascio, 2005, van Zeijl et al., 2007).

A number of biological and chemical substances affect the function of gap junctions. For example junctions can be inhibited following the phosphorylation of connexin proteins or following exposure to agents that disrupt the accumulation of connexin or mediate local damage to cellular membranes. The function of membrane channels also require the presence of particular species of lipid in the surrounding membrane. Locke and Harris were the first to identify endogenous phospholipids tightly associated with connexin channels and these results suggested that specific phospholipids are associated with different connexin isoforms to form connexin-specific regulatory networks and/or structural interactions with lipid membranes. Ongoing studies of connexin channel function and cell biology to characterize lipid-protein interactions and membrane biophysics are providing valuable insight into these processes (Locke & Harris, 2009).

Phenomena associated with changes in cell membranes are suspected to play an important role during the cancer transformation. At physiological pH, the cell membrane surface is negatively charged, which is determined based on the number of negative and positive charge carriers present (i.e., phosphates, carboxyl and amino groups of proteins and phospholipids). Furthermore, electrical properties of a membrane are determined by acid-base and complex formation equilibria at the membrane and in response to surrounding medium components. For example, membrane components including - proteins, phospholipids, and free fatty acids contribute to this equilibria. Correspondingly, we hypothesis that the electrical charge of tumor cells can indirectly represent changes that have occurred during cell transformation and may indicate tumor cell status.

2. The cell membrane

Biological membranes are essential boundaries within a living cell. The cell membranes separate the interior of the cell from its microenvironment and also participate in intercellular communication.

2.1 Electric properties of cell membranes

For a biological membrane, its electrical charge and difference in potential between the membrane and surrounding solution are key properties. Cell membrane charge has been found to increase during tumorigenesis and decrease during necrosis (Dołowy, 1984). Correspondingly, investigations of factors that influence membrane electric charge during cancer transformation have been performed. These factors include determining pH, acidic (C_{TA}) and basic (C_{TB}) functional group concentrations and their average association constants with hydrogen (K_{AH}) or hydroxyl (K_{BOH}) ions (Dobrzyńska et al., 2006).
The electrical properties of a membrane are determined by acid-base and complex formation equilibria. Both membrane and surrounding medium components contribute to this equilibria, with the former including proteins, phospholipids and fatty acids (Gennis, 1989; Tien, 1974). As a result, we hypothesise that the electrical charge of tumor cells can be indirectly estimated from changes detected in tumor cells that are concomitant with their transformation during tumorigenesis.

2.1.1 Surface charge density cell membrane

Surface charge density dependence on pH of normal and tumor large intestine cell membrane are similarly shaped (Fig. 1). For example, an increase in positive surface charge density is observed at low pH values until a plateau is reached. Conversely, at high pH values, the proportion of negative charges present increases until it reaches a plateau. Overall, an increase in negative charge at low pH values as well as in positive charge at high pH is observed in human large intestine tumor cells compared to unaffected cells (Szachowicz-Petelska et al., 2002).

2.1.2 Theory

The dependence of surface charge density of a cell membrane on pH of electrolyte solution can be described according to four equilibria factors. Two equilibria concern negative groups and involve sodium and hydrogen ions, and two other equilibria refer to positive groups and involve hydroxide and chloride ions. These factors can then be expressed as follows written in the form:

$$A^- + H^+ \Leftrightarrow AH \qquad (1)$$

$$A^- + Na^+ \Leftrightarrow ANa \quad (2)$$

$$B^+ + OH^- \Leftrightarrow BOH \quad (3)$$

$$B^+ + Cl^- \Leftrightarrow BCl \quad (4)$$

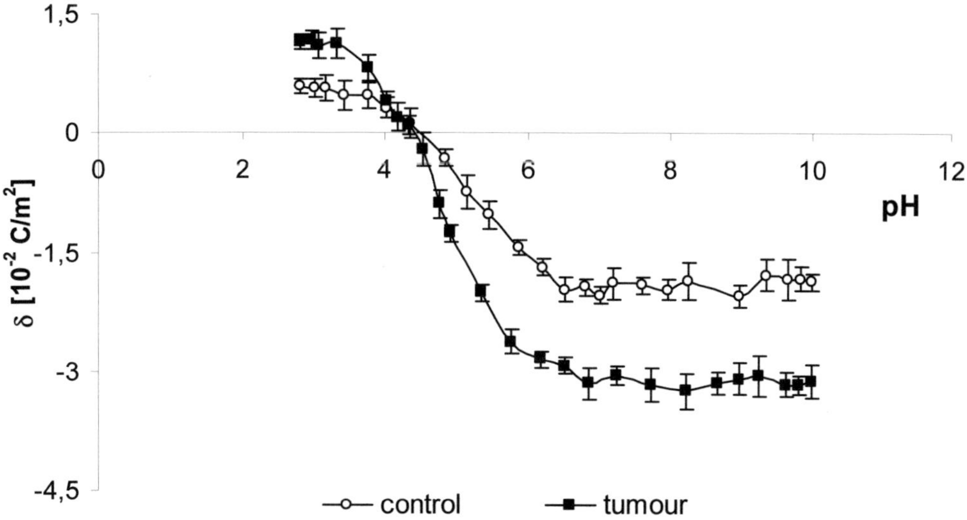

Fig. 1. The dependence of surface charge density on pH for normal and colorectal cancer cell membranes from several patients.

An association constant of the H^+ Na^+, OH^- and Cl^- ions with functional groups can be expressed according to the following equations:

$$K_{AH} = \frac{a_{AH}}{a_{A^-} \cdot a_{H^+}} \quad (5)$$

$$K_{ANa} = \frac{a_{ANa}}{a_{A^-} \cdot a_{Na^+}} \quad (6)$$

$$K_{BOH} = \frac{a_{BOH}}{a_{B^+} \cdot a_{OH^-}} \quad (7)$$

$$K_{BCl} = \frac{a_{BCl}}{a_{B^+} \cdot a_{Cl^-}} \quad (8)$$

Here:

K_{AH}, K_{ANa}, K_{BOH} and K_{BCl} represent association constants,

a_{A^-}, a_{AH}, a_{ANa}, a_{B^+}, a_{BOH} and a_{BCl} represent surface concentrations, that are present on the membrane surface,

and a_{H^+}, a_{Na^+}, a_{OH^-} and a_{Cl^-} represent corresponding concentrations in solution.

Surface charge density (δ) is expressed as follows:

$$\delta = (a_{B^+} - a_{A^-}) \cdot F \tag{9}$$

where F=96487 [C/mol] - Faraday constant.
And functional group concentration balances can be expressed as follows:

$$C_{TA} = a_{A^-} + a_{AH} + a_{ANa} \tag{10}$$

$$C_{TB} = a_{B^+} + a_{BOH} + a_{BCl} \tag{11}$$

where C_{TA} and C_{TB} represent the total surface concentrations functional groups.
Elimination of a_{A^-}, a_{AH}, a_{B^+}, and a_{BOH} values from above equations yields the following formula:

$$\frac{\delta}{F} = \frac{C_{TB} \cdot a_{H^+}}{a_{H^+}(1 + K_{BCl} \cdot a_{Cl^-}) + K_{BOH} \cdot K_w} - \frac{C_{TA}}{K_{AH} \cdot a_{H^+} + K_{ANa} \cdot a_{Na^+} + 1} \tag{12}$$

It is difficult to carry out the regression function of Eqn. (12) to determine the C_{TA}, C_{TB}, K_{AH} and K_{BOH} constants.
Simplifying to one fraction and making transformations described in this work (Dobrzyńska et al., 2006), we can receive the equation of a straight line for high and low ion concentration H^+, from which C_{TA}, C_{TB}, K_{AH} and K_{BOH} values can be established.
The coefficients could be determined using linear regression and C_{TA}, C_{TB}, K_{AH} and K_{BOH} values could be calculated. However, in determining each values, there are points that would need to be considered in the regression, both for high and low H^+ concentration ranges.

2.1.3 Parameters characterizing the cell membrane

In this study C_{TA}, C_{TB} and K_{BOH} values for a cell membrane were found to be affected by cancer cell transformation, and were higher than the same parameters assayed in unmodified cells (Figs. 2-4). Meanwhile K_{AH} was found to decrease in cancer cells versus normal cells (Fig. 3).
In normal cells, the aminophospholipids such as phoshatidylserine (PS) and phosphatidylethanolamine (PE) are asymmetrically distributed across the plasma membrane e.g., they primarily localize to the cell's inner membrane leaflet (Stafford & Thorpe, 2011; Marconescu & Thorpe, 2008). This membrane lipid asymmetry is maintained by a group of P-type ATPases known as aminophospholipid translocases (APTLs). These APTLs catalyze the active transport of PS and PE from the external side to the internal side of the leaflet of the plasma membrane (Devaux, 1992). The distribution of PS, a component of the skeleton, has been shown to undergo changes, which could cause an increase in the proportion of negatively charged groups present at high pH values. As a result, anionic phospholipids present on tumor vessels could potentially represent tumor-specific markers for targeting and imaging (Ran et al., 2002).
Hypoxia/reoxygenation and acidity-induced exposure of anionic phospholipids, most likely phosphatidylserine and phosphatidylethanolamine (Zhao et al., 1998; Ran et al., 2002). According to previous studies both hypoxia and acidity can exist in a tumor. In particular,

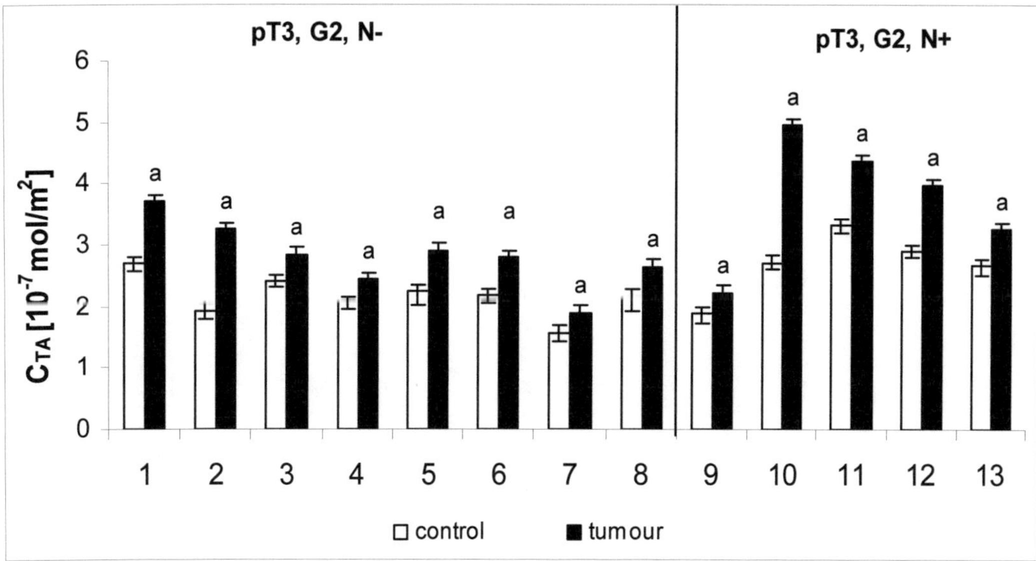

Fig. 2. The concentration of acidic functional groups present on pT3 stage, G2 grade human colorectal cancer cell membranes associated with metastasis (N+) and not associated with metastasis (N-). [a] $p<0.05$, compared with control.

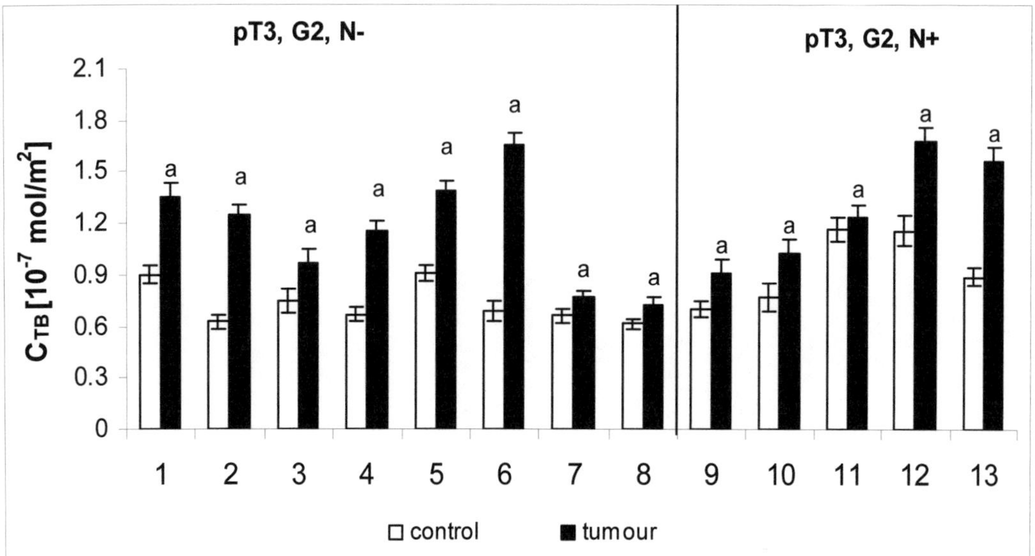

Fig. 3. The concentration of basic functional groups present on pT3 stage, G2 grade human colorectal cancer cell membranes associated with metastasis (N+) and not associated with metastasis (N-). [a] $p<0.05$, compared with control.

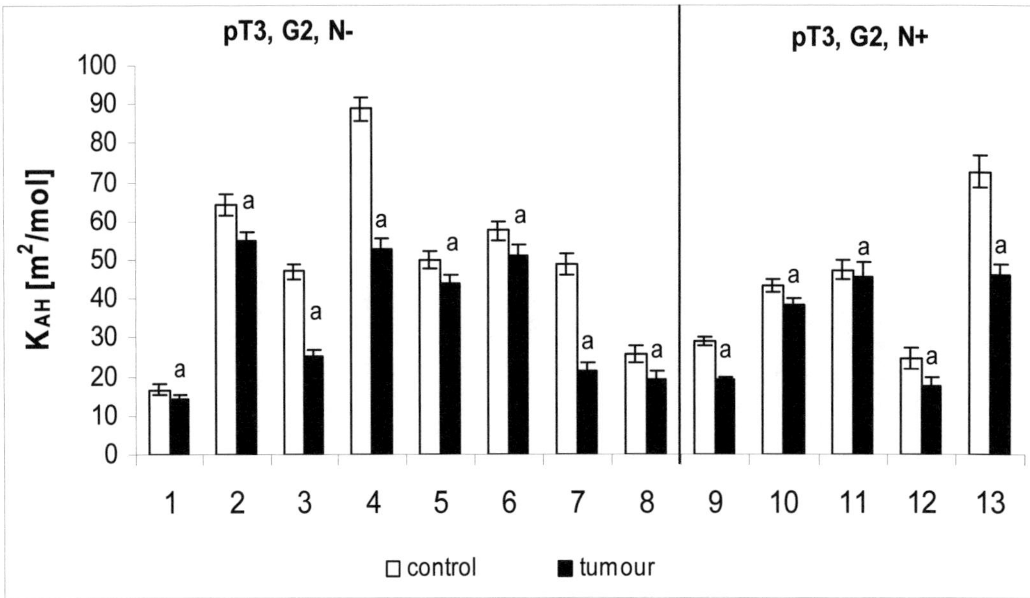

Fig. 4. The average association constant for hydrogen ions associated with pT3 stage, G2 grade human colorectal cancer cell membranes associated with metastasis (N+) and not associated with metastasis (N-). [a] $p<0.05$, compared with control.

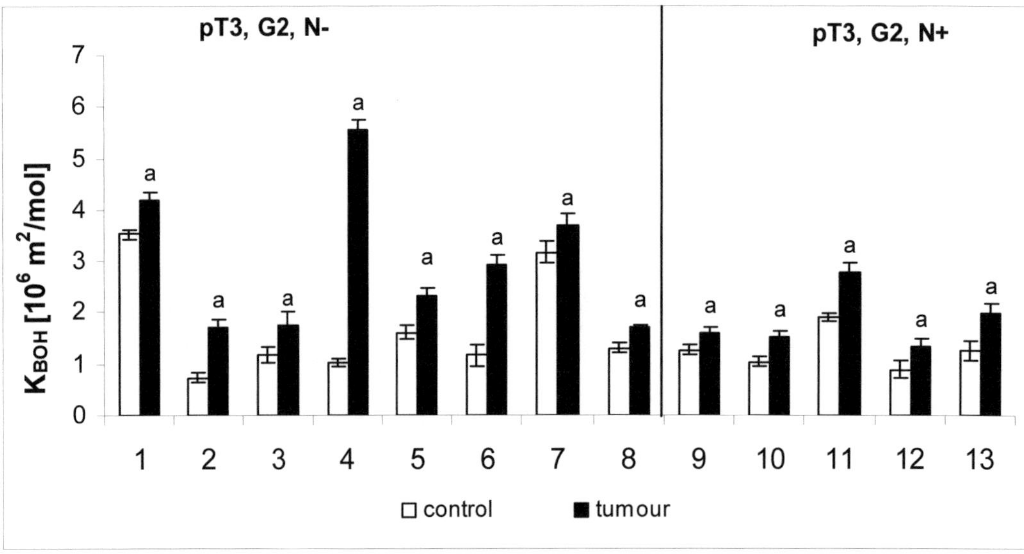

Fig. 5. The average association constant for hydroxyl ions associated with pT3 stage, G2 grade human colorectal cancer cell membranes associated with metastasis (N+) and not associated with metastasis (N-). [a] $p<0.05$, compared with control.

hypoxia represents an important cellular stressor that can trigger a survival program by which cells attempt to adapt to a new environment. Typically, these adaptations will largely affect cell metabolism and/or stimulation of oxygen delivery (Bos et al., 2004).
Cell membrane charge is also affected by sialic acid present in glycolipids and glycoproteins. It has previously been hypothesized that sialic acid influences the concentrations of acid and basic groups present on the cell surface as well as association constants of positively and negatively charged groups during cancer transformation. An increase in the content of sialic acid in glycolipids and glycoproteins has been confirmed in, and increased sialic acid content has been found to provoke an increase in the surface concentration of acid groups (Erbil et al., 1986; Narayanan, 1994; Wang, 2005).

2.2 The compounds present in the cell membranes of human colorectal cancer

Neoplasms produce and secrete agents at trace levels inside of cells. These agents can include carcinogenic antigens, hormones, metabolites, growth factors, enzymes and cytokines (Skrzydlewska et al., 2005; Koda et al., 2004). In malignant cells, the ultrastructural architecture of the cell membrane is altered, partially as a result of changes in the quantities of membrane components present. Correspondingly, the transport of agents through the cell membrane is affected, thereby altering the biological properties of a cell. In many cases, expression levels of proteins, phospholipids and free unsaturated fatty acids are also affected due to enzyme disorders associated with biosynthesis processes that are altered. It is hypothesized that quantitation of the changes in the levels of phospholipids and structural proteins at the cell surface can reflect the extent of disintegration and impairment of genomic functioning that has occurred as a result of mutations associated with malignant transformation (Baldassarre et al., 2004; Tsunada et al., 2003).
Changes in membrane composition have the potential to affect cell growth and interactions between cells (including cells of the immune system), as well as the function of proteins and other components present at the cell membrane. For example, the immune system depends on interactions between different cell types for its function and these interactions are mediated by the membrane composition of the cells involved (Yaqoob, 2003). Moreover, immune cell activation (e.g., cell proliferation, phagocytosis) and tumor growth (malignancy) are processes associated with an increased rate of *de novo* synthesis and turnover of membrane phospholipids (Field & Schley, 2004).

2.2.1 Changes in the phospholipids composition of human colorectal cancer cell membranes

Phospholipids are an integral part of a cell membrane and determine its structure. Accordingly, different biological conditions are associated with differences in membrane phospholipids composition particularly during cancer transformation (Dobrzyńska et al., 2005; Szachowicz-Petelska et al., 2007).
For example, most cases of colorectal cancer involve an increase in the concentration of all phospholipid types at the cell membrane, including: phosphatidylinositol (PI), phosphatidylserine (PS), phosphatidylethanolamine (PE) and phosphatidylcholine (PC) (Table 1).
Previous studies have shown that an increase in the concentration of phospholipids in the cell membrane is associated with human colon cancer cells (Dueck et al., 1996) and murine mammary tumor cells (Monteggia et al., 2000). Moreover, this increase has been proposed to be the result of enhanced cell membrane synthesis related to accelerated neoplasm cell replication (Ruiz-Cabello & Cohen, 1992). Furthermore, the mechanisms involved can vary

Patient no	Type of phospholipid	Phospholipid content detected (mg/g tissue)	
		Control	Tumor
1.	PI	0.010 ± 0.002	0.225 ± 0.020[a]
	PS	0.016 ± 0.003	0.100 ± 0.010[a]
	PE	0.550 ± 0.010	0.890 ± 0.030[a]
	PC	0.675 ± 0.011	1.100 ± 0.061[a]
2.	PI	0.012 ± 0.003	0.239 ± 0.040[a]
	PS	0.028 ± 0.002	0.151 ± 0.022[a]
	PE	0.510 ± 0.020	0.740 ± 0.081[a]
	PC	0.116 ± 0.010	1.237 ± 0.099[a]
3.	PI	0.074 ± 0.008	0.081 ± 0.007
	PS	0.086 ± 0.006	0.131 ± 0.010[a]
	PE	0.494 ± 0.021	0.902 ± 0.051[a]
	PC	0.648 ± 0.024	1.240 ± 0.085[a]
4.	PI	0.087 ± 0.009	0.248 ± 0.020[a]
	PS	0.097 ± 0.007	0.097 ± 0.006
	PE	0.901 ± 0.050	0.932 ± 0.050
	PC	1.139 ± 0.061	1.245 ± 0.089[a]
5.	PI	0.064 ± 0.005	0.109 ± 0.010[a]
	PS	0.086 ± 0.004	0.114 ± 0.015[a]
	PE	0.498 ± 0.012	0.768 ± 0.080[a]
	PC	0.677 ± 0.018	1.054 ± 0.095[a]
6.	PI	0.020 ± 0.002	0.056 ± 0.006[a]
	PS	0.024 ± 0.002	0.096 ± 0.009[a]
	PE	0.432 ± 0.012	0.951 ± 0.092[a]
	PC	0.707 ± 0.019	1.368 ± 0.101[a]
7.	PI	0.009 ± 0.001	0.030 ± 0.015[a]
	PS	0.010 ± 0.011	0.021 ± 0.010
	PE	0.419 ± 0.023	0.828 ± 0.052[a]
	PC	0.675 ± 0.034	1.182 ± 0.065[a]
8.	PI	0.036 ± 0.012	0.136 ± 0.016[a]
	PS	0.042 ± 0.015	0.103 ± 0.050[a]
	PE	0.468 ± 0.028	0.895 ± 0.039[a]
	PC	0.686 ± 0.039	1.287 ± 0.070[a]

Table 1. The phospholipid content of pT3 stage, G2 grade human colorectal cancer cell membranes not associated with metastasis (N-). [a] $p<0.05$, compared with control.

depending on the cell type, cell growth phase and malignancy status. For example, the greatest changes in the content of PC and PE have been observed in the G_1 phase of the cell cycle, during which activity of the enzymes controlling biosynthesis, catabolism and metabolism of phospholipids is maximal (Jackowski et al., 1996; Jackowski et al., 1994). As shown in Table 1 the PC content detected in normal mucosa in lesions of colorectal cancer cells and in other cancer cells was found to be higher than that of other phospholipids. These observations are consistent with the results of previous studies.

Patient no	Type of phospholipid	Phospholipid content detected (mg/g tissue)	
		Control	Control
9.	PI PS PE PC	0.044 ± 0.002 0.043 ± 0.002 0.642 ± 0.011 0.783 ± 0.012	0.225 ± 0.011[a] 0.145 ± 0.009[a] 0.909 ± 0.019[a] 1.406 ± 0.025[a]
10.	PI PS PE PC	0.150 ± 0.009 0.055 ± 0.003 0.540 ± 0.012 0.925 ± 0.022	0.160 ± 0.008 0.055 ± 0.003 0.545 ± 0.013 1.555 ± 0.028[a]
11.	PI PS PE PC	0.044 ± 0.002 0.025 ± 0.001 0.381 ± 0.018 0.475 ± 0.020	0.144 ± 0.009[a] 0.075 ± 0.005[a] 0.396 ± 0.011 1.281 ± 0.016[a]
12.	PI PS PE PC	0.018 ± 0.001 0.031 ± 0.003 0.551 ± 0.018 0.698 ± 0.021	0.113 ± 0.008[a] 0.110 ± 0.007[a] 0.592 ± 0.013[a] 0.933 ± 0.026[a]
13.	PI PS PE PC	0.026 ± 0.003 0.013 ± 0.001 0.433 ± 0.019 0.770 ± 0.030	0.039 ± 0.003[a] 0.026 ± 0.002[a] 0.546 ± 0.014[a] 1.240 ± 0.019[a]

Table 2. The phospholipid content of pT3 stage, G2 grade human colorectal cancer cell membranes associated with metastasis (N+). [a] $p<0.05$, compared with control.

Differences in membrane phospholipid content can also affect the potential for metastasis (Podo, 1999; Dobrzyńska et al., 2005). For example, malignant neoplasm cells associated with a greater number of metastases were characterized by a higher PC/PE ratio than malignant neoplasm cells with fewer metastases (Table 2).

2.2.2 Changes in the membrane free unsaturated fatty acid composition of human colorectal cancer cells

Free fatty acids are present in cell membranes, with the former present at low levels and the latter having a strong influence on the structure, properties and functions of the cell membrane. Polyunsaturated free fatty acids (PUFAs) also participate in the normal functioning of a cell, particularly by contributing to intracellular cell signaling. In addition, PUFAs represent nutritional components of a human diet and can indirectly affect tumorigenesis. For example, long-chain n-3 fatty acids have been shown to alter co-stimulatory molecules and activation markers, as well as calcium signaling and protein kinase C translocation at the cell membrane of immune cells (Hughes & Pinder, 2000). Similarly, the incorporation of n-3 fatty acids in the membrane of other cell types has been shown to alter membrane permeability, membrane fluidity and hormone and growth factor binding (Hashimoto et al., 1999; Lund et al., 1999). In colorectal cancer cells, reduced levels of PUFAs have been detected in the membrane, concomitant with increased levels of arachidonic and oleic acids, and lower levels of linoleic and α-linolenic acids (Table 3) (Szachowicz-Petelska et al., 2002, 2007).

Moreover, decreased levels of linoleic and α-linolenic acids have been detected in the plasma and erythrocytes of colorectal cancer patients. These changes are probably due to metabolic alterations caused by the illness and not necessarily by malnutrition (Baro et al., 1998). In addition, two clinical investigations have reported a significant increase in plasma and tissue concentrations of arachidonic acid (AA) in colorectal cancer patients compared with control patients (Neoptolemos et al., 1991; Hendrickse et al., 1994). This increase may be related to an enhancement of lipid peroxidation, which is a feature of rapidly growing cells (Skrzydlewska et al., 2001, 2005). Alternatively, increased AA levels could be due to elevated desaturase activity involving linoleic acid (LA) and α-linolenic acid (ALA), possibly leading to increased formation of prostaglandins and other lipoxygenase products (Dommels et al., 2002).

Other classes of unsaturated fatty acids include the palmitoleic (n-7) and oleic (n-9) family, both of which can be produced by most cells in humans and, thus, are not essential (Pandian et al., 1999). Levels of oleic acids have been found to be increased in colon cancer cells (Table 3). Furthermore, a significant elevation in the concentration of oleic acid has been detected in the plasma of colorectal cancer patients (Baro et al., 1998). Correspondingly, an almost statistically significant increase in the intake of oleic acid was found in another study of high-risk subjects for colorectal cancer (Schloss et al., 1997). These results may be due to changes in oleic acid metabolism as part of the pathogenic process. It has also been shown that human colon tumor growth is promoted by oleic acid (Calder et al., 1998) via mechanisms of increased fatty acid oxidation and a disturbance of membrane enzymes (Suziki et al., 1997).

Work by Rakheja et al., demonstrated that an overall reduction in free unsaturated fatty acids was associated with cancer cell membranes, while another recent report detected an elevated proportion of saturated versus unsaturated total fatty acids in colonic adenocarcinoma (Rakheja et al., 2005). In the latter case, the increase in saturated total fatty acids was attributed to elevated levels of the enzyme fatty acid synthase (Rashid et al., 1997). Furthermore, saturated fatty acids may be targeted to lipid raft microdomains, which are rich in cholesterol, sphingolipids and phospholipids with saturated fatty acid side chains (Swinnen et al., 2003; Rakheja et al., 2005). Recently, an increased intake of dietary n-3 fatty acids has been shown to decrease levels of sphingomyelin, cholesterol and caveolin-1 collectively, suggesting that n-3 fatty acids can modulate the composition of lipid rafts (Martin et al., 2005). Moreover, polyunsaturated fatty acids have been proposed to play a role in cancer therapy and to perturb membrane lipids rafts, thereby affecting cell functions (Hardman, 2004; Ma et al., 2004).

Under pathological conditions, such as hypoxia/reoxygenation, byproducts of AA that are generated can reduce gap junction-mediated coupling (Martinez & Saez, 2000). Dommels et. al., demonstrated that short-term incubation with LA, α-ALA or AA did not influence gap junctional intercellular communication (GJIC), yet long-term incubation with LA and α-ALA did inhibit GJIC of colon cells. Although the exact mechanisms mediating the inhibition of GJIC remain unclear, it is hypothesized that the associated cytotoxicity releated to the disruption of gap junctions is mediated by lipid peroxidation products. This hypothesis is supported by the observation that incubation with PUFAs, such as AA, can completely abolish GJIC (Dommels et. al., 2002).

Patient no	Type of fatty acid	Fatty acid content detected (mg/g tissue)	
		Control	Control
1.	18:2n-6	0.059 ± 0.005	0.014 ± 0.002[a]
	18:3n-3	0.045 ± 0.002	0.032 ± 0.005[a]
	16:1	0.032 ± 0.009	0.027 ± 0.007
	20:4n-6	0.036 ± 0.008	0.050 ± 0.010
2.	18:2n-6	0.028 ± 0.005	0.014 ± 0.005[a]
	18:3n-3	0.086 ± 0.010	0.071 ± 0.011
	16:1	0.021 ± 0.005	0.028 ± 0.005
	20:4n-6	0.064 ± 0.007	0.071 ± 0.008
3.	18:2n-6	0.033 ± 0.006	0.011 ± 0.003[a]
	18:3n-3	0.055 ± 0.005	0.039 ± 0.008[a]
	16:1	0.022 ± 0.003	0.022 ± 0.004
	20:4n-6	0.044 ± 0.009	0.061 ± 0.007[a]
4.	18:2n-6	0.022 ± 0.004	0.003 ± 0.001[a]
	18:3n-3	0.034 ± 0.006	0.028 ± 0.005
	16:1	0.016 ± 0.003	0.016 ± 0.003
	20:4n-6	0.028 ± 0.005	0.031 ± 0.006
5.	18:2n-6	0.014 ± 0.004	0.007 ± 0.001[a]
	18:3n-3	0.034 ± 0.006	0.017 ± 0.003[a]
	16:1	0.010 ± 0.002	0.014 ± 0.002
	20:4n-6	0.027 ± 0.004	0.041 ± 0.006[a]
	18:1	0.058 ± 0.007	0.075 ± 0.008[a]
6.	18:2n-6	0.016 ± 0.004	0.003 ± 0.001[a]
	18:3n-3	0.024 ± 0.005	0.019 ± 0.004
	16:1	0.005 ± 0.001	0.008 ± 0.001[a]
	20:4n-6	0.024 ± 0.004	0.035 ± 0.005[a]
	18:1	0.011 ± 0.002	0.027 ± 0.004[a]
7.	18:2n-6	0.009 ± 0.002	0.002 ± 0.001[a]
	18:3n-3	0.019 ± 0.004	0.009 ± 0.002[a]
	16:1	0.005 ± 0.001	0.005 ± 0.001
	20:4n-6	0.015 ± 0.003	0.026 ± 0.005[a]
	18:1	0.009 ± 0.002	0.019 ± 0.004[a]
8.	18:2n-6	0.057 ± 0.008	0.007 ± 0.001[a]
	18:3n-3	0.071 ± 0,009	0.036 ± 0.005[a]
	16:1	0.028 ± 0.005	0.043 ± 0.004[a]
	20:4n-6	0.064 ± 0.007	0.071 ± 0.007
	18:1	0.019 ± 0.004	0.056 ± 0.006[a]

18:2n-6, linoleic acid;18:3n-3, α-linolenic acid;16:1, palmitoleic acid;20:4n-6, arachidonic acid;18:1, oleic acid.

Table 3. PUFA content of pT3 stage, G2 grade human colorectal cancer cells not associated with metastasis (N-). [a] $p<0.05$, compared with control.

2.2.3 Changes in membrane proteins of human colorectal cancer cells

Currently, membrane proteins are classified into five groups according to their putative functions. These include: 1) receptor proteins associated with various extracellular ligands such as growth factors and hormones, 2) channel proteins that mediate the transportation of ions and small molecules across the membrane, 3) various enzyme proteins such as phospholipases and phosphatases, 4) regulatory proteins associated with functional proteins such as p21 and 5) cellular adhesion proteins such as cell - CAMs. In the latter case, most CAMs belong to one of four protein families: immunoglobulin (Ig), superfamily (IgSF), integrins, cadherins or selectins.

Structural changes in membrane proteins are associated with changes in the electrical potential of tumor cell membranes. These changes also correspond with altered biological properties exhibited by tumor cells. For example, a decrease in levels of E-cadherin expression in colorectal cancer cells has been shown to affect the diversification of cells in a tumor as well as the probability that tumor cells will contribute to distant metastasis.

While characterization of membrane proteins of tumor cells has made progress and provided valuable insight into the role of the cell membrane in tumorigenesis, additional studies are still needed to elucidate tumor-specific mechanisms associated with these changes (Kojima, 1993).

3. Conclusions

A higher proportion of phospholipids present in cell membranes results in a larger number of functional groups present at the cell surface and these can include: amino, carboxy and phosphate functional groups. Correspondingly, in acidic medium (e.g., a low pH), the charge associated with the phospholipid population at the cell surface is mainly determined by the amino groups present. In contrast, carboxy and phosphate groups present in a basic medium (e.g., a high pH) are key. For large intestine cell membranes, the main component of the outer layer is PC and at higher concentrations, PC can provoke an increase in both C_{TA} and C_{TB} values. In addition, when cells undergo transformation the association constant of negatively charged groups present (e.g., K_{AH}) decreases while the association constant of positively charged groups (e.g., K_{BOH}) increases.

Anionic phospholipids associated with tumor vessels also potentially represent markers for tumor vessel targeting and imaging (Ran et al., 2002). In addition, alterations in the distribution of PS, a component of the skeleton, can cause an increase in C_{TA} values.

Therefore, an evaluation of the membrane status of tumor cells may be an important consideration in future studies of tumor biology.

4. References

Baro, L.; Hermoso, J.C.; Nunez, M.C.; Jimenez-Rios, J.A. & Gil, A. (1998). Abnormalities in plasma and red cell fatty acid profiles of patients with colorectal cancer. *British Journal of Cancer* Vol.77, No.11, pp. 1978-1983, ISSN 0007-0920

Bos, R.; van Diest, P.J.; van der Groep, P.; Shvarts, A.; Greijer, A.E. & van der Wall, E. (2004). Expression of hypoxia-inducible factor-1α and cell cycle proteins in invasive breast cancer are estrogen receptor related. *Breast Cancer Research*. Vol.6, No.4, (June 2004), pp. R450-R459, ISSN 1465-5411

Calder, P.C.; Davis, J.; Yaqoob, P.; Pala, H.; Thies, F. & Newsholme, E.A. (1998). Dietary fish oil suppresses human colon tumour growth in athymic mice. *Clinical Science* Vol.94, No.3, (March 1998), pp. 303-311, ISSN 0143-5221

Cascio, M. (2005). Connexins and their environment: effects of lipids composition on ion channels. *Biochimica et Biophysica Acta.* Vol.1711, (December 2004), pp. 142-153, ISSN 0006-3002

Contreras, J.E.; Sanchez, H.A.; Eugenin, E.A.; Speidel, D.; Theis, M.;Willecke, K.; Bukauskas, F.F.; Bennett, M.V.L. & Saez, J.C. (2002). Metabolic inhibition induces opening of unopposed connexin 43 gap junction hemichannels and reduces gap junctional communication in cortical astrocytes in culture. *Proceedings of the National Academy of Sciences of the United States of America.* Vol.99, No.1, (November 2001), pp. 495-500, ISSN 0027-8424

Devaux, P.F. (1992). Protein involvement in transmembrane lipid asymmetry. *Annual Review of Biophysics and Biomolecular Structure.* Vol.21, (June 1992), pp. 417-439, ISSN 1056-8700

Dobrzyńska, I., Skrzydlewska, E. Figaszewski, Z. (2006). Parameters characterizing acid-base equilibria between cell membrane and solution and their application to monitoring the effect of various factors on the membrane. *Bioelectrochemistry.* Vol.69, No.2, (February 2006), pp. 142-147, ISSN 1567-5394

Dobrzyńska, I.; Szachowicz-Petelska, B.; Figaszewski, Z. & Sulkowski, S. (2005). Changes in electric charge and phospholipid composition in human colorectal cancer cells. *Molecular and Cellular Biochemistry.* Vol.276, No.1-2, (August 2005), pp. 113-119, ISSN: 0300-8177

Dołowy, K. (1984). Bioelectrochemistry of cell surface. *Progress in Surface Science.* Vol.15, No.3, pp. 245-368, ISSN 0079-6816

Dommels, Y.E.M.; Alink, G.M.; Linssen, J.P. & van Ommen, B. (2002). Effects of n-6 and n-3 polyunsaturated fatty acids on gap junctional intercellular communication during spontaneous differentiation of the human colon adenocarcinoma cell line Caco-2. *Nutrition and Cancer.* Vol.42, No.1, pp. 125-130, ISSN 0163-5581

Dueck, D.A.; Chan, M.; Tran, K.; Wong, J.T.; Jay, F.T.; Littman, C.; Stimpson, R. & Choy, P.C. (1996). The modulation of choline phosphoglyceride metabolism in human colon cancer. *Molecular and Cellular Biochemistry.* Vol.162, No.2, pp. 97-103, ISSN: 0300-8177

Erbil, K.M.; Sen, S.E.; Zincke, H. & Jones, J.D. (1986). Significance of serum protein and lipid-bound sialic acid as a marker for genitourinary malignancies. *Cancer.* Vol.57, No.7, (April 1986), pp. 1389-1394, ISSN 1097-0142

Field, C.J. & Schley, P.D. (2004). Evidence for potential mechanisms for the effect of conjugated linoleic acid on tumor metabolism and immune function: lessons from n-3 fatty acids. *American Journal of Clinical Nutrition.* Vol.79, No.6, (June 2004), 1190S-1198S, ISSN 0002-9165

Gennis, R.B. (1989). *Biomembranes: Molecular structure and functions.* Springer-Verlag, ISBN 0-387-96760-5, New York, USA.

Hardman, W.E. (2004). (n-3) fatty acids and cancer therapy. *Journal of Nutrition.* Vol.134, No.12, (December 2004), 3427S-3430S, ISSN 0022-3166

Hashimoto, M.; Hossain, S.; Yamasaki, H.; Yazawa, K. & Masumura, S. (1999). Effects of eicosapentaenoic acid and docosahexaenoic. acid on plasma membrane fluidity of aortic endothelial cells. *Lipids* Vol.34, No.12, (December 1999), pp. 1297-1304, ISSN 0024-4201

Hendrickse, C.W.; Kelly, R.W.; Radley, S.; Donovan, I.A.; Keighley, M.R. & Neoptolemos, J.P. (1994). Lipid peroxidation and prostaglandins in colorectal cancer. *British Journal of Surgery.* Vol.81, No.8, (August 1994), pp. 1219-1223, ISSN 0007-1323

Hughes, D.A. & Pinder, A.C. (2000). n-3 polyunsaturated fatty acids inhibit the antigen-presenting function of human monocytes. *American Journal of Clinical Nutrition.* Vol.71, No.1, (January 2000), 357S-360S, ISSN 0002-9165

Jackowski, S. (1996). Cell cycle regulation of membrane phospholipids metabolism. *Journal of Biological Chemistry.* Vol.271, (August 1996), pp. 20219-20222, ISSN 0021-9258

Jackowski, S. (1994). Coordination of membrane phospholipids synthesis with the cell cycle. *Journal of Biological Chemistry.* Vol.269, (February 1994), pp. 3858-3867, ISSN 0021-9258

Koijma, K. (1993). Molecular aspects of the plasma membrane in tumor cells. *Nagoya Journal of Medical Science* Vol.56, No.1-4, (November 1993), pp.1-18 , ISSN 00277622

Locke, D. & Harris, A.L. (2009). Connexin channels and phospholipids: association and modulation. *BMC Biology.* Vol.7, (August 2009), pp. 52-76, ISSN 1741-7007

Lund, E.K.; Harvey, L.J.; Ladha, S.; Clark, D.C. & Johnson, I.T. (1999). Effects of dietary fish oil supplementation on the phospholipid composition and fluidity of cell membranes from human volunteers. *Annals of Nutrition and Metabolism.* Vol.43, No.5, pp. 290-300, ISSN 0250-6807

Ma, D.W.; Seo, J.; Switzer, K.C.; Fan, Y.Y.; McMurray, D.N.; Lupton, J.R. & Chapkin, R.S. (2004). n-3 PUFA and membrane microdomains: a new frontier in bioactive lipid research. *The Journal of Nutritional Biochemistry.* Vol.15, No.11, (November 2004), pp. 700-706, ISSN 0955-2863

Marconescu, A. & Thorpe, P.E. (2008). Coincident exposure of phosphatidylethanolamine and anionic phospholipids on the surface of irradiated cells. *Biochimica et Biophysica Acta.* Vol.1778, pp. 2217-2224, ISSN 0006-3002

Martin, R.E.; Elliott, M.H.; Brush, R.S. & Anderson, R.E. (2005). Detailed characterization of the lipid composition of detergent-resistant membranes from photoreceptor rod outer segment membranes. *Investigative Ophthalmology & Visual Science.* Vol.46, No.4, (April 2005), pp. 1147-1154, ISSN 0146-0404

Monteggia, E.; Colombo, I.; Guerra, A. & Berra, B. (2000). Phospholipid distribution in murine mammary adenocacinomas induced by activated neu oncogene. *Cancer Detection and Prevention.* Vol.24, No.3, pp.207-211, ISSN 0361-090X

Narayanan, S. (1994). Sialic acid as a tumor marker. Annals of Clinical and Laboratory Science. Vol.24, No.4, (July-August 1994), pp. 376-384, ISSN 0091-7370

Neoptolemos, J.P.; Husband, D.; Imray, C.; Rowley, S. & Lawson, N. (1991). Arachidonic acid and docosahexaenoic acid are increased in human colorectal cancer. *Gut.* Vol.32, No.3, (March 1991), pp. 278-281, ISSN 0017-5749

Podo, F. (1999). Tumour phospholipid metabolism. *NMR in Biomedicine.* Vol.12, No.7, (November 1999), pp. 413-439, ISSN 0952-3480

Rakheja, D.; Kapur, P.; Hoang, M.P.; Roy, L.C. & Bennett, M.J. (2005). Increased ratio of saturated to unsaturated C18 fatty acids in colonic adenocarcinoma: implications for cryotherapy and lipid raft function. *Medical Hypotheses.* Vol.65, No.6, (August 2005), pp. 1120-1123, ISSN 0306-9877

Ran, S.; Downes, A. & Thorpe, P.E. (2002). Increased exposure of anion phospholipids on the surface of tumor blood vessels. *Cancer Research.* Vol.62, (November 2002), pp. 6132-6140, ISSN 0008-5472

Rashid, A.; Pizer, E.S.; Moga, M.; Milgraum, L.Z.; Zahurak, M.; Pasternack, G.R.; Kuhajda, F.P. & Hamilton, S.R. (1997). Elevated expression of fatty acid synthase and fatty acid synthetic activity in colorectal neoplasia. *The American Journal of Pathology.* Vol.150, No.1, (January 1997), pp. 201-208, ISSN 0002-9440

Ruiz-Cabello, J. & Cohen, J.S. (1992). Phospholipids metabolites as indicators of cancer cell function. *NMR in Biomedicine.* Vol.5, No.5, (September-October 1992), pp. 226-233, ISSN 0952-3480

Schloss, I.; Kidd, M.S.G.; Young, G.O. & O'Keefe, S.J. (1997). Dietary factors associated with a low risk of colon cancer in coloured west coast fishermen. *South African Medical Journal.* Vol.87, No.2, (February 1997), pp. 152-8, ISSN 0256-9574

Skrzydlewska, E.; Stankiewicz, A.; Sulkowska, M.; Sulkowski, S. & Kasacka, I, (2001). Antioxidant status and lipid peroxidation in colorectal cancer. *Journal of Toxicology and Environmental Health A.* 12, Vol.64, No.3, (October 2001), pp. 213-22, ISSN 1528-7394

Skrzydlewska, E.; Sulkowski, S.; Koda, M.; Zalewski, B.; Kanczuga-Koda, L. & Sulkowska, M. (2005). Lipid Peroxidation and antioxidant status in colorectal cancer. *World Journal of Gastroenterology* Vol.11, No.3, (January 2005), pp. 403-406, ISSN 1007-9327

Stafford, J.H. & Thorpe P.E. (2011). Increased exposure of phosphatidylethanolamine on the surface of tumor vascular endothelium. *Neoplasia.*Vol.13, No.4, pp. 299-308, ISSN 0004-3664

Suziki, I.; Iigo, M.; Ishikawa, C.; Kuhara, T.; Asamoto, M.; Kunimoto, T.; Moore, M.A.; Yazawa, K.; Araki, E. & Tsuda, H. (1997). Inhibitory effects of oleic acid and DHA on lung metastasis by colon-carcinoma-26 cells are associated with reduced matrix metalloproteinase-2 and -9 activities. *International Journal of Cancer.* Vol.73, pp. 607-612, ISSN 0020-7136

Swinnen, J.V.; van Veldhoven, P.P.; Timmermans, L.; Schrijver, E.D.; Brusselmans, K.; Vanderhoydonc, F.; Van de Sande, T.; Heemers, H.; Heyns, W. & Verhoeven, G. (2003). Fatty acid synthase drives the synthesis of phospholipids partitioning into detergent-resistant membrane microdomains. *Biochemical and Biophysical Research Communications.* Vol.302, No.4, (March 2003), pp. 898-903, ISSN 0006-291X

Szachowicz-Petelska, B.; Dobrzyńska, I.; Sulkowski, S. & Figaszewski, Z. (2010). Characterization of the cell membrane during cancer transformation. *Journal of Environmental Biology.* Vol.31, (September 2010), pp. 845-850, ISSN: 0254-8704

Szachowicz-Petelska, B.; Sulkowski, S. & Figaszewski, Z. (2007). Altered membrane free unsaturated fatty acid composition in human colorectal cancer tissue. *Molecular and Cellular Biochemistry.* Vol.294, No.1-2, (January 2007), pp. 237-242, ISSN: 0300-8177

Szachowicz-Petelska, B.; Dobrzyńska, I.; Sulkowski, S. & Figaszewski, Z. (2002). Changes in physico-chemical properties of human large intestine tumour cells membrane. *Molecular and Cellular Biochemistry.* Vol.238, No.1-2, (September 2002), pp. 41-47, ISSN: 0300-8177

Tien, H.T. (1974). *Bilayer Lipid Membranes (BLM): Theory and Practice.* Marcel Dekker Inc., ISBN 0-8247-6048-4, New York, USA

Wang, P.H. (2005). Altered glycosylation in cancer: sialic acid and sialyltransferases. *Journal of Cancer Molecules*. Vol.1, No.2, pp. 73-81, ISSN 1817-4256

Van Zeijl, L.; Ponsioen, B.; Giepmans, B.N.C.; Ariaens, A.; Postma, F.R.; Varnai, P.; Balla, T.; Divecha, N.; Jalink, K. & Moolenaar, W.H. (2007). Regulation of connexin43 gap junctional communication by phosphatidylinositol 4,5-bisphosphate. *The Journal of Cell Biology*. Vol.177, No.5, (June 2007), pp. 881-891, ISSN 0021-9525

Zhao, J.; Zhou, Q.; wiedmer, T. & Sims, P.J. (1998). Level of expression of phospholipid scramblase regulates induced movement of phosphotidylserine to the cell surface. *Journal of Biological Chemistry*. Vol.273, No.12, (March 1998), pp. 6603-6606, ISSN 0021-9258

12

Emergent Concepts from the Intestinal Guanylyl Cyclase C Pathway

Mehboob Ali and Giovanni M. Pitari
Division of Clinical Pharmacology,
Thomas Jefferson University, Philadelphia, PA,
USA

1. Introduction

Cancer is one of the world's top killers accounting for 7.4 million deaths, or 13% of all deaths (World Health Organization [WHO], 2011). Colorectal cancer is the third most common and deadly cancer worldwide (Jemal et al., 2011). An unequal geographic distribution of the disease burden exists, with less developed areas of the world exhibiting the lowest incidence and mortality (Pitari et al., 2003). In contrast, populations dwelling in western countries are at increased risk to develop and die of colorectal cancer. In the US, 141,210 new cases are estimated to be diagnosed in 2011 and 49,380 patients are expected to die for this disease, representing an intolerable socio-economical toll (Siegel et al., 2011).

Promises derive from substantial advancements in early detection and prevention strategies, which have contributed to reduce colorectal cancer incidence and mortality rates in recent years (Siegel et al., 2011). However, new chemotherapeutic approaches have not emerged and terminal clinical stages of the disease remain incurable. Specifically, invasion and metastatic disease progression, traditionally unnameable to surgical resection, are largely refractory to pharmacological therapy. About 90% of patients with distant metastasis die of the disease within 5 years from diagnosis (Siegel et al., 2011). Moreover, racial and educational health-disparities exist in which minorities and less educated individuals of the affected population exhibit the worst clinical prognosis and the highest mortality, in part reflecting their more advanced stages at diagnosis compared to other patient segments (Siegel et al., 2011). Together, these considerations underscore the enormous impact that therapeutic target discovery might have on western societies, especially if they would translate into innovative, curative pharmacological approaches that will prolong the survival of patients with colorectal cancer.

Crucial systems regulating the intestinal crypt-villus axis are also important determinants of the carcinogenetic process (Aoki et al., 2003; Fodde et al., 2001; Korinek et al., 1998). Among these, the signalling pathway orchestrated by the surface receptor guanylyl cyclase C (GCC) has recently emerged as both an integral component of intestinal mucosa homeostasis and a negative regulator of the malignant cell phenotype. GCC, expressed in the epithelial layer of the gastrointestinal wall, and its endogenous ligands guanylin and uroguanylin control fluid balance and renewal crypt dynamics by operating sophisticated biochemical circuits in both the small and large intestine. Intriguingly, a bacterial mimicry of endogenous hormones exists, the E. coli heat-stable enterotoxin (ST), which may confer both harmful (watery diarrhea) and beneficial (colorectal cancer resistance) effects to exposed individuals (Lucas et al., 2000; Pitari et al., 2001). In this model, the uneven epidemiological distribution of colon cancer incidence across different geographic areas of the world reflect, in part, inverse differences in the prevalence of enterotoxigenic E. coli infections (Pitari et al., 2003). Moreover, an unexplained mutation early in colorectal tumorigenesis leads to the loss of guanylin and uroguanylin expression, producing a dormant GCC pathway in neoplastic cells (Fig. 1) (Pitari et al., 2007).

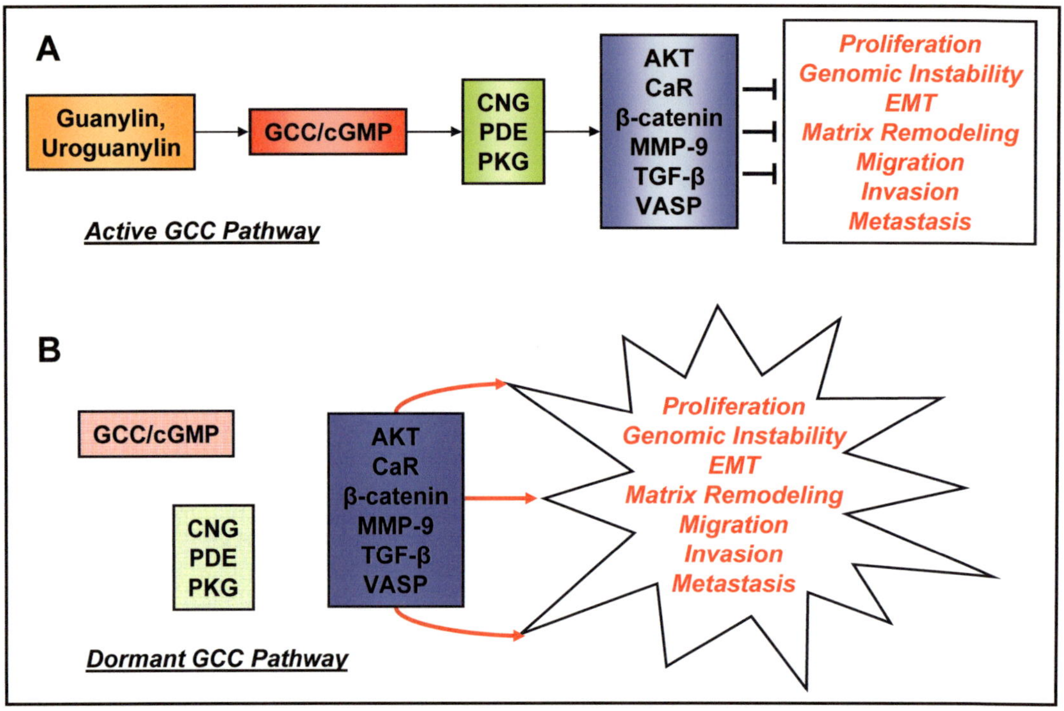

Fig. 1. Significance of the dormant guanylyl cyclase C (GCC) pathway for colorectal carcinogenesis.
Selected GCC signalling components with reported impact on tumorigenesis are depicted. A) In normal intestinal physiology, the GCC pathway is constitutively activated by paracrine hormonal regulation with the endogenous GCC agonists guanylin and uroguanylin. The active GCC pathway promotes signalling by proximal cGMP effectors cyclic nucleotide-gated channel (CNG), phosphodiesterases (PDE) and protein kinase G (PKG) that, in turn, affect the function of key distal effectors, including the v-akt murine thymoma viral oncogene homolog (AKT), Ca^{2+}-sensing receptor (CaR), β-catenin, matrix metalloproteinase 9 (MMP-9), transforming growth factor β (TGF-β), and vasodilator-stimulated phosphoprotein (VASP). As a result, tumorigenic forces are restrained and normal intestinal mucosa homeostasis is maintained. B) During neoplastic transformation the GCC pathway becomes dormant, principally because of the loss of endogenous hormone expression. Loss of signalling between GCC and the proximal cGMP effectors deregulates the distal components of the pathway, thereby producing an oncogenic system favouring colorectal cancer progression and metastasis. EMT, epithelial-mesenchymal transition.

This chapter will details the consequences at the functional and cellular level of the silenced GCC signalling for colorectal tumor formation and progression. Key molecular effectors comprising the GCC pathway with high clinical translational significance will be presented and their potential impacts for both diagnostic and therapeutic advances discussed.

2. GCC and the intestinal crypt-villus axis

GCC is a member of membrane-bound guanylyl cyclases (GCA to GCG), enzymes which catalyze the formation of cyclic guanosine monophosphate (cGMP) from GTP. Although they exhibit unique physicochemical and antigenic properties, particulate guanylyl cyclases are homodimeric transmembrane domain proteins sharing conserved cytoplasmic portions with tyrosine kinase-like and cyclase catalytic domains (Lucas et al., 2000). The amino acid sequence of GCC considerably diverges from the other isoforms in the extracellular domain, which represents the ligand binding domain for the E. coli heat-stable enterotoxin ST and the endogenous peptides guanylin and uroguanylin (Lucas et al., 2000). Beyond selected dopaminergic neurons in the central nervous system (Gong et al., 2011), in mammals GCC expression is principally restricted to brush-border membranes of epithelial cells lining the intestinal inner surface from the duodenum to the rectum, uniformly distributed along the crypt-villus axis (Lucas et al., 2000). This unique anatomical distribution subserves the functional role of GCC as a critical regulator of the intestinal mucosa homeostasis. In particular, the signalling pathway regulated by GCC and its second messenger cGMP contributes to the control of epithelial self-renewal and maturation dynamics underlying the integrity of the crypt-villus axis (Pitari et al., 2007).

2.1 The GCC pathway

Modulation of intracellular cGMP concentrations represents the fundamental event of a variety of signal transduction circuits shaping cellular behaviour. Synthesis (by guanylyl cyclases) and breakdown (by phosphodiesterases) are recognized as the major mechanisms defining cGMP levels in tissues. In intestinal epithelial cells, GCC is the principle source of cGMP (Lucas et al., 2000). GCC activity defines the type, intensity and duration of biological responses mediated by cGMP through unique physical, spatial and temporal dynamics at intestinal mucosal surfaces. The most important modality to regulate GCC activity is by ligand binding to its extracellular domain, which induces an intramolecular conformational change that is transmitted down to the cytoplasmic C-terminus catalytic domain. In this way, cellular cGMP levels can be raised numerous folds over basal states (Lucas et al., 2000; Schulz et al., 1989). Furthermore, the three ligand peptides know to induce GCC activation in mammalian cells exhibit different affinities and potencies for GCC, resulting in different patterns of cGMP concentrations/effects. The exogenous ligand ST, produced by E. coli and responsible for life-threatening diarrhoeagenic syndromes, is the most potent GCC agonist and consists of 18 amino acids with three intrachain disulfide bonds (Guarino et al., 1989). In contrast the endogenous paracrine hormones, guanylin and uroguanylin, are 15-16 amino acid long with two intrachain disulfide bonds and uneven tissue distributions and physico-chemical characteristics. Thus, while uroguanylin is a more potent (~100 fold) and abundant GCC agonist at acidic pH of proximal intestinal tracts, guanylin is more potent (~4 fold) as a GCC agonist at basic pH and is highly expressed in the colon and rectum (Forte, 1999; Hamra et al., 1997). Finally, elegant spatio-temporal constrains along the crypt-villus axis

represent additional determinants of cGMP signalling by GCC. At the tissue level, maximal GCC activity and the dependant cGMP functions are imposed at the epithelial crypt/villus interface by increased GCC ligand expression (Cohen et al., 1995; Whitaker et al., 1997). In addition at the cellular level, compartmentalization of GCC-ligand interactions at luminal membrane borders establishes an increasing baso-apical cGMP gradient, wherein highest nucleotide concentrations are ensured at microvillus cell domains (Lucas et al., 2000).
Beyond GCC activation, the functional consequences of cGMP rises in intestinal epithelial cells reflect the specific expression and compartmentalization of downstream target molecules. Two evolutionarily distinct allosteric binding sites for cGMP exist in eukaryotic cells: one is present in cGMP- (PKG) and cAMP- (PKA) dependent protein kinases and in the cyclic nucleotide gated (CNG) cation channels, while the other is expressed in cGMP-regulated phoshodiesterases (PDEs). These proteins represent the intracellular receptors for cGMP and permit the selective transmission of information in a cell-(and subcellular-) specific manner. PKGs are Ser/Thr protein kinases comprising the soluble type I, widely distributed across tissues and including the isoforms Iα and Iβ, and the particulate type II, mainly expressed in the intestine (Pfeifer et al., 1999). PKA is a tetrameric kinase preferentially activated by cAMP (Chao et al., 1994). CNG channels are heterotetrameric proteins of α- and β-subunits, which mediate membrane Na^+ and Ca^{2+} influx by cGMP in intestine as well as different other tissues (Bielet al., 1999). Further, cGMP-regulated PDEs (eg, PDE2, PDE5) are hydrolytic enzymes specialized in cleaving the cyclic nucleotide phosphodiester bond, thereby terminating correspondent biological activities (Corbin & Francis, 1999; Francis et al., 2011). Cyclic GMP binding to the consensus site of these intracellular targets results in regulation of important downstream effectors which control specific biochemical networks and cellular functions. Molecules distal to cGMP with paramount significance for intestinal cell biology include ions, ion channels, cytoskeleton regulators and enzymes. For instance, cGMP binding to two allosteric sites present at the amino-terminal region of PKG II fully activates the enzyme and induces phosphorylation and opening of the cystic fibrosis transmembrane conductance regulator (CFTR), a pivotal mechanism underlying control of intestinal fluid homeostasis (Pfeifer et al., 1999). For an in depth discussion on the regulation of the various biochemical cGMP-dependent targets, such as the CFTR channel, the reader is referred to other comprehensive reviews (Browning et al., 2010; Lucas et al., 2000; Steinbrecher & Cohen, 2011). Here, the focus will be on those molecular elements of the GCC and cGMP pathway that affect the epithelial cell phenotype, including its proliferative, morphogenetic and migratory attributes that greatly influence the crypt-villus homeostasis and the process of neoplastic transformation.

2.2 Regulation of the intestinal epithelial cell phenotype

The human intestinal mucosa is characterized by minute tubular invaginations called crypts, of maximal length in large intestinal tracts. In addition, the small intestinal mucosa exhibits lumenal protrusions of multi- (villi) and sub-cellular (microvilli) dimensions devoted to digestive activities. As a result, the inner intestinal surface is enormously expanded to optimally serve fundamental processes, from food processing and absorption to pathogen protection and immune system control (Montgomery et al., 1999). In this context, the complexity of those processes, constantly exposing the organism to potentially harmful external factors, is reflected by the sophisticated functional organization adopted by the columnar monolayer of epithelial cells lining the intestine. First, a self-renewal epithelial ability is conferred by multipotent stem cells located at crypt bottoms, ensuring weekly cycles of cellular replacement to eliminate damaged or aging cells worn out by the demanding intestinal functions (Potten & Loeffler, 1990). Also, intriguing maturation dynamics are operating that turn proliferating progenitor cells into differentiated, cell cycle-arrested epithelial cells with specialized functions, mostly populating the upper crypt and villus areas. They include a) the enterocytes, absorptive cells with food digestive functions (Montgomery et al., 1999), b) goblet cells, mucus-producing cells with detergent activities (Koldovsky et al., 1995), c) enteroendocrine cells, hormone-secreting cells comprising an intestinal endocrine system (Koldovsky et al., 1995), and d) Paneth cells, which secrete antimicrobial peptides and growth factors and are uniquely located at crypt bases (Bry et al., 1994). Further, incompletely understood check-up mechanisms constantly detect genetic or epigenetic defects and direct epithelial cells to the appropriate maintenance (e.g., cell resistance), self-repair (e.g., DNA excision repair) or death (e.g., apoptosis, autophagy) program (Potten & Loeffler, 1990). Finally, the spatio-temporal coordination of this variety of processes is ensured by the migratory nature of the epithelial monolayer that physically maps the proliferation-differentiation transition at crypt/villus (small intestine) or lower/upper crypt (colon) interfaces, and drives the shedding of senescent cells at mucosal tips (Montgomery et al., 1999).

The GCC signalling pathway represents one of the elaborate homeostatic mechanisms evolved to direct the integration of each component supporting the intestinal epithelial cell phenotype. Indeed, targeted deletion of guanylin expression induces expansion of the proliferating crypt compartment and accelerated cell migration in mouse colon, presumably as a consequence of reduced GCC activation and cGMP-dependent signalling (Steinbrecher et al., 2002). In agreement with this notion, elimination of GCC in mice produces hyperplastic colonic crypts, populated by a higher number of fast-cycling and fast-migrating progenitor cells, associated with impaired cell maturation and death dynamics, with fewer Paneth and goblet cells but increased apoptotic events (Li et al., 2007a). Moreover, compound mice in which the expression of uroguanylin or GCC has been disrupted exhibit similar structural alterations in the crypt-villus axis, with loss of tight junction-mediated intestinal barrier function and increased mucosal permeability (Han et al., 2011). Of relevance, intestine-specific expression of GCC is under the control of the caudal homeobox gene Cdx2, a transcriptional factor regulating development and cell fate specification of intestinal epithelial cells (Park et al., 2000). The Cdx2 gene product binds a consensus site present in the GCC proximal promoter and stimulates GCC transcription in an intestine-specific fashion (Di Guglielmo et al., 2001). Thus, it is tempted to speculate that GCC expression and the dependant cGMP signalling are part of the universal developmental program supporting the integrity of the intestinal crypt-villus axis.

Molecular mechanisms underlying effects of the GCC pathway on the intestinal cell phenotype have only recently been investigated. In one paradigm, lumenal Ca^{2+} is the key distal mediator of GCC activity (Pitari et al., 2003, 2008). The role of dietary Ca^{2+} as antiproliferative agent and promoter of differentiation and cell death along the epithelial crypt-villus axis is well defined (Lipkin & Newmark, 1995; Whitfield, 1992), and Ca^{2+}-deficient diets induce larger proliferative compartments in mouse colonic crypts (Rozen et al., 1989). One key molecular target for antiproliferative effects by dietary Ca^{2+} is the Ca^{2+}-sensing receptor (CaR), a G protein-coupled receptor present at apical membranes of intestinal epithelial cells (Sheinin et al., 2000). Binding of Ca^{2+} to the N-terminal extracellular domain of CaR initiates discreet intracellular events mediated by the second messengers inositol 1,4,5-triphosphate (IP3) and diacylglycerol (DAG), which result in mobilization of intracellular Ca^{2+} and protein kinase C (PKC) activation, respectively (Berridge et al., 2000; Gama et al., 1997; Rhee, 2001). Intriguingly, elimination of GCC expression in mice is associated with loss of CaR from enterocyte brush borders (Pitari et al., 2008). Moreover, expression of CaR and GCC ligands is maximal at upper-crypt areas (Chakrabarty et al., 2005; Cohen et al., 1995; Whitaker et al., 1997), where epithelial cells stop proliferation and enter the maturation program, suggesting that CaR activity may be subordinated to GCC signalling along the crypt–villus axis (Pitari et al., 2008). Further, lumenal Ca^{2+} (1-3 mM) triggering cell cycle arrest at colonic mid-crypts (Whitfield et al., 1995) opposes pro-proliferative β–catenin activity and favour p21- and p27-mediated differentiation (Chakrabarty et al., 2003, 2005), molecular effectors also regulated by cGMP signalling in the intestine (Lin et al., 2010; Liu et al., 2001). Thus, GCC signalling may promote the proliferation-differentiation transition of intestinal epithelial cells through CaR regulation (Pitari et al., 2008). This is important as CaR is also the receptor for other polyvalent cations (i.e., Gd^{3+}, Mg^{2+}, Ni^{2+}) and polyamines (i.e., spermine, spermidine, putrescine) produced by commensal colonic bacteria (Hofer & Brown, 2003), pointing to a crucial role of the GCC-CaR pathway as regulator of a variety of antiproliferative signals in intestine (Pitari et al., 2008). In addition, lumenal Ca^{2+} may mediate intestinal GCC actions through CaR-independent mechanisms, including ionic currents by CNG channels (Biel et al., 1999; Pitari et al., 2003, 2008). Cyclic GMP-gated Ca^{2+} current through CNG is a major regulator of signal generation and transmission in excitable cells (Ames et al., 1999; Zufall et al., 1997). Of relevance, in colon cancer cells GCC signalling slows cell cycle progression, in part, by inducing cGMP-dependent CNG channel activation, intracellular Ca^{2+} influx and cytosolic Ca^{2+} rises (Pitari et al., 2003).

Another model proposes the v-akt murine thymoma viral oncogene homolog (AKT) as the master biological effector of the GCC pathway (Lin et al., 2010). AKT regulates survival and metabolic circuits in proliferating intestinal cells, and AKT over activation promotes crypt hyperplasia and tumorigenesis in mouse intestine (Sakatani et al., 2005). Importantly, elimination of GCC expression in mice results in hyperactivation of AKT signalling pathways, associated with expanded crypt compartments populated by glycolytic cells with accelerated G_1-S cell cycle transition (Lin et al., 2010). Conversely, loss of GCC and cGMP signalling restricts the differentiated villus compartment and diminishes mitochondria-dependent oxidative metabolism in intestinal epithelial cells (Lin et al., 2010). Investigations employing genetic and pharmacologic manipulation of AKT confirmed that GCC signalling through cGMP control the proliferative cell metabolism by decreasing the function of AKT (Lin et al., 2010). Thus, AKT-dependent regulation of cell survival and glycolytic metabolism along the crypt-villus axis, at the basis of intestinal mucosa development and homeostasis, may be conditionally regulated by the activity of the GCC pathway, whose increasing crypt-villus gradient directly correlates with differentiation and oxidative phosphorylation.

2.3 Regulation of epithelium-stroma interactions

Beyond the epithelium, the intestinal wall also encompasses mesenchymal and a smooth muscle layers. The intestinal mesenchymal compartment comprises mucosal and submucosal layers of connective tissues, composed of both acellular (e.g., glycoproteins, hyaluronic acid, proteoglycans, collagen I and III) and cellular components (e.g., fibroblasts, myofibroblasts, leukocytes, endothelial cells). The basement membrane, a balanced mix of matrix components (e.g., nidogen, laminin, collagen IV, perlecan), physically separates the enterocytes from the underlying mesenchyme. The basement membrane and all the other mesenchymal components significantly contribute to the dynamic renewal of intestinal epithelial cells. Indeed, intestinal epithelium-stroma interactions contribute to maintain the crypt-villus homeostasis through direct cell-matrix and cell-cell contacts or paracrine signalling (Montgomery et al., 1999; Pinchuk et al., 2010). In contrast, corrupted epithelium-stroma interactions promote the initiation and progression of an array of intestinal pathologies (Kraus & Arber, 2009; Suzuki et al., 2011).

Studies with targeted deletion of GCC in mice revealed striking morphogenetic alterations affecting the extra-epithelial layers of the intestine (Gibbons et al., 2009). Indeed, the intestinal wall of these mice is significantly enlarged compared to mice with normal GCC expression. The mesenchymal compartment exhibits hypertrophy as a result of both exaggerated activation of its cellular elements and increased deposition of its interstitial matrix components (Gibbons et al., 2009). In particular, an increased ratio of activated myofibroblasts over quiescent fibroblasts is present in mice with loss of GCC signalling, an alteration which contributes to the establishment of a reactive stromal environment characterized by overexpression of collagen I, tenascin C and matrix metalloproteinase 9 (MMP-9) (Gibbons et al., 2009). In part, these alterations appear to be the consequence of an increased interstitial activity of the profibrinogenic transforming growth factor β (TGF-β), as GCC signalling through cGMP inhibits TGF-β secretion and function in intestinal epithelial cells and opposes stromal remodelling underlying inflammatory processes (Gibbons et al., 2009). Further, intestinal smooth muscle layers of mice lacking GCC signalling exhibit hyperplasia and hypertrophy, which represent important contributors of the transmural gut enlargement in these animals (Gibbons et al., 2009). Thus, the GCC pathway operating in intestinal mucosal cells exerts strong developmental and functional influences on the underlying stroma, presumably by regulating discreet hormonal circuits supporting epithelial-mesenchymal crosstalk (Pitari et al., 2007). Given the established role of the intestinal mesenchyme in inflammation and tumorigenesis (Kraus & Arber, 2009; Pinchuk et al., 2010; Suzuki et al., 2011), it is possible to speculate that dysregulation of GCC signalling in intestinal epithelial cells may favour the emergence of a reactive stromal environment promoting pathological processes.

3. GCC and intestinal transformation

Colorectal carcinogenesis comprises a pathological continuum turning pre-cancerous lesions into invasive malignant tumors. The process begins with single (epi)genetic mutations driven by carcinogenic insults that disrupt the physiological epithelial cell phenotype (Gryfe et al., 1997; van Engeland et al., 2011). As a result, the balance of migration, proliferation, differentiation and cell death along the colonic crypt-surface axis is perturbed and neoplastic cells with limitless replicative potential emerge. Remodelling of the surrounding stroma also participates to the promotion and progression of transformation, imposing cell non-autonomous drivers of tumorigenesis such us angiogenesis and inflammation (Kraus & Arber, 2009; Suzuki et al., 2011). Ultimately, malignant cells lose their epithelial characteristics and acquire a mesenchymal phenotype that enables them to translocate and establish new colonies at distant sites, such as the liver, lung and peritoneum (Nicolson, 1988; Polyak & Weinberg 2009; Suzuki et al., 2011).

The paracrine hormone hypothesis of colorectal cancer suggests that sporadic intestinal tumorigenesis is a process initiated by loss of endogenous GCC ligand expression, which induces a state of guanylinopenia and uroguanylinopenia (Pitari et al., 2007). Indeed, extensive studies have demonstrate that early in transformation intestinal epithelial cells acquire a mysterious mutation that renders pre-cancerous adenomatous lesions devoid of guanylin and uroguanylin (Birkenkamp-Demtroder et al., 2002; Cohen et al., 1998; Notterman et al., 2001; Steinbrecher et al., 2000). Those reports suggest that guanylin and uroguanylin, organized in a tail-to-tail configuration on human chromosome 1p, are the most commonly lost gene products in colorectal cancer in both animals and humans, exhibiting mutational frequency rates comparable to that of APC. Conversely, GCC is retained in colorectal cancer cells, which often exhibit higher GCC expression levels compared to normal epithelial tissues (Schulz et al., 2006; Witek et al., 2005). Increased GCC in the context of reduced guanylin and uroguanylin expression probably reflects the common pharmacological paradigm of receptor upregulation following specific ligand deprivation. More importantly, dysregulation of GCC signalling with an intact, but silent (for failure of ligand-dependent activation), intracellular molecular pathway produces a dormant cGMP-regulated system, which might be pathognomonically associated with neoplastic disease progression (Pitari et al., 2007). In this model, colorectal carcinogenesis following paracrine GCC ligand insufficiency reflects the central role of GCC in coordinating processes maintaining epithelial cell homeostasis and the crypt-villus axis, including the proliferation-differentiation balance, migration, metabolic programming and mesenchymal development (Li et al., 2007a; Pitari et al., 2007).

3.1 Regulation of the colon cancer cell phenotype

Neoplastic cell transformation ensues from the stepwise accumulation of mutations that produce hyper functioning oncogenes and silenced tumor suppressors (Bishop & Weinberg, 1996). Universally, the final combination of all the mutations and signalling deregulations occurring in cancers has similar functional consequences, the promotion of tumor cell growth and dissemination, and the evasion of host mechanisms of elimination (e.g., immuno-surveillance) (Hanahan & Weinberg, 2000). In intestinal tumorigenesis, acquisition of these malignant traits resembles a pathological amplification of the crypt stem cell phenotype, which self-perpetuates through relentless rounds of cell proliferation and migration (Montgomery et al., 1999; Potten & Loeffler, 1990). Conversely, invasive cancer cells progressively lose the morphology and metabolism of the differentiated epithelium, acquiring the ancestral functional plasticity of pluripotent stem cells. Indeed, overexpression of molecules (Wnt, β-catenin, Tcf) that support the crypt cell compartment (Gregorieff & Clevers, 2005; Korinek et al., 1998), or disruption of gene products (the adenomatous polyposis coli gene APC, Smad, CDX-2) restricting it (Aoki et al., 2003; Fodde et al., 2001; Tang et al., 2005) promotes intestinal tumorigenesis in animal models. In close agreement with these observations, the majority of sporadic human colorectal cancers exhibits a perturbed APC signalling as the initial mutational event, which crystallizes crypt-like nuclear proliferative programs driven by the β-catenin/Tcf complex (Fodde et al., 2001).

Since it regulates crypt compartments and the proliferation-differentiation balance along the crypt-villus axis (Li et al., 2007a; Pitari et al., 2007), dormancy of the GCC signalling pathway contributes to neoplastic transformation in the intestine (Li et al., 2007a; Pitari et al., 2007). Indeed, the increased migration and proliferation induced by loss of GCC signalling in mucosal colonocytes (Li et al., 2007a) represents a significant oncogenic stress (Aoki et al., 2003; Spruck et al., 1999) that creates the pre-neoplastic intestinal crypt (Pitari et al., 2007). Accordingly, cell cycle progression and growth of human colon cancer cells, experimental mimicry of the GCC dormancy characterizing the human disease because they express GCC but not the endogenous ligands (Lucas et al., 2000; Pitari et al., 2001), are greatly impaired upon reactivation of GCC signalling with exogenous supplementation of its specific agonists (Pitari et al., 2001, 2003, 2005, 2008). Ligand-dependent GCC activation restores lost cGMP-regulated circuits and imposes cancer cytostasis by reducing nuclear DNA synthesis and the G_1/S transition (Lin et al., 2010; Pitari et al., 2001). Antiproliferation by GCC, in part, is mediated by extracellular Ca^{2+} actions at cancer cell membrane surfaces, through its dependant effects on CaR activation and CNG channel-mediated Ca^{2+} influx (Pitari et al., 2003; Pitari et al., 2008). In addition, reactivation of GCC signalling through cGMP opposes the Wnt/β-catenin/Tcf4 signalling axis, the regulator of the proliferative crypt phenotype and tumor promoter in intestine (Pinto & Clevers 2005; Reya & Clevers 2005; van Es et al., 2005), by directly inhibiting β-catenin stability (Liu et al., 2001; Thompson et al., 2000). Underscoring the significance of the dormant GCC pathway in colon cancer, elimination of GCC in mice significantly enhances intestinal tumor initiation and progression (Li et al., 2007b). Mice deficient of GCC signalling exhibit enhanced sensitivity to tumorigenesis induced by $Apc^{Min/+}$ and the carcinogen azoxymethane, reflected by increased tumor incidence, multiplicity, and burden (Li et al., 2007b). A principal mechanism by which GCC promotes colorectal tumorigenesis is the perturbation of regulators of G_1/S cell cycle transition, including increased expression of oncogenes cyclin D_1 and pRb, and decreased activity of tumor suppressor p27 (Li et al., 2007b). Beyond hyperproliferation, GCC-deficient mice also exhibit increased genomic instability in their intestinal mucosa cells. In particular, an increased incidence of DNA breaks, loss of heterozygosity and point mutations in genes central to tumorigenesis, including APC and β-catenin, are observed along the crypt-villus axis (Li et al., 2007b). Although it remains unclear, the molecular mechanism mediating maintenance of the genome by GCC, including damage detection or mutational repair, appears to be distinct from that regulating proliferation (Li et al., 2007b). Rather, proliferative restriction and genomic quality control reflect two reinforcing systems by which the GCC pathway opposes intestinal carcinogenesis (Li et al., 2007b; Pitari et al., 2007). While accelerated G_1/S cell cycle transition favours inheritance and amplification of genetic mutations (Aoki et al., 2003; Spruck et al., 1999), instability involving tumor suppressors or oncogenes further deregulates the cancer cell cycle (Spruck et al., 1999).

Another consequence of a dormant GCC pathway in colorectal transformation is the promotion of the cancer cell metabolism (Lin et al., 2010). As discussed above, intestinal crypt stem cells principally rely on glycolysis to produce ATP and support their metabolism. Activation of GCC signalling restricts the glycolytic crypt compartment and favours the acquisition of mitochondria-mediated oxidative phosphorylation by differentiated epithelial cells in villi (Lin et al., 2010). Importantly, neoplastic cells utilize glycolytic ATP as their source of energy, even in the context of optimal environmental oxygen levels (Capuano et al., 1997; Kroemer, 2006; Pelicano et al., 2006). Dr. Otto Warburg first described this malignant paradox suggesting that cancer cells undergo metabolic reprogramming, wherein they switch from oxidative phosphorylation to aerobic glycolysis to produce ATP (Warburg, 1956). This malignant transition provides a competitive advantage to cancer cells that have a readily accessible supply of energy and substrates to support proliferation, adapt to the hypoxic tumor microenvironment, and promote invasion. Of relevance, restoration of GCC signalling by exogenous ligand administration increases the number, size and function of mitochondria in human colon cancer cells (Lin et al., 2010). Tumor reversion to mitochondria-dependent oxidative metabolism is associated with concurrent reduction in rate-limiting glycolytic enzymes, and reflects modulation of AKT and its downstream effectors (e.g., mTOR) by GCC signalling reactivation (Lin et al., 2010). Thus, while GCC signalling in human colon cancer cells induces expression of critical transcription factors required for mitochondrial biogenesis (PGC1α, mtTFA, NRF1), inhibition of glycolysis by GCC results in a reduced ability of tumors to uptake glucose and produce lactate (Lin et al., 2010). Importantly, elimination of AKT rescues the tumorigenic intestinal phenotype of mice deficient in GCC signalling (Lin et al., 2010), underscoring the central role of metabolic circuits in mediating inhibition of colorectal carcinogenesis by GCC. Together, these observations suggest that the dormant GCC pathway, produced by hormone deprivation early in transformation (Birkenkamp-Demtroder et al., 2002; Cohen et al., 1998; Notterman et al., 2001; Steinbrecher et al., 2000), can be envisioned as a loss-of-function mutation of a tumor suppressor system, which promotes crypt stem-like proliferation and metabolism and favours genomic instability and the development of the colon cancer cell phenotype.

3.2 Regulation of the colon tumor microenvironment

The tumor microenvironment is recognized as a major determinant of cancer formation, growth and dissemination (Fidler, 2001; Kraus & Arber, 2009; Suzuki et al., 2011). Both cellular and acellular components comprising the tumor stroma contribute to intestinal transformation, reflecting the intimate crosstalk between tumor epithelial cells and the underneath mesenchyme (Kraus & Arber, 2009; Suzuki et al., 2011; Witz & Levy-Nissenbaum, 2006). Thus, interstitial matrix remodelling, secretion of paracrine factors by stromal cells, lymphocyte-mediated immunoresponses, and neo-angiogenesis significantly influence cancer development (Fidler, 2001; Kraus & Arber, 2009; Suzuki et al., 2011). Among the molecular mediators of cancer-mesenchyme interactions, the matrix metalloproteinases (MMPs) play an essential role (Zucker & Vacirca, 2004). MMPs are a family of zinc-dependent metalloendopeptidases that cleave interstitial matrix components, growth factors, chemokines and cell surface receptors creating a nurturing niche for cancer growth and invasion (Cox & O'Byrne, 2001; Curran & Murray, 2000; McCawley & Matrisian, 2001). Depending on their substrate specificities, MMPs are divided into collagenases, gelatinases, stromelysins, and matrilysins (Stamenkovic, 2003).
The soluble collagenase MMP-9 has been conclusively linked with colorectal carcinogenesis (Chu et al., 2011; Lubbe et al., 2006; Nascimento et al., 2010; Zucker & Vacirca 2004; Zuzga et al., 2008). Structurally, MMP-9 (92-kDa protein) consists of a pro-peptide sequence, a catalytic domain containing the zinc binding site and fibronectin type II-like repeats, which promote MMP-9 binding to gelatin and elastin (Fridman et al., 2003; Shipley et al., 1996). Although enzymatic-independent signalling also has been reported (Bjorklund et al., 2004; Librach et al., 1991), the catalytic activity of MMP-9 is the principal mediator of tumor

matrix remodelling (Fridman et al., 2003; Lubbe et al., 2006). In this way, MMP-9 degrades basement membrane collagen type IV, allowing intestinal tumor epithelial cells to invade the adjacent stromal compartment (Fridman et al., 2003). Moreover, MMP-9 promotes tumor angiogenesis by specifically processing and releasing TGF-β and VEGF from cancer cell surfaces and the interstitial matrix, respectively (Bergers et al., 2000; Qian et al., 1997; Yu & Stamenkovic, 2000). Given its crucial role in those pathological processes, MMP-9-dependent proteolytic activity is considered a driving force conferring the migratory and invasive phenotype to cancer cells and favouring tumor progression (Bergers et al., 2000; Fridman et al., 2003; Lubbe et al., 2006; Yu & Stamenkovic, 2000). Consequently, MMP-9 activity needs to be tightly controlled in biological tissues. Indeed, normally MMP-9 is a silent protease, secreted by cancer cells as a pro-zymogen that is activated only upon cleavage of its 10-kDa N-terminal pro-peptide by various proteases (e.g., MMP-2, MMP-3, MMP-13, plasmin, thrombin) (Ahmed et al., 2003; Fridman et al., 2003; Ramos-DeSimone et al., 1999). Endogenous inhibitors of MMP-9 also exists (e.g., the tissue inhibitor of matrix metalloproteinase 1) which bind to both the pro- and the active-form of MMP-9 and neutralize its proteolytic activity (Goldberg et al., 1992; Stamenkovic, 2003).

Beyond inhibition of catalytic activity, regulation of zymogen expression and secretion represents additional effective modalities to contain tumorigenic MMP-9 functions (St-Pierre et al., 2003; Zhang et al., 2006). Cyclic GMP inhibits the synthesis and secretion of MMP-9 in various cell systems (Akool el et al., 2003; Gurjar et al., 1999). Accordingly, restoration of ligand-dependent GCC signalling though cGMP induces a compartmental redistribution of colon cancer cell MMP-9, in which intracellular retention results in reciprocal extracellular depletion of that collagenase (Lubbe et al., 2009). As a consequence, MMP-9 proteolytic activities at the pericellular tumor space are suppressed, with abrogation of MMP-9-dependent interstitial matrix remodelling and cell spreading (Lubbe et al., 2009). Conversely, mutational dormancy of the GCC pathway early in transformation (Birkenkamp-Demtroder et al., 2002; Cohen et al. 1998; Notterman et al., 2001; Steinbrecher et al., 2000) may permit the emergence of a pro-tumorigenic stromal environment characterized by increased MMP-9 secretion, break-down of epithelial basement membranes by MMP-9 catalytic activity and disruption of homeostatic epithelial-mesenchymal interactions. It has been proposed that GCC effect on spatiotemporal MMP-9 dynamics in colon cancer cells has a profound impact on the overall tumor phenotype, because by disrupting its surface localization, membrane anchoring and focal catalytic activity it suppresses oncogenic MMP-9 functions (Lubbe et al., 2009).

4. GCC and colorectal cancer metastasis

Cancer metastasis consists in the dissemination of tumor cells to distant locations (Fidler, 2003). Clinically, metastasis coincides with the most terminal disease stages, incurable conditions associated with poor prognosis and survival (Mehlen & Puisieux, 2006; Siegel et al., 2011). Pathogenetically, it comprises a sequence of distinct, individual processes including cancer cell invasion of the primary site, intravasation and distribution through blood or lymphatic vessels, and colonization of target organs (Fidler, 2003; Folkman, 1986; Nicolson, 1988). Following organ seeding, tumor cells have to migrate into and invade tissue parenchyma (Wanget al., 2004; Steeg, 2006), resist to local immune defences and establish a nurturing micro-environment to develop and growth (Fidler, 2003; Folkman, 1986). In colon cancer, preferred organs of metastatic colonization include the liver, lung and peritoneum.

Once colorectal cancer has spread to these organs, the risk of mortality increases dramatically, and ~90% of patients diagnosed with distant metastasis die within 5 years from diagnosis (Siegel et al., 2011). Indeed, the management of patients with colorectal cancer metastasis is characterized by the highest incidence of therapeutic failure, in which surgery is not practicable (Pihlet al., 1981; Shapiro, 1992) and adjuvant chemotherapy is ineffective (increasing median survival only few months) (Meyerhardt & Mayer, 2005).
The functional phenotype of metastatic cells is unique and very selective. It has been calculated that of intravasated tumor cells, only a minute fraction remains viable after 24 hour, and >99.99% are eliminated before reaching their target organ (Fidler, 1970). This metastatic inefficiency reflects the scarcity of cancer cell clones exhibiting the full molecular machinery to execute all the individual steps comprising the metastatic process (Fidler, 1970; Weiss, 1990). In that context, since its inception primary colorectal cancer consists of biologically heterogeneous cell subpopulations, among which are present those possessing the ability to migrate and spread to distant parenchyma (Fidler, 2003; Heppner, 1984). Intriguingly as demonstrated by extensive immune detection and mRNA analyses of clinical specimens, GCC is uniformly expressed in metastatic colon tumors regardless of anatomical location (Carrithers et al., 1994; Carrithers et al., 1996; Waldman et al., 1998). Moreover, the structural and functional integrity of GCC and its principal downstream effectors appears to be preserved in metastasis, as colorectal cancer cells at extra-intestinal sites exhibit identical binding characteristics to, and signalling activation by, the exogenous ligand ST to those of normal intestinal cells (Carrithers et al., 1994; Schulz et al., 2006; Witek et al., 2005). However away from its primary organ, GCC is a ligand-starved receptor with an intracellular dormant pathway, as normal mucosal cells in intestine are the principal producers of endogenous hormones guanylin and uroguanylin (Forte, 1999). Thus, the loss of GCC ligand expression early in transformation (Birkenkamp-Demtroder et al., 2002; Cohen et al., 1998; Notterman et al., 2001; Steinbrecher et al., 2000) may be part of the exclusive phenotypic mutations conferring a pro-metastatic evolutionary advantage to selected colon cancer clones (Lubbe et al., 2009; Pitari et al., 2007; Zuzga et al., 2011).

4.1 Control of invasive cell shape

To successfully execute the metastatic program, transformed cells require a dynamic actin cytoskeleton. Thus, a hallmark of metastasis is the abandon of the static epithelial cell polarity and the acquisition of plastic membrane borders with specialized actin-based organelles promoting locomotion and invasion (Fidler, 2003; Steeg, 2006). Similarly to lymphocytes or neutrophils at inflammatory sites, cancer cells constantly remodel their actin to assume atypical morphological architectures, a process often referred to as epithelial-mesenchymal transition (Polyak & Weinberg, 2009). Changes in cell shapes reflect profound molecular rearrangements at tumor surfaces, including loss of E-cadherin-dependent cell-cell contacts and transient assembly of integrin-driven cell-matrix adhesions (Avizienyte et al., 2004, 2005; Polyak & Weinberg, 2009). These processes permit *de novo* development of membrane protrusions, such as filopodia and lamellipodia for probing the matrix during spreading and migration, and invadopodia for focal proteolytic matrix degradation in invasion (Linder, 2007; Yamaguchi & Condeelis, 2007).
In general, common molecular regulators coordinate tumor cytoskeletal remodelling by transducing external signals into actin processes. In colon cancer cells, tyrosine kinase receptors (e.g., EGF receptor, Eph receptors, Met receptors), G protein-coupled receptors

(e.g., cholecystokinin receptors) and cytokine receptors (e.g., chemokine receptors, TGF-β receptor) have been established as important inducers of the metastatic cell morphology (Dienstmann & Tabernero 2010; Dong et al., 2009; Fulton, 2009; Kitamura et al., 2010; Larsen & Dashwood, 2010; Ongchin et al., 2009; Yuet al., 2006). They activate the intracellular signalling system controlling cytoskeletal actin (e.g., focal adhesion kinases, rho-GTPases, Arp2/3 complex), which assembles the membrane protrusive structures mediating invasion (Linder, 2007; Yamaguchi & Condeelis, 2007). Normally restricted at intestinal epithelial brush borders (Lucas et al., 2000), GCC is ideally positioned to affect those molecular networks and exert spatio-temporal control of actin remodelling. Indeed, ligand-dependent GCC signalling through cGMP appears to act as a suppressor of metastatic cell morphology in intestine (Lubbe et al., 2009; Zuzga et al., 2011). Thus, colon cancer cells assume a rounded shape upon GCC signalling activation, with elimination of F-actin rich filopodia and lamellipodia (Lubbe et al., 2009). The number and length of cancer cell invadopodia also significantly decreases after activation of the GCC pathway (Zuzga et al., 2011). Importantly, failure to form protrusive structures forces tumor cells to aggregate into compact colonies devoid of spreading and invading abilities (Lubbe et al., 2009; Zuzga et al., 2011). Together, these observations suggest that the GCC pathway is one of the intrinsic homeostatic systems that maintain the stable epithelial cell polarity, shape and tight junctions, which form the essential mucosal barrier between the intestine and the external environment (Han et al., 2011). This notion is further supported by the inhibitory role that GCC signalling exerts on known inducers of epithelial-mesenchymal transition (Polyak & Weinberg, 2009), including the reactive stromal environment (with enhanced TGF-β and MMP-9 activities) (Gibbons et al., 2009) and the stem cell-promoting PI3K/AKT system (Lin et al., 2010). Hence, dysregulation of GCC signalling in intestinal tumorigenesis may enable the epithelial-mesenchymal transition required for cancer cell dissemination (Lubbe et al., 2009).

A key intracellular effector of the GCC pathway that regulates colon cancer cell shape is the vasodilator-stimulated phosphoprotein (VASP) (Zuzga et al., 2011). Ena/VASP family proteins control F-actin geometry supporting cell motility (Krause et al., 2003). VASP promotes filopodia and lamellipodia formation and extension by organizing molecular complexes comprising G-actin, F-actin and actin regulatory proteins (Krause et al., 2003). It functions by protecting actin barbed ends from binding to capping proteins, thereby permitting filament elongation (Bear et al., 2002; Mejillano et al., 2004). Three critical domains enable VASP to intimately interact with the actin cytoskeleton (Krause et al., 2003), including 1) the N-terminus Ena/VASP homology 1 (EVH1), which binds to focal adhesion proteins vinculin and zyxin, 2) the central prolin-rich region, which contains a consensus binding motif for the G-actin-binding protein profilin, and 3) the C-terminus EVH2, which binds to both G- and F-actin and mediates VASP oligomerization. Importantly, Ser239 within the EVH2 VASP domain is a preferred phosphorylation site for PKG, functioning as a biological marker for cGMP signalling in intestinal (Deguchi et al., 2002) and other cells (Krause et al., 2003; Yaroslavskiy et al., 2005). Cyclic GMP-dependent VASP phosphorylation inhibits membrane protrusion formation in normal cells (Krause et al., 2003; Lindsay et al., 2007). Accordingly, in colorectal cancer cells VASP Ser239 phosphorylation induced by ligand activation of GCC signalling through cGMP and PKG induces rapid disassembly (less than 10 minutes) of invasive and migratory membrane organelles (Zuzga et al., 2011). Herein, GCC promotes VASP removal from tumor membrane protrusions with subsequent collapse of the F-actin infrastructure supporting filopodia and invadopodia (Zuzga et al., 2011). However, colorectal cancer cells expressing a mutant VASP construct not-phosphorylatable at Ser239 are resistant to GCC effects on VASP intracellular distribution and membrane protrusions (Zuzga et al., 2011). These findings are the most significant because they uncover the novel paradigm of a single intracellular biochemical reaction, VASP Ser239 phosphorylation, as an invasion suppressive mechanism for colon cancer (Zuzga et al., 2011). Hence, the loss of this mechanism during colorectal tumorigenesis, reflecting silencing of the GCC-cGMP-VASP system following hormonal deprivation (Birkenkamp-Demtroder et al., 2002; Cohen et al., 1998; Notterman et al., 2001; Steinbrecher et al., 2000), may favour the acquisition of the metastatic cell morphology, characterized by dissolution of normal cell-matrix and cell-cell contacts, increased actin polymerization dynamics, and enhanced formation of membrane protrusions (Zuzga et al., 2011).

4.2 Control of cancer cell dissemination

Relocation of cancer cells to distant sites requires acquisition of novel motor abilities, enabling them to spread through remodelled matrix surfaces at both primary and secondary tissues. In primary tumors, cancer cell spreading in the direction of blood vessels initiates the migratory journey of the intravasation process (Fidler et al., 1978; Fidler, 2003). In secondary organs, tumor cell adhesion and spreading onto vascular endothelial surfaces starts cancer invasion of target parenchyma (Im et al., 2004; Wang et al., 2004). In this context, polarized cell spreading drives cancer cell migration in the direction of invasion by permitting the establishment of specialized cell-matrix contacts at membrane protrusions, which mediates actin cytoskeleton-driven anchorage and traction of the cell body (Small et al., 1996). Thus, regulators of the cytoskeleton, adhesion receptors and extracellular proteases, which universally control spreading and migration in cells, are key players underlying cancer dissemination (Yamaguchi & Condeelis, 2007). Since its signalling through cGMP and VASP controls actin cytoskeletal dynamics and membrane protrusions in colon cancer cells (Zuzga et al., 2011), the GCC pathway may exert substantial impacts on those processes underlying formation of distant metastasis. Consistent with this hypothesis, elimination of GCC signalling in mice accelerates cell migration along the intestinal crypt-villus axis (Li et al., 2007a). Of relevance, basal GCC activity appears insufficient to restraining epithelial cell motility, as demonstrated by the increased migration of intestinal mucosa cells in mice with targeted ligand (guanylin) deletion (Steinbrecher et al., 2002). These observations suggest a model in which loss of hormone expression at the beginning of colorectal tumorigenesis (Birkenkamp-Demtroder et al., 2002; Cohen et al., 1998; Notterman et al., 2001; Steinbrecher et al., 2000) results in the acquisition of increased migratory abilities by transformed cells, driven by the accelerated formation of locomotory organelles mediating cell spreading and invasion (Zuzga et al., 2011).

A significant regulator of colorectal cancer cell migration and dissemination is the MMP-9 secreted by tumor epithelial cells (Lubbe et al., 2006). Beyond matrix degradation, this MMP-9 promotes the spreading and migration of colon cancer cells along two dimensional surfaces (Lubbe et al., 2006). Moreover, the catalytic activity of cancer cell MMP-9 is required for optimal colon tumor cell seeding of target mouse organs (Lubbe et al., 2006), an effect probably reflecting remodelling of the tumor pericellular microenvironment by MMP-9 (Fridman et al., 2003). Accordingly, inhibitors of MMP-9 suppress the formation of colorectal liver metastasis in an animal model (Aparicio et al., 1999). The significance of

MMP-9 for colon cancer metastasis is further underscored by its universal role in regulating migration and invasion across different cell types (Buisson et al., 1996; Leppert et al., 1995; Sanceau et al., 2003; Schultz et al., 1988; Yu & Stamenkovic, 1999). Importantly, ligand-dependent GCC signalling through cGMP suppresses the function of the MMP-9 produced by colorectal cancer cells (Lubbe et al., 2009). Activation of the GCC pathway suppresses tumor cell spreading, migration and dissemination by specifically inhibiting the secretion of cancer cell MMP-9 in the extracellular space (Lubbe et al., 2009). Further, colon tumor cells treated with GCC ligands fail to form metastatic colonies on mouse diaphragms following intraperitoneal injections (Lubbe et al., 2009). This effect also depends on the ability of GCC to inhibit cancer cell MMP-9, as demonstrated by the resistance of cells overexpressing MMP-9 to GCC-mediated inhibition of peritoneal metastasis (Lubbe et al., 2009). Conceivably, a silent GCC pathway in colorectal carcinogenesis (Birkenkamp-Demtroder et al., 2002; Cohen et al., 1998; Notterman et al., 2001; Steinbrecher et al., 2000) facilitates colon tumor invasion and metastatic dissemination by removing a key inhibitory mechanism restraining the oncogenic activity of cancer cell MMP-9.

5. The GCC pathway as a source of novel clinical targets

As discussed above, the loss of ligand-dependent GCC signalling produces a dormant GCC/cGMP pathway, which has significant impacts on the initiation, progression and metastasis of colorectal cancer. Conversely, deregulation of that pathway and its individual molecular components uncovers novel targets with unexploited clinical potential for improved diagnosis and therapy of patients. Thus, detection of hormone downregulation in colon biopsies could indicate presence of intestinal carcinogenesis and demand appropriate follow-up (Cohen et al., 1998; Notterman et al., 2001). The selective expression of GCC in colorectal tumor cells at metastatic sites (Carrithers et al., 1994, 1996; Waldman et al., 1998), suggests its utility as a diagnostic marker and specific target for delivering imaging and therapeutic agents *in vivo* (Gali et al., 2001; Wolfe et al., 2002). Indeed, clinical trials are confirming the value of GCC as a diagnostic marker for molecular staging of patients and prognostic indicator of colorectal cancer recurrence (Mejia et al., 2010; Waldman et al., 2009). Moreover, the structural preservation of GCC and its intracellular effectors offers the GCC hormone replacement therapy as a novel clinical paradigm for the prevention and treatment of colorectal cancer (Pitari et al., 2007). In this context, oral administration of uroguanylin prevents polyp formation in an animal model of intestinal tumorigenesis (Shailubhai et al., 2000). Further, the resistance to colon cancer initiation and progression exhibited by populations living in the developing world (Pitari et al., 2003; Shailubhai et al., 2000), where enterotoxigenic infections are highest, suggests that replacement therapy with the exogenous GCC ligand ST, the enterotoxin produced by E. coli, might be an effective treatment for colorectal cancer patients (Pitari et al., 2007). This latter consideration is supported by observations that ST is the most potent GCC agonist available (Lucas et al., 2000), and the only ligand successfully investigated to fully restore the tumor suppressor activities of the GCC pathway in colorectal cancer cells (Lubbe et al., 2009; Pitari et al., 2001, 2003, 2005, 2007; Zuzga et al.,2011).

Distal components of the GCC pathway also could be exploited in original clinical applications against colon cancer. As expected for its significance in intestinal mucosa homeostasis, the intracellular GCC signalome comprises a complex molecular network

(Pitari et al., 2007), probably still incomplete and in which each of the molecular elements may deserve critical translational evaluations. For some of these, preclinical testing is currently ongoing that is revealing emerging features as promising colorectal cancer bio-targets (Table 1). One model is the CaR, whose surface expression in colon cancer cells is conditionally regulated by activation of GCC signalling (Pitari et al., 2008). The dormant GCC pathway probably contributes to the reduced CaR expression observed in colorectal tumors (Chakrabarty et al., 2003; Kallay et al., 2003), a mutational event with clinical potential as a diagnostic marker of disease progression (Pitari et al., 2008). Moreover, CaR activation by extracellular Ca^{2+} inhibits cell proliferation (Chakrabarty et al., 2003), and dietary Ca^{2+} supplementation has been proposed as a chemopreventive strategy for colon cancer (Cho et al., 2004). Since restoration of the GCC pathway with exogenous ST administration potentiates antitumorigenic CaR signalling in human colon carcinoma cells (Pitari et al., 2008), combinatorial therapies including dietary Ca^{2+} and GCC ligand replacement may represent promising clinical regimens for the prevention and treatment of colorectal cancer.

Protein	*Alteration in Colorectal Tumorigenesis*	*Diagnostic Target*	*Therapeutic Target*	*Ref.*
CaR	Reduced expression	Tumor formation	Inhibition of tumor growth	(Chakrabarty et al., 2003; Kallay et al., 2003; Pitari et al., 2008)
MMP-9	Increased cancer cell secretion	Distant metastasis	Metastasis prevention	(Lubbe et al., 2009; Zuzga et al., 2008)
VASP	Loss of Ser phosphorylation	Invasion, metastasis	Local invasion prevention	(Zuzga et al., 2011)

Table 1. Examples of emergent colon cancer molecular targets from the GCC pathway.

Another intriguing effector of the GCC pathway is MMP-9, whose cancer cell compartmentalization depends on intracellular cGMP signalling (Lubbe et al., 2009). A silent GCC network may favour increased release and proteolytic activity of MMP-9 at the tumor pericellular space (Lubbe et al., 2009), thereby promoting matrix remodelling and invasion (Curran & Murray, 1999). Importantly, colon cancer cell MMP-9 behaves as a selective prognostic and predictive biomarker for disease stage stratification and therapeutic regimen selection in patients (Bendardaf et al., 2010; Zuzga et al., 2008). Reactivation of the GCC pathway with ST, in turn, is one successful strategy to specifically inhibit MMP-9 in tumor epithelial cells, without collateral damage in normal tissue, that has been suggested for the chemoprevention of colorectal cancer metastasis (Lubbe et al., 2009). Further, recent studies are indicating VASP as yet another GCC target with attractive translational applications for patients with colon cancer (Zuzga et al., 2011). VASP is a crucial actin-binding protein controlling membrane protrusion geometry, cell adhesion and migration (Bear et al., 2002; Krause et al., 2003; Mejillano et al., 2004). Dormancy of the GCC pathway in tumorigenesis depletes colon cancer cells of the cGMP-dependent VASP Ser phosho-species, molecular regulators of VASP activity at dynamic membrane regions (Krause et al., 2003). Thus, loss of VASP Ser phosphorylation may represent a novel prognostic biomarker of colon cancer progression (Zuzga et al., 2011). Conversely, reconstitution of VASP Ser phosphorylation could be exploited as an original paradigm for the chemoprevention of cancer migration and invasion, because the potent GCC ligand ST suppresses the malignant cell morphology and its pathological functions in colon cancer (Zuzga et al., 2011).

6. Conclusion

A novel paradigm is emerging in which colorectal cancer, one of the top cancer killers in the world, is pathogenetically conditioned by a dormant GCC pathway, developed early in tumorigenesis following specific ligand downregulation. Indeed, GCC and its paracrine hormones restrict the proliferative crypt phenotype and promote the normal epithelial cell morphology by orchestrating an articulated intracellular network comprising interconnected, but functionally distinct molecular effectors. Silencing of the pathway for loss of agonist-induced GCC/cGMP signalling alters the activity of those molecules with profound consequences for the initiation and progression of colorectal transformation (Fig. 1). Virtually all the key processes underlying carcinogenesis and metastasis are enhanced by dysregulation of the GCC pathway components, including proliferation, survival, genetic instability, migration, matrix remodelling and invasion. At the same time, the dormant pathway creates unexplored opportunities for novel diagnostic applications. This is because the biochemical deregulation that ensues from the silent cGMP-dependent machinery can be traced by analysis of the single pathway components at the molecular level. As a result, novel molecular fingerprints of colorectal carcinogenesis are emerging from the GCC pathway that can be exploited as clinical prognostic or predictive indicators of disease.
Restoration of the lost function by the GCC pathway in colorectal tumors also is proving its great translational value. Preclinical studies indicate that, though dormant, the pathway is largely intact and can be reconstituted simply by ligand replacement. Thus, administration of bacterial enterotoxin STs, potent GCC agonists, suppresses proliferation, migration, matrix degradation, invasion and metastasis by colorectal cancer cells. Altogether, these findings support the notion that oral replacement therapy with GCC ligands could represent a novel strategy for both the chemoprevention and cure of colorectal cancer. Additional therapies targeting the individual pathway components, either alone or in combination, also are being developed with the goal to improve clinical efficacy and selectivity. However, information from clinical testing is still missing and important questions remain to be addressed before this knowledge could be applied to the patient bed. In particular, general gastrointestinal toxicity worries need to be dissipated as GCC ligands such as ST are known for their potent diarrheagenic effects. Also, the temporal profile of GCC-targeted therapy will require complete characterization, including estimation of duration of treatments and effects. Finally, pharmacokinetics evaluation will need to be performed to accurately define dosing and timing regimens. In summary, the intestinal GCC pathway is an exciting potential source of novel diagnostic and therapeutic targets that could significantly affect the clinical management and disease outcome of patients with colorectal cancer.

7. Acknowledgment

This work was supported by grants to GMP from the National Institute of Health (R03CA133950), the Elsa U. Pardee Foundation and the American Institute for Cancer Research. The National Institute of Health specifically disclaims responsibility for any analyses, interpretations or conclusions.

8. References

Ahmed, N., Oliva, K., Wang, Y., Quinn M., & Rice, G. (2003). Downregulation of urokinase plasminogen activator receptor expression inhibits Erk signalling with concomitant suppression of invasiveness due to loss of uPAR-beta1 integrin complex in colon cancer cells. *Br J Cancer,* Vol.89, No.2, (July 2003), pp. 374-384, PMID 12865932

Akool el, S., Kleinert, H., Hamada, F.M., Abdelwahab, M.H., Forstermann, U., Pfeilschifter, J., & Eberhardt, W. (2003). Nitric oxide increases the decay of matrix metalloproteinase 9 mRNA by inhibiting the expression of mRNA-stabilizing factor HuR. *Mol Cell Biol,* Vol.23, No.14, (July 2003), pp. 4901-4916, PMID 12832476

Ames, J.B., Dizhoor, A.M., Ikura, M., Palczewski, K., & Stryer, L. (1999). Three-dimensional structure of guanylyl cyclase activating protein-2, a calcium-sensitive modulator of photoreceptor guanylyl cyclases. *J Biol Chem,* Vol.274, No.27, (July 1999), pp. 19329-19337, PMID 10383444

Aoki, K., Tamai, Y., Horiike, S., Oshima, M., & Taketo, M. M. (2003). Colonic polyposis caused by mTOR-mediated chromosomal instability in Apc+/Delta716 Cdx2+/- compound mutant mice. *Nat Genet,* Vol.35, No.4, (Dec 2003), pp. 323-330, PMID 14625550

Aparicio, T., Kermorgant, S., Dessirier, V., Lewin, M & Lehy T. (1999). Matrix metalloproteinase inhibition prevents colon cancer peritoneal carcinomatosis development and prolongs survival in rats. *Carcinogenesis,* Vol.20, No.8, (Aug 1999), pp. 1445-1451, PMID 10426790

Avizienyte, E., Fincham, V.J., Brunton, V.G., & Frame, M.C. (2004). Src SH3/2 domain-mediated peripheral accumulation of Src and phospho-myosin is linked to deregulation of E-cadherin and the epithelial-mesenchymal transition. *Mol Biol Cell,* Vol.15, No.6, (June 2004), pp. 2794-2803, PMID 15075377

Avizienyte, E., Brunton, V.G., Fincham, V.J., & Frame M.C. (2005). The SRC-induced mesenchymal state in late-stage colon cancer cells. *Cells Tissues Organs,* Vol.179, No.1-2, (June 2005), pp. 73-80, PMID 15942195

Bear, J.E., Svitkina, T.M., Krause, M., Schafer, D.A., Loureiro, J.J., Strasser, G.A., Maly, I.V., Chaga, O.Y., Cooper, J.A., Borisy, G.G., & Gertler, F.B. (2002). Antagonism between Ena/VASP proteins and actin filament capping regulates fibroblast motility. *Cell,* Vol.109, No.4, (May 2002) pp. 509-521, PMID 12086607

Bendardaf, R., Buhmeida, A., Hilska, M., Laato, M., Syrjanen, S., Syrjanen, K., Collan Y., & Pyrhonen S. (2010). MMP-9 (gelatinase B) expression is associated with disease-free survival and disease-specific survival in colorectal cancer patients. *Cancer Invest,* Vol.28, No.1, (Jan 2010), pp. 38-43, PMID 20001295

Bergers, G., Brekken, R., McMahon, G., Vu, T.H., Itoh, T., Tamaki, K., Tanzawa, K., Thorpe, P., Itohara, S., Werb, Z., & Hanahan, D. (2000). Matrix metalloproteinase-9 triggers the angiogenic switch during carcinogenesis. *Nat Cell Biol,* Vol.2, No.10, (Oct 2000), pp. 737-744, PMID 11025665

Berridge, M.J., Lipp, P., & Bootman, M.D. (2000). The versatility and universality of calcium signalling. *Nat Rev Mol Cell Biol,* Vol.1, (Oct 2000), pp. 11-21, PMID 11413485

Biel, M., Zong, X., Ludwig, A., Sautter, A., & Hofmann, F. (1999). Structure and function of cyclic nucleotide-gated channels. *Rev Physiol Biochem Pharmacol,* Vol.135, pp. 151-171, PMID 9932483

Birkenkamp-Demtroder, K., Christensen, L.L., Olesen, S.H., Frederiksen, C.M., Laiho, P., Aaltonen, LA., Laurberg, S., Sorensen, F.B., Hagemann, R., & TF, O.R. (2002). Gene expression in colorectal cancer. *Cancer Res*, Vol.62, No.15, (Aug 2002), pp. 4352-4363, PMID 12154040

Bishop, JM.,&Weinberg, RA. (Eds.). (1996). *Molecular Oncology*, SA Inc., New York

Bjorklund, M., Heikkila, P., & Koivunen, E. (2004). Peptide inhibition of catalytic and noncatalytic activities of matrix metalloproteinase-9 blocks tumor cell migration and invasion. *J Biol Chem*, Vol.279, No.28, (July 2004), pp. 29589-29597, PMID 15123665

Browning, D.D., Kwon, I.K., & Wang, R. (2010). cGMP-dependent protein kinases as potential targets for colon cancer prevention and treatment. *Future Med Chem*, Vol.2, No.1, (Jan 2010), pp. 65-80, PMID21426046

Bry, L., Falk, P., Huttner, K., Ouellette, A., Midtvedt, T., & Gordon, J.I. (1994). Paneth cell differentiation in the developing intestine of normal and transgenic mice. *Proc Natl Acad Sci U S A*, Vol.91, No.22, (Oct 1994), pp. 10335-10339, PMID 7937951

Buisson, A.C., Zahm, J.M., Polette, M., Pierrot, D., Bellon, G., Puchelle, E., Birembaut, P., & Tournier, J.M. (1996). Gelatinase B is involved in the in vitro wound repair of human respiratory epithelium. *J Cell Physiol*, Vol.166, No.2, (Feb 1996), pp. 413-426, PMID 8592002

Capuano, F., Guerrieri, F., & Papa, S. (1997). Oxidative phosphorylation enzymes in normal and neoplastic cell growth. *J Bioenerg Biomembr*, Vol.29, No.4, (Aug 1997), pp. 379-384, PMID 9387098

Carrithers, S.L., Parkinson, S.J., Goldstein S., Park, P., Robertson, D.C., & Waldman, S.A. (1994). Escherichia coli heat-stable toxin receptors in human colonic tumors. *Gastroenterology*, Vol.107, No.6, (Dec 1994) pp. 1653-1661, PMID 7958675

Carrithers, S.L., Barber, M.T., Biswas, S., Parkinson, S.J., Park, P.K., Goldstein, S.D., & Waldman, S.A. (1996). Guanylyl cyclase C is a selective marker for metastatic colorectal tumors in human extraintestinal tissues. *Proc Natl Acad Sci U S A*, Vol.93, No.25, (Dec 1996), pp. 14827-14832, PMID 8962140

Chakrabarty, S., Radjendirane, V., Appelman, H., & Varani, J. (2003). Extracellular calcium and calcium sensing receptor function in human colon carcinomas: promotion of E-cadherin expression and suppression of beta-catenin/TCF activation. *Cancer Res*, Vol.63, No.1, (Jan 2003), pp. 67-71, PMID 12517779

Chakrabarty, S., Wang, H., Canaff, L., Hendy, G.N., Appelman, H. & Varani, J. (2005). Calcium sensing receptor in human colon carcinoma: interaction with Ca(2+) and 1,25-dihydroxyvitamin D(3). *Cancer Res*, Vol. 65, No.2, (Jan 2005), pp. 493-498, PMID 15695393

Chao, A.C., de Sauvage, F.J., Dong, Y.J., Wagner, J.A., Goeddel, D.V., and Gardner, P. (1994). Activation of intestinal CFTR Cl- channel by heat-stable enterotoxin and guanylin via cAMP-dependent protein kinase. *EMBO J*, Vol.13, No.5, (March 1994), pp. 1065-1072, PMID 7510634

Cho, E., Smith-Warner, S.A., Spiegelman, D., Beeson, W.L., van den Brandt, P.A., Colditz, G.A., Folsom, A.R., Fraser, G.E., Freudenheim, J.L., Giovannucci, E., Goldbohm, R.A., Graham, S., Miller, A.B., Pietinen, P., Potter, J.D., Rohan, T.E., Terry, P., Toniolo, P., Virtanen, M.J., Willett, W.C., Wolk, A., Wu, K., Yaun, S.S., Zeleniuch-Jacquotte A., & Hunter, D.J. (2004). Dairy foods, calcium, and colorectal cancer: a pooled analysis of 10 cohort studies. *J Natl Cancer Inst*, Vol.96, No.13, (July 2004) pp. 1015-1022, PMID 15240785

Chu, D., Zhao, Z., Zhou, Y., Li, Y., Li, J., Zheng, J., Zhao, Q., & Wang, W. (2011). Matrix Metalloproteinase-9 Is Associated with Relapse and Prognosis of Patients with Colorectal Cancer. *Ann Surg Oncol*, (Epub ahead of print), PMID 21455597

Cohen, M.B., Witte, D.P., Hawkins J.A., & Currie, M.G. (1995). Immunohistochemical localization of guanylin in the rat small intestine and colon. *Biochem Biophys Res Commun,* Vol.209, No.3, (April 1995), pp. 803-808, PMID 7733972

Cohen, M.B., Hawkins, J.A., & Witte, D.P. (1998). Guanylin mRNA expression in human intestine and colorectal adenocarcinoma. *Lab Invest*, Vol.78, No.1, (Jan 1998), pp. 101-108, PMID 9461126

Corbin, J.D., & Francis, S.H. (1999). Cyclic GMP phosphodiesterase-5: target of sildenafil. *J Biol Chem,* Vol.274, No.20, (May 1999), pp. 13729-13732, PMID 10318772

Cox, G., & O'Byrne, K.J. (2001). Matrix metalloproteinases and cancer. *Anticancer Res,* Vol.21, No.6B, (Nov-Dec 2001), pp. (4207-4219), PMID 11908674

Curran, S., & Murray, G.I. (1999). Matrix metalloproteinases in tumour invasion and metastasis. *J Pathol*, Vol.189, No.3, (Nov 1999) pp. 300-308, PMID 10547590

Curran, S., & Murray, G.I. (2000). Matrix metalloproteinases: molecular aspects of their roles in tumour invasion and metastasis. *Eur J Cancer,* Vol.36, No.13 Spec no, (Aug 2000), pp. 1621-1630, PMID 10959048

Deguchi, A.J., Soh, W., Li, H., Pamukcu, R., Thompson, W.J., & Weinstein, I.B. (2002). Vasodilator-stimulated phosphoprotein (VASP) phosphorylation provides a biomarker for the action of exisulind and related agents that activate protein kinase G. *Mol Cancer Ther*, Vol.1, No.10, (Aug 2001), pp. 803-809, PMID 12492114

Di Guglielmo, M.D., Park, J., Schulz, S., & Waldman, S.A. (2001). Nucleotide requirements for CDX2 binding to the cis promoter element mediating intestine-specific expression of guanylyl cyclase C. *FEBS Lett*, Vol.507, No.2, (Oct 2001), pp. 128-132, PMID 11684084

Dienstmann, R. ,& Tabernero, J. (2010). Necitumumab, a fully human IgG1 mAb directed against the EGFR for the potential treatment of cancer. *Curr Opin Investig Drugs,* Vol.11, No.12, (Dec 2010), pp. 1434-1441, PMID 21154125

Dong, Y., Wang, J., Sheng, Z., Li, G., Ma, H., Wang, X., Zhang, R., Lu, G., Hu, Q., Sugimura, H., & Zhou, X. (2009). Downregulation of EphA1 in colorectal carcinomas correlates with invasion and metastasis. *Mod Pathol*, Vol.22, No.1, (Jan 2009) pp. 151-160, PMID 19011600

Fidler, I.J. (1970). Metastasis: guantitative analysis of distribution and fate of tumor embolilabeled with 125 I-5-iodo-2'-deoxyuridine. *J Natl Cancer Inst*, Vol.45, No.4, (Oct1 970), pp. 773-782, PMID 5513503

Fidler, I.J., Gersten, D.M., & Hart, I.R. (1978). The biology of cancer invasion and metastasis. *Adv Cancer Res,* Vol.28, pp. (149-250), PMID 360795.

Fidler, I.J. (2001). Seed and soil revisited: contribution of the organ microenvironment to cancer metastasis. *Surg Oncol Clin N Am*, Vol.10, No.2, (April 2001), pp. 257-269, PMID 11382586

Fidler, I.J. (2003). The pathogenesis of cancer metastasis: the 'seed and soil' hypothesis revisited. *Nat Rev Cancer*, Vol.3, No.6, (Jun 2003), pp. 453-458, PMID 12778135

Fodde, R., Kuipers, J., Rosenberg, C., Smits, R., Kielman, M., Gaspar, C., van Es, J.H., Breukel, C., Wiegant, J., Giles, R.H., & Clevers, H. (2001). Mutations in the APC tumour suppressor gene cause chromosomal instability. *Nat Cell Biol*, Vol.3, No.4, (April 2001), pp. 433-438, PMID 11283620

Folkman, J. (1986). How is blood vessel growth regulated in normal and neoplastic tissue? G.H.A. Clowes memorial Award lecture. *Cancer Res*, Vol.46, No.2, (Feb 1986), pp. 467-473, PMID 2416426

Forte, L.R. (1999). Guanylin regulatory peptides: structures, biological activities mediated by cyclic GMP and pathobiology. *Regul Pept*, Vol.81, No.1-3, (May 1999), pp. 25-39, PMID 10395405

Francis, S.H., Blount M.A., & Corbin, J.D. (2011). Mammalian cyclic nucleotide phosphodiesterases: molecular mechanisms and physiological functions. *Physiol Rev*, Vol.91, No.2, (Apr 2011), pp. 651-690, PMID 21527734

Fridman, R., Toth, M., Chvyrkova, I., Meroueh, S.O., & Mobashery, S. (2003). Cell surface association of matrix metalloproteinase-9 (gelatinase B). *Cancer Metastasis Rev*, Vol.22, No.2-3, (Jun-Sep 2003), pp. 153-166, PMID 12784994

Fulton, A.M. (2009). The chemokine receptors CXCR4 and CXCR3 in cancer. *Curr Oncol Rep*, Vol.11, No.2, (Mar 2009), pp. 125-131, PMID 19216844

Gali, H., Sieckman, G.L., Hoffman, T.J., Owen, N.K., Chin, D.T., Forte, L.R., & Volkert, W.A. (2001). In vivo evaluation of an 111In-labeled ST-peptide analog for specific-targeting of human colon cancers. *Nucl Med Biol*, Vol.28, No.8, (Nov 2001), pp. 903-909, PMID 11711309

Gama, L., Baxendale-Cox, L.M., & Breitwieser, G.E. (1997). Ca2+-sensing receptors in intestinal epithelium. *Am J Physiol*, Vol.273, No.4Pt1, (Oct 1997), pp. C1168-C1175, PMID 9357760

Gibbons, A.V., Snook, A.E., Li, P., Lin, J.E., DeGodoy, M., Rattan, S.C., Dasgupta, A., Schulz, S., Pitari, G.M., & Waldman, S.A. (2009). The intestinal tumor susceptibility gene product GUCY2C coordinates epithelial-mesenchymal interactions opposing the tumorigenic stromal niche through TGF-β_1, *Proceedings of American Association for Cancer Research Annual Meeting*, Denver (CO), Apr 2009

Goldberg, G.I., Strongin, A., Collier, I.E., Genrich, L.T., & Marmer, B.L. (1992). Interaction of 92-kDa type IV collagenase with the tissue inhibitor of metalloproteinases prevents dimerization, complex formation with interstitial collagenase, and activation of the proenzyme with stromelysin. *J Biol Chem*, Vol.267, No.7, (March 1992), pp. 4583-4591, PMID 1311314

Gong, R., Ding, C., Hu, J., Lu, Y., Liu, F., Mann, E., Xu, F., Cohen, MB., & Luo M. (2011). Role for the Membrane Receptor Guanylyl Cyclase-C in Attention Deficiency and Hyperactive Behavior. *Science*, (Epub ahead of print), PMID 21835979

Gregorieff, A., & Clevers, H. (2005). Wnt signaling in the intestinal epithelium: from endoderm to cancer. *Genes Dev*, Vol. 19, No.8, (April 2005), pp. 877-890, PMID 15833914

Gryfe, R., Swallow, C., Bapat, B., Redston, M., Gallinger, S., & Couture, J. (1997). Molecular biology of colorectal cancer. *Curr Probl Cancer*, Vol.21, No.5, (Sept-Oct 1997), pp. 233-300, PMID 9438104

Guarino, A., Guandalini,S., Alessio,M., Gentile,F., Tarallo,L., Capano,G., Migliavacca,M., & Rubino,A. (1989). Characteristics and mechanism of action of a heat-stable enterotoxin produced by Klebsiella pneumoniae from infants with secretory diarrhea. *Pediatr Res*, Vol.25, No.5, (May 1989), pp. 514-518, PMID 2470015

Gurjar, M.V., Sharma, R.V., & Bhalla, R.C. (1999). eNOS gene transfer inhibits smooth muscle cell migration and MMP-2 and MMP-9 activity. *Arterioscler Thromb Vasc Biol*, Vol.19, No.12, (Dec 1999) pp. 2871-2877, PMID 10591663

Hamra, F.K., Eber, S.L., Chin, D.T., Currie, M.G., & Forte, L.R. (1997). Regulation of intestinal uroguanylin/guanylin receptor-mediated responses by mucosal acidity. *Proc Natl Acad Sci U S A*, Vol.94, No.6, (March 1997), pp. 2705-2710, PMID 9122260

Han, X., Mann, E., Gilbert, S., Guan, Y., Steinbrecher, K.A., Montrose, M.H., & Cohen, M.B. (2011). Loss of guanylyl cyclase C (GCC) signaling leads to dysfunctional intestinal barrier. *PLoS One*, Vol.6, No.1, (Jan 2011), pp. e16139, PMID 21305056

Hanahan, D., & Weinberg, R.A. (2000). The hallmarks of cancer. *Cell*, Vol.100, No.1, (Jan 2000), pp. 57-70, PMID 10647931

Heppner, G.H. (1984). Tumor heterogeneity. *Cancer Res*, Vol.44, No.6, (Jun 2000), pp. 2259-2265, PMID 6372991

Hofer, A.M., & Brown, E.M. (2003). Extracellular calcium sensing and signalling. *Nat Rev Mol Cell Biol*, Vol.4, No.7, (July 2003), pp. 530-538, PMID, 12838336

Im, J.H., Fu, W., Wang, H., Bhatia, S.K., Hammer, D.A., Kowalska, M.A., & Muschel, R.J. (2004). Coagulation facilitates tumor cell spreading in the pulmonary vasculature during early metastatic colony formation. *Cancer Res*, Vol.64, No.23, (Dec 2004), pp. 8613-8619, PMID 15574768

Jemal, A., Bray, F., Center, M.M., Ferlay, J., Ward, E. & Forman, D. (2011). Global cancer statistics. *CA Cancer J Clin*, Vol.61, No.2, (March-Apr 2011), pp. 69-90, PMID 21296855

Kallay, E., Bonner, E., Wrba, F., Thakker, R.V., Peterlik, M., & Cross, H.S. (2003). Molecular and functional characterization of the extracellular calcium-sensing receptor in human colon cancer cells. *Oncol Res*, Vol.13, No.12, pp. 551-559, PMID 12899245

Kitamura, T., Fujishita, T., Loetscher, P., Revesz, L., Hashida, H., Kizaka-Kondoh, S., Aoki, M., & Taketo, M.M. (2010). Inactivation of chemokine (C-C motif) receptor 1 (CCR1) suppresses colon cancer liver metastasis by blocking accumulation of immature myeloid cells in a mouse model. *Proc Natl Acad Sci U S A*, Vol.107, No.29, (July 2010), pp. 13063-13068, PMID

Koldovsky, O., Dobiasova, M., Hahn, P., Kolinska, J., Kraml, J., & Pacha, J. (1995). Development of gastrointestinal functions. *Physiol Res*, Vol.44, No.6, pp. 341-348, PMID 20616008

Korinek, V., Barker, N., Moerer, P., van Donselaar, E., Huls, G., Peters, P.J., & Clevers, H. (1998). Depletion of epithelial stem-cell compartments in the small intestine of mice lacking Tcf-4. *Nat Genet*, Vol. 19, No.4, (Aug 1998), pp. 379-383, PMID 8798267

Kraus, S., & Arber, N. (2009). Inflammation and colorectal cancer. *Curr Opin Pharmacol*, Vol.9, No.4, (Aug 2009), pp. 405-410, PMID 19589728

Krause, M., Dent, E.W., Bear, J.E., Loureiro, J.J., & Gertler, F.B. (2003). Ena/VASP proteins: regulators of the actin cytoskeleton and cell migration. *Annu Rev Cell Dev Biol*, Vol.19, pp. 541-564, PMID 14570581

Kroemer, G. (2006). Mitochondria in cancer. *Oncogene*, Vol.25, No.34, (Aug 2003) pp. 4630-4632, PMID 16892077

Larsen, C.A., & Dashwood, R.H. (2010). (-)-Epigallocatechin-3-gallate inhibits Met signaling, proliferation, and invasiveness in human colon cancer cells. *Arch Biochem Biophys*, Vol.501, No.1, (Sep 2010), pp. 52-57, PMID 20361925

Leppert, D., Hauser, S.L., Kishiyama, J.L., An, S., Zeng, L., & Goetzl, E.J. (1995). Stimulation of matrix metalloproteinase-dependent migration of T cells by eicosanoids. *FASEB J*, Vol.9, No.14, (Nov 1995), pp. 1473-1481, PMID 7589989

Li, P., Lin, J.E., Chervoneva, I., Schulz, S., Waldman, S.A., & Pitari, G.M. (2007a). Homeostatic control of the crypt-villus axis by the bacterial enterotoxin receptor guanylyl cyclase C restricts the proliferating compartment in intestine. *Am J Pathol*, Vol.171, No.6, (Dec 2007), pp. 1847-1858, PMID 17974601

Li, P., Schulz, S., Bombonati, A., Palazzo, J.P., Hyslop, T.M., Xu, Y., Baran, A.A., Siracusa, L.D., Pitari, G.M., & Waldman, S.A. (2007b). Guanylyl cyclase C suppresses intestinal tumorigenesis by restricting proliferation and maintaining genomic integrity. *Gastroenterology*, Vol.133, No.2, (Aug 2007), pp. 599-607, PMID

Librach, C.L., Werb, Z., Fitzgerald, M.L., Chiu, K., Corwin, N.M., Esteves, R.A., Grobelny, D., Galardy, R., Damsky, C.H., & Fisher, S.J. (1991). 92-kD type IV collagenase mediates invasion of human cytotrophoblasts. *J Cell Biol*, Vol.113, No.2, (April 1991), pp. 437-449, PMID 1849141

Lin, J.E., Li, P., Snook, A.E., Schulz, S., Dasgupta, A., Hyslop, T.M., Gibbons, A.V., Marszlowicz, G., Pitari, G.M., & Waldman, S.A. (2010). The hormone receptor GUCY2C suppresses intestinal tumor formation by inhibiting AKT signaling. *Gastroenterology*, Vol.138, No.1, (Jan 2010), pp. 241-254, PMID 19737566

Linder, S. (2007). The matrix corroded: podosomes and invadopodia in extracellular matrix degradation. *Trends Cell Biol*, Vol.17, No.3, (March 2007), pp. 107-117, PMID 17275303

Lindsay, S.L., Ramsey, S., Aitchison, M., Renne, T., & Evans, T.J. (2007). Modulation of lamellipodial structure and dynamics by NO-dependent phosphorylation of VASP Ser239. *J Cell Sci*, Vol.120, No.Pt17, (Sep 2007), pp. 3011-3021, PMID 17684063

Lipkin, M., & Newmark, H. (1995). Calcium and the prevention of colon cancer. *J Cell Biochem Suppl*, Vol.22, pp. 65-73, PMID 8538212

Liu, L., Li, H., Underwood, T., Lloyd, M., David, M., Sperl, G., Pamukcu, R., & Thompson, W.J. (2001). Cyclic GMP-dependent protein kinase activation and induction by exisulind and CP461 in colon tumor cells. *J Pharmacol Exp Ther*, Vol.299, No.2, (Nov 2001), pp. 583-592, PMID 11602670

Lubbe, W.J., Zhou, Z.Y., Fu, W., Zuzga, D., Schulz, S., Fridman, R., Muschel, R.J., Waldman, S.A., & Pitari, G.M. (2006). Tumor epithelial cell matrix metalloproteinase 9 is a target for antimetastatic therapy in colorectal cancer. *Clin Cancer Res*, Vol.12, No.6, (March), pp. 1876-1882, PMID 16551873

Lubbe, W.J., Zuzga, D.S., Zhou, Z., Fu, W., Pelta-Heller, J., Muschel, R.J., Waldman, S.A., & Pitari, G.M. (2009). Guanylyl cyclase C prevents colon cancer metastasis by regulating tumor epithelial cell matrix metalloproteinase-9. *Cancer Res*, Vol.69, No.8, (April 2009), pp. 3529-3536, PMID 19336567

Lucas, K.A., Pitari, G.M., Kazerounian, S., Ruiz-Stewart, I., Park, J., Schulz, S., Chepenik, K.P., & Waldman, S.A. (2000). Guanylyl cyclases and signaling by cyclic GMP. *Pharmacol Rev*, Vol.52, No.3, (Sep 2000), pp. 375-414, PMID 10977868

McCawley, L.J., & Matrisian, L.M. (2001). Tumor progression: defining the soil round the tumor seed. *Curr Biol*, Vol.11, No.1, (Jan 2001), pp. R25-R27, PMID 11166192

Mehlen, P., & Puisieux, A. (2006). Metastasis: a question of life or death. *Nat Rev Cancer*, Vol.6, No.6, (Jun 2006), pp. 449-458, PMID 16723991

Mejia, A., Schulz, S., Hyslop, T., Weinberg, D.S., & Waldman, S.A. (2010). Molecular staging estimates occult tumor burden in colorectal cancer. *Adv Clin Chem*, Vol.52, pp. 19-39, PMID 21275338

Mejillano, M.R., Kojima, S., Applewhite, D.A., Gertler, F.B., Svitkina, T.M., & Borisy, G.G. (2004). Lamellipodial versus filopodial mode of the actin nanomachinery: pivotal role of the filament barbed end. *Cell*, Vol.118, No.3, (Aug 2004), pp. 363-373, PMID 15294161

Meyerhardt, J.A., & Mayer, R.J. (2005). Systemic therapy for colorectal cancer. *N Engl J Med*, Vol.352, No.5, (Feb 2005), pp. 476-487, PMID 15689586

Montgomery, R.K., Mulberg, A.E., & Grand, R.J. (1999). Development of the human gastrointestinal tract: twenty years of progress. *Gastroenterology*, Vol.116, No.3, (March 1999), pp. 702-731, PMID 10029630

Nascimento, C.F., Gama-De-Souza, L.N., Freitas, V.M., & Jaeger, R.G. (2010). Role of MMP9 on invadopodia formation in cells from adenoid cystic carcinoma. Study by laser scanning confocal microscopy. *Microsc Res Tech*, Vol.73, No.2, (Feb), pp. 99-108, PMID 19658178

Nicolson, G.L. (1988). Cancer metastasis: tumor cell and host organ properties important in metastasis to specific secondary sites. *Biochim Biophys Acta*, Vol.948, No.2, (Nov 1998), pp. 175-224, PMID 3052592

Notterman, D.A., Alon, U., Sierk, A.J., & Levine, A.J. (2001). Transcriptional gene expression profiles of colorectal adenoma, adenocarcinoma, and normal tissue examined by oligonucleotide arrays. *Cancer Res*, Vol.61, No.7, (April 2001), pp. 3124-3130, PMID 11306497

Ongchin, M., Sharratt, E., Dominguez, I., Simms, N., Wang, J., Cheney, R., LeVea, C., Brattain, M., & Rajput, A. (2009). The effects of epidermal growth factor receptor activation and attenuation of the TGF beta pathway in an orthotopic model of colon cancer. *J Surg Res*, Vol.156, No.2, (Oct 2009), pp. 250-256, PMID 19524264

Park, J., Schulz, S., & Waldman, S.A. (2000). Intestine-specific activity of the human guanylyl cyclase C promoter is regulated by Cdx2. *Gastroenterology*, Vol.119, No.1, (July 2000) pp. 89-96, PMID 10889158

Pelicano, H., Martin, D.S., Xu, R.H., & Huang, P. (2006). Glycolysis inhibition for anticancer treatment. *Oncogene*, Vol.25, No.34, (Aug 2006), pp. 4633-4646, PMID 16892078

Pfeifer, A., Ruth, P., Dostmann, W., Sausbier, M., Klatt, P., & Hofmann, F. (1999). Structure and function of cGMP-dependent protein kinases. *Rev Physiol Biochem Pharmacol*, Vol.135, pp. 105-149, PMID 9932482

Pihl, E., Hughes, E.S., McDermott, F.T., Milne, BJ., & Price, A.B. (1981). Disease-free survival and recurrence after resection of colorectal carcinoma. *J Surg Oncol*, Vol.16, No.4, pp. 333-341, PMID 7253653

Pinchuk, I.V., Mifflin, R.C., Saada, J.I., and Powell, D.W. (2010). Intestinal mesenchymal cells. *Curr Gastroenterol Rep*, Vol.12, No.5, (Oct 2010), pp. 310-318, PMID 20690004

Pinto, D., and Clevers, H. (2005). Wnt, stem cells and cancer in the intestine. *Biol Cell*, Vol.97, No.3, (Mar 2005), pp. 185-196. PMID 15715524

Pitari, G.M., Di Guglielmo, M.D., Park, J., Schulz, S., and Waldman, S.A. (2001). Guanylyl cyclase C agonists regulate progression through the cell cycle of human colon carcinoma cells. *Proc Natl Acad Sci U S A*. Vol.98, No.14, (July 2001), pp. 7846-7851, PMID 11438734

Pitari, G.M., Zingman, L.V., Hodgson, D.M., Alekseev, A.E., Kazerounian, S., Bienengraeber, M., Hajnoczky, G., Terzic, A., & Waldman, S.A. (2003). Bacterial enterotoxins are associated with resistance to colon cancer. *Proc Natl Acad Sci U S A*, Vol.100, No.5, (March 2003), pp. 2695-2699, PMID 12594332

Pitari, G.M., Baksh, R.I., Harris, D.M., Li, P., Kazerounian, S., and Waldman, S.A. (2005). Interruption of homologous desensitization in cyclic guanosine 3',5'-monophosphate signaling restores colon cancer cytostasis by bacterial enterotoxins. *Cancer Res*, Vol.65, No.23, (Dec 2005), pp. 11129-11135, PMID 16322263

Pitari, G.M., Li, P., Lin, J.E., Zuzga, D., Gibbons, A.V., Snook, A.E., Schulz, S., & Waldman, S.A. (2007). The paracrine hormone hypothesis of colorectal cancer. *Clin Pharmacol Ther*, Vol.82, No.4, (Oct 2007) pp. 441-447, PMID 17687268

Pitari, GM., Lin, J.E., Shah, F.J., Lubbe, W.J., Zuzga, D.S., Li, P., Schulz, S., and Waldman, S.A. (2008). Enterotoxin preconditioning restores calcium-sensing receptor-mediated cytostasis in colon cancer cells. *Carcinogenesis*, Vol.29, No.8, (Aug 2008), pp. 1601-1607, PMID 18566015

Polyak, K., & Weinberg, R.A. (2009). Transitions between epithelial and mesenchymal states: acquisition of malignant and stem cell traits. *Nat Rev Cancer*, Vol.9, No.4, (April 2009), pp. 265-273, PMID 19262571

Potten, C.S., & Loeffler, M. (1990). Stem cells: attributes, cycles, spirals, pitfalls and uncertainties. Lessons for and from the crypt. *Development*, Vol.110, No.4, (Dec 1990), pp. 1001-1020, PMID 2100251

Qian, X., Wang, T.N., Rothman, V.L., Nicosia, R.F., & Tuszynski, G.P. (1997). Thrombospondin-1 modulates angiogenesis in vitro by up-regulation of matrix metalloproteinase-9 in endothelial cells. *Exp Cell Res*, Vol.235, No.2, (Sep 1997), pp. 403-412, PMID 9299165

Ramos-DeSimone, N., Hahn-Dantona, E., Sipley, J., Nagase, H., French, D.L., & Quigley, J.P. (1999). Activation of matrix metalloproteinase-9 (MMP-9) via a converging plasmin/stromelysin-1 cascade enhances tumor cell invasion. *J Biol Chem*, Vol.274, No.19, (May 1999), pp. 13066-13076, PMID 10224058

Reya, T., and Clevers, H. (2005). Wnt signalling in stem cells and cancer. *Nature*, Vol.434, No.7035, (April 2005) pp. 843-850, PMID 15829953

Rhee, S.G. (2001). Regulation of phosphoinositide-specific phospholipase C. *Annu Rev Biochem*, Vol.70, pp. 281-312, PMID 11395409

Rozen, P., Fireman, Z., Fine, N., Wax, Y., & Ron, E. (1989). Oral calcium suppresses increased rectal epithelial proliferation of persons at risk of colorectal cancer. *Gut*, Vol.30, No.5, (May 1989), pp. 650-655, PMID 2731758

Sakatani, T., Kaneda, A., Iacobuzio-Donahue, C.A., Carter, M.G., de Boom Witzel, S., Okano, H., Ko, M.S., Ohlsson, R., Longo, D.L., & Feinberg, A.P. (2005). Loss of imprinting of Igf2 alters intestinal maturation and tumorigenesis in mice. *Science*, Vol.307, No.5717, (March 2005), pp. 1976-1978, PMID 15731405

Sanceau, J., Truchet, S., & Bauvois, B. (2003). Matrix metalloproteinase-9 silencing by RNA interference triggers the migratory-adhesive switch in Ewing's sarcoma cells. *J Biol Chem*, Vol.278, No.38, (Sep 2003), pp. 36537-36546, PMID 12847101

Schulz, S., Singh, S., Bellet, R.A., Singh, G., Tubb, D.J., Chin, H., & Garbers, D.L. (1989). The primary structure of a plasma membrane guanylate cyclase demonstrates diversity within this new receptor family. *Cell*, Vol.58, No.6, (Sep 1989), pp. 1155-1162, PMID 2570641

Schulz, S., Hyslop, T., Haaf, J., Bonaccorso, C., Nielsen, K., Witek, M.E., Birbe, R., Palazzo, J., Weinberg, D., & Waldman, S.A. (2006). A validated quantitative assay to detect occult micrometastases by reverse transcriptase-polymerase chain reaction of guanylyl cyclase C in patients with colorectal cancer. *Clin Cancer Res*, Vol.12, No.15, (Aug 2006), pp. 4545-4552, PMID 16899600

Schultz, R.M., Silberman, S., Persky, B., Bajkowski, A.S., & Carmichael, D.F. (1988). Inhibition by human recombinant tissue inhibitor of metalloproteinases of human amnion invasion and lung colonization by murine B16-F10 melanoma cells. *Cancer Res*, Vol.48, No.19, (Oct 1988), pp. 5539-5545, PMID 3416307

Shailubhai, K., Yu, H.H., Karunanandaa, K., Wang, J.Y., Eber, S.L., Wang, Y., Joo, N.S., Kim, H.D., Miedema, B.W., Abbas, S.Z., Boddupalli, S.S., Currie, M.G., & Forte, L.R. (2000). Uroguanylin treatment suppresses polyp formation in the Apc(Min/+) mouse and induces apoptosis in human colon adenocarcinoma cells via cyclic GMP. *Cancer Res,* Vol.60, No.18, (Sep 2000), pp. 5151-5157, PMID 11016642

Shapiro, S. (1992). Goals of screening. *Cancer,* Vol.70, No.5, (Sep 1992), pp. 1252-1258, PMID 1511372

Sheinin, Y., Kallay, E., Wrba, F., Kriwanek, S., Peterlik, M., & Cross, H.S. (2000). Immunocytochemical localization of the extracellular calcium-sensing receptor in normal and malignant human large intestinal mucosa. *J Histochem Cytochem,* Vol.48, No.5, (May 2000), pp. 595-602, PMID 10769043

Shipley, J.M., Doyle, G.A., Fliszar, C.J., Ye, Q.Z., Johnson, L.L., Shapiro, S.D., Welgus, H.G., & Senior, R.M. (1996). The structural basis for the elastolytic activity of the 92-kDa and 72-kDa gelatinases. Role of the fibronectin type II-like repeats. *J Biol Chem,* Vol.271, No.8, (Feb 1996), pp. 4335-4341, PMID 8626782

Siegel, R., Ward, E., Brawley, O., & Jemal, A. (2011). Cancer statistics, 2011: The impact of eliminating socioeconomic and racial disparities on premature cancer deaths. *CA Cancer J Clin,* Vol.61, No.4, (July-Aug 2011), pp. 212-236, PMID 21685461

Small, J.V., Anderson, K., & Rottner, K. (1996). Actin and the coordination of protrusion, attachment and retraction in cell crawling. *Biosci Rep,* Vol.16, No.5, (Oct 1996), pp. 351-368, PMID 8913526

Spruck, C.H., Won, K.A., & Reed, S.I. (1999). Deregulated cyclin E induces chromosome instability. *Nature,* Vol.401, No.6750, (Sep 1999) pp. 297-300, PMID 10499591

St-Pierre, Y., Van Themsche, C., & Esteve, P.O. (2003). Emerging features in the regulation of MMP-9 gene expression for the development of novel molecular targets and therapeutic strategies. *Curr Drug Targets Inflamm Allergy,* Vol.2, No.3 (Sep 2003), pp. 206-215, PMID 14561155

Stamenkovic, I. (2003). Extracellular matrix remodelling: the role of matrix metalloproteinases. *J Pathol,* Vol.200, No.4, (July 2003), pp. 448-464, PMID12845612

Steeg, P.S. (2006). Tumor metastasis: mechanistic insights and clinical challenges. *Nat Med,* Vol.12, No.8, (Aug 2006), pp. 895-904, PMID 16892035

Steinbrecher, K.A., Tuohy, T.M., Heppner Goss, K., Scott, M.C., Witte, D.P., Groden, J., & Cohen, MB. (2000). Expression of guanylin is downregulated in mouse and human intestinal adenomas. *Biochem Biophys Res Commun,* Vol.273, No.1, (Jun 2000), pp. (225-230), PMID 10873591

Steinbrecher, K.A., Wowk, S.A., Rudolph, J.A., Witte, D.P., & Cohen, M.B. (2002). Targeted inactivation of the mouse guanylin gene results in altered dynamics of colonic epithelial proliferation. *Am J Pathol,* Vol.161, No.6, (Dec 2002), pp. 2169-2178, PMID 12466132

Steinbrecher, K.A., & Cohen, M.B. (2011). Transmembrane guanylate cyclase in intestinal pathophysiology. *Curr Opin Gastroenterol,* Vol.27, No.2, (March 2011), pp. 139-145, PMID 21102322

Suzuki, K., Sun, R., Origuchi, M., Kanehira, M., Takahata, T., Itoh, J., Umezawa, A., Kijima, H., Fukuda, S.,& Saijo, Y. (2011). Mesenchymal Stromal Cells Promote Tumor Growth through the Enhancement of Neovascularization. *Mol Med,* Vol.17, No.7-8, pp. 579-587, PMID 21424106

Tang, Y., Katuri, V., Srinivasan, R., Fogt, F., Redman, R., Anand, G., Said, A., Fishbein, T., Zasloff, M., Reddy, E.P., Mishra, B., & Mishra, L. (2005). Transforming growth factor-beta suppresses nonmetastatic colon cancer through Smad4 and adaptor protein ELF at an early stage of tumorigenesis. *Cancer Res*, Vol.65, No.10, (May 2005), pp. 4228-4237, PMID 15899814

Thompson, W.J., Piazza, G.A., Li, H., Liu, L., Fetter, J., Zhu, B., Sperl, G., Ahnen, D., & Pamukcu, R. (2000). Exisulind induction of apoptosis involves guanosine 3',5'-cyclic monophosphate phosphodiesterase inhibition, protein kinase G activation, and attenuated beta-catenin. *Cancer Res*, Vol.60, No.13, (July 2000), pp. 3338-334, PMID 10910034

van Engeland, M., Derks, S., Smits, K.M., Meijer, G.A., & Herman, J.G. (2011). Colorectal cancer epigenetics: complex simplicity. *J Clin Oncol*, Vol.29, No.10, (April 2011), pp. 1382-1391, PMID 21220596

van Es, J.H., Jay, P., Gregorieff, A., van Gijn, M.E., Jonkheer, S., Hatzis, P., Thiele, A., van den Born, M., Begthel, H., Brabletz, T., Taketo, M.M., & Clevers, H.(2005). Wnt signalling induces maturation of Paneth cells in intestinal crypts. *Nat Cell Biol*, Vol.7, No.4, (April 2005), pp. 381-386, PMID 15778706

Waldman, S.A., Cagir, B., Rakinic, J., Fry, R.D., Goldstein, S.D., Isenberg, G., Barber, M., Biswas, S., Minimo, C., Palazzo, J., Park, PK., & Weinberg, D. (1998). Use of guanylyl cyclase C for detecting micrometastases in lymph nodes of patients with colon cancer. *Dis Colon Rectum*, Vol.41, No.3, (March 1998), pp. 310-315, PMID 9514425

Waldman, S.A., Hyslop, T., Schulz, S., Barkun, A., Nielsen, K., Haaf, J., Bonaccorso, C., Li, Y., & Weinberg, DS. (2009). Association of GUCY2C expression in lymph nodes with time to recurrence and disease-free survival in pN0 colorectal cancer. *JAMA*, Vol.301, No.7, (Feb 2009), pp. 745-752, PMID 19224751

Wang, H., Fu, W., Im, J.H., Zhou, Z., Santoro, S.A., Iyer, V., DiPersio, C.M., Yu, Q.C., Quaranta,V., Al-Mehdi, A., & Muschel, R.J. (2004). Tumor cell alpha3beta1 integrin and vascular laminin-5 mediate pulmonary arrest and metastasis. *J Cell Biol*, Vol.164, No.6, (March 2004), pp. 935-941, PMID 2172296

Warburg, O. (1956). On the origin of cancer cells. *Science*, Vol.123, No.3191, (Feb 1956), pp. 309-314, PMID 13298683

Weiss, L. (1990). Metastatic inefficiency. *Adv Cancer Res*, Vol.54, pp. (159-211), PMID 1688681

Whitaker, T.L., Witte, D.P., Scott, M.C., & Cohen, M.B. (1997). Uroguanylin and guanylin: distinct but overlapping patterns of messenger RNA expression in mouse intestine. *Gastroenterology*, Vol.113, No.3, (Sep), pp. 1000-1006, PMID 9287995

Whitfield, J.F. (1992). Calcium signals and cancer. *Crit Rev Oncog*, Vol.3, No.1-2, pp. 55-90, PMID 1550862

Whitfield, J.F., Bird, R.P., Chakravarthy, B.R., Isaacs, R.J., & Morley, P. (1995). Calcium-cell cycle regulator, differentiator, killer, chemopreventor, and maybe, tumor promoter. *J Cell Biochem Suppl*, Vol.22, pp. 74-91, PMID 8538213

Witek, M.E., Nielsen, K., Walters, R., Hyslop, T., Palazzo, J., Schulz, S., & Waldman, S.A. (2005). The putative tumor suppressor Cdx2 is overexpressed by human colorectal adenocarcinomas. *Clin Cancer Res*, Vol.11, (Dec 2005), pp. 8549-8556, PMID 16361536

Witz, I.P., & Levy-Nissenbaum, O. (2006). The tumor microenvironment in the post-PAGET era. *Cancer Lett*, Vol.242, No.1, (Oct 2006), pp. 1-10, PMID 16413116

Wolfe, H.R., Mendizabal, M., Lleong, E., Cuthbertson, A., Desai, V., Pullan, S., Fujii, D.K., Morrison, M., Pither, R. and Waldman, S.A. (2002). In vivo imaging of human colon cancer xenografts in immunodeficient mice using a guanylyl cyclase C--specific ligand. *J Nucl Med*, Vol.43, No.3, (March 2002), pp. 392-399, PMID 11884500

World Health Organization (WHO). (February 2011). Cancer, In: *WHO fact sheet N°297*, 29.07.2011, Available from: http://www.who.int/mediacentre/factsheets/fs297/

Yamaguchi, H., & Condeelis, J. (2007). Regulation of the actin cytoskeleton in cancer cell migration and invasion. *Biochim Biophys Acta*, Vol.1773, No.5, (May 2007), pp. 642-652, PMID 16926057

Yaroslavskiy, B.B., Zhang, Y., Kalla, S.E., Garcia Palacios,V., Sharrow, A.C., Li, Y., Zaidi, M., Wu, C., & Blair, HC. (2005). NO-dependent osteoclast motility: reliance on cGMP-dependent protein kinase I and VASP. *J Cell Sci*, Vol.118, No.Pt23, (Dec 2005), pp. 5479-5487, PMID 16291726

Yu, H.G., Tong, S.L., Ding, Y.M., Ding, J., Fang, X.M., Zhang, X.F., Liu, Z.J., Zhou, Y.H., Liu, Q.S., Luo, H.S., & Yu, J.P. (2006). Enhanced expression of cholecystokinin-2 receptor promotes the progression of colon cancer through activation of focal adhesion kinase. *Int J Cancer*, Vol.119, No.12, (Dec 2006), pp. 2724-2732, PMID 16998832

Yu, Q., & Stamenkovic, I. (1999). Localization of matrix metalloproteinase 9 to the cell surface provides a mechanism for CD44-mediated tumor invasion. *Genes Dev*, Vol.13, No.1, (Jan 1999), pp. 35-48, PMID 9887098

Yu, Q., & Stamenkovic I. (2000). Cell surface-localized matrix metalloproteinase-9 proteolytically activates TGF-beta and promotes tumor invasion and angiogenesis. *Genes Dev*, Vol.14, No.2, (Jan), pp. 163-176, PMID 10652271

Zhang, Q., Furukawa, K., Chen, H.H., Sakakibara,T., & Urano T. (2006). Metastatic potential of mouse Lewis lung cancer cells is regulated via ganglioside GM1 by modulating the matrix metalloprotease-9 localization in lipid rafts. *J Biol Chem*, Vol.281, No.26, (Jun 2006), pp. 18145-18155, PMID 16636068

Zucker, S., & Vacirca, J. (2004). Role of matrix metalloproteinases (MMPs) in colorectal cancer. *Cancer Metastasis Rev*, Vol.23, No.1-2, (Jan-Jun 2004), pp. 101-117, PMID 15000152

Zufall, F., Shepherd, GM., & Barnstable, CJ. (1997). Cyclic nucleotide gated channels as regulators of CNS development and plasticity. *Curr Opin Neurobiol*, Vol.7, No.3, (Jun 1997), pp. 404-412, PMID 9232810

Zuzga, D.S., Gibbons, A.V., Li, P., Lubbe, W.J., Chervoneva, I. & Pitari, G.M. (2008). Overexpression of matrix metalloproteinase 9 in tumor epithelial cells correlates with colorectal cancer metastasis. *Clin Transl Sci*, Vol.1, No.2, (Sep 2008), pp. 136-141, PMID 20443834

Zuzga, D.S., Pelta-Heller, J., Li, P., Bombonati, A., Waldman, S.A., & Pitari, GM. (2011). Phosphorylation of vasodilator-stimulated phosphoprotein Ser239 suppresses filopodia and invadopodia in colon cancer. *Int J Cancer*, (Epub ahead of printing), PMID 21702043

13

Molecular Mechanisms of Lymphatic Metastasis

M.C. Langheinrich[1], V. Schellerer[1], K. Oeckl[1],
M. Stürzl[2], E. Naschberger[2] and R.S. Croner[1]
[1]Department of Surgery, University Hospital Erlangen,
[2]Division of Molecular and Experimental Surgery, Department of Surgery, University Hospital Erlangen,
Germany

1. Introduction

Colorectal cancer (CRC) is the third most common cancer worldwide. Considering the high rate of incidence and mortality of CRC it is critical to determine the mechanisms of its dissemination. Although one of the better characterised tumours the prognosis of patients decreases dramatically when lymphatic metastasis occurs. In addition, the main important prognostic factor of CRC is the stage of tumour at the time of diagnosis, which is defined by the TNM system from the American Joint Committee on Cancer and the International Union Against Cancer. Therefore, during surgical treatment not only the primary tumour but also the draining lymph nodes have to be removed. From multivariate analysis it is known, that the number of examined lymph nodes is an independent prognostic factor. In this context, a prognostic relevance has been demonstrated not only for N0-, but also for N1- and N2-status. Adjuvant chemotherapy is recommended for stage UICC III colon cancer. It has been shown to reduce tumour recurrence and improve overall survival (Schmiegel, Reinacher-Schick et al. 2008). The five-year survival rate drops significantly from the UICC stage I to IV (Table 1). Patients with an early stage tumour (UICC I) have an excellent prognosis and a five-year survival rate of 90%, compared to those with advanced tumours and lymph node metastasis, who have a five-year survival rate of 30-60%. Patients with distant metastasis have a five-year survival rate below 10%.
Thus the prognosis of CRC is significantly influenced by the occurrence of lymph node metastasis and in addition to its value as a prognostic indicator it also affects the therapeutically management of patients. The understanding of molecular mechanisms involved in lymphatic metastases may open the door for future treatment strategies.

2. The lymphatic system

2.1 Development of the lymphatic system

Aspects of the lymphatic fluid and the associated transport system were already mentioned by the ancient Greeks, but it was poorly considered until the 17th century. In 1622 the Italian physician Gasparo Asselli re-identified lymphatic vessels as "milky veins" in the gut of a

Stage			5-year survival rate
UICC	TNM	Dukes	
I a b	T1N0M0 T2N0M0	A	>90%
II a b	T3N0M0 T4N0M0	B	60-80%
III a b c	T1/2N1M0 T3/4N1M0 T1-4N2M0	C	30-60%
IV	T1-4N1-2M1	D	<10%

Table 1. UICC stage and 5-year cancer related survival of patients with CRC.

dog. The embryonic origin of lymphatic vessels remains further unclear. Since the beginning of the 20th century, two developmental theories -the centrifugal and the centripetal- have been controversial debated. The centrifugal theory by Sabin based upon dye and ink injection experiments in pigs. According to her view, lymphatic vessel formation occurs early during embryonic development from isolated primitive lymph sacs that originate from endothelial cells that bud from the veins. The peripheral lymphatic system originates from these primary lymph sacs by endothelial sprouting into the surrounding tissues and organs, where local capillaries are formed (Oliver and Detmar 2002). Simultaneously Huntington and McClure suggested an alternative model, the centripetal theory. In their opinion primary lymph sacs arise from mesenchymal precursor cells, independent of the veins and secondarily establish venous connections.

To date, the development of the lymphatic vasculature system has not been ultimately resolved. Recent molecular analyses describe a polarized expression of the homeobox transcription factor Prox-1 in anterior cardinal vein endothelial cells, which is required for specification of lymphatic endothelial cells (LECs). Prox-1 is a master regulator which drives the transcription of a variety of genes whose expression is associated with key LEC characteristics (Tammela, Petrova et al. 2005).

2.2 Structure and function of the lymphatic system

The lymphatic vascular system is a hierarchical network comprising blind-ended capillaries, collecting vessels, lymph nodes, lymphoid organs and circulation lymphocytes. A number of important physiological functions have been described. It maintains fluid homeostasis by absorbing and draining e.g. interstitial fluids, plasma proteins and cells extravasated from blood vessels and returning them back into the blood circulation (Butler, Isogai et al. 2009). Furthermore, the lymphatic system is also known to be an important part of the body´s immunological surveillance system (Wiig, Keskin et al. 2010). Lymphatic vessels are distributed to most organs, with the exceptions of the central nervous system, bone marrow, cartilage, cornea and epidermis. Due to its dual role, fluid absorption and lymph transport, the structure of lymphatic vessels differ from blood vessels (Schulte-Merker, Sabine et al.

2011). Lymph capillaries are characterized by loose intercellular junctions, no or an incomplete basement membrane. The wall of lymphatic endothelial cells (LECs) is joined to the extracellular matrix by anchoring filaments. These filaments help the vessels open and function. Collecting lymphatic vessels consist of pericytes, which reduce lymphatic fluid extravasation and they are surrounded by smooth muscle cells (Figure 1) (Shayan, Achen et al. 2006).

Tumour cells can take advantage of these structural characteristics to promote their dissemination to lymph nodes or other organs by the process of permeation into peritumoural lymphatics. In addition, LECs secrete chemotactic agents, which can attract tumours cells toward lymphatics, such as CCL21, whose receptor (CCR7) is expressed on some tumour cells (Shields, Emmett et al. 2007). Chemokines may mediate the tumour LEC interaction by increasing the interactive surface area (Ji 2006).

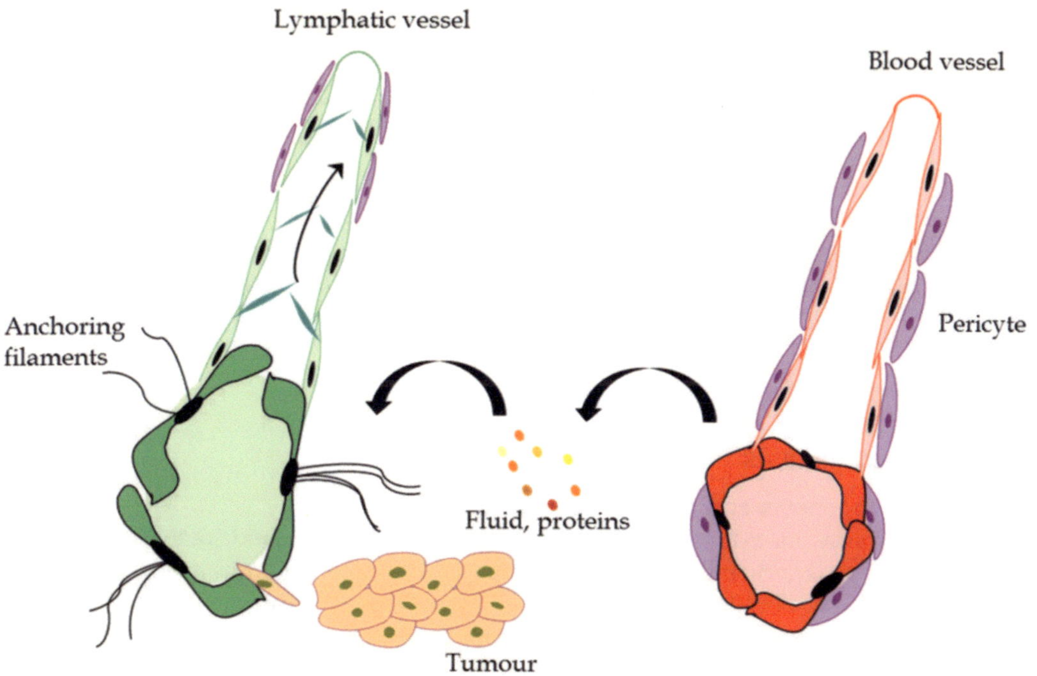

Fig. 1. Structure of lymphatic vessels compared against blood vessels. The initial lymphatics have no or an incomplete basement membrane and no pericytes, which makes them suitable for the uptake of tumour cells. Anchoring filaments attach LECs to the extracellular matrix (ECM) and prevent vessel collapse.

Gene expression profiles of LECs and blood endothelial cells (BECs) have been analysed and compared (Figure 2). The most obvious differences were detected in genes coding for pro-inflammatory cytokines/chemokines and their receptors, cytoskeletal and cell matrix organisation (Saharinen, Tammela et al. 2004). For example Interleukin (IL)-8, IL-6, the chemokine receptor CXCR4, ICAM-1, Integrin α5 are expressed in higher levels in the BECs.

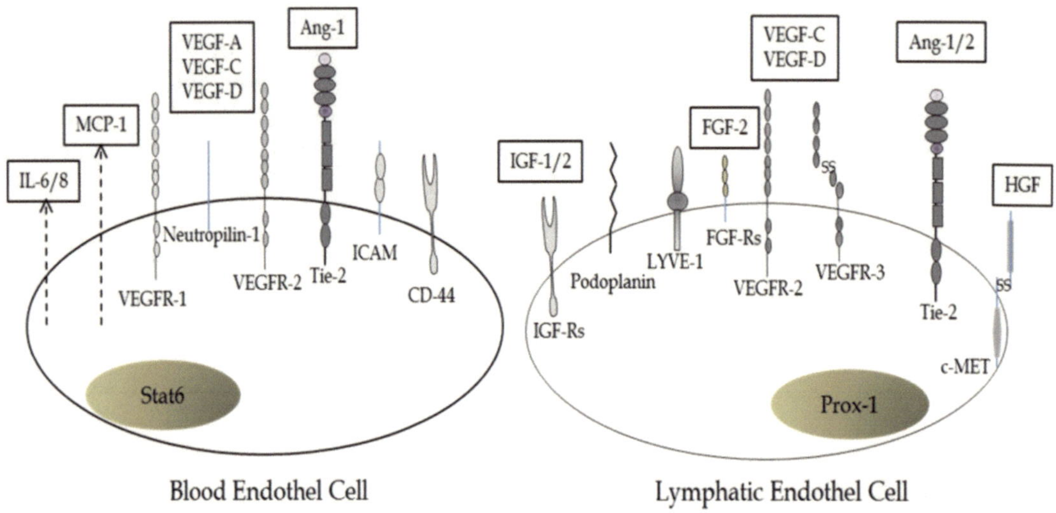

Abbreviations: Stat6 (signal transducer and activator of transcription 6), MCP-1 (monocyte chemotactic protein-1), IL-6/8 (Interleukin-6/-8), ICAM (intracellular adhesion molecule), Ang-1 (Angiopoietin-1), VEGF/ R (Vascular endothelial growth factor/receptor), CD-44 (Cluster of Differentiation 44), IGF-1/2 (Insulin like growth factor 1/2), FGF-2 (Fibroblast growth factor 2), HGF (Hepatocyte growth factor), c-MET (mesenchymal epithelial transition factor), Tie-2 (angiopoietin receptor 2). Note that not all molecular markers are shown.

Fig. 2. Molecular characteristics of BECs and LECs.

3. Lymphangiogenesis

3.1 Lymphangiogenesis and cancer metastasis

Lymphangiogenesis takes place in a variety of physiological and pathophysiological processes, such as embryonic development, regeneration and wound healing on the one hand, and in lymph vascular malformations, inflammation and cancer on the other hand (Witte, Jones et al. 2006). Carcinogenesis is a complex multi-step process and despite the importance, that the lymphatic system provided one of the main routes for cancer progression, little information has been available about the molecular mechanisms by which the tumour cells gain access to the lymph system and are able to spread.

Traditionally, lymphatic metastasis of tumours was considered to be a passive process, where tumour cells metastasized to lymph nodes by utilizing pre-existing lymphatic vessels via open junctions or that lymphatic vessel entry occurred by tumour eroding. The process of new lymphatic formation (lymphangiogenesis) does not occur.

This view has been challenged (Achen and Stacker 2008). The identification of lymphatic specific markers, lymphangiogenic growth factors and their ligand receptor pathways, the

isolation of lymphatic endothelial cells and the development of specific in vitro culture systems in the past decades led to a broader understanding of the molecular mechanisms that control lymphatic metastasis.
Yet there is mounting evidence that lymphangiogenesis does occur in tumours and that it promotes cancer progression. A shift in the balance between lymphangiogenic and anti-lymphangiogenic signalling, like in the process of angiogenesis, might lead to lymphangiogenesis. Therefore a wide range of interactions at the tumour host interface have to take place, which support tumour proliferation, migration and survival. These processes are controlled by growth factors, adhesion molecules, fibroblasts, blood vessels, cytokines and chemo attractants (Figure 3) (Cueni and Detmar 2006; Ji 2006). In the following section the most widely studied molecular mediators of lymphangiogenesis are reviewed.

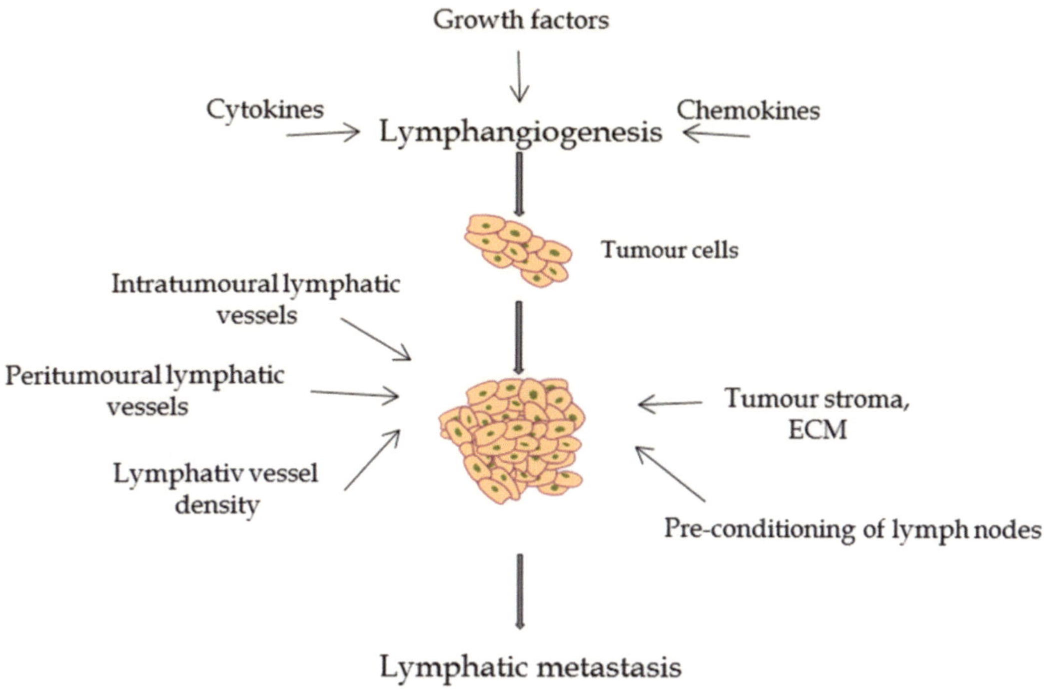

Fig. 3. Schematic overview of processes involved in tumour lymphangiogenesis and metastasis. Growth factors, cytokines, chemokines and tumour stroma contributes to tumour formation, growth, lymphangiogenesis and cancer progress. The tumour stroma consists of fibroblasts, ECM (extracellular matrix), blood vessels, lymphatic vessels and immune cells.

3.2 Molecular players in tumour lymphangiogenesis

3.2.1 Vascular endothelial growth factor

The human VEGF family of growth factors includes VEGF-A, -B, -C, -D and placental growth factor (PIGF). They bind with different specificity to three tyrosine kinase receptors: VEGFR-1 (fms-like tyrosine kinase 1), VEGFR-2 (human kinase insert domain receptor),

VEGFR-3 (fms-like tyrosine kinase 4) and two non-protein kinase co-receptors (neuropilin-1 and neuropilin-2). All VEGFRs have an extracellular binding region containing seven immunoglobulin-like domains (excepted VEGFR-3 who has only 6 domains), a single transmembrane helix and a conserved cytoplasmic domain that contains the catalytic core and regulatory sequences (Lohela, Bry et al. 2009). Activation of VEGFR by its ligands leads to receptor dimerization, autophosphorylation of tyrosine residues and initiation of signalling pathways (Roskoski 2008).

VEGF-C, VEGF-D and their ligand VEGFR-3 were the first discovered and most exensively studied lymphangiogenic factors (Baldwin et al. 2002; Nagy et al. 2002). After activation of VEGFR-3 by its ligands, autophosphorylation of tyrosine residues results in binding of the signalling adaptor proteins Shc (adaptor protein p66), Grb-2 (growth factor receptor-bound protein) and in activation of the ERK 1/2 (extracellular signal regulated kinase) signal transduction cascade in a protein kinase C dependent manner and via PI3K-Akt (phosphatidylinositol 3-kinase protein kinase B) signalling cascade (Figure 4). Binding of the adaptor protein CRK 1/2 initiates the MKK4-JNK 1/2 (mitogen-activated protein kinase kinase 4- Jun N-terminal kinase) pathway and results in induction of c-JNK (c-Jun N-terminal kinase) expression. The VEGFR-3 pathway mediates lymph endothelial growth, survival and migration (Wissmann and Detmar 2006).

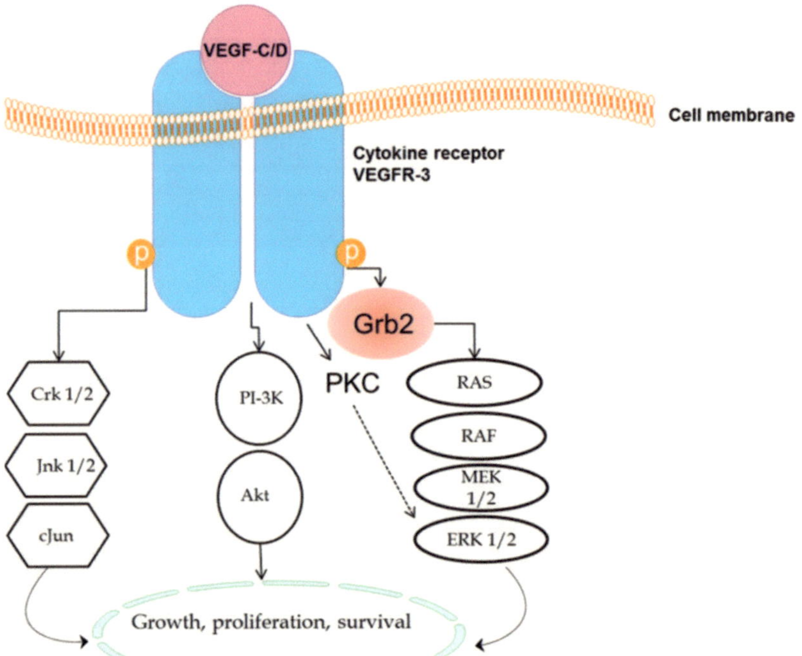

Fig. 4. The VEGF-C and VEGF-D pathways via VEGFR-3. Proteolytic processing, signal adaptor binding and activation of downstream signalling molecules results in lymph endothelial growth, proliferation and survival.

There are several studies, which suggested a correlation between the expression level of VEGF-C and lymph node metastasis (LNM) in e.g. CRC, gastric, prostate, esophageal and lung cancers (Achen and Stacker 2008). The mechanisms regulating the VEGF-C/VEGF-D expression in tumours are not fully revealed. It is known, that pro-inflammatory cytokines such as tumour necrosis factor (TNF) and Interleukins induce the expression of VEGF-C in tumour cells. The local ECM environment is assumed to trigger different VEGF receptors, resulting in signalling pathways which promote lymphangiogenesis.

In fact, the results of some studies showed that the expression levels of VEGF-D and VEGFR-3 in colorectal carcinoma tissues are significantly higher than in normal tissues (Omachi, Kawai et al. 2007). Furthermore, recent reports have linked the VEGF-C/VEGF-D expression to lymphatic metastasis and poor patient outcome (Nagahashi, Ramachandran et al. 2010; Lin, Lin et al. 2011). Our histopathological examination also revealed that VEGF-C was present in CRC tissue, whereas the surrounding tissue was negative.

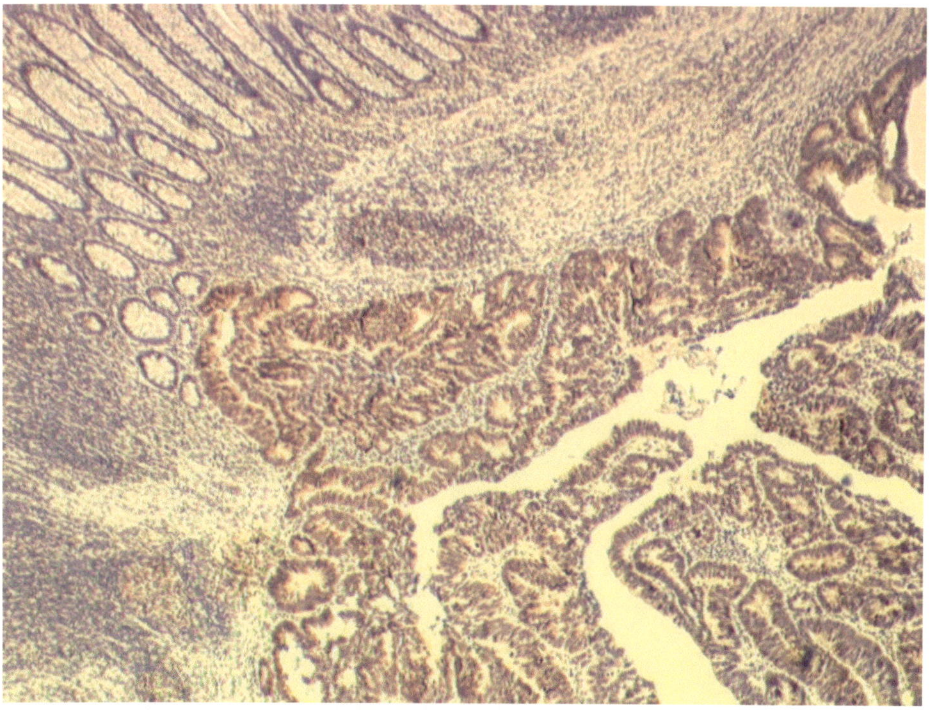

Fig. 5. CRC immunohistochemically staining for VEGF-C expression. The strong VEGF-C expression appears in the colon carcinoma tissue, while the surrounding tissue is negative.

VEGF-A is associated with angiogenesis, but it may also contribute to lymphangiogenesis. During angiogenesis VEGF-A induces proliferation and migration of endothelial cells, protease production and promotes cell survival. Fibroblasts, macrophages and endothelial cells are cells in the tumour microenvironment which are known to secrete VEGF-A. Evidence indicates that transforming growth factor α (TGFα) plays a role in regulating VEGF-A expression. The biological activity of VEGF-A is mainly mediated direct via activating of VEGFR-2 and indirectly by recruiting monocytes and neutrophils, which express VEGFR-1 and produce VEGF-C/VEGF-D.

A number of reports describe in CRC a correlation between VEGF-A expression levels and lymph node metastasis (Sundlisaeter, Dicko et al. 2007).

3.2.2 Prox-1

Prox-1 is a homeobox transcription factor. In several tissues, such as liver and pancreas Prox-1 is an important regulator of cell differentiation and oncogenesis. As mentioned before, the expression of Prox-1 is also essential for the lymphatic development and downstream signalling results in up-regulation of e.g. LYVE-1, VEGFR-3 and other lymphatic endothelial specific molecules.

Prox-1 expression is revealed to be significantly increased in CRC (Parr and Jiang 2003). The precise function must be further clarified.

3.2.3 Podoplanin

Podoplanin is a 38-kDa single transmembrane mucin-type glycoprotein and in normal human tissue it is expressed e.g. by osteoblasts, kidney podocytes and lung alveolar type 1 cells (Cueni, Hegyi et al. 2010). Due to its expression on lymphatic endothelial cells but not on blood vessels it is used as a specific marker for LECs.

Under normal conditions podoplanin is involved in the regulation of the shape of podocytes, LV formation and it is supposed to be involved in platelet aggregation. The expression of podoplanin is regulated by Prox-1 (Raica, Cimpean et al. 2008).

Since podoplanin expression is up-regulated in a number of different carcinomas such as vascular tumours, mesotheliomas and in squamous cell carcinomas, it is suggested that podoplanin is involved in carcinogenesis (Yamanashi et al. 2009). In addition, recent data in numerous of squamous cell carcinomas indicated that podoplanin is expressed at the invasive edge (Wicki and Christofori 2007). Podoplanin might favour tumour invasion via

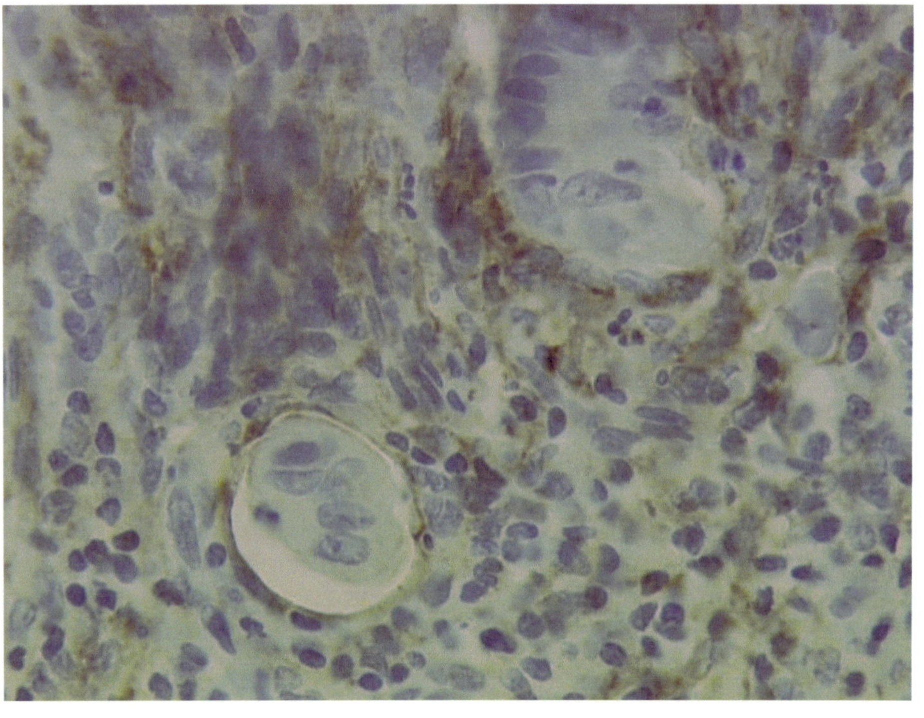

Fig. 6. Immunohistochemical detection of podoplanin positive lymphatic vessels, filled with cancer cells, in CRC.

its ability to remodel the cytoskeleton (Cueni, Hegyi et al. 2010). About the role of podoplanin in CRC little information is available. Lu et al. revealed, that the expression of podoplanin was significantly higher in patients with lymph node metastasis than in those without metastasis (Lu, Yang et al. 2007). While the group of Yamanashi suggested, that a positive podoplanin expression in stromal fibroblasts in patients with CRC is a significant indicator for a good prognosis (Yamanashi, Nakanishi et al. 2009). Figure 6 shows a lymphatic vessel stained with podoplanin and filled with a tumour cell embolus

3.2.4 LYVE-1

LYVE-1 is a homologue of the blood vascular endothelium specific hyaluronan receptor CD 44 and accordingly a member of the Link protein family. CD44 is directly involved in leucocyte migration (Jackson 2009). Lyve-1 is one of the most specific and widely used lymphatic endothelial markers (Hirakawa 2011). During embryogenesis it is expressed in cardinal vein endothelium and is involved in vascular development. On LECs LYVE-1 is expressed on the luminal and ab-luminal surface and functional studies demonstrated that it is able to act as an endocytic receptor for hyaluronan (Al-Rawi, Mansel et al. 2005). Hyaluronan is an important component of the extracellular matrix with versatile features for the interaction of cells during embryogenesis and woundhealing. LYVE-1 is also expressed by sinusoidal endothelial cells in the liver, spleen and by macrophages. Its exact function remains unclear.

3.2.5 Hepatocyte growth factor

Hepatocyte growth factor (HGF) belongs to the plasminogen-prothrombin gene superfamily. C-Met, the HGF receptor is a tyrosine kinase receptor and composed of an extracellular α chain and a transmembrane β chain. HGF activity has been reported to play a role in embryogenesis and organogenesis (Lee et al. 2010).

HGF is also supposed to be a potent lymphangiogenic factor. In this context HGF is involved in proliferation, migration, and tube formation of LECs (Cueni and Detmar 2006). The HGF downstream pathway is mediated via ERK 1/2 and PI3K and resulted in cell growth and inhibition of apoptosis. In many solid tumours c-Met is differently expressed. Novel investigations in CRC revealed an over expression of HGF and c-Met, and increased expression is associated with advanced disease stage and poor outcome (Kammula, Kuntz et al. 2007; Organ, Tong et al. 2011).

3.2.6 Fibroblast growth factors

The fibroblast growth factor family consists of structurally related ligands and four receptors (FGFR-1, FGFR-2, FGFR-3, FGFR-4), which consist the classical receptor tyrosine kinase structure: a extracellular Immunglobulin-like domain, a transmembrane domain and a intracellular tyrosine kinase domain, which initiated downstream signalling. The FGFs are involved in multi biological processes such as proliferation, survival, migration and differentiation during organogenesis and in adult life. A deregulation in human cancer has been found e.g. in breast cancer, prostate cancer, bladder cancer and cancer of the lung (Wesche, Haglund et al. 2011). FGF-2 is able to induce angiogenesis and lymphangiogenesis. Recent studies suggest that in LECs lymphangiogenic signalling is mediated through the

Akt-mammalian target of rapamycin (mTOR)-p70S6 kinase pathway (Matsuo, Yamada et al. 2007).

3.2.7 Angiopoietins

Ang-1 and Ang-2 are the more intensive analysed members of the angiopoietin family. Both bind to the Tie-2 receptor, which is expressed on the surface of LECs. The expression of Ang-1 and Ang-2 differs in human tissue. While Ang-1 is widely expressed in adult tissues, where it promotes vessel maturation and stabilization, Ang-2 expression occurs during vascular remodelling and via acting in conjugation with VEGF-A Ang-2 is supposed to be a stimulator of angiogenesis (Makinen, Norrmen et al. 2007).

About the role and function of the angiopoietins Ang-1/Ang-2 in lymphangiogenesis little information is known. Ang-1 is involved in LEC proliferation and lymphatic vessel sprouting. From analysis of pancreatic cancer, we know that Ang-2 drives lymphatic metastasis via a Tie-2 dependent manner and in a Tie-2 independent manner through enhancing the capacity of tumour cells for adherence to endothelial cells (Schulz, Fischer et al. 2011).

3.2.8 Insulin like growth factors

The insulin like growth factor system consists of the ligands insulin, insulin like growth factor 1 (IGF-1) and insulin like growth factor 2 (IGF-2) and acts via four receptors: the insulin receptor (IR), the type I IGF receptor, the type II IGF receptor and the hybrid IR/IGF-1R receptor. The IGF-IR receptor consists of two α and two β chains. IGF-IR ligand binding induces multiple downstream signal transduction pathways such as the MAPK, ERK and PI3-K pathway. It is well known, that IGF family members are frequently expressed in many solid tumours like CRC and breast cancer (Werner, Roberts et al. 1996; Reinmuth, Liu et al. 2002). In addition IGF-1R contributes to cancer development by regulation cell proliferation, differentiation and by preventing apoptosis. Other researchers investigated that IGF-1 and IGF-2 induce lymphangiogenesis (Bjorndahl, Cao et al. 2005) in a VEGFR-3 independent signalling pathway.

3.2.9 Chemokines

The chemokines, are a super family of chemotactic cytokines. They are key regulators of leukocyte, endothelial and epithelial cell migration and play a functional role in embryogenesis. Chemokines are low molecular weight proteins with cysteins at well conserved domains. According to the position of the cystein residue 4 chemokine subfamilies (CXC, CXC_3, CC, C) have been identified so far. The chemokine CXCL12 is supposed to be involved in lymphogenesis via its receptor CXCR4 and CCL21 mediates homing of lymphocytes and migration of dendritic cells into lymphatic vessel.

Nonetheless, it has been reported that chemokines and their receptors are expressed in a variety of human cancers such as melanoma, breast cancer, gastric cancer or prostate cancer (Hoon, Kitago et al. 2006). Recent findings about the direct role of chemokines in LNM in CRC, suggested an involvement of CXCR3, CXCL12/CXCR4 and CCL21/CCR7 (Kawada and Taketo 2011; Singh et al. 2011; Raman et al. 2010). In addition CXCL12 is supposed to be a prognostic factor for local recurrence and liver metastasis and CXCR4 expression was significantly positive in CRCs with high tumour stage and LNM.

Taken together, Table 2 summarizes factors which are involved in lymphangiogenesis.

Factor	Function during lymphangiogenesis
VEGF-C/VEGF-D via VEGFR-3	Growth factor/receptor: proliferation, migration, survival
VEGF-A via VEGFR-2	Activating VEGF-C/VEGF-D/VEGFR-3 signaling pathway
Prox-1	Transcription factor: LEC identity
Podoplanin	Cell motility
LYVE-1	Hyaluronan receptor
HGF	Growth factor: proliferation, migration, tube formation of LECs
FGF	LEC migration, proliferation
Ang-1/2	Growth factor
IGF	Growth factor: proliferation, differentiation and preventing apoptosis
Chemokines CCL21	Lymphocytes homing

Table 2. Molecules which are involved in lymphangiogenesis

3.3 Lymphatic vessel density and tumour progression

Since, microvessel density (MVD), a parameter for the ability of angiogenesis in tumours, is a prognostic marker in numerous cancers, the quantification of lymphatic vessel density (LVD) is of growing interest. Screening the literature, the prognostic significance of LVD in tumours remains controversial (Royston and Jackson 2009). Some studies reported that high LVD was associated with lymph node metastasis and patient outcome, while others could not confirm these findings (Gao, Knutsen et al. 2009). Furthermore, there is a debate about the dominant role of intratumoural vs. peitumoural lymphatic vessels. By some researchers it has been demonstrated that LVD in the intratumoural areas but not in peritumoural areas were associated with lymph node metastasis and poor outcome. Others reported that LVD in peritumoural areas was correlated to advanced tumour stage (Longatto-Filho, Pinheiro et al. 2008). In patients with colorectal cancer, a significant correlation between the number of intratumoural and peritumoural lymphatic vessels with the occurrence of lymph node metastases was evaluated (Matsumoto, Nakayama et al. 2007). These findings again underline the hypothesis of active lymphatic vessel formation within the tumour. These new lymphatic vessels may facilitate the drainage of tumour cells to regional lymph nodes.

3.4 Future perspectives

Further characterization of the exact molecular pathways which are involved in lymphatic metastasis is needed and essential for the development of new forecast estimates and individually oriented therapies. Gene expression profiling by microarray technique, which allows the investigation of thousands of differentially expressed genes, provide therefore a promising tool to further clarify the molecular signature for lymphatic metastasis in CRC. These signatures can provide new players which are responsible for lymphatic metastasis or identify patients with a high risk for the development of lymph node metastases. New treatment targets could be evaluated and high risk patients can be selected for individual treatment regiments. (Croner, Peters et al. 2005; Croner, Fortsch et al. 2008; Croner, Schellerer et al. 2010).

4. Conclusion

Metastasis via tumour cell invasion into lymphatic vessels and lymph nodes is a common feature of various carcinomas. Our knowledge of the mechanisms controlling lymphatic metastasis has increased significantly in the last decades since the identification of LEC specific markers such as LYVE-1, podoplanin and Prox-1. The visualisation of the lymphatic system led to a new understanding of tumour activities involved in lymphatic vessel differentiation and growth. Take together, lymphangiogenesis is a complex multi step process, which is regulated by numerous molecular players and additional studies are needed to devise new and more efficient strategies against CRC.

5. References

Achen, M. G. and S. A. Stacker (2008). "Molecular control of lymphatic metastasis." Ann N Y Acad Sci 1131: 225-234.

Al-Rawi, M. A., R. E. Mansel, et al. (2005). "Lymphangiogenesis and its role in cancer." Histol Histopathol 20(1): 283-298.

Bjorndahl, M., R. Cao, et al. (2005). "Insulin-like growth factors 1 and 2 induce lymphangiogenesis in vivo." Proc Natl Acad Sci U S A 102(43): 15593-15598.

Butler, M. G., S. Isogai, et al. (2009). "Lymphatic development." Birth Defects Res C Embryo Today 87(3): 222-231.

Croner, R. S., T. Fortsch, et al. (2008). "Molecular signature for lymphatic metastasis in colorectal carcinomas." Ann Surg 247(5): 803-810.

Croner, R. S., A. Peters, et al. (2005). "Microarray versus conventional prediction of lymph node metastasis in colorectal carcinoma." Cancer 104(2): 395-404.

Croner, R. S., V. Schellerer, et al. (2010). "One step nucleic acid amplification (OSNA) - a new method for lymph node staging in colorectal carcinomas." J Transl Med 8: 83.

Cueni, L. N. and M. Detmar (2006). "New insights into the molecular control of the lymphatic vascular system and its role in disease." J Invest Dermatol 126(10): 2167-2177.

Cueni, L. N., I. Hegyi, et al. (2010). "Tumor lymphangiogenesis and metastasis to lymph nodes induced by cancer cell expression of podoplanin." Am J Pathol 177(2): 1004-1016.

Gao, J., A. Knutsen, et al. (2009). "Clinical and biological significance of angiogenesis and lymphangiogenesis in colorectal cancer." Dig Liver Dis 41(2): 116-122.

Hirakawa, S. (2011). "Regulation of pathological lymphangiogenesis requires factors distinct from those governing physiological lymphangiogenesis." J Dermatol Sci 61(2): 85-93.

Hoon, D. S., M. Kitago, et al. (2006). "Molecular mechanisms of metastasis." Cancer Metastasis Rev 25(2): 203-220.

Jackson, D. G. (2009). "Immunological functions of hyaluronan and its receptors in the lymphatics." Immunol Rev 230(1): 216-231.

Ji, R. C. (2006). "Lymphatic endothelial cells, lymphangiogenesis, and extracellular matrix." Lymphat Res Biol 4(2): 83-100.

Ji, R. C. (2006). "Lymphatic endothelial cells, tumor lymphangiogenesis and metastasis: New insights into intratumoral and peritumoral lymphatics." Cancer Metastasis Rev 25(4): 677-694.

Kammula, U. S., E. J. Kuntz, et al. (2007). "Molecular co-expression of the c-Met oncogene and hepatocyte growth factor in primary colon cancer predicts tumor stage and clinical outcome." Cancer Lett 248(2): 219-228.

Lin, M., H. Z. Lin, et al. (2011). "Vascular endothelial growth factor-A and -C: expression and correlations with lymphatic metastasis and prognosis in colorectal cancer." Med Oncol 28(1): 151-158.

Lohela, M., M. Bry, et al. (2009). "VEGFs and receptors involved in angiogenesis versus lymphangiogenesis." Curr Opin Cell Biol 21(2): 154-165.

Longatto-Filho, A., C. Pinheiro, et al. (2008). "Peritumoural, but not intratumoural, lymphatic vessel density and invasion correlate with colorectal carcinoma poor-outcome markers." Virchows Arch 452(2): 133-138.

Lu, Y., Q. Yang, et al. (2007). "Expression analysis of lymphangiogenic factors in human colorectal cancer with quantitative RT-PCR." Cancer Invest 25(6): 393-396.

Makinen, T., C. Norrmen, et al. (2007). "Molecular mechanisms of lymphatic vascular development." Cell Mol Life Sci 64(15): 1915-1929.

Matsumoto, K., Y. Nakayama, et al. (2007). "Lymphatic microvessel density is an independent prognostic factor in colorectal cancer." Dis Colon Rectum 50(3): 308-314.

Matsuo, M., S. Yamada, et al. (2007). "Tumour-derived fibroblast growth factor-2 exerts lymphangiogenic effects through Akt/mTOR/p70S6kinase pathway in rat lymphatic endothelial cells." Eur J Cancer 43(11): 1748-1754.

Nagahashi, M., S. Ramachandran, et al. (2010). "Lymphangiogenesis: a new player in cancer progression." World J Gastroenterol 16(32): 4003-4012.

Oliver, G. and M. Detmar (2002). "The rediscovery of the lymphatic system: old and new insights into the development and biological function of the lymphatic vasculature." Genes Dev 16(7): 773-783.

Omachi, T., Y. Kawai, et al. (2007). "Immunohistochemical demonstration of proliferating lymphatic vessels in colorectal carcinoma and its clinicopathological significance." Cancer Lett 246(1-2): 167-172.

Organ, S. L., J. Tong, et al. (2011). "Quantitative Phospho-Proteomic Profiling of Hepatocyte Growth Factor (HGF)-MET Signaling in Colorectal Cancer." J Proteome Res 10(7): 3200-3211.

Parr, C. and W. G. Jiang (2003). "Quantitative analysis of lymphangiogenic markers in human colorectal cancer." Int J Oncol 23(2): 533-539.

Raica, M., A. M. Cimpean, et al. (2008). "The role of podoplanin in tumor progression and metastasis." Anticancer Res 28(5B): 2997-3006.

Reinmuth, N., W. Liu, et al. (2002). "Blockade of insulin-like growth factor I receptor function inhibits growth and angiogenesis of colon cancer." Clin Cancer Res 8(10): 3259-3269.

Royston, D. and D. G. Jackson (2009). "Mechanisms of lymphatic metastasis in human colorectal adenocarcinoma." J Pathol 217(5): 608-619.

Saharinen, P., T. Tammela, et al. (2004). "Lymphatic vasculature: development, molecular regulation and role in tumor metastasis and inflammation." Trends Immunol 25(7): 387-395.

Schmiegel, W., A. Reinacher-Schick, et al. (2008). "[Update S3-guideline "colorectal cancer" 2008]." Z Gastroenterol 46(8): 799-840.

Schulte-Merker, S., A. Sabine, et al. (2011). "Lymphatic vascular morphogenesis in development, physiology, and disease." J Cell Biol 193(4): 607-618.

Schulz, P., C. Fischer, et al. (2011). "Angiopoietin-2 drives lymphatic metastasis of pancreatic cancer." FASEB J.

Shayan, R., M. G. Achen, et al. (2006). "Lymphatic vessels in cancer metastasis: bridging the gaps." Carcinogenesis 27(9): 1729-1738.

Shields, J. D., M. S. Emmett, et al. (2007). "Chemokine-mediated migration of melanoma cells towards lymphatics--a mechanism contributing to metastasis." Oncogene 26(21): 2997-3005.

Sundlisaeter, E., A. Dicko, et al. (2007). "Lymphangiogenesis in colorectal cancer--prognostic and therapeutic aspects." Int J Cancer 121(7): 1401-1409.

Tammela, T., T. V. Petrova, et al. (2005). "Molecular lymphangiogenesis: new players." Trends Cell Biol 15(8): 434-441.

Werner, H., C. T. Roberts, Jr., et al. (1996). "Regulation of insulin-like growth factor I receptor gene expression by the Wilms' tumor suppressor WT1." J Mol Neurosci 7(2): 111-123.

Wesche, J., K. Haglund, et al. (2011). "Fibroblast growth factors and their receptors in cancer." Biochem J 437(2): 199-213.

Wicki, A. and G. Christofori (2007). "The potential role of podoplanin in tumour invasion." Br J Cancer 96(1): 1-5.

Wiig, H., D. Keskin, et al. (2010). "Interaction between the extracellular matrix and lymphatics: consequences for lymphangiogenesis and lymphatic function." Matrix Biol 29(8): 645-656.

Wissmann, C. and M. Detmar (2006). "Pathways targeting tumor lymphangiogenesis." Clin Cancer Res 12(23): 6865-6868.

Witte, M. H., K. Jones, et al. (2006). "Structure function relationships in the lymphatic system and implications for cancer biology." Cancer Metastasis Rev 25(2): 159-184.

Yamanashi, T., Y. Nakanishi, et al. (2009). "Podoplanin expression identified in stromal fibroblasts as a favorable prognostic marker in patients with colorectal carcinoma." Oncology 77(1): 53-62.

Part 4

Tumor Microenvironment

14

Modulation of Tumor Angiogenesis by a Host Anti-Tumor Response in Colorectal Cancer

N. Britzen-Laurent[1], V.S. Schellerer[2], R.S. Croner[2], M. Stürzl[1] and E. Naschberger[1]
[1]*Division of Molecular and Experimental Surgery, Department of Surgery, University Medical Center Erlangen, Erlangen,*
[2]*Department of Surgery, University Medical Center Erlangen, Erlangen, Germany*

1. Introduction

Colorectal carcinoma (CRC) is the second most frequently occurring cancer in industrialized countries, in both men and women. The cumulative lifetime risk of developing colorectal carcinoma is about 6%, and the cancer-related five year survival rate is 62% (Smith et al., 2002). Malignant transformation of CRC occurs in a multistep process via three different pathways: the chromosomal instability pathway, the microsatellite instability pathway (Vogelstein et al., 1988) and the methylation pathway (Jass, 2002). Moreover, putative tumor-initiating cells with increased malignancy were isolated from CRC (O'Brien et al., 2007; Ricci-Vitiani et al., 2007). These cells exhibited stem cell-like characteristics; however, their role in CRC pathogenesis is still controversial (Shmelkov et al., 2008). Tumor development and metastasis require the presence of a newly formed vasculature. Tumor cells can directly promote angiogenesis but the tumor microenvironment plays also a crucial role in this process. The tumor microenvironment consists of a variety of conjunctive tissue components and cells, as well as infiltrating immune cells. It is inflammatory and undergoes constant remodelling. Immune cells are not only recruited in order to eliminate the tumor, they can also be attracted by tumor cells in order to support a tumor-promoting inflammation. In CRC, the type of immune cells infiltrating the tumor has been shown to influence tumor growth and patient survival (Galon et al., 2007; Tosolini et al., 2011). In addition, immune cells have been shown to exert antagonistic effects on tumor angiogenesis. In this chapter, we focus on the modulation of tumor angiogenesis by tumor infiltrating immune cells and on its implications in terms of diagnosis and prognosis in CRC.

2. Tumor angiogenesis and tumor vessels

Tumor growth beyond two to three millimeters in diameter and metastasis requires angiogenesis, the formation of new blood vessels. Angiogenesis plays a crucial role in the development and progression of CRC, and this has been convincingly documented in the literature. It has been shown that microvessel density is increased in primary tumors compared to normal mucosa or adenoma tissues (Bossi et al., 1995), and this is a strong independent predictor of poor outcome (Takebayashi et al., 1996). A high microvessel density is associated with a more than threefold increased relative risk of cancer-related death from CRC (Choi et al., 1998). Moreover, the expression of vascular endothelial growth factor (VEGF), a potent angiogenesis-promoting factor, is significantly increased in all stages of colorectal carcinoma (Kumar et al., 1998). The major sources of VEGF are either the tumor cells themselves or monocytes/macrophages recruited into the tumor tissue through paracrine signalling. Intratumor expression of VEGF was also found to increase the relative risk of cancer-related death from CRC by twofold (Kang et al., 1997; Ishigami et al., 1998; Kahlenberg et al., 2003).

The recruitment and growth of tumor vessels is a critical adaption step that has to be achieved during the development of clinically relevant solid tumors such as the CRC. This process has been termed "angiogenic switch" (Folkman, 1995) and the "induction of angiogenesis" has been included in the eight hallmarks of cancer defined by Hanahan and Weinberg (Hanahan & Weinberg, 2000; Hanahan & Weinberg, 2011). New vessels may arise through different ways in the organism under physiological and/or pathological conditions. During embryonic development angioblasts differentiate into endothelial cells in a process called vasculogenesis whereas new vessels in adults are generated through angiogenesis (Risau, 1997). The major driving molecules for angiogenic processes are VEGF, VEGF-C, angiopoietin-2, fibroblast growth factors and chemokines (Carmeliet & Jain, 2011). Active angiogenesis is achieved either by vessel sprouting, non-sprouting intussusception (splitting of existing vessels), vessel co-option (tumor cells hijack vasculature), vascular mimicry (tumor cells line vessels), luminal incorporation of bone marrow-derived endothelial progenitor cells or a recently described non-VEGF-dependent biomechanical mechanism (Risau, 1997; Kilarski et al., 2009; Carmeliet & Jain, 2011).

The role of so called "tumor stem cells" in tumor angiogenesis is currently heavily discussed. Cancer stem cells might not only have an impact on the growth and assembly of the CRC tumor cells themselves (O'Brien et al., 2007; Ricci-Vitiani et al., 2007) but also on the formation of tumor vessels (Ricci-Vitiani et al., 2010; Wang et al., 2010). The two latter studies described for the first time the differentiation of putative cancer stem cells not only into functional tumor cells but also into tumor endothelial cells. However, these findings were demonstrated for the brain tumor glioblastoma. Of note, normal neuronal stem cells are able to differentiate into endothelial cells under physiological conditions, which questions whether these findings can be also applied to non-brain tumors such as colorectal carcinoma.

Tumor vessels are structurally and functionally abnormal compared to vessels in healthy tissues (Carmeliet & Jain, 2000; Hida et al., 2008). In contrast to normal vessels, they show a deficient support provided by only few perivascular cells with loose connections to the endothelium and the vessels maintain an immature structure. The tumor vasculature is commonly disorganized and heterogenous, with excessive branching and shunts, reduced interendothelial cell contacts, reduced barrier function and uneven vessel lumen. This disturbs the blood flow in the tumors, leads to hypoxia and acidification as well as high fluid pressure concomitant with increased resistance to the application of systemic drugs [reviewed in (Carmeliet & Jain, 2000; Hida et al., 2008; Carmeliet & Jain, 2011)]. Tumor cells attempt to overcome this issue by the expression of more pro-angiogenic factors such as VEGF resulting in amplified formation of abnormal vessels. However, tumor hypoxia cannot be rescued by the formation of abnormal vessels (Leite de Oliveira et al., 2011).

When anti-angiogenic treatment was initially developed, tumor endothelial cells (TECs) were thought to be similar in all tumor types and, in contrast to tumor cells, genetically stable. However, subsequent studies showed that TECs are different in tumors from different organs and are actually genetically instable. It has been suggested that this is due to the involvement of endothelial cells (ECs) from different vascular beds. In addition, tumor cells and TECs interact strongly with each other and with additional cells present in the stroma via paracrine and possibly also juxtacrine pathways. Importantly, these interactions might induce microenvironment-dependent abnormalities in TECs that could differentiate them from normal endothelial cells. Recently, studies in mice and humans showed that abnormalities observed in TECs are maintained over long periods in cell culture, and include chromosomal abnormalities (Streubel et al., 2004; Hida & Klagsbrun, 2005; Akino et al., 2009), resistance to apoptosis (Bussolati et al., 2003), increased adhesiveness for tumor cells (Bussolati et al., 2003), drug resistance (Xiong et al., 2009), abnormal angiogenic capability (Ghosh et al., 2008; Xiong et al., 2009), and pronounced growth in the absence of serum (Bussolati et al., 2003).

TECs have been isolated from numerous animal models and from a limited number of human tumors mentioned above (Bussolati et al., 2003; Streubel et al., 2004; Buckanovich et al., 2007; Xiong et al., 2009). Until recently, no viable, pure TEC cultures from human colorectal carcinomas were available, and the biological phenotype of these cells was not characterized at the functional level. We have developed the first protocol for the routine isolation of both CRC TECs and the corresponding ECs from normal colon tissue (NECs) by collagenase II-digestion followed by multiple CD31-MACS selections (Schellerer et al., 2007). It was demonstrated that the cells were of endothelial blood cell origin (CD31-, CD105-, VE-cadherin-positive; E-selectin-, VCAM-1-, ICAM-1-positive after stimulation with inflammatory cytokines; capability to form capillaries in matrigel, take up acetylated LDL and bind *ulex europaeus*; CD45-, CD68-, CK-20-, podoplanin-negative). Moreover, the isolated TECs maintained differences from NECs during long-term culture for example by decreased von Willebrand factor (vWF) levels in the isolated tumor endothelial cells as well as in the original cancer tissue biopsies compared to the corresponding normal endothelial cells and normal colon biopsy (Schellerer et al., 2007). Meanwhile, we could show that the TEC isolated from CRC differ from each other also at the transcriptome and genome level (data unpublished).

TEC-specific markers were isolated from CRC by serial analysis of gene expression after laser-microdissection of tumor vessels (St Croix et al., 2000). The identified genes were designated as tumor endothelial markers (TEMs) (St Croix et al., 2000; Nanda et al., 2004). However, out of the nine different TEMs initially described, five were not pursued in future studies and two were shown to be expressed by other cells rather than tumor endothelial cells (Lee et al., 2006; Christian et al., 2008). These results indicated that the initial samples were most likely contaminated with non-endothelial cells such as pericytes that cover the mature vessel. Up to now, no widely accepted specific marker for tumor vessel endothelial cells in the CRC or other human tumors has been identified. Accordingly, a superior approach would be to specifically isolate pure, viable TEC cultures from CRC and then use these cells to identify TEC-specific markers.

In summary, the described results indicate that the induction and maintenance of tumor angiogenesis is an important feature in CRC growth and progression and that the interaction of TECs with tumor cells and other stromal cells changes the TEC phenotype.

Furthermore, pure viable TEC cultures isolated from CRC might be a valuable tool, allowing functional analysis of the TEC phenotype in CRC and the identification of TEC-specific markers. Pure CRC-derived TEC cultures will shed light on the manifold interactions between tumor and endothelial cells and their impact on the pathogenesis and prognosis of this tumor. This understanding will lead to improved anti-angiogenic treatment strategies in the CRC.

3. Host anti-tumor response and angiogenesis in colorectal cancer

3.1 Tumor infiltrating immune cells and angiogenesis in CRC

In CRC, tumor progression is tightly associated with and partly promoted by the tumor microenvironment. The tumor microenvironment consists of extracellular matrix, the vasculature and tumor-infiltrating cells. Infiltrating cells are recruited through inflammation and chemoattractants produced by the tumor cells or by cells of the stroma. Tumor infiltrating cells comprise cancer-associated fibroblasts (CAFs), endothelial cells, platelets, mesenchymal stem cells and various types of immune cells. Initial studies addressing the prognostic role of intratumoral immune cells infiltrates in colorectal cancer were partly contradictory. Some studies supported a protective role of inflammatory infiltrates (Jass, 1986; Harrison et al., 1994; Ropponen et al., 1997; Naito et al., 1998; Leo et al., 2000; Guidoboni et al., 2001; Galon et al., 2006) but other reports did not (Roncucci et al., 1996; Nielsen et al., 1999).

It is now clear that the type, the subtype and the localization of the infiltrating immune cells determine their effects on the tumor cells and the tumor microenvironment. Both the innate and the adaptive immune responses are involved in this process. For instance, the infiltration of cytotoxic T cells and type I helper T cells (Th1 cells) in CRC correlates with a prolonged disease-free survival, whereas the presence of infiltrating Th17 cells is of poor prognosis (Galon et al., 2006). In the same way, polarization of tumor-associated macrophages towards either M1 or M2 subpopulation results in anti-tumorigenic (M1) or pro-tumorigenic (M2) effects (Mantovani & Sica, 2010). Some forms of inflammatory infiltrates participate to the anti-tumor immune response while other immune cells are actively recruited by the tumor to exploit their pro-angiogenic and pro-metastatic effects (Balkwill & Mantovani, 2001; Coussens & Werb, 2001).

In addition, there is a growing body of evidence that tumor infiltrating immune cells can modulate tumor angiogenesis in cancer and particularly in CRC as summarized in table 1 and discussed in more detail below.

Pro-angiogenic	**Anti-angiogenic**
Tumor-associated macrophages (M2)	Lymphocytes (Th1)
TIE-2 expressing monocytes	NK cells
Mast cells	NKT cells
Neutrophils	Dendritic cells
MDSCs	
Immature DCs	
Th17 lymphocytes	
Immature dendritic cells	

Table 1. Pro-angiogenic or anti-angiogenic features of tumor infiltrating immune cells.

3.1.1 Tumor-associated macrophages

The recruitment of tumor-associated macrophages (TAMs) is mediated by various factors such as colony-stimulating factor-1 (CSF-1), which is produced by colon carcinoma cells, or the chemokines CCL2, CCL3, CCL4 and CCL5 (Sica et al., 2008a; Sica et al., 2008b). Tumors are predominantly infiltrated by TAMs with M2 polarization and high TAM infiltration in CRC is associated with a poor prognosis (Bacman et al., 2007). TAMs express pro-angiogenic factors including VEGF, basic fibroblast growth factor (bFGF), TNF-α, IL-8, IL-1β or platelet derived growth factor-β (PDGF-β) (Figure 1) (Barbera-Guillem et al., 2002; Sica et al., 2008a; Sica et al., 2008b). In addition, TAMs secrete matrix metalloproteases (MMP-7, MMP12) which participate in tumor angiogenesis by remodelling the extracellular matrix (Peddareddigari et al., 2010).

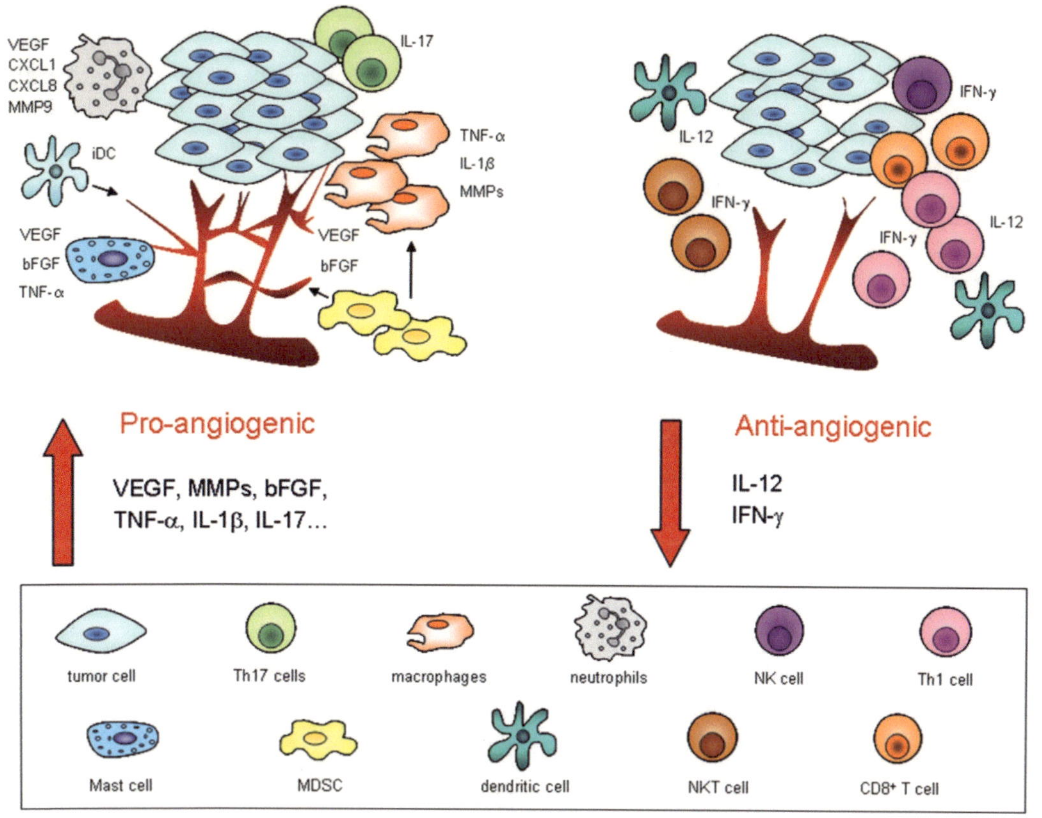

Fig. 1. Tumor-infiltrating immune cells exert opposite effects on angiogenesis.

3.1.2 TIE-2 expressing monocytes

TIE-2 expressing monocytes (TEMs) represent a subset of monocytes differing from the classical inflammatory monocytes (De Palma et al., 2005). The number of TEMs is increased in the blood of cancer patients and the tumor stroma of various types of cancers including CRC (De Palma et al., 2007; Venneri et al., 2007). TIE-2 is an angiopoietin receptor which is normally found at the surface of endothelial cells or haematopoietic stem cells. TEM recruitment in tumors is mediated by the chemokines CCL3, CCL5 and CCL8, and the expression of angiopoietin-2 by tumor cells or tumor endothelial cells (De Palma & Naldini, 2009; De Palma & Naldini, 2011). TEMs have been shown to promote tumor angiogenesis and tumor growth in tumor mouse models (De Palma & Naldini, 2011).

3.1.3 Mast cells

Mast cells are myeloid-derived cells which contain numerous granules rich in histamine and heparin. They are resident in tissues and represent key effectors of allergic reactions. Mast cells can also infiltrate tumors where they localize in the vicinity of blood vessels (Maltby et al., 2009). A high mast cell infiltration is usually associated with increased tumor growth, invasion and vascularisation. It has been shown that low mast cell numbers in CRC samples correlate with a better patient survival and hypovascularization (Gulubova & Vlaykova, 2009). Mast cells are able to produce numerous pro-angiogenic factors such as VEGF, bFGF, angiopoietin-1, TNF-α, heparin, histamine or various proteases (Maltby et al., 2009). It has been suggested that mast cell infiltration triggers the "angiogenic switch" during tumor growth: mast cells might be involved in angiogenesis at early stages of tumor growth, while at late stages the tumor cells control growth and angiogenesis in a mast cell-independent manner (Coussens et al., 1999).

3.1.4 Neutrophils

Infiltrates of neutrophils have been observed in various cancers including CRC (Roncucci et al., 2008; Tazzyman et al., 2009). In addition, neutrophils are involved in the pathogenesis of inflammatory bowel disease (Roessner et al., 2008). The recruitment of neutrophils is mediated by the chemokines CXCL1 and CXCL8 (Eck et al., 2003). Neutrophils stimulate tumor angiogenesis by releasing proteins including VEGF, CXCL1, CXCL8 or MMP9. The latter induces the release of VEGF from the extracellular matrix by cleavage of heparan sulfates (Hawinkels et al., 2008; Tazzyman et al., 2009).

3.1.5 Tumor infiltrating lymphocytes

Recent studies have highlighted the prognostic importance of tumor infiltrating lymphocytes (TILs) in colorectal carcinoma (Galon et al., 2006; Katz et al., 2009). The type, density and localization of T-cells in colorectal tumors have been found to be a better predictor of patient survival than the classical histopathological staging (Galon et al., 2006). T-cells can be divided in different subtypes. Naïve CD4+ T-cells differentiate in T helper (Th) cells of type 1 (Th1) in the presence of IL-12 or of type 2 (Th2) in the presence of IL-4 (Zhou et al., 2009). Th1 and Th2 cells inhibit each other. The presence of a Th1 adaptive immune response in CRC correlates with a better survival and an anti-angiogenic phenotype (Galon et al., 2006; Naschberger et al., 2008). Th1 cells facilitate the recruitment and the action of CD8+ cytotoxic T cells (Zhang et al., 2009). In CRC, CD8+ infiltrating T cells are the cell type most strongly associated with an improved survival (Galon et al., 2006). Th1 cells and CD8+ T-cells produce IL-12 and IFN-γ, both anti-angiogenic cytokines (Figure 1) (Zhu & Paul, 2010; Briesemeister et al., 2011). IL-12 promotes the production of IFN-γ by CD8+ T-cells and reduces the production of pro-angiogenic proteases such as MMP-9 by endothelial cells (Tartour et al., 2011). IFN-γ induces the production of angiostatic chemokines (CXCL9 and CXCL10) by endothelial cells and blocks the production of both VEGF and bFGF (Tartour et al., 2011).

Besides Th1 and Th2 cells, two other populations of T-cells have been shown to be involved in cancer, namely the regulatory T-cells (Treg) and the Th17 cells. In CRC, the infiltration of Treg, as well as of Th2 cells, seems to have no influence on patient survival (Tosolini et al., 2011). However, a direct association was found between the presence of a Th17 response and a worse prognosis (Tosolini et al., 2011). Th17 cells differentiate from naïve CD4+ T-cells upon exposure to IL-6 or TGF-β, and produce IL-17, IL-17F and IL-22 (Zhou et al., 2009). IL-17 promotes angiogenesis by inducing the production of angiogenic growth factors and chemokines by tumor cells and fibroblasts (Figure 1). Furthermore, IL-17 exerts a direct effect on endothelial cells, increasing migration and tube formation. Finally, IL-17 can indirectly promote angiogenesis by recruiting neutrophils to the tumor site (Tartour et al., 2011).

3.1.6 Myeloid-derived suppressor cells

Myeloid-derived suppressor cells (MDSCs) are immature myeloid cells including progenitors of macrophages, granulocytes and DCs. The number of MDSCs has been shown to be increased in the blood of CRC patients (Mandruzzato et al., 2009). MDSCs are immunosuppressive and in particular inhibit T-cells (Condamine & Gabrilovich, 2011). In addition, they modulate the action of NK cells and induce Treg cells. MDSCs exert their functions through up-regulation of NO, arginase or ROS (Gabrilovich & Nagaraj, 2009). In mouse models, MDSCs have been shown to promote angiogenesis, tumor cell invasion and metastasis (Youn & Gabrilovich, 2010). MDSCs are very heterogenic but one can distinguish two different subtypes: the granulocytic (G)-MDSCs and the monocytic (M)-MDSCs (Youn & Gabrilovich, 2010). G-MDSCs are found in the spleen or in peripheral lymphoid organs, use primarily ROS for immune suppression, require cell-cell contact with T cells and are dependent on antigen-specific interactions (Youn & Gabrilovich, 2010). M-MDSCs are found in tumors, use primarily iNOS, arginase and cytokines for immune suppression, their action does not require direct cell-cell contact. M-MDSCs exert a non-specific suppression and are more potent (Youn & Gabrilovich, 2010). M-MDSCs are able to differentiate towards TAMs under hypoxic conditions (Corzo et al., 2010). Some MDSCs express endothelial markers such as CD31 or VEGFR2 and are able to incorporate into the tumor endothelium (Figure 1) (Yang et al., 2004).

3.1.7 Dendritic cells

Dendritic cells (DCs) are bone-marrow derived cells and represent the most important antigen-presenting cells (Salama & Platell, 2008). In CRC, DCs localize at the invasive margin of the tumor and in lymph nodes (Ambe et al., 1989; Suzuki et al., 2002). The presence of a high number of DCs in CRC correlates with a better prognosis, in particular when DCs infiltrate the intra-epithelial compartment of the tumor (Dadabayev et al., 2004; Sandel et al., 2005). Mature DCs are able to produce IL-12 which induces the polarization of immune cells towards the Th1 anti-tumorigenic and anti-angiogenic phenotype. Tumors are in addition able to recruit immature DCs (iDCs) which have been shown in ovarian cancer to secrete pro-angiogenic factors and to be capable of incorporating in newly formed vessels (Figure 1) (Curiel et al., 2004).

3.1.8 NK and NKT cells

NK cells are lymphocytes from the innate immune system which are able to recognize tumor cells as target. The immune infiltration of NK cells represents a positive prognostic marker in various solid tumors including CRC (Coca et al., 1997). They represent together with CD8+ T cells the most likely effectors of the anti-tumor immunity. NK cells exert their anti-tumorigenic effects notably through the production of IFN-γ and participate therefore in the anti-angiogenic immune response (Levy et al., 2011).

NKT cell are a small population of T cells which also exhibit NK cells markers. They have the property to modulate immune responses and to link the innate and the adaptive immune responses. NKT cells are able to recognize lipid antigens that are not recognized by other T cell subsets (Terabe & Berzofsky, 2008). Two subtypes of NKT cells have been described. The most frequent type of NKT cells, called type I, has a very restricted T-cell receptor (TCR) repertoire and expresses the invariant Vα24Jα18 TCR. On the contrary, the type II NKT cells express different TCRs (Terabe & Berzofsky, 2008). NKT type I cells exert anti-tumor effects through IFN-γ but independently of perforin (van der Vliet et al., 2008). In addition, they activate DCs to produce IL-12. In colorectal carcinoma, a high infiltration of type I NKT cells, which are Vα24 positive, correlates with a better overall and disease-free survival (Tachibana et al., 2005). Through their production of IFN-γ and their activation of DCs, type I NKT cells participate in the Th1 anti-angiogenic immune response in CRC (Figure 1). While type I NKT cells enhance anti-tumor immunity, mouse models showed that type II NKT cells repress it (Terabe & Berzofsky, 2008).

Tumor angiogenesis is promoted by the production of VEGF from the tumor cells but also from mast cells, M2 macrophages and neutrophils. In addition, macrophages and mast cells produce IL-1β and TNF-α, which can promote a local pro-angiogenic inflammation through the further recruitment of macrophages *in vivo*, even if their direct action on endothelial cells *in vitro* is anti-angiogenic. Neutrophils and macrophages produce MMPs, inducing a matrix remodeling necessary for angiogenesis. Th17 cells directly promote angiogenesis through the secretion of IL-17, which enhances the recruitment of neutrophils. Immature MDSCs can differentiate towards M2 macrophages or, like immature dendritic cells, can be incorporated into newly formed vessels. On the contrary, a Th1 dominated immune response exerts anti-angiogenic effects, mainly through the production of IFN-γ by Th1 cells, $CD8^+$ T cells, NK or NKT cells. Th1 cells are activated by IL-12, notably produced by some DCs.

3.2 Markers for the interplay of angiogenesis and a host anti-tumor response in CRC

The impact of angiogenesis on colorectal tumor growth and progression described in the previous paragraphs was convincingly supported by a clinical phase III study in which an anti-VEGF antibody (bevacizumab) was added to fluorouracil-based combination chemotherapy. The combination therapy led to a statistically significant and clinically meaningful improvement in overall survival (20.3 months vs. 15.6 months for the control group) and progression-free survival among patients with metastatic CRC (Hurwitz et al., 2004). Based on these results bevacizumab was approved as the first solely anti-angiogenic drug used as anti-cancer agent by the FDA in 2004. Moreover, two additional anti-angiogenic drugs for the same molecular target have been approved for the clinics meanwhile: sunitinib and sorafenib. These drugs are both broad-spectrum receptor tyrosine kinase (RTK) inhibitors that target VEGFR1, VEGFR2, VEGFR3 or PDGFR-α/β among other RTKs (Escudier et al., 2007; Motzer et al., 2007).

However, in all of the clinical studies employing anti-angiogenic treatment for human tumors including CRC, only a fraction of the treated patients responded completely or partially to the therapy (10-49.3% maximum partial response rates) (Hurwitz et al., 2004;

Demetri et al., 2006; Escudier et al., 2007; Motzer et al., 2007; Sobrero et al., 2009). Additionally, in some cases, severe side effects such as cardiovascular damage, perforation of the colon or venous thromboembolic events have been observed (Hurwitz et al., 2004; Sobrero et al., 2009). Furthermore, anti-angiogenic treatment is very expensive and puts a significant cost burden on the health system. This raises important questions: (1) which subset of patients will benefit most from these therapies? (2) How can these patients be preselected? (3) Can the side effects be decreased by patient preselection?

From these questions it becomes obvious that valid biomarkers able to indicate different angiogenic or angiostatic tumor microenvironments, and in consequence patients who will benefit most from anti-angiogenic therapy, are urgently required. Numerous efforts have been undertaken to identify predictive and/or prognostic biomarkers and this research field is rapidly expanding. By definition a predictive biomarker is able to foretell the response of the patient to a certain treatment whereas a prognostic biomarker predicts the potential outcome of the disease independently of the applied therapy. Promising results have been reported in the last few years, however, none of the proposed markers has been accepted widely (Asghar et al., 2010; Gerger et al., 2011).

Different kinds of potential biomarkers for anti-angiogenic treatment have been reported in the literature in the past few years: serum, tissue and genetic markers. Initially, for obvious reasons, VEGF tissue and serum levels were heavily investigated but surprisingly did not make it into the clinics due to the inability to predict response at the tissue level (Jubb et al., 2006) and contradictory results at the serum level (Loupakis et al., 2007; Willett et al., 2009). Efforts have also been undertaken to investigate the impact of genetic polymorphisms of VEGF and VEGFR-2 as potential biomarkers (Schneider et al., 2008). Many other potential biomarkers were reported in the last few years in the literature to be measured either at the tissue or serum/plasma level. Examples for these markers are tissue CD31 and PDGFR-β expression in breast cancer (Yang et al., 2008), soluble angiopoietin-2 (Goede et al., 2010), circulating endothelial cells (Ronzoni et al., 2010), TNF-α, MMP-9 (Perez-Gracia et al., 2009), soluble KIT (Deprimo et al., 2009) as well as IL-8 (Kopetz et al., 2010). However, all of these potential markers require confirmation in larger cohorts and unfortunately lack either prognostic or predictive value.

From these results it becomes clear that very likely different biomarkers will be required for the different kinds of anti-angiogenic treatments and the different kinds of cancers. In addition, as discussed in the section 3 of this review, a broad range of immune cells can infiltrate tumors and have been detected in CRC samples. These cells interact with tumor endothelial cells during their extravasation and some of them are able to modulate tumor angiogenesis (Figure 1). While tumor infiltrating macrophages, mast cells, Th17 lymphocytes and neutrophils are recognized to exert pro-angiogenic effects in CRC, Th1 lymphocytes are associated with an anti-angiogenic microenvironment. On the other end, tumor vessels can be more or less permissive for the infiltration of immune cells. Therefore, the interplay between immune cells and tumor endothelial cells represents an important issue with implications for the anti-tumor host response and angiogenesis.

3.2.1 GBP-1 as a marker for the anti-angiogenic Th1 immune response in CRC

As mentioned above, the presence of a Th1 microenvironment is associated with a significantly improved prognosis in CRC (Galon et al., 2006). A Th-1 microenvironment is characterized by increased IFN-γ expression, often combined with the increased expression of pro-inflammatory cytokines IL-1β and TNF-α (Dayer, 2002b; Dayer, 2002a; Cui et al., 2007). The guanylate-binding protein 1 (GBP-1) has been identified as a marker of the Th1 microenvironment in CRC (Naschberger et al., 2008). GBP-1 expression is induced upon stimulation by IFN-γ but also by other pro-inflammatory cytokines such as IL-1β and/or TNF-α (Guenzi et al., 2001; Lubeseder-Martellato et al., 2002). In CRC, GBP-1 is strongly expressed in infiltrating cells and in the vasculature. Its expression correlates with expression of IFN-γ-induced genes, chemokines and immune reaction-associated genes (Naschberger et al., 2008). Among them, three anti-angiogenic chemokines known to play a role in tumors (CXCL9, CXCL10, CXCL11) could also be detected (Romagnani et al., 2004). GBP-1 expression in CRC stroma is associated with an increase of the cancer-related five-year survival rate and GBP-1 represents an independent prognostic factor indicating a reduction of the relative risk of cancer-related death by the half (Naschberger et al., 2008). In tumor-associated endothelial cells the presence of GBP-1 is associated with a decreased angiogenic activity (Naschberger et al., 2008; Guenzi et al., 2001; Guenzi et al., 2003). GBP-1 is presently the only marker available to specifically indicate whether endothelial cells in tissues are exposed to an angiostatic Th-1-like tumor microenvironment.

3.2.2 Modulation of lymphocytes infiltration by endothelial cells

The relationship between tumor angiogenesis and immunity is actually bidirectional. As described above, infiltrating immune cells can positively or negatively regulate angiogenesis in tumors. On the other hand, tumor endothelial cells are able to regulate extravasation of immune cells, notably through the expression of surface molecules. Among the potential molecular effectors identified, endothelin, endothelin receptor and CD137 seem to play a prominent role.

The endothelin-endothelin receptor axis

The endothelin (ET) family comprises four members designated ET-1 to -4 (Kandalaft et al., 2009). ETs derive from precursor proteins after cleavage by membrane-bound metalloproteinases. ET-1 is the most potent ligand and the most widely expressed in endothelial cells (Kandalaft et al., 2009). In addition, ET-1 is overexpressed in many tumor cell lines and many tumors, including CRC (Kusuhara et al., 1990; Arun et al., 2004; Bagnato & Rosano, 2008). Two endothelin receptors have been identified: the endothelin A and the endothelin B receptor, respectively ET_AR and ET_BR (Kandalaft et al., 2009). In normal tissues, ET_AR and ET_BR regulate vasoconstriction and are also involved in inflammation. Both receptors exert opposite effects. In particular, ET_AR promote T-cell adhesion to endothelial cells, whereas ET_BR inhibits it. In tumor cells, concomitant up-regulation of ET-1 and ET_AR inhibits apoptosis and promotes cell proliferation, invasion and metastasis (Kedzierski & Yanagisawa, 2001; Kandalaft et al., 2009). In a study comparing the expression profiles of tumor associated endothelial cells (TECs) in ovarian cancer with or without TILs, ET_BR has been associated with the absence of TILs and short patient survival time (Buckanovich et al., 2008). Of note, in this study, GBP-1 expression in TECs correlated with the presence of TILs. The inhibition of T cells homing in tumor by ET_BR is mediated by an increase of NO synthase and NO release and by a decrease in the expression of the adhesion molecule ICAM-1. In CRC, ET-1 and ET_AR are expressed by the tumor cells, generating a stimulatory loop, while ET_BR expression in TECs is reduced as compared to normal colon blood vessels (Ali et al., 2000a; Ali et al., 2000b; Asham et al., 2001; Hoosein et al., 2007).

Investigation of the expression of ET_BR in TECs in relation to TILs infiltration might provide further insights into the molecular regulation of immune cells extravasation by endothelial cells in CRC.

CD137 (TNFRSF9)

CD137 is a surface glycoprotein of the TNF-α receptor family involved in T-cell co-stimulation (Shao & Schwarz, 2011). CD137 is expressed on the surface of activated T cells, NK cells, DCs, macrophages or B cells, while its ligand, CD137L is expressed by APCs (Shao & Schwarz, 2011). CD137 is induced under hypoxia and by TNF-α, LPS or IL-1β. CD137 is however also expressed in human tumor capillaries, notably in CRC (Broll et al., 2001; Wang et al., 2008). In tumors, CD137 is expressed on the vessel walls whereas CD137L is expressed on tumor cells (Salih et al., 2000; Broll et al., 2001). The effects of CD137 are mediated by the up-regulation of V-CAM, I-CAM and E-selectin, inducing thereby the recruitment of T lymphocytes (Palazon et al., 2011). In addition, it has been shown that the ligation of CD137L on lung squamous carcinoma cells with CD137 on T cells induced IFN-γ production by T cells (Salih et al., 2000). Therefore, expression of CD137 by TECs might promote the recruitment of T cells in CRC and their polarization towards the anti-tumorigenic and anti-angiogenic Th1 subtype.

4. Conclusions

In this review we tried to shed light on the current understanding of tumor angiogenesis and its modulation by a potential host anti-tumor response with a specific focus on colorectal carcinoma. Our major aim was to point out the connection of these two processes. A host anti-tumor response does not only have a direct effect on the tumor cells but also a major impact on the development and function of the tumor vasculature. Different tumor microenvironments, which can either inhibit or foster angiogenesis, are established during a specific immune response. These various microenvironments are achieved by different means: (1) immune cells such as Th1-T-cells are attracted into the tumor tissue within the context of a specific host anti-tumor response that secrete soluble mediators (e.g. IFN-γ) directly acting on tumor endothelial cells in an anti-angiogenic manner. (2) The tumor cells themselves also attract immune cells such as M2 macrophages or Th17-T-cells that might release mediators which modulate the microenvironment in a pro-angiogenic manner. (3) Endothelial cells can also modulate the stromal composition of infiltrating leukocytes which alters the soluble mediator profile to which the tumor and its vasculature are exposed. Therefore, biomarkers are required in order to characterize the specific angiogenic phenotype of each CRC patient. Moreover, these biomarkers should have prognostic and/or predictive potential for anti-angiogenic treatment and at best also give information about the presence of a host anti-tumor immune response. A potential candidate for such a biomarker might be the guanylate binding protein-1 (GBP-1).

5. References

Akino, T.; Hida, K.; Hida, Y.; Tsuchiya, K.; Freedman, D.; Muraki, C.; Ohga, N.; Matsuda, K.; Akiyama, K.; Harabayashi, T.; Shinohara, N.; Nonomura, K.; Klagsbrun, M. & Shindoh, M. (2009). Cytogenetic abnormalities of tumor-associated endothelial cells in human malignant tumors. *Am J Pathol*, Vol.175, No.6, (Dec 2009), pp. 2657-2667

Ali, H.; Dashwood, M.; Dawas, K.; Loizidou, M.; Savage, F. & Taylor, I. (2000a). Endothelin receptor expression in colorectal cancer. *J Cardiovasc Pharmacol*, Vol.36, No.5 Suppl 1, (Nov 2000a), pp. S69-71

Ali, H.; Loizidou, M.; Dashwood, M.; Savage, F.; Sheard, C. & Taylor, I. (2000b). Stimulation of colorectal cancer cell line growth by ET-1 and its inhibition by ET(A) antagonists. *Gut*, Vol.47, No.5, (Nov 2000b), pp. 685-688

Ambe, K.; Mori, M. & Enjoji, M. (1989). S-100 protein-positive dendritic cells in colorectal adenocarcinomas. Distribution and relation to the clinical prognosis. *Cancer*, Vol.63, No.3, (Feb 1 1989), pp. 496-503

Arun, C.; London, N. J. & Hemingway, D. M. (2004). Prognostic significance of elevated endothelin-1 levels in patients with colorectal cancer. *Int J Biol Markers*, Vol.19, No.1, (Jan-Mar 2004), pp. 32-37

Asghar, U.; Hawkes, E. & Cunningham, D. (2010). Predictive and prognostic biomarkers for targeted therapy in metastatic colorectal cancer. *Clin Colorectal Cancer*, Vol.9, No.5, (Dec 2010), pp. 274-281

Asham, E.; Shankar, A.; Loizidou, M.; Fredericks, S.; Miller, K.; Boulos, P. B.; Burnstock, G. & Taylor, I. (2001). Increased endothelin-1 in colorectal cancer and reduction of tumour growth by ET(A) receptor antagonism. *Br J Cancer*, Vol.85, No.11, (Nov 30 2001), pp. 1759-1763

Bacman, D.; Merkel, S.; Papadopoulos, T.; Croner, R. S.; Brueckl, W. M. & Dimmler, A. (2007). TGF-beta receptor 2 downregulation in tumour-associated stroma worsens prognosis and high-grade tumours show more tumour-associated macrophages and lower TGF-beta1 expression in colon carcinoma: a retrospective study. *BMC Cancer*, Vol.7, No.1, (Aug 10 2007), pp. 156

Bagnato, A. & Rosano, L. (2008). The endothelin axis in cancer. *Int J Biochem Cell Biol*, Vol.40, No.8, 2008), pp. 1443-1451

Balkwill, F. & Mantovani, A. (2001). Inflammation and cancer: back to Virchow? *Lancet*, Vol.357, No.9255, (Feb 17 2001), pp. 539-545

Barbera-Guillem, E.; Nyhus, J. K.; Wolford, C. C.; Friece, C. R. & Sampsel, J. W. (2002). Vascular endothelial growth factor secretion by tumor-infiltrating macrophages essentially supports tumor angiogenesis, and IgG immune complexes potentiate the process. *Cancer Res*, Vol.62, No.23, (Dec 1 2002), pp. 7042-7049

Bossi, P.; Viale, G.; Lee, A. K.; Alfano, R.; Coggi, G. & Bosari, S. (1995). Angiogenesis in colorectal tumors: microvessel quantitation in adenomas and carcinomas with clinicopathological correlations. *Cancer Res*, Vol.55, No.21, (Nov 1 1995), pp. 5049-5053

Briesemeister, D.; Sommermeyer, D.; Loddenkemper, C.; Loew, R.; Uckert, W.; Blankenstein, T. & Kammertoens, T. (2011). Tumor rejection by local interferon gamma induction in established tumors is associated with blood vessel destruction and necrosis. *Int J Cancer*, Vol.128, No.2, (Jan 15 2011), pp. 371-378

Broll, K.; Richter, G.; Pauly, S.; Hofstaedter, F. & Schwarz, H. (2001). CD137 expression in tumor vessel walls. High correlation with malignant tumors. *Am J Clin Pathol*, Vol.115, No.4, (Apr 2001), pp. 543-549

Buckanovich, R. J.; Facciabene, A.; Kim, S.; Benencia, F.; Sasaroli, D.; Balint, K.; Katsaros, D.; O'Brien-Jenkins, A.; Gimotty, P. A. & Coukos, G. (2008). Endothelin B receptor mediates the endothelial barrier to T cell homing to tumors and disables immune therapy. *Nat Med*, Vol.14, No.1, (Jan 2008), pp. 28-36

Buckanovich, R. J.; Sasaroli, D.; O'Brien-Jenkins, A.; Botbyl, J.; Hammond, R.; Katsaros, D.; Sandaltzopoulos, R.; Liotta, L. A.; Gimotty, P. A. & Coukos, G. (2007). Tumor vascular proteins as biomarkers in ovarian cancer. *J Clin Oncol*, Vol.25, No.7, (Mar 1 2007), pp. 852-861

Bussolati, B.; Deambrosis, I.; Russo, S.; Deregibus, M. C. & Camussi, G. (2003). Altered angiogenesis and survival in human tumor-derived endothelial cells. *FASEB J*, Vol.17, No.9, (Jun 2003), pp. 1159-1161

Carmeliet, P. & Jain, R. K. (2000). Angiogenesis in cancer and other diseases. *Nature*, Vol.407, No.6801, (Sep 14 2000), pp. 249-257

Carmeliet, P. & Jain, R. K. (2011). Molecular mechanisms and clinical applications of angiogenesis. *Nature*, Vol.473, No.7347, (May 19 2011), pp. 298-307

Choi, H. J.; Hyun, M. S.; Jung, G. J.; Kim, S. S. & Hong, S. H. (1998). Tumor angiogenesis as a prognostic predictor in colorectal carcinoma with special reference to mode of metastasis and recurrence. *Oncology*, Vol.55, No.6, (Nov-Dec 1998), pp. 575-581

Christian, S.; Winkler, R.; Helfrich, I.; Boos, A. M.; Besemfelder, E.; Schadendorf, D. & Augustin, H. G. (2008). Endosialin (Tem1) is a marker of tumor-associated myofibroblasts and tumor vessel-associated mural cells. *Am J Pathol*, Vol.172, No.2, (Feb 2008), pp. 486-494

Coca, S.; Perez-Piqueras, J.; Martinez, D.; Colmenarejo, A.; Saez, M. A.; Vallejo, C.; Martos, J. A. & Moreno, M. (1997). The prognostic significance of intratumoral natural killer cells in patients with colorectal carcinoma. *Cancer*, Vol.79, No.12, (Jun 15 1997), pp. 2320-2328

Condamine, T. & Gabrilovich, D. I. (2011). Molecular mechanisms regulating myeloid-derived suppressor cell differentiation and function. *Trends Immunol*, Vol.32, No.1, (Jan 2011), pp. 19-25

Corzo, C. A.; Condamine, T.; Lu, L.; Cotter, M. J.; Youn, J. I.; Cheng, P.; Cho, H. I.; Celis, E.; Quiceno, D. G.; Padhya, T.; McCaffrey, T. V.; McCaffrey, J. C. & Gabrilovich, D. I. (2010). HIF-1alpha regulates function and differentiation of myeloid-derived suppressor cells in the tumor microenvironment. *J Exp Med*, Vol.207, No.11, (Oct 25 2010), pp. 2439-2453

Coussens, L. M.; Raymond, W. W.; Bergers, G.; Laig-Webster, M.; Behrendtsen, O.; Werb, Z.; Caughey, G. H. & Hanahan, D. (1999). Inflammatory mast cells up-regulate angiogenesis during squamous epithelial carcinogenesis. *Genes Dev*, Vol.13, No.11, (Jun 1 1999), pp. 1382-1397

Coussens, L. M. & Werb, Z. (2001). Inflammatory cells and cancer: think different! *J Exp Med*, Vol.193, No.6, (Mar 19 2001), pp. F23-26

Cui, G.; Goll, R.; Olsen, T.; Steigen, S. E.; Husebekk, A.; Vonen, B. & Florholmen, J. (2007). Reduced expression of microenvironmental Th1 cytokines accompanies adenomas-carcinomas sequence of colorectum. *Cancer Immunol Immunother*, Vol.56, No.7, (Jul 2007), pp. 985-995

Curiel, T. J.; Cheng, P.; Mottram, P.; Alvarez, X.; Moons, L.; Evdemon-Hogan, M.; Wei, S.; Zou, L.; Kryczek, I.; Hoyle, G.; Lackner, A.; Carmeliet, P. & Zou, W. (2004). Dendritic cell subsets differentially regulate angiogenesis in human ovarian cancer. *Cancer Res*, Vol.64, No.16, (Aug 15 2004), pp. 5535-5538

Dadabayev, A. R.; Sandel, M. H.; Menon, A. G.; Morreau, H.; Melief, C. J.; Offringa, R.; van der Burg, S. H.; Janssen-van Rhijn, C.; Ensink, N. G.; Tollenaar, R. A.; van de Velde, C. J. & Kuppen, P. J. (2004). Dendritic cells in colorectal cancer correlate with other tumor-infiltrating immune cells. *Cancer Immunol Immunother*, Vol.53, No.11, (Nov 2004), pp. 978-986

Dayer, J. M. (2002a). Evidence for the biological modulation of IL-1 activity: the role of IL-1Ra. *Clin Exp Rheumatol*, Vol.20, No.5 Suppl 27, (Sep-Oct 2002a), pp. S14-20

Dayer, J. M. (2002b). Interleukin 1 or tumor necrosis factor-alpha: which is the real target in rheumatoid arthritis? *J Rheumatol Suppl*, Vol.65, (Sep 2002b), pp. 10-15

De Palma, M.; Murdoch, C.; Venneri, M. A.; Naldini, L. & Lewis, C. E. (2007). Tie2-expressing monocytes: regulation of tumor angiogenesis and therapeutic implications. *Trends Immunol*, Vol.28, No.12, (Dec 2007), pp. 519-524

De Palma, M. & Naldini, L. (2009). Tie2-expressing monocytes (TEMs): Novel targets and vehicles of anticancer therapy? *Biochim Biophys Acta*, (Apr 10 2009),

De Palma, M. & Naldini, L. (2011). Angiopoietin-2 TIEs Up Macrophages in Tumor Angiogenesis. *Clin Cancer Res*, (May 16 2011),

De Palma, M.; Venneri, M. A.; Galli, R.; Sergi Sergi, L.; Politi, L. S.; Sampaolesi, M. & Naldini, L. (2005). Tie2 identifies a hematopoietic lineage of proangiogenic monocytes required for tumor vessel formation and a mesenchymal population of pericyte progenitors. *Cancer Cell*, Vol.8, No.3, (Sep 2005), pp. 211-226

Demetri, G. D.; van Oosterom, A. T.; Garrett, C. R.; Blackstein, M. E.; Shah, M. H.; Verweij, J.; McArthur, G.; Judson, I. R.; Heinrich, M. C.; Morgan, J. A.; Desai, J.; Fletcher, C. D.; George, S.; Bello, C. L.; Huang, X.; Baum, C. M. & Casali, P. G. (2006). Efficacy and safety of sunitinib in patients with advanced gastrointestinal stromal tumour after failure of imatinib: a randomised controlled trial. *Lancet*, Vol.368, No.9544, (Oct 14 2006), pp. 1329-1338

Deprimo, S. E.; Huang, X.; Blackstein, M. E.; Garrett, C. R.; Harmon, C. S.; Schoffski, P.; Shah, M. H.; Verweij, J.; Baum, C. M. & Demetri, G. D. (2009). Circulating levels of soluble KIT serve as a biomarker for clinical outcome in gastrointestinal stromal tumor patients receiving sunitinib following imatinib failure. *Clin Cancer Res*, Vol.15, No.18, (Sep 15 2009), pp. 5869-5877

Eck, M.; Schmausser, B.; Scheller, K.; Brandlein, S. & Muller-Hermelink, H. K. (2003). Pleiotropic effects of CXC chemokines in gastric carcinoma: differences in CXCL8 and CXCL1 expression between diffuse and intestinal types of gastric carcinoma. *Clin Exp Immunol*, Vol.134, No.3, (Dec 2003), pp. 508-515

Escudier, B.; Eisen, T.; Stadler, W. M.; Szczylik, C.; Oudard, S.; Siebels, M.; Negrier, S.; Chevreau, C.; Solska, E.; Desai, A. A.; Rolland, F.; Demkow, T.; Hutson, T. E.; Gore, M.; Freeman, S.; Schwartz, B.; Shan, M.; Simantov, R. & Bukowski, R. M. (2007). Sorafenib in advanced clear-cell renal-cell carcinoma. *N Engl J Med*, Vol.356, No.2, (Jan 11 2007), pp. 125-134

Folkman, J. (1995). Angiogenesis in cancer, vascular, rheumatoid and other disease. *Nat Med*, Vol.1, No.1, (Jan 1995), pp. 27-31

Gabrilovich, D. I. & Nagaraj, S. (2009). Myeloid-derived suppressor cells as regulators of the immune system. *Nat Rev Immunol*, Vol.9, No.3, (Mar 2009), pp. 162-174

Galon, J.; Costes, A.; Sanchez-Cabo, F.; Kirilovsky, A.; Mlecnik, B.; Lagorce-Pages, C.; Tosolini, M.; Camus, M.; Berger, A.; Wind, P.; Zinzindohoue, F.; Bruneval, P.;

Cugnenc, P. H.; Trajanoski, Z.; Fridman, W. H. & Pages, F. (2006). Type, density, and location of immune cells within human colorectal tumors predict clinical outcome. *Science*, Vol.313, No.5795, (Sep 29 2006), pp. 1960-1964

Galon, J.; Fridman, W. H. & Pages, F. (2007). The adaptive immunologic microenvironment in colorectal cancer: a novel perspective. *Cancer Res*, Vol.67, No.5, (Mar 1 2007), pp. 1883-1886

Gerger, A.; LaBonte, M. & Lenz, H. J. (2011). Molecular predictors of response to antiangiogenesis therapies. *Cancer J*, Vol.17, No.2, (Mar-Apr 2011), pp. 134-141

Ghosh, K.; Thodeti, C. K.; Dudley, A. C.; Mammoto, A.; Klagsbrun, M. & Ingber, D. E. (2008). Tumor-derived endothelial cells exhibit aberrant Rho-mediated mechanosensing and abnormal angiogenesis in vitro. *Proc Natl Acad Sci U S A*, Vol.105, No.32, (Aug 12 2008), pp. 11305-11310

Goede, V.; Coutelle, O.; Neuneier, J.; Reinacher-Schick, A.; Schnell, R.; Koslowsky, T. C.; Weihrauch, M. R.; Cremer, B.; Kashkar, H.; Odenthal, M.; Augustin, H. G.; Schmiegel, W.; Hallek, M. & Hacker, U. T. (2010). Identification of serum angiopoietin-2 as a biomarker for clinical outcome of colorectal cancer patients treated with bevacizumab-containing therapy. *Br J Cancer*, Vol.103, No.9, (Oct 26 2010), pp. 1407-1414

Guenzi, E.; Töpolt, K.; Cornali, E.; Lubeseder-Martellato, C.; Jörg, A.; Matzen, K.; Zietz, C.; Kremmer, E.; Nappi, F.; Schwemmle, M.; Hohenadl, C.; Barillari, G.; Tschachler, E.; Monini, P.; Ensoli, B. & Stürzl, M. (2001). The helical domain of GBP-1 mediates the inhibition of endothelial cell proliferation by inflammatory cytokines. *Embo J*, Vol.20, No.20, 2001), pp. 5568-5577.

Guenzi, E.; Töpolt, K.; Lubeseder-Martellato, C.; Jörg, A.; Naschberger, E.; Benelli, R.; Albini, A. & Stürzl, M. (2003). The guanylate binding protein-1 GTPase controls the invasive and angiogenic capability of endothelial cells through inhibition of MMP-1 expression. *Embo J*, Vol.22, No.15, (Aug 1 2003), pp. 3772-3782

Guidoboni, M.; Gafa, R.; Viel, A.; Doglioni, C.; Russo, A.; Santini, A.; Del Tin, L.; Macri, E.; Lanza, G.; Boiocchi, M. & Dolcetti, R. (2001). Microsatellite instability and high content of activated cytotoxic lymphocytes identify colon cancer patients with a favorable prognosis. *Am J Pathol*, Vol.159, No.1, (Jul 2001), pp. 297-304

Gulubova, M. & Vlaykova, T. (2009). Prognostic significance of mast cell number and microvascular density for the survival of patients with primary colorectal cancer. *J Gastroenterol Hepatol*, Vol.24, No.7, (Jul 2009), pp. 1265-1275

Hanahan, D. & Weinberg, R. A. (2000). The hallmarks of cancer. *Cell*, Vol.100, No.1, (Jan 7 2000), pp. 57-70

Hanahan, D. & Weinberg, R. A. (2011). Hallmarks of cancer: the next generation. *Cell*, Vol.144, No.5, (Mar 4 2011), pp. 646-674

Harrison, J. C.; Dean, P. J.; el-Zeky, F. & Vander Zwaag, R. (1994). From Dukes through Jass: pathological prognostic indicators in rectal cancer. *Hum Pathol*, Vol.25, No.5, (May 1994), pp. 498-505

Hawinkels, L. J.; Zuidwijk, K.; Verspaget, H. W.; de Jonge-Muller, E. S.; van Duijn, W.; Ferreira, V.; Fontijn, R. D.; David, G.; Hommes, D. W.; Lamers, C. B. & Sier, C. F. (2008). VEGF release by MMP-9 mediated heparan sulphate cleavage induces colorectal cancer angiogenesis. *Eur J Cancer*, Vol.44, No.13, (Sep 2008), pp. 1904-1913

Hida, K.; Hida, Y. & Shindoh, M. (2008). Understanding tumor endothelial cell abnormalities to develop ideal anti-angiogenic therapies. *Cancer Sci*, Vol.99, No.3, (Mar 2008), pp. 459-466

Hida, K. & Klagsbrun, M. (2005). A new perspective on tumor endothelial cells: unexpected chromosome and centrosome abnormalities. *Cancer Res*, Vol.65, No.7, (Apr 1 2005), pp. 2507-2510

Hoosein, M. M.; Dashwood, M. R.; Dawas, K.; Ali, H. M.; Grant, K.; Savage, F.; Taylor, I. & Loizidou, M. (2007). Altered endothelin receptor subtypes in colorectal cancer. *Eur J Gastroenterol Hepatol*, Vol.19, No.9, (Sep 2007), pp. 775-782

Hurwitz, H.; Fehrenbacher, L.; Novotny, W.; Cartwright, T.; Hainsworth, J.; Heim, W.; Berlin, J.; Baron, A.; Griffing, S.; Holmgren, E.; Ferrara, N.; Fyfe, G.; Rogers, B.; Ross, R. & Kabbinavar, F. (2004). Bevacizumab plus irinotecan, fluorouracil, and leucovorin for metastatic colorectal cancer. *N Engl J Med*, Vol.350, No.23, (Jun 3 2004), pp. 2335-2342

Ishigami, S. I.; Arii, S.; Furutani, M.; Niwano, M.; Harada, T.; Mizumoto, M.; Mori, A.; Onodera, H. & Imamura, M. (1998). Predictive value of vascular endothelial growth factor (VEGF) in metastasis and prognosis of human colorectal cancer. *Br J Cancer*, Vol.78, No.10, (Nov 1998), pp. 1379-1384

Jass, J. R. (1986). Lymphocytic infiltration and survival in rectal cancer. *J Clin Pathol*, Vol.39, No.6, (Jun 1986), pp. 585-589

Jass, J. R. (2002). Pathogenesis of colorectal cancer. *Surg Clin North Am*, Vol.82, No.5, (Oct 2002), pp. 891-904

Jubb, A. M.; Hurwitz, H. I.; Bai, W.; Holmgren, E. B.; Tobin, P.; Guerrero, A. S.; Kabbinavar, F.; Holden, S. N.; Novotny, W. F.; Frantz, G. D.; Hillan, K. J. & Koeppen, H. (2006). Impact of vascular endothelial growth factor-A expression, thrombospondin-2 expression, and microvessel density on the treatment effect of bevacizumab in metastatic colorectal cancer. *J Clin Oncol*, Vol.24, No.2, (Jan 10 2006), pp. 217-227

Kahlenberg, M. S.; Sullivan, J. M.; Witmer, D. D. & Petrelli, N. J. (2003). Molecular prognostics in colorectal cancer. *Surg Oncol*, Vol.12, No.3, (Nov 2003), pp. 173-186

Kandalaft, L. E.; Facciabene, A.; Buckanovich, R. J. & Coukos, G. (2009). Endothelin B receptor, a new target in cancer immune therapy. *Clin Cancer Res*, Vol.15, No.14, (Jul 15 2009), pp. 4521-4528

Kang, S. M.; Maeda, K.; Onoda, N.; Chung, Y. S.; Nakata, B.; Nishiguchi, Y. & Sowa, M. (1997). Combined analysis of p53 and vascular endothelial growth factor expression in colorectal carcinoma for determination of tumor vascularity and liver metastasis. *Int J Cancer*, Vol.74, No.5, (Oct 21 1997), pp. 502-507

Katz, S. C.; Pillarisetty, V.; Bamboat, Z. M.; Shia, J.; Hedvat, C.; Gonen, M.; Jarnagin, W.; Fong, Y.; Blumgart, L.; D'Angelica, M. & DeMatteo, R. P. (2009). T cell infiltrate predicts long-term survival following resection of colorectal cancer liver metastases. *Ann Surg Oncol*, Vol.16, No.9, (Sep 2009), pp. 2524-2530

Kedzierski, R. M. & Yanagisawa, M. (2001). Endothelin system: the double-edged sword in health and disease. *Annu Rev Pharmacol Toxicol*, Vol.41, 2001), pp. 851-876

Kilarski, W. W.; Samolov, B.; Petersson, L.; Kvanta, A. & Gerwins, P. (2009). Biomechanical regulation of blood vessel growth during tissue vascularization. *Nat Med*, Vol.15, No.6, (Jun 2009), pp. 657-664

Kopetz, S.; Hoff, P. M.; Morris, J. S.; Wolff, R. A.; Eng, C.; Glover, K. Y.; Adinin, R.; Overman, M. J.; Valero, V.; Wen, S.; Lieu, C.; Yan, S.; Tran, H. T.; Ellis, L. M.; Abbruzzese, J. L. & Heymach, J. V. (2010). Phase II trial of infusional fluorouracil, irinotecan, and bevacizumab for metastatic colorectal cancer: efficacy and circulating angiogenic biomarkers associated with therapeutic resistance. *J Clin Oncol*, Vol.28, No.3, (Jan 20 2010), pp. 453-459

Kumar, H.; Heer, K.; Lee, P. W.; Duthie, G. S.; MacDonald, A. W.; Greenman, J.; Kerin, M. J. & Monson, J. R. (1998). Preoperative serum vascular endothelial growth factor can predict stage in colorectal cancer. *Clin Cancer Res*, Vol.4, No.5, (May 1998), pp. 1279-1285

Kusuhara, M.; Yamaguchi, K.; Nagasaki, K.; Hayashi, C.; Suzaki, A.; Hori, S.; Handa, S.; Nakamura, Y. & Abe, K. (1990). Production of endothelin in human cancer cell lines. *Cancer Res*, Vol.50, No.11, (Jun 1 1990), pp. 3257-3261

Lee, H. K.; Kang, D. S.; Seo, I. A.; Choi, E. J.; Park, H. T. & Park, J. I. (2006). Expression of tumor endothelial marker 7 mRNA and protein in the dorsal root ganglion neurons of the rat. *Neurosci Lett*, Vol.402, No.1-2, (Jul 10 2006), pp. 71-75

Leite de Oliveira, R.; Hamm, A. & Mazzone, M. (2011). Growing tumor vessels: More than one way to skin a cat - Implications for angiogenesis targeted cancer therapies. *Mol Aspects Med*, Vol.32, No.2, (Apr 2011), pp. 71-87

Leo, E.; Belli, F.; Andreola, S.; Gallino, G.; Bonfanti, G.; Ferro, F.; Zingaro, E.; Sirizzotti, G.; Civelli, E.; Valvo, F.; Gios, M. & Brunelli, C. (2000). Total rectal resection and complete mesorectum excision followed by coloendoanal anastomosis as the optimal treatment for low rectal cancer: the experience of the National Cancer Institute of Milano. *Ann Surg Oncol*, Vol.7, No.2, (Mar 2000), pp. 125-132

Levy, E. M.; Roberti, M. P. & Mordoh, J. (2011). Natural killer cells in human cancer: from biological functions to clinical applications. *J Biomed Biotechnol*, Vol.2011, 2011), pp. 676198

Loupakis, F.; Falcone, A.; Masi, G.; Fioravanti, A.; Kerbel, R. S.; Del Tacca, M. & Bocci, G. (2007). Vascular endothelial growth factor levels in immunodepleted plasma of cancer patients as a possible pharmacodynamic marker for bevacizumab activity. *J Clin Oncol*, Vol.25, No.13, (May 1 2007), pp. 1816-1818

Lubeseder-Martellato, C.; Guenzi, E.; Jörg, A.; Töpolt, K.; Naschberger, E.; Kremmer, E.; Zietz, C.; Tschachler, E.; Hutzler, P.; Schwemmle, M.; Matzen, K.; Grimm, T.; Ensoli, B. & Stürzl, M. (2002). Guanylate-Binding Protein-1 Expression Is Selectively Induced by Inflammatory Cytokines and Is an Activation Marker of Endothelial Cells during Inflammatory Diseases. *Am J Pathol*, Vol.161, No.5, (Nov 2002), pp. 1749-1759

Maltby, S.; Khazaie, K. & McNagny, K. M. (2009). Mast cells in tumor growth: angiogenesis, tissue remodelling and immune-modulation. *Biochim Biophys Acta*, Vol.1796, No.1, (Aug 2009), pp. 19-26

Mandruzzato, S.; Solito, S.; Falisi, E.; Francescato, S.; Chiarion-Sileni, V.; Mocellin, S.; Zanon, A.; Rossi, C. R.; Nitti, D.; Bronte, V. & Zanovello, P. (2009). IL4Ralpha+ myeloid-derived suppressor cell expansion in cancer patients. *J Immunol*, Vol.182, No.10, (May 15 2009), pp. 6562-6568

Mantovani, A. & Sica, A. (2010). Macrophages, innate immunity and cancer: balance, tolerance, and diversity. *Curr Opin Immunol*, Vol.22, No.2, (Apr 2010), pp. 231-237

Motzer, R. J.; Hutson, T. E.; Tomczak, P.; Michaelson, M. D.; Bukowski, R. M.; Rixe, O.; Oudard, S.; Negrier, S.; Szczylik, C.; Kim, S. T.; Chen, I.; Bycott, P. W.; Baum, C. M. & Figlin, R. A. (2007). Sunitinib versus interferon alfa in metastatic renal-cell carcinoma. *N Engl J Med*, Vol.356, No.2, (Jan 11 2007), pp. 115-124

Naito, Y.; Saito, K.; Shiiba, K.; Ohuchi, A.; Saigenji, K.; Nagura, H. & Ohtani, H. (1998). CD8+ T cells infiltrated within cancer cell nests as a prognostic factor in human colorectal cancer. *Cancer Res*, Vol.58, No.16, (Aug 15 1998), pp. 3491-3494

Nanda, A.; Buckhaults, P.; Seaman, S.; Agrawal, N.; Boutin, P.; Shankara, S.; Nacht, M.; Teicher, B.; Stampfl, J.; Singh, S.; Vogelstein, B.; Kinzler, K. W. & St Croix, B. (2004). Identification of a binding partner for the endothelial cell surface proteins TEM7 and TEM7R. *Cancer Res*, Vol.64, No.23, (Dec 1 2004), pp. 8507-8511

Naschberger, E.; Croner, R. S.; Merkel, S.; Dimmler, A.; Tripal, P.; Amann, K. U.; Kremmer, E.; Brueckl, W. M.; Papadopoulos, T.; Hohenadl, C.; Hohenberger, W. & Stürzl, M. (2008). Angiostatic immune reaction in colorectal carcinoma: Impact on survival and perspectives for antiangiogenic therapy. *Int J Cancer*, Vol.123, No.9, (Nov 1 2008), pp. 2120-2129

Nielsen, H. J.; Hansen, U.; Christensen, I. J.; Reimert, C. M.; Brunner, N. & Moesgaard, F. (1999). Independent prognostic value of eosinophil and mast cell infiltration in colorectal cancer tissue. *J Pathol*, Vol.189, No.4, (Dec 1999), pp. 487-495

O'Brien, C. A.; Pollett, A.; Gallinger, S. & Dick, J. E. (2007). A human colon cancer cell capable of initiating tumour growth in immunodeficient mice. *Nature*, Vol.445, No.7123, (Jan 4 2007), pp. 106-110

Palazon, A.; Teijeira, A.; Martinez-Forero, I.; Hervas-Stubbs, S.; Roncal, C.; Penuelas, I.; Dubrot, J.; Morales-Kastresana, A.; Perez-Gracia, J. L.; Ochoa, M. C.; Ochoa-Callejero, L.; Martinez, A.; Luque, A.; Dinchuk, J.; Rouzaut, A.; Jure-Kunkel, M. & Melero, I. (2011). Agonist anti-CD137 mAb act on tumor endothelial cells to enhance recruitment of activated T lymphocytes. *Cancer Res*, Vol.71, No.3, (Feb 1 2011), pp. 801-811

Peddareddigari, V. G.; Wang, D. & Dubois, R. N. (2010). The tumor microenvironment in colorectal carcinogenesis. *Cancer Microenviron*, Vol.3, No.1, 2010), pp. 149-166

Perez-Gracia, J. L.; Prior, C.; Guillen-Grima, F.; Segura, V.; Gonzalez, A.; Panizo, A.; Melero, I.; Grande-Pulido, E.; Gurpide, A.; Gil-Bazo, I. & Calvo, A. (2009). Identification of TNF-alpha and MMP-9 as potential baseline predictive serum markers of sunitinib activity in patients with renal cell carcinoma using a human cytokine array. *Br J Cancer*, Vol.101, No.11, (Dec 1 2009), pp. 1876-1883

Ricci-Vitiani, L.; Lombardi, D. G.; Pilozzi, E.; Biffoni, M.; Todaro, M.; Peschle, C. & De Maria, R. (2007). Identification and expansion of human colon-cancer-initiating cells. *Nature*, Vol.445, No.7123, (Jan 4 2007), pp. 111-115

Ricci-Vitiani, L.; Pallini, R.; Biffoni, M.; Todaro, M.; Invernici, G.; Cenci, T.; Maira, G.; Parati, E. A.; Stassi, G.; Larocca, L. M. & De Maria, R. (2010). Tumour vascularization via endothelial differentiation of glioblastoma stem-like cells. *Nature*, Vol.468, No.7325, (Dec 9 2010), pp. 824-828

Risau, W. (1997). Mechanisms of angiogenesis. *Nature*, Vol.386, No.6626, (Apr 17 1997), pp. 671-674

Roessner, A.; Kuester, D.; Malfertheiner, P. & Schneider-Stock, R. (2008). Oxidative stress in ulcerative colitis-associated carcinogenesis. *Pathol Res Pract*, Vol.204, No.7, 2008), pp. 511-524

Romagnani, P.; Lasagni, L.; Annunziato, F.; Serio, M. & Romagnani, S. (2004). CXC chemokines: the regulatory link between inflammation and angiogenesis. *Trends Immunol*, Vol.25, No.4, (Apr 2004), pp. 201-209

Roncucci, L.; Fante, R.; Losi, L.; Di Gregorio, C.; Micheli, A.; Benatti, P.; Madenis, N.; Ganazzi, D.; Cassinadri, M. T.; Lauriola, P. & Ponz de Leon, M. (1996). Survival for colon and rectal cancer in a population-based cancer registry. *Eur J Cancer*, Vol.32A, No.2, (Feb 1996), pp. 295-302

Roncucci, L.; Mora, E.; Mariani, F.; Bursi, S.; Pezzi, A.; Rossi, G.; Pedroni, M.; Luppi, D.; Santoro, L., Monni, S., Manenti, A.; Bertani, A.; Merighi, A.; Benatti, P.; Di Gregorio, C. & de Leon, P. M. (2008). Myeloperoxidase-positive cell infiltration in colorectal carcinogenesis as indicator of colorectal cancer risk. *Cancer Epidemiol Biomarkers Prev*, Vol.17, No.9, (Sep 2008), pp. 2291-2297

Ronzoni, M.; Manzoni, M.; Mariucci, S.; Loupakis, F.; Brugnatelli, S.; Bencardino, K.; Rovati, B.; Tinelli, C.; Falcone, A.; Villa, E. & Danova, M. (2010). Circulating endothelial cells and endothelial progenitors as predictive markers of clinical response to bevacizumab-based first-line treatment in advanced colorectal cancer patients. *Ann Oncol*, Vol.21, No.12, (Dec 2010), pp. 2382-2389

Ropponen, K. M.; Eskelinen, M. J.; Lipponen, P. K.; Alhava, E. & Kosma, V. M. (1997). Prognostic value of tumour-infiltrating lymphocytes (TILs) in colorectal cancer. *J Pathol*, Vol.182, No.3, (Jul 1997), pp. 318-324

Salama, P. & Platell, C. (2008). Host response to colorectal cancer. *ANZ J Surg*, Vol.78, No.9, (Sep 2008), pp. 745-753

Salih, H. R.; Kosowski, S. G.; Haluska, V. F.; Starling, G. C.; Loo, D. T.; Lee, F.; Aruffo, A. A.; Trail, P. A. & Kiener, P. A. (2000). Constitutive expression of functional 4-1BB (CD137) ligand on carcinoma cells. *J Immunol*, Vol.165, No.5, (Sep 1 2000), pp. 2903-2910

Sandel, M. H.; Dadabayev, A. R.; Menon, A. G.; Morreau, H.; Melief, C. J.; Offringa, R.; van der Burg, S. H.; Janssen-van Rhijn, C. M.; Ensink, N. G.; Tollenaar, R. A.; van de Velde, C. J. & Kuppen, P. J. (2005). Prognostic value of tumor-infiltrating dendritic cells in colorectal cancer: role of maturation status and intratumoral localization. *Clin Cancer Res*, Vol.11, No.7, (Apr 1 2005), pp. 2576-2582

Schellerer, V. S.; Croner, R. S.; Weinländer, K.; Hohenberger, W.; Stürzl, M. & Naschberger, E. (2007). Endothelial cells of human colorectal cancer and healthy colon reveal phenotypic differences in culture. *Lab Invest*, Vol.87, No.11, (Nov 2007), pp. 1159-1170

Schneider, B. P.; Wang, M.; Radovich, M.; Sledge, G. W.; Badve, S.; Thor, A.; Flockhart, D. A.; Hancock, B.; Davidson, N.; Gralow, J.; Dickler, M.; Perez, E. A.; Cobleigh, M.; Shenkier, T.; Edgerton, S. & Miller, K. D. (2008). Association of vascular endothelial growth factor and vascular endothelial growth factor receptor-2 genetic polymorphisms with outcome in a trial of paclitaxel compared with paclitaxel plus bevacizumab in advanced breast cancer: ECOG 2100. *J Clin Oncol*, Vol.26, No.28, (Oct 1 2008), pp. 4672-4678

Shao, Z. & Schwarz, H. (2011). CD137 ligand, a member of the tumor necrosis factor family, regulates immune responses via reverse signal transduction. *J Leukoc Biol*, Vol.89, No.1, (Jan 2011), pp. 21-29

Shmelkov, S. V.; Butler, J. M.; Hooper, A. T.; Hormigo, A.; Kushner, J.; Milde, T.; St Clair, R.; Baljevic, M.; White, I.; Jin, D. K.; Chadburn, A.; Murphy, A. J.; Valenzuela, D. M.; Gale, N. W.; Thurston, G.; Yancopoulos, G. D.; D'Angelica, M.; Kemeny, N.; Lyden, D. & Rafii, S. (2008). CD133 expression is not restricted to stem cells, and both CD133+ and CD133- metastatic colon cancer cells initiate tumors. *J Clin Invest*, Vol.118, No.6, (Jun 2008), pp. 2111-2120

Sica, A.; Allavena, P. & Mantovani, A. (2008a). Cancer related inflammation: the macrophage connection. *Cancer Lett*, Vol.267, No.2, (Aug 28 2008a), pp. 204-215

Sica, A.; Larghi, P.; Mancino, A.; Rubino, L.; Porta, C.; Totaro, M. G.; Rimoldi, M.; Biswas, S. K.; Allavena, P. & Mantovani, A. (2008b). Macrophage polarization in tumour progression. *Semin Cancer Biol*, Vol.18, No.5, (Oct 2008b), pp. 349-355

Smith, R. A.; Cokkinides, V.; von Eschenbach, A. C.; Levin, B.; Cohen, C.; Runowicz, C. D.; Sener, S.; Saslow, D. & Eyre, H. J. (2002). American Cancer Society guidelines for the early detection of cancer. *CA Cancer J Clin*, Vol.52, No.1, (Jan-Feb 2002), pp. 8-22

Sobrero, A.; Ackland, S.; Clarke, S.; Perez-Carrion, R.; Chiara, S.; Gapski, J.; Mainwaring, P.; Langer, B. & Young, S. (2009). Phase IV study of bevacizumab in combination with infusional fluorouracil, leucovorin and irinotecan (FOLFIRI) in first-line metastatic colorectal cancer. *Oncology*, Vol.77, No.2, 2009), pp. 113-119

St Croix, B.; Rago, C.; Velculescu, V.; Traverso, G.; Romans, K. E.; Montgomery, E.; Lal, A.; Riggins, G. J.; Lengauer, C.; Vogelstein, B. & Kinzler, K. W. (2000). Genes expressed in human tumor endothelium. *Science*, Vol.289, No.5482, (Aug 18 2000), pp. 1197-1202

Streubel, B.; Chott, A.; Huber, D.; Exner, M.; Jager, U.; Wagner, O. & Schwarzinger, I. (2004). Lymphoma-specific genetic aberrations in microvascular endothelial cells in B-cell lymphomas. *N Engl J Med*, Vol.351, No.3, (Jul 15 2004), pp. 250-259

Suzuki, A.; Masuda, A.; Nagata, H.; Kameoka, S.; Kikawada, Y.; Yamakawa, M. & Kasajima, T. (2002). Mature dendritic cells make clusters with T cells in the invasive margin of colorectal carcinoma. *J Pathol*, Vol.196, No.1, (Jan 2002), pp. 37-43

Tachibana, T.; Onodera, H.; Tsuruyama, T.; Mori, A.; Nagayama, S.; Hiai, H. & Imamura, M. (2005). Increased intratumor Valpha24-positive natural killer T cells: a prognostic factor for primary colorectal carcinomas. *Clin Cancer Res*, Vol.11, No.20, (Oct 15 2005), pp. 7322-7327

Takebayashi, Y.; Aklyama, S.; Yamada, K.; Akiba, S. & Aikou, T. (1996). Angiogenesis as an unfavorable prognostic factor in human colorectal carcinoma. *Cancer*, Vol.78, No.2, (Jul 15 1996), pp. 226-231

Tartour, E.; Pere, H.; Maillere, B.; Terme, M.; Merillon, N.; Taieb, J.; Sandoval, F.; Quintin-Colonna, F.; Lacerda, K.; Karadimou, A.; Badoual, C.; Tedgui, A.; Fridman, W. H. & Oudard, S. (2011). Angiogenesis and immunity: a bidirectional link potentially relevant for the monitoring of antiangiogenic therapy and the development of novel therapeutic combination with immunotherapy. *Cancer Metastasis Rev*, Vol.30, No.1, (Mar 2011), pp. 83-95

Tazzyman, S.; Lewis, C. E. & Murdoch, C. (2009). Neutrophils: key mediators of tumour angiogenesis. *Int J Exp Pathol*, Vol.90, No.3, (Jun 2009), pp. 222-231

Terabe, M. & Berzofsky, J. A. (2008). The role of NKT cells in tumor immunity. *Adv Cancer Res*, Vol.101, 2008), pp. 277-348

Tosolini, M.; Kirilovsky, A.; Mlecnik, B.; Fredriksen, T.; Mauger, S.; Bindea, G.; Berger, A.; Bruneval, P.; Fridman, W. H.; Pages, F. & Galon, J. (2011). Clinical impact of different classes of infiltrating T cytotoxic and helper cells (Th1, th2, treg, th17) in patients with colorectal cancer. *Cancer Res*, Vol.71, No.4, (Feb 15 2011), pp. 1263-1271

van der Vliet, H. J.; Wang, R.; Yue, S. C.; Koon, H. B.; Balk, S. P. & Exley, M. A. (2008). Circulating myeloid dendritic cells of advanced cancer patients result in reduced activation and a biased cytokine profile in invariant NKT cells. *J Immunol*, Vol.180, No.11, (Jun 1 2008), pp. 7287-7293

Venneri, M. A.; De Palma, M.; Ponzoni, M.; Pucci, F.; Scielzo, C.; Zonari, E.; Mazzieri, R.; Doglioni, C. & Naldini, L. (2007). Identification of proangiogenic TIE2-expressing monocytes (TEMs) in human peripheral blood and cancer. *Blood*, Vol.109, No.12, (Jun 15 2007), pp. 5276-5285

Vogelstein, B.; Fearon, E. R.; Hamilton, S. R.; Kern, S. E.; Preisinger, A. C.; Leppert, M.; Nakamura, Y.; White, R.; Smits, A. M. & Bos, J. L. (1988). Genetic alterations during colorectal-tumor development. *N Engl J Med*, Vol.319, No.9, (Sep 1 1988), pp. 525-532

Wang, Q.; Zhang, P.; Zhang, Q.; Wang, X.; Li, J.; Ma, C.; Sun, W. & Zhang, L. (2008). Analysis of CD137 and CD137L expression in human primary tumor tissues. *Croat Med J*, Vol.49, No.2, (Apr 2008), pp. 192-200

Wang, R.; Chadalavada, K.; Wilshire, J.; Kowalik, U.; Hovinga, K. E.; Geber, A.; Fligelman, B.; Leversha, M.; Brennan, C. & Tabar, V. (2010). Glioblastoma stem-like cells give rise to tumour endothelium. *Nature*, Vol.468, No.7325, (Dec 9 2010), pp. 829-833

Willett, C. G.; Duda, D. G.; di Tomaso, E.; Boucher, Y.; Ancukiewicz, M.; Sahani, D. V.; Lahdenranta, J.; Chung, D. C.; Fischman, A. J.; Lauwers, G. Y.; Shellito, P.; Czito, B. G.; Wong, T. Z.; Paulson, E.; Poleski, M.; Vujaskovic, Z.; Bentley, R.; Chen, H. X.; Clark, J. W. & Jain, R. K. (2009). Efficacy, safety, and biomarkers of neoadjuvant bevacizumab, radiation therapy, and fluorouracil in rectal cancer: a multidisciplinary phase II study. *J Clin Oncol*, Vol.27, No.18, (Jun 20 2009), pp. 3020-3026

Xiong, Y. Q.; Sun, H. C.; Zhang, W.; Zhu, X. D.; Zhuang, P. Y.; Zhang, J. B.; Wang, L.; Wu, W. Z.; Qin, L. X. & Tang, Z. Y. (2009). Human hepatocellular carcinoma tumor-derived endothelial cells manifest increased angiogenesis capability and drug resistance compared with normal endothelial cells. *Clin Cancer Res*, Vol.15, No.15, (Aug 1 2009), pp. 4838-4846

Yang, L.; DeBusk, L. M.; Fukuda, K.; Fingleton, B.; Green-Jarvis, B.; Shyr, Y.; Matrisian, L. M.; Carbone, D. P. & Lin, P. C. (2004). Expansion of myeloid immune suppressor Gr+CD11b+ cells in tumor-bearing host directly promotes tumor angiogenesis. *Cancer Cell*, Vol.6, No.4, (Oct 2004), pp. 409-421

Yang, S. X.; Steinberg, S. M.; Nguyen, D.; Wu, T. D.; Modrusan, Z. & Swain, S. M. (2008). Gene expression profile and angiogenic marker correlates with response to neoadjuvant bevacizumab followed by bevacizumab plus chemotherapy in breast cancer. *Clin Cancer Res*, Vol.14, No.18, (Sep 15 2008), pp. 5893-5899

Youn, J. I. & Gabrilovich, D. I. (2010). The biology of myeloid-derived suppressor cells: the blessing and the curse of morphological and functional heterogeneity. *Eur J Immunol*, Vol.40, No.11, (Nov 2010), pp. 2969-2975

Zhang, S.; Zhang, H. & Zhao, J. (2009). The role of CD4 T cell help for CD8 CTL activation. *Biochem Biophys Res Commun*, Vol.384, No.4, (Jul 10 2009), pp. 405-408

Zhou, L.; Chong, M. M. & Littman, D. R. (2009). Plasticity of CD4+ T cell lineage differentiation. *Immunity*, Vol.30, No.5, (May 2009), pp. 646-655

Zhu, J. & Paul, W. E. (2010). Heterogeneity and plasticity of T helper cells. *Cell Res*, Vol.20, No.1, (Jan 2010), pp. 4-12

15

Adaptive and Innate Immunity, Non Clonal Players in Colorectal Cancer Progression

Lucia Fini, Fabio Grizzi and Luigi Laghi
Laboratory of Molecular Gastroenterology and Department of Gastroenterology, IRCCS Istituto Clinico Humanitas, Rozzano, Milan, Italy

1. Introduction

The progression of colorectal cancer (CRC), like that of other solid tumors, has been first conceptualized by pathological staging (initially according to Dukes and later by the AJCC/UICC TNM staging system) as a step-wise invasion of bowel layers, followed by lymph-node involvement, to culminate into distant organ metastasis [1]. Additionally, the recognition of pre-cancerous lesions (*i.e.*, adenoma) set up the notion that cancer develops from a benign lesion, according to an adenoma-to-adenocarcinoma sequence. In the last two decades, the anatomic frame of progression has been embraced by the molecular genetic model of CRC, according to which accumulation of gene damage drives progression from adenoma to cancer, subsequently leading to the emergence of invasive and spreading clones [2]. Gene damage is known to be driven from two types of genetic instabilities: microsatellite (MSI) and chromosomal (CIN) instability. More recently, the epigenetic silencing of tumor suppressor genes, namely CpG island methylator phenotype (CIMP), has been claimed as a distinct pathway of colorectal carcinogenesis **(Table 1)** [3].
Moving from this cornerstone, current research is exploring non-clonal determinants of tumor progression **(Table 1)**[4,5]. Collectively referred to as "tumor microenvironment" these factors can restrain or fuel tumor development and fate, and comprise infiltrating immune cells, neo-vessels, activated fibroblasts, and mesenchymal stem cells [6]. Not acting like a tumor scaffold, rather actively signaling with neoplastic cells, microenvironment influences the selection and emergence of aggressive clones, as well as their dissemination. In a bi-directional way, tumor molecular features influence the nearby environment by expressing tumor antigens, while tumor microenvironment influences the molecular changes, controlling the tumor growth. Additionally, chemokines and their receptors can be expressed as well by cancer cells and by non-neoplastic cells, influencing clonal expansion and cancer spread [4]. The role of microenvironment in cancer promoting dynamics is well established, providing cancer cells with oxygen, growth factors and nutrients, which can impact on tumor growth, progression and dissemination. However, the contribution of persistent inflammation in the carcinogenesis process encourages anti-inflammatory drug administration as the most effective chemopreventive strategy. More recently, a growing body of evidence suggests a dual role of immunity in cancer pathogenesis **(Figure 1)**, including tumor protective functions, tightly linked to patient's prognosis. Endogenous responses may inhibit tumor growth and modulate the clinical course of disease [7,8].

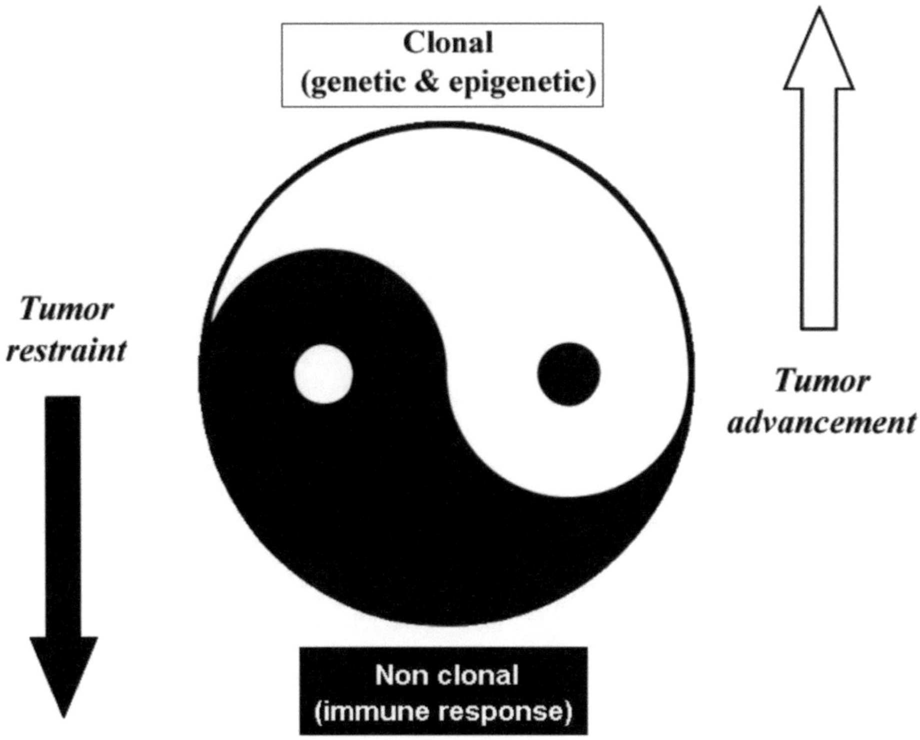

Fig. 1. Elements fueling and braking colorectal cancer progression

Genetic or Clonal Determinants	
Genetic Instability	
	Microsatellite Instability (MSI)
	Chromosomal Instability (CIN)
	CpG Island Methylator Phenotype (CIMP)
Non-Clonal Determinants	
Adaptive Immunity	
	$CD4^+$ lymphocytes
	$CD8^+$ lymphocytes
	T regulatory lymphocytes
	B lymphocytes
Innate Immunity	
	Macrophages
	Mast Cells
	Neutrophils
	Natural Killer cells
	Dendritic Cells

Table 1. Sub-anatomical determinants of colorectal carcinogenesis

We review the builders of the CRC microenvironment, focusing on innate immunity and adaptive immunity. Although there is enormous heterogeneity of results and many open issues in methodological standardization strongly limit definitive conclusions, promising evidences support the clinical utility of tumor infiltrating subpopulations, in particular as prognostic biomarkers and potential therapeutic targets.

2. The players

2.1 Innate immunity

It is well known that innate immunity, not involving specific recognition of immunogenic peptides, represents the first defense to pathological stresses, including cancer. Innate immune cells orchestrate an inflammatory response that may stimulate or inhibit cancer growth. A number of innate immune cells have been implicated in CRC development and progression, including macrophages, mast cells (MC), neutrophils, natural killer (NK) cells and dendritic cells (DC) [9-12].

Macrophages. They are a heterogeneous cell population of the myeloid linage derived from monocytes. These cells show two different polarization states, M1 and M2, in response to different micro environmental signals [13]. M1-macrophages, involved in cancer protecting mechanism, interface susceptible target cells through several different mechanisms, including secretion of tumor necrosis factor-α (TNF-α), nitric oxide, interleukin-1β (IL-1β) and reactive oxygen intermediates. Additionally, M1s can support T-helper 1 (Th1) adaptive immunity. Conversely, M2 macrophages can secrete factors stimulating the growth and migration of tumor cells, such as platelet-derived growth factor (PDGF), epidermal growth factor (EGF), and transforming growth factor-β (TGF- β), and angiogenesis-promoting factors like vascular endothelial growth factor (VEGF) and TNF-α, as well as produce proteases (such as metalloproteinases, MMPs) that potentially could facilitate tumor invasion and metastasis [13-16].

In patients with CRC, tumor associated macrophages (TAM) are usually found located around necrotic areas and the advancing tumor margin. It was originally thought that the main function of TAMs was a direct cytotoxic effect on tumor cells, phagocytosis apoptotic/necrotic *cell debris*, and present *tumor-associated antigens* to T lymphocytes. Current associative evidence is in line with this view, as a high density of TAM at the CRC invasion front, particularly the highest TAM density scored as a "hot-spot", is associated with a better patient outcome [17]. More data are likely still needed as to TAM role in CRC, as well as on the state of their activation (M1 *versus* M2) [10].

Among the M2 population, TAMs have been shown as capable of secreting proteases that enhance invasion and metastases, together with a range of cytokines inhibiting an adaptive tumor-specific immune response, and angiogenic factors that increase neovascularity. The pro-angiogenetic ability of M2-macrophages has been well characterized and it is mediated by secretion of specific factors, including VEGF, IL-1β, TNF-α, angiogenin or, indirectly, by the release of MMPs. MMPs are responsible for extracellular matrix degradation and invasiveness through the connective tissue. They are released by TAMs after cancer cell stimulation and they can act locally or be recruited to cancer cell membrane for their trip toward progression and invasion [6]. Increased frequencies of intra-tumoural TAMs have mainly been associated with high levels of MMP type 2 and 9 expression in CRC cells. These findings are in accord with a previous cell-line study showing that co-culturing of tumor cells with macrophages enhances cancer cell migration, invasiveness, and MMP-2 and MMP-9 secretion [18].

Several authors have also shown that macrophages can release various cytokines. Kaler *et al.* have recently established that macrophages promote Wnt signaling pathway in CRC cells and enhance their proliferation, and demonstrated that macrophages exert their protumorigenic activity mainly through the release of IL-1β. The same authors demonstrated that Tumor Necrosis Factor Related Apoptosis Inducing Ligand (TRAIL) induced apoptosis of CRC cells is inhibited by macrophage derived IL-1β, and showed that macrophages and recombinant IL-1β counteract TRAIL-induced apoptosis through activation of Wnt signaling and stabilization of the nuclear transcription factor Snail in tumor cells [19]. Li *et al.* first reported that IL-6 released by macrophage directly promotes CRC cell progression, also suggesting that the interaction between IL-6 and IL-10 released from macrophages is involved in CRC progression and prognosis [20]. The above findings suggest that TAMs might play a regulatory role in the tumor microenvironment, supporting cancer cells to manipulate their microenvironment and facilitate cancer growth.

Among M1 population, TAM secreting IL-12 and IL-23, infiltrating the tumor invasive front are positively correlated with a favorable outcome. As mentioned above, Forssell *et al.* showed that the higher $CD68^+$ macrophage infiltration along the tumor invasive front correlated with improved survival in colon cancer compared to rectal cancer. They concluded that a dense macrophage infiltration at the tumor invasive front positively influences prognosis in colon cancer and that the degree of cell-to-cell contact may influence the balance between pro-tumorigenic and anti-tumorigenic properties of macrophages [17]. High levels of tissue macrophages have been also associated with earlier disease stage, absence of nodal and lympho-vascular metastases and an overall better prognosis. Zhou *et al.* by analyzing the relationship between the density of TAMs and the potential of hepatic metastasis and survival have shown that a higher density of macrophages along the tumor invasive front of CRC was associated with a higher 5-year survival rate [21]. In addition, according to Forssell's scoring system that defines CD68 *hot-spots* as small areas among which the infiltration of macrophages is above the average level of CD68-positive cells, the highest CD68 hot-spot is associated with the lowest incidence of hepatic metastasis and a long interval between colon resection and the occurrence of hepatic metastasis [17, 21].

The mechanisms behind the anti-tumor effects of TAMs have still not been fully elucidated, and seem to potentially be ascribed to the M1 phenotype, which is in part controlled by the $CD4^+$T-lymphocytes and the death of cancer cells [22]. It has been ascertained that recruitment of TAMs contributes to the development of an adaptive immune response against cancer, and the balance between antigen availability and clearance through phagocytosis and subsequent degradation of senescent or apoptotic cells.

Mast Cells (MC) originate from the bone-marrow hematopoietic progenitors and migrate to peripheral tissue close to the blood vessels, nerves and mucosal surfaces, in order to provide a quick defense against any external attack. They participate in tissue remodeling, wound healing and angiogenesis, but also they are responsible for pathological conditions such as acute and chronic allergic disorders or autoimmune disorders. Recently, increasing evidences in animal models and humans support their involvement in cancer. In APC deficient and Kit^{W}-Kit^{W-v} mice, polyps contain significantly higher amount of MC [23], while depletion of MC, either pharmacologically or in MC deficient mice, correspond to tumor suppression[24]. In accordance, MC infiltration has been reported in human CRC. MC are involved in angiogenesis as well as in tumor microenvironment remodeling. Based on the close association between MC and vasculature, their role in angiogenesis is intuitive, and it is supported by the evidence of increasing densities of MC during tumor growth, which goes with neo-vessels. Although MC tryptase has been claimed as the major player in this association, human MC also constitutively expresses VEGF isoforms. Beyond the angiogenesis, MC can play other functions in tumor microenvironment, mainly through stimulatory signals, such as Fc receptors and Toll-like receptors (TLR). When activated MC release mediators involved in inflammation, matrix destruction and tissue remodeling, promoting cancer invasion and metastasis [10, 25, 26]. Accordingly, it has been reported that the increase in MC count correlated with a worse prognosis in patients. Gulubova and Vlaykova proposed the MCs density along the tumor invasive front as a helpful tool for prognosis of patients after surgical therapy, showing a correlation between high MCs density and poor prognosis [27]. Moreover, interactions between MC and regulatory T cells (Treg) have been reported [28]. MCs have been reported to mobilize T cells and antigen-presenting dendritic cells. They modulate Treg-induced tolerance, shifting the local balance of immune surveillance toward pro-inflammatory Treg activation and cancer progression[29]. In light of these evidences, modulating mast cell recruitment, viability, activity, or mediator release patterns could also have important implication in cancer therapy strategies.

However, some conflicting data still need to be solved. Analyzing a old large cohort of patients, MC infiltration resulted an independent prognostic marker of favorable outcome [30], and in a recent report by *Xia et al.* there was no association between MC and prognosis in stage IIIB CRCs [24]. More studies are required to solve contradictions and validate the role of MC as potential prognostic markers and therapeutic target.

Neutrophils may form up to 15% of the inflammatory infiltrate associated with CRCs (tumor associated neutrophils, TAN) and this proportion increases within areas of tumor necrosis. Neutrophils secrete substances such as reactive oxygen species and proteinases that are capable of altering cell behavior and tumor microenvironment, with both pro-host and pro-tumor effects.

In patients with rectal cancer a high density of neutrophils has been shown as an independent predictor of improved prognosis, especially when microscopic abscesses form [10, 31]. On the other hand, an elevated neutrophil/lymphocyte ratio was found by Halazun *et al.* to contribute to a poorer survival time and higher rate of recurrence in CRC patients undergoing surgery for liver metastasis [10, 32]. It has been proposed that TANs impact on tumor growth depends on their activation state. When moderately activated, they promote tumor growth and remodel extra cellular matrix *via* Reactive Oxygen Species (ROS) and proteinases. In contrast, when TANs are highly activated they release higher concentrations of the same mediators with toxic consequences on tumor cells[31].

Natural killer (NK) cells are granular lymphocytes that form part of the innate cellular immune response. In CRC, high numbers of NK cells in the inflammatory infiltrate are associated with better prognosis. The number of NK cells decreases with increasing cancer stage [10]. Similarly, low preoperative levels of NK cell activity in patients undergoing curative resections are associated with disease recurrence. Because of these effects, it has been suggested that NK cells can rapidly eliminate tumor cells without prior exposure, whereas cytotoxic T cells require prior sensitization and therefore more time to become effective [10]. The ratio of NK cells in the peripheral blood has also been proposed as a prognostic indicator in patients with colon cancer and it is of interest to note that 5-fluorouracil (FU)-based chemotherapy increases the numbers of NK cells [33].

Dendritic cells (DCs), antigen-presenting cells (APCs) that are critical to the stimulation of effective anti-tumor adaptive immune responses, can become defective in the tumor microenvironment and aid in tumor immune evasion by failing to stimulate T lymphocytes.

It has been suggested that the presence of DCs may be of significant benefit in patients with CRC [34]. Xie *et al.* also demonstrated that the presence of DCs was found predominantly in early compared to later disease stages and mostly located in tumor surrounding tissue [35].

2.2 Adaptive immunity

It is well known that the adaptive, or specific, immunity, occurs several days after the exposure to a particular antigen, and it is distinct from the innate immunity with respect to: *a)* the specificity towards the different macromolecules, *b)* the immunological memory, *c)* the ability to respond in a more powerful and effective way in case of repeated exposure to a single pathogen, and *d)* immunological tolerance *i.e.* the ability to discriminate between *self* and *non-self.*

The adaptive immunity consists of a cellular component represented by T- and B-lymphocytes, and soluble components represented by the immunoglobulin (Ig) or *antibodies*. From a functional point of view, it can be distinguished between an adaptive humoral immunity and a cell-mediated immunity. The antibodies represent the humoral effectors and are produced following the activation of specific bone marrow derived B-lymphocytes, while cell-mediated effectors are represented by T-lymphocytes.

T-lymphocytes participate in inflammation, cancer development and progression, as well as in anticancer immunity [4, 9]. In colitis-associated tumors (CAC) the adaptive immune system seems to have mainly a pro-tumorigenic role, while in CRC it may play a double-faced role, being the balance between *immune-surveillance* (carried out by $CD8^+$ and $CD4^+$ T-lymphocytes) and tumor-promoting inflammation (by various sub-types of T-lymphocytes) to change over time, and eventually dictating disease progression.

Cytotoxic T lymphocytes ($CD8^+$ T-lymphocytes, or CTL) constitute one of the leading effectors of antitumor immunity. In order for $CD8^+$ T cells to recognize antigens, these need to be exposed on the tumor cells in association with the human leukocyte antigen (HLA) class I proteins [36]. Upon encounter of a tumor cell antigen/HLA I complex for which their T cell receptor (TCR) is specific, $CD8^+$ T-lymphocytes clonally expand and differentiate [36]. Once activated, cytotoxic T-lymphocytes can mediate specific destruction of tumor cells through the release of lytic components via cell-cell interaction [36, 37]. Perforin, a cytolytic protein found in the granules of $CD8^+$ T-lymphocytes and NK cells, and enzymatic proteases, including granzyme B, are secreted determining cell death by disruption of the cell membrane and activation of the apoptotic pathway respectively.

$CD4^+$ T-lymphocytes, which only respond to antigens presented by the HLA class II proteins expressed by DCs, are important for antitumor immunity. $CD4^+$ T-lymphocytes are mainly subdivided into T helper-1 (Th1) or -2 (Th2) lymphocytes [38]. Th1 cells secrete cytokines such as interferon-gamma (IFN-γ) and TNF-α, and support cytotoxic T-lymphocytes by producing IL-2, required for $CD8^+$ T cells proliferation. Conversely, Th2 cells principally secrete IL-10, IL-4, and IL-5, and limit cytotoxic T-lymphocytes proliferation.

Regulatory T cells (Treg cells) have been defined as a T-cell population that functionally suppresses an immune response by influencing the activity of another cell type. Treg cells have been mainly categorized into two classes based on their ontogeny: naturally occurring Treg (nTreg), which develop in the thymus and are present in mice and healthy humans from an early postnatal period, and Treg which can arise in the periphery (or *in vitro*). nTreg are characterized by their high expression of CD25 ($CD4^+CD25^+$) and co-expression of the FoxP3 [39].

Although the role of **B-lymphocytes** in cancer has been overshadowed by the interest in developing T-cell-mediated cellular responses, it is now apparent that B-lymphocytes can play a complementary role in the host response against tumor. B-lymphocytes represent a cell population that express clonally diverse cell surface Ig receptors recognizing specific antigenic epitopes [40]. In addition to the role of B-lymphocytes in antibody production, these cells mediate/regulate several other functions fundamental for immune homeostasis. Of significant importance is the antigen-presenting role of B-lymphocytes in the initiation of T-cell immune responses. Moreover, B-lymphocytes can play a significant role in infection and autoimmunity as regulatory cells (indicated as Breg) via the elaboration of suppressive cytokines, such as IL-10, TGF-β, or IL-4. The role played by B cells in cancer immunology remains still complex and somewhat controversial. Depending upon their state of activation, B-lymphocytes have had divergent roles on T-cell differentiation and effector function. Oversimplifying, *resting B-lymphocytes* have been reported to suppress T-cell-mediated antitumor immunity, by acting on both $CD4^+$ and $CD8^+$ T-lymphocytes. In contrast, a number of reports suggest the efficacy of *activated B-lymphocytes* in cellular immunotherapy of malignancies. In particular, activated B-lymphocytes have been reported to enhance the ability to generate tumor-infiltrating lymphocytes *in vitro* involving anti-CD3 and IL-2.
The therapeutic targeting of tumors or components of the immune system with molecule-specific monoclonal antibodies (mAb) is now considered a viable treatment option for cancer patients [41]. One of the currently applied antibodies in clinics is represented by rituximab (Rituxan) that targets B cells for elimination by binding the B cell-associated marker CD20. Interestingly, Haynes *et al.* have recently developed a C57BL/6 TRAIL-sensitive tumor model with the aim of being able to use gene-targeted mice to better evaluate the innate and adaptive immune cells contributing to the tumoricidal activity of the MD5-1 mAb (*i.e.* an anti-mDR5 mAb) in more clinically relevant established tumors. C57BL/6 gene-targeted or immune cell-depleted mice were used to examine the antitumor activity of MD5-1 against the TRAIL-sensitive mouse MC38 colon adenocarcinoma. They found that an intact B cell compartment was critical for the therapeutic activity of MD5-1 against established tumors. B cells were confirmed to trigger tumor cell apoptosis by FcR-mediated cross-linking of the MD5-1 mAb *in vitro* and *in vivo* B lymphocytes were critical for directly triggering MD5-1–mediated tumor cell apoptosis.
Although the role of B-cells in human CRCs is still not completely characterized, B-cell-deficient mice exhibit spontaneous regression of MC38 colon carcinoma cells. Studies involving BCR transgenic mice indicated that B-cells might inhibit antitumor T-lymphocytes responses by antigen-nonspecific mechanisms. Shah *et al.* investigated the role of B cells in tumor immunity by studying immune responses of mice genetically lacking B cells to primary tumors. They highlight that although the effects of B-lymphocytes on anti-tumor response warrant further study, adoptive transfer of CD40(-/-) B cells into B cell-deficient mice resulted in restored growth of MC38 colon carcinoma cells suggesting additional factors other than CD40 are involved in dampening anti-tumor responses [42].

3. Immune cells in the colorectal cancer playground

Nowadays, it is well accepted that the host mounts both an innate and adaptive immune response against the cancer with variable effects. The strength of this response can be measured and has prognostic significance [43]. Dendritic cells, M1 macrophages, Th1 $CD4^+$ T lymphocytes, cytotoxic $CD8^+$ T-lymphocytes and NK cells are associated with a tumor protective behavior, while M2 macrophages, neutrophils, Th2 and Th17 CD4+ T cells, and Treg stimulate cancer progression [34] **(Table 2)**.

	PRO-TUMORIGENIC IMMUNITY	ANTI-TUMORIGENIC IMMUNITY
Cell sub-population	M2-polarized macrophages Myeloid-derived suppressor cells Moderately activated neutrophils FOXP3+ T-regulatory lymphocytes	M1-polarized macrophages Dendritic cells Highly activated neutrophils Cytotoxic T-lymphocytes Natural Killer cells
Cytokine profiles	T-lymphocytes helper-2 T-lymphocytes helper-17	T-lymphocytes helper-1 CX3CL1 CX3CL9 CX3CL10
Tissue distrution	Peritumoral	Intratumoral Close to cancer cells Invasive tumor front
Associated features	STAT 3 phosphorylation	High endothelial venules
Clinical impact	Negative *prognostic* impact	Positive *prognostic* and *predictive* impact

Table 2. Dula role of immunity in colorectal cancer

Chronic inflammation, mediated by infections, autoimmune disorders or inflammatory disease (*i.e.* Inflammatory Bowel Disease, IBD), is a well recognized cancer-trigger and represents the conceptual basis for using anti inflammatory drugs in CRC prevention. Macrophages (M2 subtype), secreting growth-, angiogenic- and chemotactic-factors, are the main determinant of this process and they are associated with poor patients' survival. Growing evidence suggests that other factors take part in this process, with negative consequences on prognosis, such as the pro-inflammatory Th17 cells or Treg [44]. However, expression of the transcription factor STAT3 was correlated with higher disease specific mortality in CRC [45]. In stage IIIB CRC, abnormal expression of the High Motility Group Box 1 protein (HMGB1) predicted poor survival [46]. It has been postulated that STAT3 and HMGB1 may have negative effects on the recruitment of anti-cancer effectors.

In contrast to chronic inflammation, immunosurveillance protects against cancer formation and progression. In this scenario, the presence of high numbers of T-lymphocytes has been reported to be a positive prognostic factor. The first reports on the beneficial effect of lymphocytic infiltration in CRC appeared already in the 1980's. They were subsequently confirmed until recent studies highlighting a prominent function for memory T-lymphocytes and CD8+ T-lymphocytes in predicting disease-free survival (DFS) and overall survival (OS) [47].

In general terms, it has been suggested that prognosis in patients with cancer is mainly positively affected by *a)* the presence of a tumor gene signature consistent with a type I adaptive immune response (*i.e.*, increased antigen presentation, IFN-γ signaling, and TCR signaling), and *b)* the presence of T cells that penetrate through tumor stroma and deeply infiltrate the parenchyma to become intra-tumoural T cells [9]. Thus, besides a Th-1 response signature, the other key feature of an effective immune response is the ability of T cells to reach the site of the tumor and to infiltrate it (Table 2).

A number of studies have reported that MSI, CIMP, BRAF mutation, PIK3CA mutation, and tumor LINE-1 hypomethylation are associated with CRC prognosis and that lymphocytic infiltration is associated with many of these molecular variables. The association of a prognostic biomarker with a given disease, strongly suggests its stage-dependency as outcome predictor. This is best exemplified by MSI CRC, whose overall prognostic advantage is associated with a low frequency of stage III and IV cases at diagnosis as compared to MSS counterpart [48]. Most MSI CRCs show a pronounced intra-tumoral inflammatory infiltrate (which remains a criterion for MSI testing), the mechanistic explanation of which, however, is still incompletely understood. Within these tumors, infiltrating lymphocytes have been identified as predominantly activated $CD8^+$ T-lymphocytes. The presence of CTLs has been attributed to the inherently greater production of abnormal peptides as a result of unreliable DNA repair in MSI-positive tumors. It is known that truncated peptides produced by frameshift mutations due to MSI may be immunogenic and contribute to the host immune response. However, the interrelationship between tumor-infiltrating T-lymphocytes, MSI status, and other tumor molecular features is still unknown. In any event, the data concerning the prognostic implications of T cells have reached now a large volume and support a clear positive correlation between the density of T cells and a better prognosis. In this respect, most seminal work has been produced by Galon *et al.* [49], who first showed that a given immunological signature was associated with the absence of pathological evidence of early metastasis and with better survival. Such signature featured a high number of $CD8^+$ T cells (including early and effector memory T cells). The presence of a high density of infiltrating memory $CD45RO^+$ cells, at immunohistochemical analysis of tumor samples, was associated with the absence of signs of early metastatic invasion, a less advanced pathological stage, and increased survival [47]. Subsequently, the same group showed that a high density of $CD3^+$ T cells at the tumor invasion front or located in the center of the tumor, once combined, can predict patient outcome better than the AJCC stage in patients with stage I to III CRC [49]. The question as to whether infiltrating T cells are such a powerful prognostic marker to overrun the prognostic predictive value of AJCC staging system was faced even by other groups. Laghi *et al.* [50] found that, in the absence of node metastasis, $CD3^+$ T infiltrating cells at the tumor invasive front were associated with a low risk of metachronous metastasis and consequent survival advantage, independently of the MS-status. This finding challenged the view that the density of the T cell infiltrate is a stage independent predictor of survival in CRC, and that the positive prognostic value of T cells is dependent upon the CRC MS-status. More relevant, is the issue of the real relevance of the adaptive immune cell infiltrate in the clinical field. Overall, one would like to know whether the density of T-cells can predict patient's outcome, and at what stage of the disease it can be safely applied, rather than whether this is a stage-dependent or independent prognostic factor. It now appears that the density of T cells, whether $CD3^+$, $CD8^+$, or $CD45RO^+$, can predict outcome in early stage CRC [49-51]. Inherently new issues arise from these data. One concerns the CD marker with the strongest prognostic value, and the other the standardization of the methods to assess T-cell density and their location with respect to CRC (*i.e.*, within the tumor or at its invasive margin). It remains controversial whether the T cells infiltration has a prognostic impact beyond the stage of lymph-node invasion, a point at which immunoevasion may overcome immunosurveillance, although recent data still support the view that even at this disease stage T-cells retain a positive prognostic impact [52].

Recently, Nosho *et al.* examined the prognostic role of tumor-infiltrating T-cell subsets in a database of 768 CRCs from two prospective cohort studies. They concurrently assessed the densities of $CD3^+$, $CD8^+$, $CD45RO^+$, and $FoxP3^+$ lymphocytes as well as other relevant molecular (including KRAS, BRAF, and PIK3CA mutations, MSI, CIMP, and LINE-1 hypomethylation) and pathological features, therefore making possible to estimate the independent effect of each T-cell subset density on patient survival. They found that the density of $CD45RO^+$ cells, but not that of $CD3^+$, $CD8^+$, or $FoxP3^+$ cells, was an independent prognostic biomarker of longer survival in CRC patients, while MSI-high and tumor LINE-1 methylation level are independent predictors of $CD45RO^+$-cell density [53]. In contrast, Salama *et al.* [54] by analyzing T-cell infiltrates in 967 CRCs including 593 stage II and 374 stage III cases, reported that $FoxP3^+$ lymphocytes density had stronger prognostic significance than $CD8^+$ and $CD45RO^+$ cells, and predicted a better outcome. $FoxP3^+$ lymphocytes were found not associated with any histopathological features. At multivariate analysis, stage, vascular invasion, and $FoxP3^+$ cell density in tumoural tissue were found to be independent prognostic indicators. These results led Salama *et al.* to conclude that the inclusion of $FoxP3^+$ cell density may help to improve the prognostication of early-stage CRC. Again, some contradiction exists, as data by other authors suggest that a high density of intraepithelial $FoxP3^+$ is associated with a worse survival [55]. It should be mentioned that in the study by Salama, tissue sampling was obtained randomly, while in the study by Sinicrope *et al.* the density of $FoxP3^+$ cells was measured within the tumor. Thus a low ratio of $CD3^+/FoxP3^+$ and a low $CD3^+$ numbers were associated with a poor outcome, underscoring that even the interplay between effector and Treg cells might be relevant for cancer progression [55]. However, it is surprising how density of $FoxP3^+$ resulted to be a positive prognostic factor when assessed in unspecified tumor regions and a negative one when assessed within the tumor. This contradiction calls for further studies aimed to re-appraise $FoxP3^+$ cells role in CRC, but also underlines the methodological issue of T cells topographic assessment [56]. More recently, Chew *et al.* investigated whether Secreted Protein Acidic and Rich in Cysteine (SPARC), a matricellular protein involved in tissue remodeling, cell migration and angiogenesis, FoxP3, CD8 and CD45RO expression levels were associated with CRC stage, disease outcome and long-term cancer specific survival (CSS) in stage II and III [57]. They found that high levels of SPARC and FoxP3 protein (which seems to have an anti-tumorigenic role in cancer progression) were associated with better disease outcome in stage II CRC and may be prognostic indicators of CSS.

As a concluding remark, it should be pointed out that the prognostic value of a given CD set likely overlaps with that of a neighbor or subset, and that the overall prognostic value is likely the sum of different action exerted by each subset, including the balance between effector and regulatory arms.

It might not exist a T-cell marker that has the highest performance, as the overlapping nature of CD includes more than one cell subset.

Targeting the immune system represents an attractive strategy for the new frontiers in colon cancer treatment. ***Strategy interfering cancer-promoting inflammation:*** it has been widely recognized that the use of anti-inflammatory agents reduces the risk of developing CRC. In randomized clinical trials, the administration of celecoxib diminished the cumulative adenoma incidence and the frequency of advanced adenomas, suggesting their efficacy in both polyp formation and progression. In patients with familial adenomatous polyposis, celecoxib and sulindac decrease the incidence of colorectal and duodenal polyps. It is unlikely that anti-inflammatory drugs alone can represent effective monotherapies for CRC patients, but they might find place in combination withchemo- or radio-therapy or in chemoprevention. The non- selective cyclooxygenase (COX) inhibitor sulindac resulted effective in CRC prevention and treatment, while aspirin, which reduces CRC risk in a dose- and time-dependent manner, is mostly considered as chemopreventive agent. However, a more complete understanding of the mechanisms underlying tumor-promoting/protecting inflammation has identified more selective targets for intervention. Among non-steroidal anti-inflammatory drugs, specific COX2 inhibitors, such as celecoxib and rofecoxib, reduced CRC risk and slowed progression of colorectal adenomatous polyps to carcinomas, interfering with the COX isoform whose increased activity is specifically associated with CRC pathogens. In the late Nineties and early 2000s, a great deal of expectations arose from COX-2 inhibitors as tools for primary prevention that were lately banned from clinical practice, due to the burden of cardiovascular side effects. Highly selective inhibitors of prostaglandin E2 (PGE2) signaling, such as ONO-8711 receptor antagonists, are expected to reduce the cardiovascular risks associated with COX inhibition but still prevent CRC [58, 59]. Recently biologic agents have been introduced in clinical practice in combination with classical chemotherapy for some subtype of disease, as a form of passive immunotherapy [60]. In contrast to traditional chemotherapeutic drugs, they target specific signaling pathways. For example, VEGF inhibition (*i.e.* bevacizumab) blocks tumor angiogenesis while the interfering with the EGF receptor signaling (*i.e.* cetuximab) reduces survival and growth of cancer cells. Bevacizumab and cetuximab are currently approved in the metastatic disease treatment [61]. Additionally, it has recently demonstrated that Bevacizumab-based therapy is able to increase B- and T-lymphocytes compartments [62]. It is known that the expansion of T lymphocytes could imply an amelioration of dendritic cell-presenting capacity. These effects correlate with a more favorable clinical outcome and could be taken into account in clinical protocols aimed at combining anti-angiogenetic-therapy with immunotherapy in metastatic CRC.

Inhibitors of pro-inflammatory cytokines might also be developed to block inflammation. A number of studies have been conducted using anti-IL6, anti-TNF, anti-IL-1, anti- IL-17, or anti-IL-23, but, although some of them have already been approved in IBD or autoimmune disorders (*i.e.* infliximab, etanercept), there is a lack of clinical trials in oncologic settings. Similarly, anti-adhesion molecules drugs, currently applied for IBD and rheumatologic disorders (*i.e.* the α (4)-integrin subunit inhibitor Natalizumab) could be potential cancer protective agents, preventing an excessive inflammatory response. A monoclonal antibody against CD3 (visilizumab), which prevents T-cell activation, had promising preliminary results in patients with active Crohn disease [10, 61, 63]. In this scenario, colitis associated cancer represents an ideal model where such drugs can be helpfully tested. Of notice, the mentioned strategies interfere with the tumor promoting inflammation. In the light of the dual role of inflammation in CRC, it is important to determine which agents block tumor-promoting inflammation without reducing antitumor immunity.

Strategy enhancing cancer-protective inflammation: the immune system in cancer patients can be stimulated by active specific immunotherapy (vaccine) in order to eradicate tumor cells. Vaccines are expected to be specific for the tumor cells, self sustaining and systemic. However a successful vaccine strategy should address and overcome the suppressor response that tumor cells are able to mount [10].

So far, vaccines to treat cancer have been largely investigated with disappointing results in terms of clinical response. In advanced CRC patients, although some measurable immune response can be registered, the current trails failed to obtain meaningful improvement in survivals. Similarly, in adjuvant setting randomized control trials did not show promising

result; in this setting, only the autologous tumor cell vaccines combined with Bacilles Calmette-Guerin (BCG) seems to significantly improve patients' survival [64].
Finally, among passive immunotherapies, a novel charming strategy consists in removing anti-tumor T cells from the body for *ex vivo* culture, followed by reinfusion (adoptive T cell transfer)[65]. Although the first trial failed mostly due to technical issues, the researcher remains optimistic that increasing competences will make this strategy a feasible form of immunotherapy in the future.

4. Open issues

Although the well established role of immune system provides concrete opportunities for clinical applications, the heterogeneity of results among studies suggest that many issues need to be solved before moving into clinical practice.
The existing discrepancies in literature may be due to a number of factors such as intra-tumor distribution of the immune cells and type of subpopulations, type of organ, tumor genetic background, and the assessment methods employed. Recent studies have reported that different macrophage phenotypes localized to different regions of the carcinoma have variable effects on tumor cells [49, 66]. Furthermore, evidence has shown that the relationship between TAMs and tumor progression is tumor type-dependent. Nevertheless, since the tumor microenvironment includes different T-cell sub-populations **(Figure 2)**, which do not display a homogeneous infiltration of tumor tissues, potential different impact on prognosis may depend on type of sub-population and peri/intra tumor distribution. Because T cell infiltration is not spatially homogeneous in CRC, attention has been focused on the predictive values of T-lymphocytes located in the center of the tumor, along the invasive margin and in lymphoid aggregate (*i.e.* tertiary lymphoid structures) mainly detectable in proximity of the tumor [43, 67]. However, the interrelationship between tumor-infiltrating T-lymphocytes, MSI status, and other tumor molecular features remains to be elucidated. It is indubitable that to define the prognostic effect of tumor-infiltrating T cells, large studies of CRC with extensive molecular characterization are needed. Additionally, caution is needed before incorporating tumor-infiltrating T cells into tumor staging. To minimize the risk of inappropriate tumor down-staging at diagnosis, survival data need to be confirmed in independent series of patients studied in the past decade. Moreover, the association has to be conclusively proven between low densities of tumor-infiltrating T cells and the clinical detection of metachronous metastases, which remains the most appropriate outcome measure for recognizing a role of the local immune response in micrometastasis suppression. Laghi *et al.* [50] investigated the relationship between the density of $CD3^+$ T infiltrating lymphocytes along the tumor invasive margin, and the occurrence of metachronous distant-organ metastases after potentially curative resection, in a large, consecutive series of patients with deeply invading (pT3 or pT4) MSI-typed CRC, and no evidence of distant organ metastasis at diagnosis. They found that large areas covered by $CD3^+$ cells at the tumor invasive front are associated with a low risk of metachronous metastasis and consequently a survival advantage, only in patients with node-negative cancers, but not in patients whose cancers involved lymph nodes. The prognostic advantage conferred by a high density of $CD3^+$ cells was independent of tumor MS-status in patients with stage II CRC. CD3-immunostaining of CRC tissue might therefore be useful for selecting stage II patients who, because they are at very low risk for cancer progression, could be spared adjuvant treatments. The usefulness in the clinical scenario of T-cell density

in patients with more advanced disease, who are subject to chemotherapy remains to be assessed. With respect to this, the relationship between T-cells and current chemotherapy regimens for CRC should be also explored, a field in which very few data are currently available.

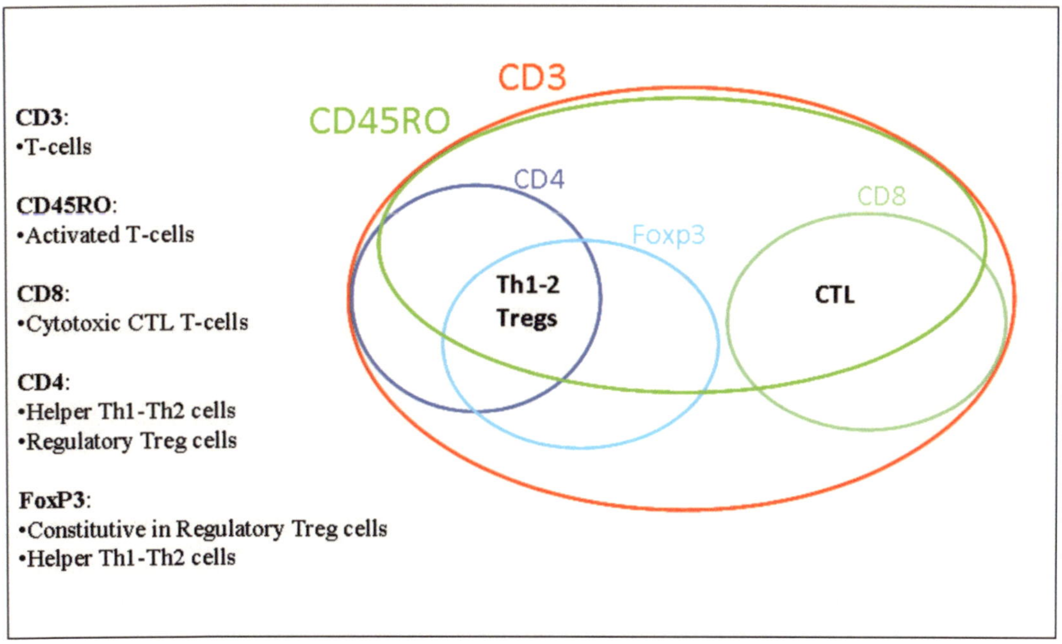

Fig. 2. Adaptive immunity: different Clusters of Differentiation (CD) are expressed by subsets of T-lymphocytes

It is clear that as tumors are heterogeneous cell populations that show distinctive genetic and epigenetic profiles, there may not be a single biomarker that will prove sufficient information for predicting treatment response and patient outcome. However, it remains to be solved, several critical issues related to the heterogeneity and complexity between the actual studies, in terms of sample size; study setting; disease stage; the presence *versus* absence of treatment data; and treatment modality (no therapy to chemotherapy, radiation therapy, or both) [8]. Laboratory methods to assess immune response (tissue microarray *versus* whole tissue; objective image analysis *versus* subjective pathologist qualitative or semi-quantitative interpretation); immunophenotyping markers; covariates and potential confounders assessed (in particular the presence versus absence of tumor molecular characteristics); and statistical method and multivariate analysis models all represent issues to take in account when comparing results from different laboratories. It is clear that to standardize research methods and appropriately evaluate evidence, we need to develop general and specific consensus on immune-cell evaluation in oncology research.

In conclusion, it can be stressed that the standardized analysis of the *type, quantity, location* and the *functions* of the immune infiltrate becomes a primary step in understanding CRC natural history, and, in a clinical perspective, its prognostic determinants. A comprehensive analysis of all components of the lymphocytic infiltrates in the context of their localization, organization and impact at various steps of tumor progression remains largely, if not entirely, to be reported to prospective studies. In parallel, understanding the mechanisms of efficient immune reactions, the place where they are initiated, the cells and key cytokines and chemokines involved, and their impact at different stages of the disease should provide new tools and goals for more effective and less toxic targeted therapies.

5. References

[1] Burke HB. Outcome prediction and the future of the TNM staging system. J Natl Cancer Inst 2004;96:1408-1409.
[2] Vogelstein B, Fearon ER, Hamilton SR, Kern SE, Preisinger AC, Leppert M, Nakamura Y, White R, Smits AM, Bos JL. Genetic alterations during colorectal-tumor development. N Engl J Med 1988;319:525-532.
[3] Grady WM, Carethers JM. Genomic and epigenetic instability in colorectal cancer pathogenesis. Gastroenterology 2008;135:1079-1099.
[4] Mantovani A, Romero P, Palucka AK, Marincola FM. Tumour immunity: effector response to tumour and role of the microenvironment. Lancet 2008;371:771-783.
[5] Ogino S, Chan AT, Fuchs CS, Giovannucci E. Molecular pathological epidemiology of colorectal neoplasia: an emerging transdisciplinary and interdisciplinary field. Gut 2011;60:397-411.
[6] Ungefroren H, Sebens S, Seidl D, Lehnert H, Hass R. Interaction of tumor cells with the microenvironment. Cell Commun Signal 2011;9:18.
[7] Ferrone C, Dranoff G. Dual roles for immunity in gastrointestinal cancers. J Clin Oncol 2010;28:4045-4051.
[8] Ogino S, Galon J, Fuchs CS, Dranoff G. Cancer immunology-analysis of host and tumor factors for personalized medicine. Nat Rev Clin Oncol 2011;8:711-719.
[9] Disis ML. Immune regulation of cancer. J Clin Oncol 2010;28:4531-4538.
[10] Salama P, Platell C. Host response to colorectal cancer. ANZ J Surg 2008;78:745-753.
[11] Saleh M, Trinchieri G. Innate immune mechanisms of colitis and colitis-associated colorectal cancer. Nat Rev Immunol 2011;11:9-20.
[12] Secher T, Gaillot O, Ryffel B, Chamaillard M. Remote control of intestinal tumorigenesis by innate immunity. Cancer Res 2010;70:1749-1752.
[13] Biswas SK, Mantovani A. Macrophage plasticity and interaction with lymphocyte subsets: cancer as a paradigm. Nat Immunol 2010;11:889-896.
[14] Mantovani A, Schioppa T, Porta C, Allavena P, Sica A. Role of tumor-associated macrophages in tumor progression and invasion. Cancer Metastasis Rev 2006;25:315-322.
[15] Mantovani A, Sica A, Locati M. New vistas on macrophage differentiation and activation. Eur J Immunol 2007;37:14-16.
[16] Sica A, Larghi P, Mancino A, Rubino L, Porta C, Totaro MG, Rimoldi M, Biswas SK, Allavena P, Mantovani A. Macrophage polarization in tumour progression. Semin Cancer Biol 2008;18:349-355.
[17] Forssell J, Oberg A, Henriksson ML, Stenling R, Jung A, Palmqvist R. High macrophage infiltration along the tumor front correlates with improved survival in colon cancer. Clin Cancer Res 2007;13:1472-1479.
[18] Kang JC, Chen JS, Lee CH, Chang JJ, Shieh YS. Intratumoral macrophage counts correlate with tumor progression in colorectal cancer. J Surg Oncol 2010;102:242-248.

[19] Kaler P, Galea V, Augenlicht L, Klampfer L. Tumor associated macrophages protect colon cancer cells from TRAIL-induced apoptosis through IL-1beta-dependent stabilization of Snail in tumor cells. PLoS One 2010;5:e11700.

[20] Li YY, Hsieh LL, Tang RP, Liao SK, Yeh KY. Interleukin-6 (IL-6) released by macrophages induces IL-6 secretion in the human colon cancer HT-29 cell line. Hum Immunol 2009;70:151-158.

[21] Zhou Q, Peng RQ, Wu XJ, Xia Q, Hou JH, Ding Y, Zhou QM, Zhang X, Pang ZZ, Wan DS, Zeng YX, Zhang XS. The density of macrophages in the invasive front is inversely correlated to liver metastasis in colon cancer. J Transl Med 2010;8:13.

[22] Umemura N, Saio M, Suwa T, Kitoh Y, Bai J, Nonaka K, Ouyang GF, Okada M, Balazs M, Adany R, Shibata T, Takami T. Tumor-infiltrating myeloid-derived suppressor cells are pleiotropic-inflamed monocytes/macrophages that bear M1- and M2-type characteristics. J Leukoc Biol 2008;83:1136-1144.

[23] Heijmans J, Büller NV, Muncan V, van den Brink GR. Role of mast cells in colorectal cancer development, the jury is still out. Biochim Biophys Acta. 2012;1822:9-13.

[24] Xia Q, Wu XJ, Zhou Q, Jing Z, Hou JH, Pan ZZ, Zhang XS. No relationship between the distribution of mast cells and the survival of stage IIIB colon cancer patients. J Transl Med 2011;9:88.

[25] Liu J, Zhang Y, Zhao J, Yang Z, Li D, Katirai F, Huang B. Mast cell: insight into remodeling a tumor microenvironment. Cancer Metastasis Rev 2011;30:177-184.

[26] Ribatti D, Crivellato E, Roccaro AM, Ria R, Vacca A. Mast cell contribution to angiogenesis related to tumour progression. Clin Exp Allergy 2004;34:1660-1664.

[27] Gulubova M, Vlaykova T. Prognostic significance of mast cell number and microvascular density for the survival of patients with primary colorectal cancer. J Gastroenterol Hepatol 2009;24:1265-1275.

[28] Blatner NR, Bonertz A, Beckhove P, Cheon EC, Krantz SB, Strouch M, Weitz J, Koch M, Halverson AL, Bentrem DJ, Khazaie K. In colorectal cancer mast cells contribute to systemic regulatory T-cell dysfunction. Proc Natl Acad Sci U S A 2010;107:6430-6435.

[29] Khazaie K, Blatner NR, Khan MW, Gounari F, Gounaris E, Dennis K, Bonertz A, Tsai FN, Strouch MJ, Cheon E, Phillips JD, Beckhove P, Bentrem DJ. The significant role of mast cells in cancer. Cancer Metastasis Rev 2011;30:45-60.

[30] Nielsen HJ, Hansen U, Christensen IJ, Reimert CM, Brunner N, Moesgaard F. Independent prognostic value of eosinophil and mast cell infiltration in colorectal cancer tissue. J Pathol 1999;189:487-495.

[31] Houghton AM. The paradox of tumor-associated neutrophils: fueling tumor growth with cytotoxic substances. Cell Cycle 2010;9:1732-1737.

[32] Halazun KJ, Aldoori A, Malik HZ, Al-Mukhtar A, Prasad KR, Toogood GJ, Lodge JP. Elevated preoperative neutrophil to lymphocyte ratio predicts survival following hepatic resection for colorectal liver metastases. Eur J Surg Oncol 2008;34:55-60.

[33] Vesely P, Touskova M, Melichar B. Phenotype of peripheral blood leukocytes and survival of patients with metastatic colorectal cancer. Int J Biol Markers 2005;20:126-133.

[34] Fridman WH, Galon J, Pages F, Tartour E, Sautes-Fridman C, Kroemer G. Prognostic and predictive impact of intra- and peritumoral immune infiltrates. Cancer Res 2011;71:5601-5605.

[35] Xie ZJ, Jia LM, He YC, Gao JT. Morphological observation of tumor infiltrating immunocytes in human rectal cancer. World J Gastroenterol 2006;12:1757-1760.

[36] Paschen A, Eichmuller S, Schadendorf D. Identification of tumor antigens and T-cell epitopes, and its clinical application. Cancer Immunol Immunother 2004;53:196-203.

[37] Loose D, Van de WC. The immune system and cancer. Cancer Biother Radiopharm 2009;24:369-376.

[38] Barnas JL, Simpson-Abelson MR, Yokota SJ, Kelleher RJ, Bankert RB. T cells and stromal fibroblasts in human tumor microenvironments represent potential therapeutic targets. Cancer Microenviron 2010;3:29-47.

[39] Saurer L, Mueller C. T cell-mediated immunoregulation in the gastrointestinal tract. Allergy 2009;64:505-519.

[40] Namm JP, Li Q, Lao X, Lubman DM, He J, Liu Y, Zhu J, Wei S, Chang AE. B lymphocytes as effector cells in the immunotherapy of cancer. J Surg Oncol 2011.

[41] Haynes NM, Hawkins ED, Li M, McLaughlin NM, Hammerling GJ, Schwendener R, Winoto A, Wensky A, Yagita H, Takeda K, Kershaw MH, Darcy PK, Smyth MJ. CD11c+ dendritic cells and B cells contribute to the tumoricidal activity of anti-DR5 antibody therapy in established tumors. J Immunol 2010;185:532-541.

[42] Shah S, Divekar AA, Hilchey SP, Cho HM, Newman CL, Shin SU, Nechustan H, Challita-Eid PM, Segal BM, Yi KH, Rosenblatt JD. Increased rejection of primary tumors in mice lacking B cells: inhibition of anti-tumor CTL and TH1 cytokine responses by B cells. Int J Cancer 2005;117:574-586.

[43] Pages F, Galon J, eu-Nosjean MC, Tartour E, Sautes-Fridman C, Fridman WH. Immune infiltration in human tumors: a prognostic factor that should not be ignored. Oncogene 2010;29:1093-1102.

[44] Tosolini M, Kirilovsky A, Mlecnik B, Fredriksen T, Mauger S, Bindea G, Berger A, Bruneval P, Fridman WH, Pages F, Galon J. Clinical impact of different classes of infiltrating T cytotoxic and helper cells (Th1, th2, treg, th17) in patients with colorectal cancer. Cancer Res 2011;71:1263-1271.

[45] Morikawa T, Baba Y, Yamauchi M, Kuchiba A, Nosho K, Shima K, Tanaka N, Huttenhower C, Frank DA, Fuchs CS, Ogino S. STAT3 expression, molecular features, inflammation patterns, and prognosis in a database of 724 colorectal cancers. Clin Cancer Res 2011;17:1452-1462.

[46] Peng RQ, Wu XJ, Ding Y, Li CY, Yu XJ, Zhang X, Pan ZZ, Wan DS, Zheng LM, Zeng YX, Zhang XS. Co-expression of nuclear and cytoplasmic HMGB1 is inversely associated with infiltration of CD45RO+ T cells and prognosis in patients with stage IIIB colon cancer. BMC Cancer 2010;10:496.

[47] Pages F, Berger A, Camus M, Sanchez-Cabo F, Costes A, Molidor R, Mlecnik B, Kirilovsky A, Nilsson M, Damotte D, Meatchi T, Bruneval P, Cugnenc PH, Trajanoski Z, Fridman WH, Galon J. Effector memory T cells, early metastasis, and survival in colorectal cancer. N Engl J Med 2005;353:2654-2666.

[48] Malesci A, Laghi L, Bianchi P, Delconte G, Randolph A, Torri V, Carnaghi C, Doci R, Rosati R, Montorsi M, Roncalli M, Gennari L, Santoro A. Reduced likelihood of metastases in patients with microsatellite-unstable colorectal cancer. Clin Cancer Res 2007;13:3831-3839.

[49] Galon J, Costes A, Sanchez-Cabo F, Kirilovsky A, Mlecnik B, Lagorce-Pages C, Tosolini M, Camus M, Berger A, Wind P, Zinzindohoue F, Bruneval P, Cugnenc PH, Trajanoski Z, Fridman WH, Pages F. Type, density, and location of immune cells within human colorectal tumors predict clinical outcome. Science 2006;313:1960-1964.

[50] Laghi L, Bianchi P, Miranda E, Balladore E, Pacetti V, Grizzi F, Allavena P, Torri V, Repici A, Santoro A, Mantovani A, Roncalli M, Malesci A. CD3+ cells at the invasive margin of deeply invading (pT3-T4) colorectal cancer and risk of post-surgical metastasis: a longitudinal study. Lancet Oncol 2009;10:877-884.

[51] Pages F, Kirilovsky A, Mlecnik B, Asslaber M, Tosolini M, Bindea G, Lagorce C, Wind P, Marliot F, Bruneval P, Zatloukal K, Trajanoski Z, Berger A, Fridman WH, Galon J. In situ cytotoxic and memory T cells predict outcome in patients with early-stage colorectal cancer. J Clin Oncol 2009;27:5944-5951.

[52] Mlecnik B, Tosolini M, Kirilovsky A, Berger A, Bindea G, Meatchi T, Bruneval P, Trajanoski Z, Fridman WH, Pages F, Galon J. Histopathologic-based prognostic factors of colorectal cancers are associated with the state of the local immune reaction. J Clin Oncol 2011;29:610-618.

[53] Nosho K, Baba Y, Tanaka N, Shima K, Hayashi M, Meyerhardt JA, Giovannucci E, Dranoff G, Fuchs CS, Ogino S. Tumour-infiltrating T-cell subsets, molecular changes in colorectal cancer, and prognosis: cohort study and literature review. J Pathol 2010;222:350-366.

[54] Salama P, Phillips M, Grieu F, Morris M, Zeps N, Joseph D, Platell C, Iacopetta B. Tumor-infiltrating FOXP3+ T regulatory cells show strong prognostic significance in colorectal cancer. J Clin Oncol 2009;27:186-192.

[55] Sinicrope FA, Rego RL, Ansell SM, Knutson KL, Foster NR, Sargent DJ. Intraepithelial effector (CD3+)/regulatory (FoxP3+) T-cell ratio predicts a clinical outcome of human colon carcinoma. Gastroenterology 2009;137:1270-1279.

[56] Laghi L, Bianchi P, Grizzi F, Malesci A. How dense, how intense? Role of tumour-infiltrating lymphocytes across colorectal cancer stages. Re: Nosho et al. Tumour-infiltrating T-cell subsets, molecular changes in colorectal cancer, and prognosis: cohort study and literature review. J Pathol 2010; 222: 350-366. J Pathol 2011;225:628.

[57] Chew A, Salama P, Robbshaw A, Klopcic B, Zeps N, Platell C, Lawrance IC. SPARC, FOXP3, CD8 and CD45 correlation with disease recurrence and long-term disease-free survival in colorectal cancer. PLoS One 2011;6:e22047.

[58] Chan AT, Ogino S, Fuchs CS. Aspirin use and survival after diagnosis of colorectal cancer. JAMA 2009;302:649-658.

[59] Keller JJ, Giardiello FM. Chemoprevention strategies using NSAIDs and COX-2 inhibitors. Cancer Biol Ther 2003;2:S140-S149.

[60] Cohen DJ, Hochster HS. Rationale for combining biotherapy in the treatment of advanced colon cancer. Gastrointest Cancer Res 2008;2:145-151.

[61] Terzic J, Grivennikov S, Karin E, Karin M. Inflammation and colon cancer. Gastroenterology 2010;138:2101-2114.

[62] Manzoni M, Rovati B, Ronzoni M, Loupakis F, Mariucci S, Ricci V, Gattoni E, Salvatore L, Tinelli C, Villa E, Danova M. Immunological effects of bevacizumab-based treatment in metastatic colorectal cancer. Oncology 2010;79:187-196.

[63] Stenson WF. Prostaglandins and epithelial response to injury. Curr Opin Gastroenterol 2007;23:107-110.
[64] Hanna MG, Jr., Hoover HC, Jr., Vermorken JB, Harris JE, Pinedo HM. Adjuvant active specific immunotherapy of stage II and stage III colon cancer with an autologous tumor cell vaccine: first randomized phase III trials show promise. Vaccine 2001;19:2576-2582.
[65] June CH. Adoptive T cell therapy for cancer in the clinic. J Clin Invest 2007;117:1466-1476.
[66] Galon J, Fridman WH, Pages F. The adaptive immunologic microenvironment in colorectal cancer: a novel perspective. Cancer Res 2007;67:1883-1886.
[67] Zlobec I, Lugli A. Invasive front of colorectal cancer: dynamic interface of pro-/anti-tumor factors. World J Gastroenterol 2009;15:5898-5906.

16

The Role of Infectious Agents in Colorectal Carcinogenesis

Hytham K. S. Hamid[1] and Yassin M. Mustafa[2]
[1]*Department of Surgery, Waterford Regional Hospital, Waterford,*
[2] *Department of Internal Medicine,*
Howard University Hospital, Washington D. C.,
[1]*Ireland*
[2]*USA*

1. Introduction

Infectious agents have been increasingly recognized as bona fide etiologic factors of human malignancies, particularly gastrointestinal cancers. The estimated total of infection-attributed malignancies per year is 1.9 million cases, accounting for 17.8% of the global cancer burden (Parkin, 2006). Given that colorectal cancer (CRC) is the third most common incident cancer worldwide (World health organization, 2003), it seems prudent to explore the role of microbial pathogens in colorectal carcinogenesis. By elucidating the probable mechanisms by which infectious agents contribute to colorectal oncogenesis, the management of CRC may one day parallel what is already in place for cancers such as gastric lymphoma and cervical cancer. Antimicrobial therapy and vaccination against some of these infections may herald a future with a curtailed role for traditional therapies of surgery and chemo-radiotherapy.

Unlike gastric cancer, which is chiefly linked to a single infectious agent, multiple organisms may contribute to the genesis of CRC. Epidemiological and experimental evidence strongly implicate several bacterial and parasitic agents in promotion of colorectal carcinogenesis. Most of these agents incite continual inflammation, which generates a procarcinogenic microenvironment (Parsonnet, 1995; Vennervald & Polman, 2009). Viruses have not attained the same status as other microorganisms as probable causative agents, though merit attention because of their inherent oncogenic properties and the increasing strength of their association with other malignancies (McLaughlin-Drubin & Munger, 2008). Yet, putative viral agents seemingly display an immense geographic variation that has led to much debate regarding the relative importance of one organism versus another. The present review summarizes the data available on the possible relationship of certain micro-organisms and CRC. These include but not limited to *Helicobacter pylori*, *Streptococcus bovis*, *Bacteroides fragilis*, JC virus (JCV), and human papillomavirus (HPV), and intestinal schistosomes. The consistency and nature of these associations are discussed, as are the mechanisms whereby each pathogen participates in the malignant transformation of the colonic mucosa.

2. Bacteria

2.1 *Helicobacter pylori*

H. pylori is a gastric microbiome that colonizes approximately 50% of the population worldwide (EUROGAST study group, 1993). Gastric infection with *H. pylori* fosters chronic inflammation and significantly increases the risk of developing peptic ulcer disease and gastric cancer. Indeed, the bacterium has been designated by the International Agency for Research in Cancer (IARC, 1994), as a class I carcinogen in human causing gastric cancer. Recently, promotion of tumour development by *H. pylori* infection in extragastric target organs, such as the colorectum, has been reported, though causal relationship is presently controversial.

Cancer in human

Numerous comparative and case-control studies have examined the relationship between *H. pylori* IgG seropositivity and colorectal neoplasia risk, but the results have been inconsistent. While some studies demonstrated positive correlations between colorectal neoplastic lesions, especially adenomas, and *H. pylori* seroprevalence (Aydin et al., 1999; Hartwich et al., 2001b; Meucci et al., 1997; Mizuno et al., 2005; Zumkeller et al., 2007), others showed null or inverse associations (Moss et al., 1995; Penman et al., 1994; Fireman et al., 2000; Shmuely et al., 2001; Siddheshwar et al., 2001; Machida-Montani et al., 2007; D'Onghia et al., 2007). Most of these studies were, however, confounded by uncontrolled extraneous variables. Breuer-Katschinski et al. (1999) compared *H. pylori* serostatus between 98 colorectal adenoma patients and age/sex-matched hospitalized and populations-based control groups. The results clearly demonstrated an increase in the risk of colorectal adenoma in association with *H. pylori* infection following adjustment for dietary and lifestyle factors. Importantly, two case-control studies nested in large population-based cohorts failed to establish any association between *H. pylori* seroprevalence and incident CRC, irrespective of adjustment for potential confounders (Thorburn et al., 1998; Limburg et al., 2002). In each study, the presence of *H. pylori* was determined in subjects who developed CRC years after serum donation. The inconclusive findings in these studies have been partially attributed to small sample size, lack of control heterogeneity, and incomplete colonoscopic evaluation (Takeda & Asaka, 2005). Besides, serologic methods may not always reflect real-time *H. pylori* infection and likely yield positive results for infections caused by *Helicobacter* species other than *H. pylori*, which commonly colonize the human colonic mucosa (Keenan et al., 2010).
Other studies have utilized more reliable diagnostic tools for detection of *H. pylori* infection. Lin et al. (2010) conducted a cross-sectional study using biopsy urease test, and demonstrated a significantly increased risk of colorectal adenoma among *H. pylori* infected-patients, particularly those with concomitant metabolic syndrome. Conversely, two case control studies, using 13^{C}-Urea breath test (UBT), did not substantiate any significant associations of *H. pylori* infection with colorectal tumours (Penman et al., 1994; Liou et al., 2006). Fujimori et al. (2005) evaluated 699 patients for *H. pylori* infection using combination of three tests; UBT, rapid urease test, and gastric biopsy histology. Their analysis revealed a significantly higher prevalence of colorectal adenoma and adenocarcinoma among *H. pylori*-positive female patients compared to their *H. pylori*-free counterparts.
Of note, in a metanalysis of 11 case-control studies, the summary odd ratio for the association of *H. pylori* infection with the risk for colorectal carcinoma or adenoma was found to be 1.4 (95% CI, 1.1–1.8). Different testing methods were, nevertheless, combined to

assess the *H. pylori* infection status in these studies (Zumkeller et al., 2006). More recently, a meta-analysis comprising 13 studies and 1709 patients with colorectal neoplasms, arrived at summary odd ration of 1.49 (95% CI 1.17–1.91). Further analysis of studies using serologic response as the sole indicator of infection revealed a higher summary odd ratio of 1.56 (95% CI, 1.14–2.14) (Y. S. Zhao et al., 2008).

Recently, Soylu et al. (2008) have investigated the presence of *H. pylori* in colorectal neoplasms using immunohistochemical methods, which allowed more accurate detection of the non-spiral forms of the bacterium. The prevalence of *H. pylori* was higher in villous type polyps than in tubular type polyps and adenocarcinomas. Contrary to this finding, Jones et al. (2007) demonstrated that villous adenoma had the lowest rate of *H. pylori* positivity compared to other premalignant and malignant colonic lesions. Their results also showed significant associations of *H. pylori* positivity with tubular and tubulovillous adenomas, and adenocarcinomas, but not with villous adenomas.

Likewise, studies employing PCR analysis for detection of *H. pylori* genomic material in the cancerous tissue have yielded conflicting results. A Swedish group detected *H. pylori* DNA in 27% of CRC specimens (Bulajic et al., 2007). In contrast, Grahn et al. (2005) identified *H. pylori* DNA in 1.2% of the malignant tissues and, unexpectedly, in 6% of normal mucosal samples among patients with CRC. Additionally, there was no statistical correlation between *H. pylori* PCR positivity and CRC. This finding was further confirmed in a later study on a separate population (Keenan et al., 2010).

Cancer in experimental animals

Studies have shown that amidated gastrins have no stimulatory effect on colon mucosal growth or progression of colon cancer in different experimental models (Hakanson et al., 1986, 1988). Others demonstrated that non-amidated gastrins, including progastrin and Gly-gastrin, have a mitogenic effect on the colonic mucosa in transgenic mice (T.C. Wang., 1996; Koh et al., 1999). Singh et al. (2000a, 2000b) reported that transgenic mice with elevated plasma progastrin, but not amidated gastrins, exhibit increased aberrant crypt foci, adenomas, and adenocarcinomas after treatment with azoxymethane, whilst no tumours developed in mice exposed to either progastrin or azoxymethane only. These results suggest that non-amidated gastrin is not a carcinogen on its own, but rather promotes oncogenic progression.

Mechanisms/Mechanistic studies

Various pathogenetic mechanisms have been suggested by which *H. pylori* exerts its oncogenic potential. First, persistent *H. pylori* exposure induces hypergastrinemia, which is a putative trophic factor for the human colorectal mucosa, thereby increasing the mutation susceptibility (Renga et al., 1997). Moreover, studies showed that most human colon cancers secrete gastrin, primarily non-amidated gastrins, which likely function in autocrine fashion (Baldwin et al., 1998). Non-amidated gastrin induces proliferation and invasiveness of human tumour cells *in vitro* (Kermorgant & Lehy, 2001). In conjunction with these findings, the overexpression of cyclooxygenase-2 (COX-2) was shown to stimulate the cancer cells to release excessive amount of prostaglandin E_2 (PGE_2), leading to further proliferation (Hartwich et al., 2001b).

Although some reports, including a well-controlled prospective study, provided statistical evidence that high fasting plasma gastrin level is associated with increased risk of colorectal adenoma and carcinoma (Hartwich et al., 2001b; Thorburn et al., 1998; Georgopoulos et al.,

2006), others showed no associations (Penman et al., 1994; Fireman et al., 2000; Machida-Montani et al., 2007; Robertson et al., 2009). In a majority of these studies only amidated gastrin was measured, which may have contributed to the discrepancy in results (Dickinson, 1995). In a recent study, circulating forms of both amidated and non-amidated gastrins were measured. Non-amidated gastrins were significantly higher in patients with colorectal carcinomas, compared with levels in control patients (Ciccotosto et al., 1995).

Second, *H. pylori*-related chronic gastritis might contribute to colorectal carcinogenesis by reducing gastric acid secretion with consequent alteration in the normal gastrointestinal flora (Kanno et al., 2009). Another possibility is that CagA protein (Fig 1.), which is produced by virulent strain of *H. pylori*, may contribute to colorectal carcinogenesis by inducing an enhanced inflammatory response and potentiating gastrin secretion (Peek et al., 1995; J.H. Kim et al., 1999). As for the correlation between colorectal neoplasia and CagA+ *H. pylori* serostatus, three studies indicated positive correlations between CagA+ *H. pylori* seropositivity and colorectal tumours (Hartwich et al., 2001b; Shmuely et al., 2001; Georgopoulos et al., 2006), while two other studies found no such correlation (Zumkeller et al., 2007; Limburg et al., 2002).

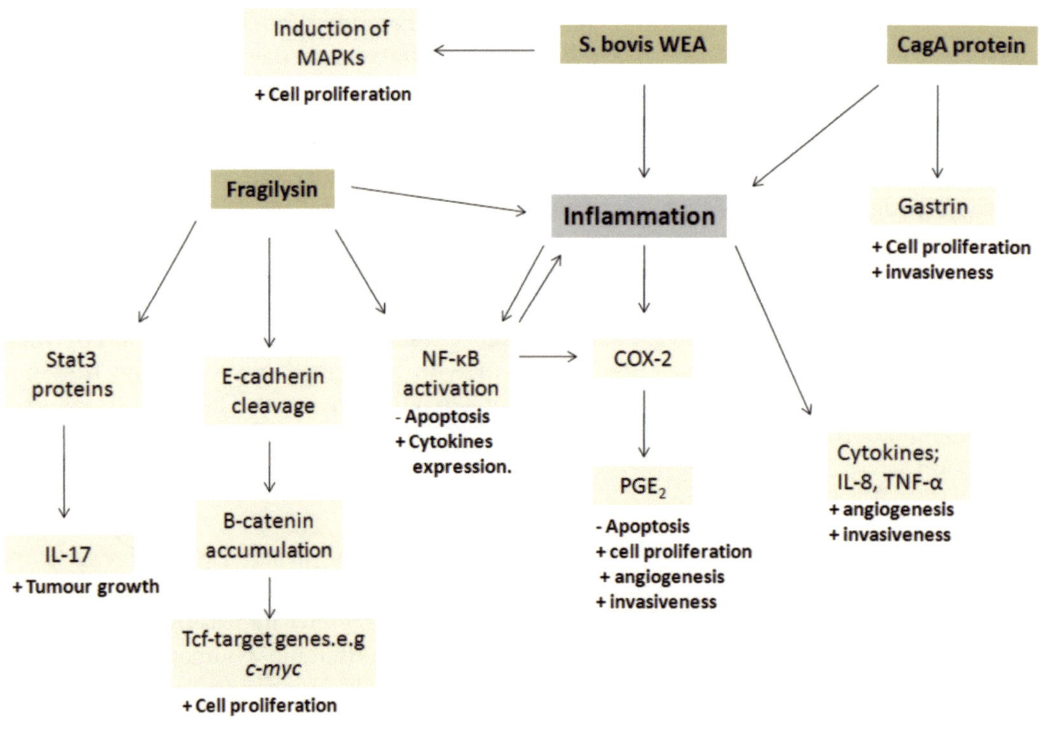

Fig. 1. Illustration of the possible mechanisms of bacterial-toxin-induced carcinogenesis.

2.2 *Streptococcus bovis*

S. bovis, a nonenterococcal lancefield group D *streptococcus*, is a transient colonic commensal with fecal carriage rate of 5 - 13 % in healthy adults (Potter et al., 1998; Dubrow et al., 1991), and accounts for 11-12% of infective endocarditis (Ballet et al., 1995; Kupferwasser et al., 1998). Traditionally, *S. bovis* has been classified into three distinct biotypes; I, II/1, and II/2, based on phenotypical and genetic characteristics (Coykendall & Gustafson, 1985). Further studies using phylogenetic analysis allowed clear and unambiguous differentiation of human clinical isolates and indicated that all strains of *S. bovis* I and II/2 be identified as *S. gallolyticus* (Schlegel et al., 2003). The latter accounts for most of the human strains isolated from blood or faeces, and is often responsible for endocarditis cases associated with colonic cancer (Schlegel et al., 2003).

Cancer in humans

The association between *S. bovis* endocarditis and colorectal carcinoma was first brought to light by Keusck (1974). Subsequent case studies showed a wide range of prevalence of colorectal neoplasms in patients with *S. bovis* bacteraemia (6 - 67%), depending on the diligence with which the diagnosis was sought (Pigrau et al., 1988; Klein et al, 1979; H.W. Murray & Roberts, 1978; Friedrich et al., 1982a; Reynolds et al., 1983; Zarkin et al., 1990; Gold et al, 2004; Alazmi et al, 2006; Beeching et al., 1985). Additionally, some patients developed new colonic tumours 2 to 4 years following the incidence of *S. bovis* endocarditis, pointing to a possible temporal relationship between the two events (Zarkin et al., 1990; Robbins & Klein, 1983; Muhlemann et al., 1999; Friedrich et al., 1982b). Other studies reported that patients with *S. bovis* endocarditis had significantly higher rates of colorectal neoplasms than those with endocarditis due to other pathogens or non-endocarditis patients (Pergola et al., 2001; Hoen et al., 1994). More particularly, Ruoff et al. (1989) showed that *S. bovis* I bacteraemia was highly correlated with malignant and premalignant colonic lesions, compared to bacteraemia due to other *S. bovis* biotypes. This conclusion was affirmed by several recent analyses, in which the incidence of colonic tumours in patients with *S. bovis* I infection ranged between 27 - 94% (Herrero et al., 2002; Tripodi et al., 2004; Corredoira et al., 2008; Vaska & Faoagali, 2009; Ruoff et al, 1999).

Several investigators have studied the association between the fecal carriage rate of *S. bovis* and both malignant and premalignant colorectal lesions, with the results being contradictory (Klein et al., 1977; Potter et al., 1998; Norfleet & Mitchell, 1993; Burns et al., 1985). Comparing the growth of *S. bovis* from tissue biopsy of adenomas or carcinomas did not show increased frequency compared to normal mucosa from the same patients or non-cancer-patients group (Potter et al., 1998; Norfleet & Mitchell, 1993). In contrast, Abdulamir et al. (2010), using bacteriological studies and molecular techniques to detect *S. gallolyticus* in tissue or faeces, revealed a significantly higher frequency of *S. gallolyticus* isolation from tumorous and non-tumorous tissue in CRC patients than from normal mucosa in control subjects. In parallel, the faecal carriage rate of *S. gallolyticus* was similar in cancer and control groups.

In another aspect, Darjee and Gibb (1993) used immunoblotting and enzyme-linked immunosorbent assay (ELISA) to compare anti-*S. bovis* IgG levels in sera of 16 colonic cancer patients and 16 age-matched controls. Immunoblot assay showed no significant difference in the serologic parameters between patients and controls, whilst ELISA demonstrated higher median *S. bovis* IgG antibody titres in patients with colonic cancer, compared to controls. Using immunocapture mass spectrometry, Tjalsma et al. (2006) showed a higher frequency of anti-*S. bovis* seropositivity in patients with colonic polyps and cancer than age-matched controls. Importantly, recent studies reported that CRC and adenoma were associated with higher levels of serum anti-*S. gallolyticus* IgG antibody in comparison with healthy and tumour-free control subjects (Abdulamir et al., 2009).

It is clear that a strong association does exist between symptomatic *S. bovis* infection and colorectal neoplasia, which has important clinical implications. Patients who have *S. bovis* bacteraemia, with or without endocarditis, require extensive endoscopic evaluation for occult premalignant and malignant colonic cancer (Konda & Duffy, 2008). Further, recent evidence indicates that serum antibodies to *S. bovis* represent a promising potential for early diagnosis and prevention of CRC (Tjalsma et al., 2006).

Cancer in experimental animals

Studies have shown that administration of *S. bovis* or *S. bovis* wall extracted antigens (WEA) to azoxymethane- treated rats resulted in almost two-fold increase in the number of aberrant colonic crypts, compared to azoxymethane-only treated control rats. Fifty percent of the rats receiving WEA developed colonic adenomas, whereas no tumour was detected in the other groups. It is noteworthy to mention that normal rats did not develop hyperplastic colonic crypts upon treatment with *S. bovis* suspension, implying that *S. bovis* proteins are involved in promoting rather than initiating oncogenesis (Ellmerich et al., 2000b). Similar results were obtained by Biarc et al., (2004) who also reported that a purified form of S. bovis WEA (S300 fraction) is even more potent inducer of neoplastic progression than WEA or the intact bacteria.

Mechanisms/Mechanistic studies

Although Klein et al. (1977) originally theorized that *S. bovis* may play a role in producing carcinogens in the large bowel, recent data showed that *S. bovis* wall proteins (Fig. 1.) have proinflammatory potential and procarcinogenic properties (Nguyen et al., 2006). *In vitro* studies indicated that activation of human colonic epithelial cell line Caco-2 by *S. bovis* cell wall proteins, especially S300 fraction, resulted in significant increase in IL-8 production, COX-2 expression, and PGE_2 release (Biarc et al., 2004), whereas binding of *S. bovis* activated human leucocytes cell line to release TNF-α (Ellmerich et al., 2000a). These results are in agreement with those obtained in *in vivo* experiments showing that *S. bovis* as well as cell wall antigens from this bacterium are able to increase the production of IL-8 and PGE_2 in the colonic mucosa of rats (Ellmerich et al., 2000b; Biarc et al., 2004). More recently, human studies have provided evidence for a strong association between *S. gallolyticus* IgG seropositivity and nuclear factor kappa B (NF-κB) and IL-8 expression in tumorous sections of both colorectal adenomas and carcinomas (Abdulamir et al., 2009). Using quantitative PCR analysis to measure bacterial count in cancerous tissue, the same group observed a positive correlation between the levels of expression of IL-1, COX-2, and IL-8 and the *S. gallolyticus* load in tumorous colorectal tissue (Abdulamir et al., 2010). Apart from its inflammatory potential, *S. bovis* cell wall proteins may activate mitogen-activated protein kinases (MAPKs), stimulating a proliferative response in the host cells and increasing the likelihood of cell transformation (Biarc et al., 2004).

Notably, the chemokine 1L-8 is potent angiogenic factor and neutrophil chemoattractant (Li et al., 2001), which as well as other cytokine such as TNF-α, IL-1β, and IL-6, trigger a chronic inflammation with resultant production of highly mutagenic reactive oxygen and nitrogen species (Ohshima & Bartsch., 1994). COX-2, through production of excessive amounts of prostaglandins, inhibits apoptosis, and promotes tumour cell proliferation, angiogenesis, and tumour invasiveness (Hartwich et al., 2001a). In addition, activation of NF-κB pathway induces the expression of downstream mediators such as COX-2, TNF-α, and IL-6, all contributing to inflammation-related tumorigenesis (S. Wang et al., 2009).

2.3 *Bacteroides fragilis*

B. fragilis is a gram-positive, anaerobic colonic microflora in most mammals, and is the leading cause of anaerobic bacteraemia and intraabdominal suppurative infection in human adults (Wexler et al., 2007). The pathogenicity of this bacterium is attributed to several virulence determinants, including a recently identified metalloprotease toxin, called fragilysin. Fragilysin-producing *B. fragilis*, termed enterotoxigenic *B. fragilis* (ETBF), causes acute inflammatory diarrheal disease and asymptomatically colonizes up to 20 -35 % of adults (Sears et al., 2008). As well, it has been recently linked to flare-ups of inflammatory bowel disease (Basset et al., 2004; Prindiville et al., 2000).

Cancer in human

The epidemiological evidence on the association *B. fragilis* infection and colorectal neoplasia is limited. Early studies by Legakis et al. (1981) indicated that the incidence of fecal *B. fragilis* in CRC patients was significantly higher than in healthy subjects, suggesting a possible role for *B. fragilis* in colon carcinogenesis. Moore et al. (1995), however, did not find any significant difference in the frequency of fecal carriage of *B. fragilis* between colorectal adenoma patients and low-risk healthy controls. Similarly, a seroepidemiological study showed lack of associations between *B. fragilis* IgG serostatus and colorectal adenoma and carcinoma (Abdulamir et al., 2009). Using PCR methods, Toprak et al. (2006) recently compared the prevalence of ETBF in stool specimens from 73 patients with CRC with 59 age-matched controls. The frequency of isolation of the organism was significantly higher in the CRC patients (38%) than in the control group (12%). These findings, however, have not been replicated in another population.

Cancer in experimental animals

Studies of murine models have demonstrated that ETBF induced persistent subclinical colonic inflammation and hyperplasia in specific pathogen-free C57BL/6 mice (Rhee et al., 2009). The same group used the adenomatous polyposis coli multiple intestinal neoplasia ($Apc^{Min/+}$) mice to model human CRC. ETBF-colonized $Apc^{Min/+}$ mice developed inflammatory colitis and unusually early onset microadenomas. In addition, *de novo* colon tumours appeared as early as 4 weeks and distributed predominantly in the distal colon, similar to those found in humans (Wu et al., 2009).

Mechanisms/Mechanistic studies

The current experimental evidence suggests a potential role of fragilysin in the oncogenic transformation of the colonic mucosa (Fig. 1.). *In vitro* studies have shown that fragilysin induces IL-8 expression and NF-κB activation in human colonic epithelial cell lines HT29 and Caco-2 (Sanfiloppo et al., 2000; J.M. Kim et al., 2001). IL-8 is a potent neutrophil chemokine, whereas NF-κB is an essential transcription factor that regulates neutrophils migration and the host epithelial cell chemokine response (J.M. Kim et al., 2002). Additionally, it was demonstrated that fragilysin binds to human colonic epithelial cell line HT29/C1 and stimulates cleavage of the tumour suppressor protein, E-cadherin. The resultant nuclear translocation of the adhesion molecule β-catenin causes increased expression of T-cell factor-target genes, including *c-myc*, with consequent persistent cellular proliferation (Wu et al., 1998, 2003).

Recent showed that all ETBF-induced tumours in $Apc^{Min/+}$ mice exhibited intense Stat3 protein activation, which in turn induces dominant colonic IL-17-producing $CD4^+$ T-cells infiltrate. Tumour formation was significantly inhibited by administration of blocking antibodies to IL-17 (Wu et al., 2009). The latter is known to promote tumour growth *in vitro* and *in vivo* through induction of IL-6 synthesis (L. Wang et al., 2009). These results emphasized the contribution of endogenous T cell immune response in ETBF infection-derived colorectal carcinogenesis.

In addition, *B. fragilis* may indirectly promote colon carcinogenesis through production of cytotoxic metabolites such as deoxycholic acid and fecapentaenes. Studies have shown that deoxycholic acid induce proliferation of colonic cells in vitro and promote colonic tumour progression in experimental animals (Peiffer et al., 1997; T. Hori et al., 1998). Several epidemiological studies found a positive association between high faecal deoxycholic acid concentration and colorectal adenoma and carcinoma risk (Little et al., 2002; Reddy & Wynder, 1977), including a prospective study assessing faecal deoxycholic acid levels before the diagnosis of colorectal tumours (Kawano et al., 2010). Fecapentaenes are other fecal mutagens synthesized by *Bacteroides* species, which were shown to be highly genotoxic in both mammalian and bacterial *in vitro* assays (Plummer et al., 1986; Curren et al., 1987). Clinical studies, however, indicated that fecal fecapentaenes levels are not associated with colorectal adenomas and inversely associated with carcinomas (de Kok et al., 1993; Schiffman et al., 1989). It was concluded that if fecapentaenes form a relevant factor in colorectal carcinogenesis, their role is more likely to be related to the transformation of late adenomas into malignant tumors.

2.4 Other bacterial species

There are very few reports on the role of enteric bacterial flora other than *B. fragilis* in colorectal tumorigenesis. Severe distal colitis, rectal dysplasia, and adenocarcinoma were observed in IL-10 knockout mice colonized with *Enterococcus faecalis* (Balish & Warner, 2002; S.C. Kim et al., 2005). *E. faecalis* has been shown to produce reactive oxygen species and induce DNA damage, aneuploidy and tetraploidy in colonic epithelial cells both *in vivo* and *in vitro* (Huycke et al., 2002; X. Wang et al., 2008). Furthermore, it was demonstrated that *E. faecalis* promotes chromosomal instability in mammalian cells, possibly through COX-2 dependent mechanism (X. Wang & Huycke, 2007). Epidemiological studies, however, could not establish any association between colonic colonization of *E. faecalis* and development of CRC (Winters et al., 1998).

Studies showed that mucosa-associated and intramucosal *Escherichia coli* were significantly associated with Crohn's disease, and colorectal adenomas and carcinomas (Swidsinski et al., 1998; Martin et al., 2004). *E. coli* stimulates IL-8 release from the I407 and HT29 cell lines (Martin, 2004), and acts synergistically with *E. faecalis* to induce aggressive pancolitis with reactive atypia in IL-10 deficient mice (S.C. Kim et al., 2007). Recently, Maddocks et al. (2009) reported that enteropathogenic *E. coli* downregulates DNA mismatch repair proteins which increases the susceptibility of colonic epithelial cells to mutations and therefore promotes colonic tumorigenesis.

3. Viruses

3.1 Human papilloma virus

Human papilloma virus is a double stranded DNA virus that is transmitted through direct contact with infected skin or mucous membrane, and causes the most common sexually transmitted disease among sexually active individuals (Koutsky, 1997). While it is well established that HPV is a necessary cause of cervical cancer, studies suggest HPV may be involved in the malignant transformation of the oropharynx and the anogenital tract (D'Souza et al., 2007; Steenbergen et al., 2005). There are more than 100 subtypes of HPV; some of these subtypes, particularly HPV-16 and HPV-18, are referred to as high risk oncogenic infections (Wiley & Masongsong, 2006; Munoz et al., 2003).

Cancer in human

Early case studies have failed to show any association between HPV infection and colorectal carcinoma in relatively small samples of colorectal carcinoma tissue (Boguszakova et al., 1988; Koulos et al., 1991; Shah et al., 1992; Shroyer et al., 1992). Subsequent studies have employed more stringent methods for HPV detection, including PCR and immunohistochemistry. Despite the variation in the control specimen, all studies confirmed an association between HPV detection rates, specifically subtypes 16 and 18, and CRC with odd ratio ranging between 2.7 (95% CI, 1.1–6.2) and 9.1 (95% CI, 3.7–22.3). (Cheng et al., 1995; Kirgan et al., 1990). Moreover, the strength of association was related to the degree of tumour dysplasia. On the contrary, two of three large prospective cohort studies, with sample sizes ranging between 21,222 and 104,760 cases of cervical cancer, reported no increased risk of subsequent CRC in patients with cervical cancer (Weinberg et al., 1999; Rex, 2000). The other study has shown increased risk of anorectal cancer among patients with cervical cancer, though with lack of clarity over whether it was due to HPV infection or radiation (Chaturvedi et al., 2007).

Mechanism/ mechanistic studies

The oncogenic property of the virus is related to early genes which encode the regulatory proteins E6 an E7. It was hypothesized that these proteins interact and inactivate suppressor genes p53 and pRb, and thus inhibiting apoptosis (Steenbergen et al., 2005). Although about 50% of all colorectal cancer has mutated *p53* (Slattery et al., 2002), Buyru et al. (2003) reported that only 3.6% of HPV-positive colorectal cancers contained mutations in *p53*, suggesting that HPV may have direct oncogenic effects independent of any *p53* mutations.

3.2 John Cunningham virus

JC virus is a widespread neurotropic polyoma virus, with seroprevalence rates of 39-90% among healthy adult population (Kean et al., 2009; Shah, 1996). Primary JCV infection typically occurs during early childhood, probably via fecal-oral route, followed by latency of the virus in the kidney and gastrointestinal tract (Khalili et al., 2003, Ricciardiello et al., 2000). The virus may be reactivated in the presence of severe immunosuppression, and replicates in the central nervous system causing a fatal demyelinating disease, progressive multifocal leukoencephalopathy. Furthermore, there is mounting evidence suggesting that JCV infection may be associated with several human malignancies including brain tumours and upper gastrointestinal cancers (Caldarelli-Stefano et al., 2000; Del Valle et al., 2001, 2005; Shin et al., 2006).

Cancer in human

The potential association between JCV infection and colorectal neoplasia has been examined using nested PCR, Southern blotting and *in situ* hybridization techniques. Ten studies, with sample sizes ranging from 18 to 186, detected JCV genomic sequences in 9-89% of colorectal carcinomas and 5-82% of adenomatous tissue (Laghi et al., 1999; Theodoropoulos et al., 2005;

R. Hori et al., 2005; Casini et al., 2005; Enam et al., 2002; Goel et al., 2006; P. Y. Lin et al., 2008, Niv et al., 2010a; Karpinski et al., 2011; Jung et al., 2008). Comparing neoplastic tissues with normal mucosa, three of these studies showed consistently higher detection rates for JCV in colorectal cancerous tissues and adenomas than in normal tissue (Theodoropoulos et al., 2005; R. Hori et al., 2005; Enam et al., 2002). As well, significantly higher viral copy numbers were observed in colorectal carcinomas and adenomas compared to adjacent normal mucosa (Laghi et al., 1999; Theodoropoulos et al., 2005). Of note, a sequence of the Mad-1 variant of JCV, which lacks 98 nucleotides repeats, has been found preferentially in colon cancers, raising the possibility that certain strains may be selectively activated in colonic epithelial cells (Ricciardello et al., 2001). Other studies have employed real-time PCR, a less sensitive molecular technique, to detect JCV genetic material in colorectal carcinomas, adenomas, normal mucosa, and urine samples from CRC patients and controls. While JCV carrier frequencies in urine were comparable to previously published reports (Agostini et al., 1999), none of the neoplastic tissues and less than 1% of the normal tissues tested positive for JCV DNA (Newcomb et al., 2004; Campello et al., 2010; Militello et al., 2009). The discordant results in previous investigations may be explained by the small sample sizes, variable prevalence of viral infection among the studied populations, inherent lack of uniformity in the sensitivity of the assay used, and possible laboratory contamination particularly in studies where Mad 1 viral sequence was used as a positive template control (Newcomb et al., 2004).

The expression pattern of JCV T-antigen has also been studied in both colorectal neoplastic and normal mucosa. About 35%-94% of CRC tissues and 5-50% of colorectal adenomas were found to host JCV T-antigen, which is often concentrated in the nucleus (Enam et al., 2002; P. Y. Lin et al., 2008; Goel et al., 2006; Link et al., 2009; Nosho et al., 2008, 2009; Ogino et al., 2009; Selgrad et al., 2008; Jung et al., 2008). The expression of JCV T-antigen was significantly higher in colorectal adenomas from liver transplant recipients compared to adenomas in normal controls, pointing to a possible etiologic role for immunosuppression (Selgrad et al., 2008). Interestingly, viral DNA has always been detected more frequently than Tag expression in both colonic adenomas and carcinomas. This suggests that either in some samples, the viral copy number is too low to determine expression of the early gene or, alternatively, that the growing tumour tends to lose viral sequences (Ricciardello et al., 2003). In another aspect, two prospective nested case-control investigated the association between JC seroprevalence and colorectal neoplasms in large groups of patients from whom blood samples were collected months or years before colorectal cancer diagnosis (Rollison et al., 2009; Lundstig et al., 2007). Although there was no association between JC seropositivity and colorectal cancer, one study showed a significantly increased risk of adenomas among seropositive male subjects (Rollison et al., 2009). More recently, Niv et al. (2010b) observed positive correlation between the presence of neoplastic colonic lesion and the titre of JCV antibody in the serum, pointing to JCV infection as an early event for the formation of colorectal adenoma.

Mechanism/ mechanistic studies

The JCV T-antigen is a potent oncogenic protein capable of transforming mammalian cells and is likely involved the early stages of colorectal carcinogenesis though "hit and run" mechanisms. These include disruption of the Wnt signalling pathway and inactivation of tumour suppressor genes such as *pRb* and *p53* (Ludlow, 1993). Both in vitro and in vivo studies have shown that coexpression of *p53* and JCV T-antigen in CRC cells (Enam et al., 2002; Nosho et al., 2009; Ricciardello et al., 2003). Similarly, colocalization of T-antigen and B-catenin was observed in the nuclei of neoplastic columnar cells (Enam et al., 2002; nosho et al., 2009). Cooperativity between B-catenin and JCV T-antigen increased in vitro transcription of *c-myc*, leading to chromosomal instability (Enam et al., 2002). Ricciardiello et al. (2003) demonstrated that JCV can induce chromosomal instability in vitro using the diploid CRC cell line, which defines loss of heterozygosity (LOH). Subsequent studies reported a significant association between JCV T-antigen expression and CRC with LOH (Nosho et al., 2009; Goel et al., 2006; Ogino et al., 2009). This deletional event probably provides the second hit at the tumour suppressor genes, and eventually leads to clonal expansion. The role of DNA hypermethylation has recently been explored in both colorectal carcinoma and adenoma, nevertheless the results were contradictory (Nosho et al., 2008, 2009; Goel et al., 2006).

3.3 Other viruses

Epstein-Barr virus (EBV) is a DNA virus with strong association with several lymphoreticular malignancies, especially Burkett's lymphoma, as well as certain epithelial tumours such as the nasopharyngeal carcinoma (Parkin, 2006). Additionally, EBV has also been reported with gastric cancer (Koriyama et al., 2001; Takada, 2000), breast (Labrecque et al., 1995; Bonnet et al., 1999; Fina et al., 2001) and lung cancer (Castro et al., 2001; Han et al., 2001; M.P. Wong et al., 1995). For colorectal cancer, although early studies have detected high rates of EBV infection in colorectal carcinoma tissue, using PCR, immunohistochemisrty and fluorescence in situ hybridization (Song et al., 2006; Liu et al., 2002, 2003), only one study reported significant difference in EBV detection rates between colorectal carcinoma tissue and adjacent normal mucosa (Song et al., 2006). Follow-up studies failed to show any evidence that EBV was detected at a significantly higher rate in colorectal carcinoma (Grinstein et al., 2002; Yuen et al., 1994), even in higher risk populations such as patients with ulcerative colitis (N.A. Wong et al., 2003).

In the case of Cytomegalovirus (CMV), early limited studies have detected CMV genome in the colon carcinoma tissue, whereas controls from normal colons and cases of Crohn disease were negative (Huang & Roche, 1978; Hashiro et al., 1979). Further studies then showed that CMV was not detected at a significantly higher rate in carcinoma tissue than normal tissue by multiple detection methods, such as FISH, immunohistochemistry, or DNA hybridization (Hart et al., 1982; Ruger & Fleckenstein, 1985). It was found that patients with colorectal cancer who were treated with chemotherapy had significantly increased CMV IgG titre (Avni et al., 1981). However, this finding appeared to be related to CMV infection or reactivation secondary to immunosuppression by chemotherapy rather than primary infection causing colorectal cancer.

4. Helminths

4.1 *Schistosoma japonicum*

The epidemiologic parallel between schistosomiasis japonica endemicity and the distribution of large bowel cancer has been noted in the eastern provinces of China in the 1970s (E. S. Zhao, 1981). Subsequently, ecological studies in the same endemic areas showed a strong geographical correlation between the prevalence of schistosomiasis japonica and CRC incidence and mortality (Xu & Su, 1984). Likewise, significant association was observed between the mortality from CRC and from schistosomiasis japonica in rural China, even after adjustment for dietary factors (Chen et al., 1990; Guo et al., 1993). The authors attributed the continuing high incidence of colorectal cancer in endemic regions to persistent large populations of chronically infected individuals. This conclusion was further bolstered by a retrospective cohort study conducted in an endemic area in Japan, where the standardized mortality ratio for colonic cancer was significantly high in females who lived in the area for 50 years or more (Inaba, 1984).

More importantly, a case-control study carried out in the endemic area of Jiangsu Province, China, showed that the risk of rectal cancer was increased among subjects with a previous diagnosis of *S. japonicum* infection with odds ratios of 4.5 and 8.3 (depending on the type of controls used), but the risk of colon cancer was not significantly increased in the same patients group (Xu & Su, 1984). A similar investigation in the same endemic area has confirmed strong associations between colon cancer and early and late-stage *S. japonicum* infection, regardless of the type of control used for comparison. When the results were adjusted to smoking and family history of colon cancer, statistically significant associations were still noted. In addition, the estimated relative risk increased with the duration of exposure to *S. japonicum* infection (Mayer & Fried, 2007). Of interest also is a recent matched case-control study which reported that patients with chronic schistosomiasis japonica have more than three times risk to develop colon cancer than those with no previous exposure to schistosomal infection. Moreover, the authors attributed 24% of colon cancer cases to long-standing schistosomal infestation (Qiu et al., 2005).

The consensus of available pathological data strongly implicates an association between *S. japonicum* infestation and induction of CRC. In a review of the literature between 1898 and 1974, 276 cases of schistosomiasis japonica associated with cancer of the large intestine were analysed. The results showed significant differences between carcinoma with schistosomiasis and ordinary carcinoma in symptoms, age range, sex ratio, and histopathologic findings, indicating that schistosomiasis may induce carcinoma (Shindo, 1976). Ming-Chai et al. (1965) reported similar findings in their study of 90 cases of simultaneous CRC and schistosomiasis, and proposed that *S. japonicum* colitis, in its late phases, is a premalignant condition not infrequently leading to cancer. Supporting their previous results and giving better insight into the pathogenesis of schistosomal colorectal carcinoma, the same group has examined the mucosal changes in the immediate vicinity of the tumours of patients with schistosomiasis, and referred to the close similarity between certain schistosome-induced lesions and those associated with long-standing ulcerative colitis. Pointing to mimicry of cancer evolution in these two clinical entities, they described presence of pseudopolyps, multiple ulcers, and hyperplastic ectopic submucosal glands, with evidence of oviposition and precancerous and cancerous transformation in these lesions (Ming-Chai et al., 1980). It was also demonstrated that the closer to the tumour the area is the more ova tend to be detected (Matsuda et al., 1999). In a following study, Ming-Chai et al. (1981) observed variable degree of colonic epithelial dysplasia in 60% of cases with *S. japonicum* colitis and regarded these changes as the transition on the way towards cancer development in schistosomal colonic disease. A similar conclusion was drawn by Yu et al. (1991) from their studies on different types of schistosomal egg polyps.

Of note, distinct clinico-pathologic characteristics of S. japonicum-related colorectal cancer seem emerge from the existing literature. Bearing in mind the early environmental exposure to schistosomal infection in childhood, schistosomal colorectal cancer was notably shown to occur in younger age group with a maximum age incidence 6 to 16 years earlier than ordinary colorectal cancer (Shindo, 1976; Ming-Chai et al., 1965, 1980). Furthermore, the gender ratio of male to female in schistosomal colorectal cancer is consistently higher than in nonschistosomal cancer (Shindo, 1976; Ming-Chai et al., 1980). This can be attributed to the fact that men are more prone to schistosomal infection through contact with cercariae-infested waters during agricultural activities.

4.2 *Schistosoma mansoni*

The epidemiological evidence associating *S. mansoni* infection with CRC is lacking, of poor quality, or conflicting. Supporting the absence of such a causal association, Parkin et al. (1986) pointed out that although there is a great disparity in the geographical distribution of *S. mansoni*, CRC occurs in the African continent with clear uniformity. In a recent hospital-based study in Uganda and Zimbabwe, Waku et al. (2005) compared 950 cases of infective gastrointestinal disease, particularly schistosomiasis and amebiasis, with 249 patient controls admitted for various diseases other than GI disease. The cases were thoroughly investigated and further stratified into three groups on the basis of the stage of the disease; cured, acute, and chronic patients group. Colorectal cancer was found in 34 patients; nearly all of them had chronic schistosomiasis or amebiasis, whereas no CRC was detected in the other patients or control groups. It was concluded that large bowel cancer is strongly associated with chronic infectious gastrointestinal diseases. This study, though, was limited by the inability to adjust for potential confounders such as age and gender. Furthermore, the issue of correspondence between the population giving rise to the cases and that sampled for the controls was not addressed. To date, there have been no epidemiological studies conducted at the population level to verify the link between *S. mansoni* infestation and large bowel cancer.

The pathological evidence supporting an association between *S. mansoni* infestation and colorectal carcinoma is rather weak. In 1956, Dimmette et al. (1956) failed to demonstrate any specific pathological changes in patients with simultaneous CRC and *S. mansoni* infestation, and considered the two conditions unrelated. Contrasting to these results, a recent study by Madbouly et al. (2007) has shown that S. mansoni-associated colorectal cancer has distinctive pathological features often similar to those of colitis-induced carcinoma (Fig. 2a,b). These include high percentage of multicentric tumours and mucinous adenocarcinoma, and the tendency of the tumour to present at an advanced stage with high risk of malignant lymph node invasion. Although direct causal inference is limited, this study indicates that *S. mansoni* infestation may exercise some influence on the prognosis of patients with CRC. Other studies have examined the pathological changes in endoscopic biopsies and cadaveric specimens from the colon of patients with *S. mansoni* colitis (Mohamed et al., 1990; Cheever et al., 1987). The gross pathological lesions were akin to those observed in patients with *S. japonicum* colitis. However, histological analysis of the specimens showed no evidence of atypism or carcinomatous changes. This discrepancy in pathologic findings may be explained by the larger number of eggs deposited by *S. japonicum* than *S. mansoni* worms, thus causing more pathological problems (Ishii et al., 1994).

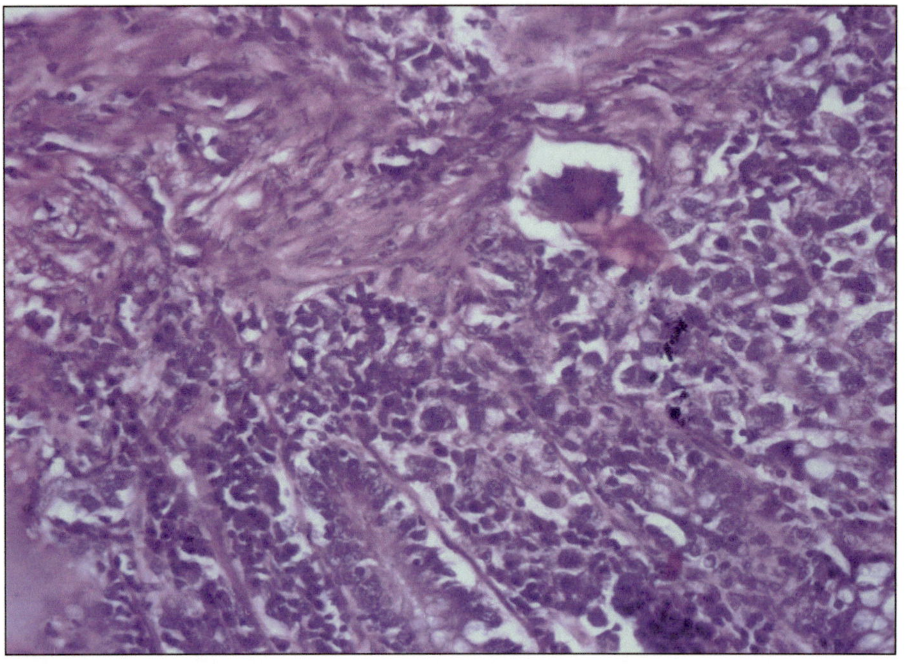

Fig. 2a. Photomicrograph showing S. mansoni egg shell in a background of mucinous adenocarcinoma. H&E × 40

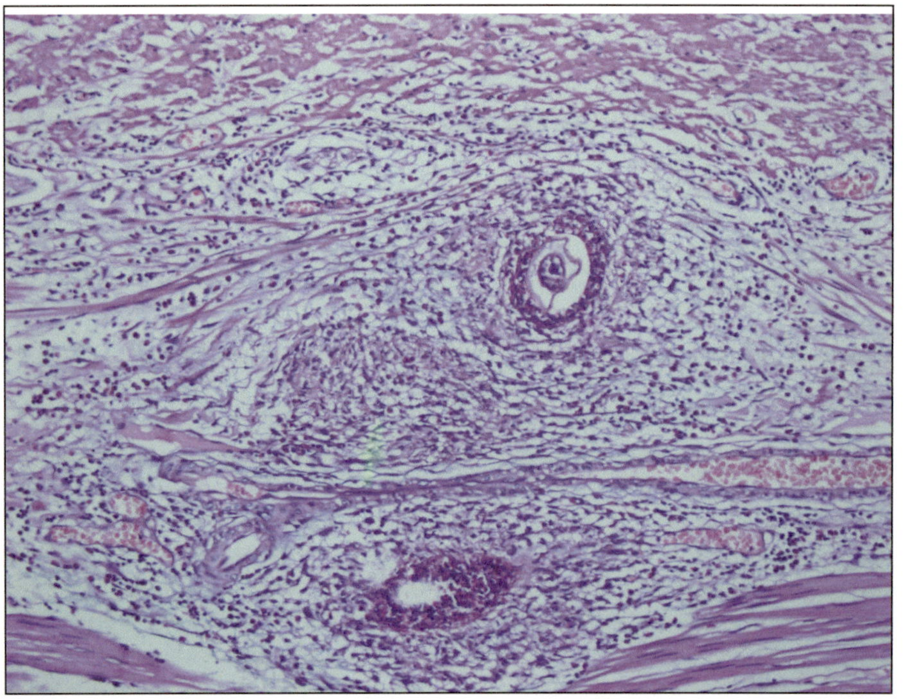

Fig. 2b. Photomicrograph showing calcified and viable S. mansoni ova with granuloma formation in the muscularis propria of the sigmoid colon. H&E × 20

4.3 Mechanisms of tumorigenesis

The exact etiopathogenesis of schistosomal colorectal cancer is enigmatic. Several explanations have been advanced for the possible role of schistosomiasis in colorectal tumorigenesis: the presence of endogenously produced carcinogens (Rosin et al., 1994), chronic immunomodulation resulting in impairment of immunological surveillance (van Riet et al., 2007), symbiotic action of other infective agents (Shindo, 1976), and the presence of schistosomal toxins (Long et al., 2004). While these factors may interact to induce carcinogenesis, chronic inflammation appears to play a central role. In support of this view are data showing that CRC tends to occur mainly in patients who had history of schistosomiasis for 10 years or more and in whom the large bowel is wholly involved (Shindo, 1976; Ming-Chai et al., 1980). Moreover, there is significantly higher rate of synchronous tumours in patients with schistosomal colorectal cancer than in patients with spontaneous colorectal cancer (Ming-Chai et al., 1980; Madbouly et al., 2007). This can be ascribed to the field effect caused by chronic schistosomal inflammation throughout the colon, a phenomenon analogous to that described in the context of colitis-associated cancer.

It has been suggested that chronic inflammatory reaction provoked by schistosome antigens provides the proliferative stimulus necessary to promote cancer growth from potentially malignant foci produced by other carcinogens (Ming-Chai et al., 1980). However, whereas increased epithelial cell proliferation likely contributes to carcinogenesis, it is insufficient to cause cancer. Rather, inflammatory cells generate potentially genotoxic mediators during the course of schistosomal infection such as reactive oxygen and nitrogen species and proinflammatory cytokines, which cause genomic instability and dysregulation of oncogenes and oncosuppresor genes (Herrera et al., 2005; Trakatelli et al., 2005). The accumulation of these molecular disturbances, in turn, drives the progression toward dysplasia and carcinoma. Another factor that may play a major role in colorectal carcinogenesis of schistosomiasis patients is the presence of concomitant enterobacterial infections. In both clinical and experimental studies, various strains of enterobacteriaceae have been described in association with schistosome infection which confers a survival advantage to bacteria by inducing immunosuppression (Chieffi, 1992; Tuazon et al., 1985). Some of these organisms are thought to promote colorectal carcinogenesis through multiple pathways such as production of reactive oxygen intermediates, dysregulation in the T cell response, and alterations in host epithelial carbohydrate expression (Hope et al., 2005).

A further explanation for the carcinogenic process of schistosomal CRC is a possible direct mutagenic effect of the schistosome soluble antigens. Evidence against this hypothesis has come from a study by Ishii et al. (1989), who evaluated the mutagenicity of *S. japonicum* extracts using the Ames *Salmonella/E. coli* test in the presence and absence of rat liver S9 mixture. They did not identify any mutagenic activity for the soluble extracts of both eggs and adult worms. Nevertheless, a weak but significant tumour-promoting activity was noted for the *S. japonicum* soluble egg antigen when tested using cultured viral genome-carrying human lymphoblastoid cells. Osada et al. (2005) tested the adult worm and egg extracts of *S. mansoni* using more reliable genetic toxicology assays, the *Salmonella* Umu test and the hypoxanthine guanine phosphoribosyltransferase (HGPRT) gene mutation assay. They could not demonstrate any mutagenic potential in either parasite extracts of *S. mansoni* before and after addition of S9 mixture.

Recent studies have thrown some light on the molecular events associated with schistosomal colorectal cancer, taking the latter as a separate clinical entity. Zhang et al. (1998) investigated the mutation pattern in the *p53* gene in S. japonicum-associated rectal carcinomas. They observed a higher proportion of base-pair substitutions at CpG dinucleotides and arginine missense mutations among schistosomal rectal cancer patients than in patients with ordinary CRC, albeit the differences were of marginal significance. Their results also indicated that the majority of mutations in *p53* gene were in exon 7 in schistosomal group compared to exon 5 in non-schistosomal group. Barrowing from the ulcerative colitis example, nitric oxide, an endogenously produced genotoxic agent, is capable of inducing similar transition mutations and activation of *p53* gene in the inflamed colonic mucosa (Goodman et al., 2004). Conceivably therefore, it seems plausible that chronic colonic inflammation induced by schistosomal infection may follow a similar pathway.

For *S. mansoni*-associated colorectal carcinomas, it was demonstrated that parasitism is strongly associated with microsatellite instability, which is a sign of defective DNA repair (Soliman et al., 2001). This genomic instability results in DNA replication errors that preferentially affect target genes such as transforming growth factor (*TGH)βRII* and insulin-like growth factor (IGF)2R, and render them incapable of normal colonocytes homeostasis resulting in malignant growth (Itzkowitz & Yio, 2004). In another aspect, Madbouly et al. (2007) evaluated the expression of *p53* in patients with *S. mansoni*-related colorectal cancer, and found that mutant *p53* overexpression was significantly more frequent in schistosomal than in non-schistosomal colorectal cancer. Moreover, *p53* overexpression in schistosomal CRC correlated well with mucinous carcinoma, nodal metastasis, and tumour multicentricity. Zalata et al. (2005) developed a more comprehensive study of the expression pattern of *p53*, *Bcl-2*, and *c-myc* in seventy five CRC cases, 24 of these had pathological evidence of *S. mansoni* infection. Although they did not find a significant association between parasitism and *p53* and *c-myc* expression, their results showed that S. mansoni-associated colorectal tumours characterized by *Bcl-2* overexpression and less apoptotic activity than ordinary colorectal tumours. This supports the contention that evasion of apoptosis through change in the expression of *Bcl-2* may be an alternative molecular pathway through which genotoxic agents can induce carcinogenesis in intestinal schistosomiasis.

5. Concluding remarks

It is clearly evident that a wide array of microbial agents is associated with colorectal cancer. Nonetheless, establishing a causal link between a certain organism and colorectal cancer is a complicated process, considering the long latency of infection during which numerous endogenous and exogenous factors interact to obscure causality. For most of these putative agents, the association has been inconsistent, and may either define subsets of the tumour, or may act to modify phenotype of an established tumour, possibly contributing to some phase of oncogenesis.

Despite the fact that *H. pylori* and *S. bovis* were discovered in colorectal tumours and linked to the malignancy by seroepidemiologic studies and molecular analyses, these pathogens are considered to be at most contributing cofactors. The two reasons for this loss of etiological status were the inconsistency in the epidemiological data regarding *H. pylori* and *S. bovis* infections and risk of colorectal cancer (Gold et al, 2004; Y. S. Zhao et al., 2008), whereas none of these agents produced *de novo* colorectal cancer in animal models (Singh et al., 2000a; Biarc et al., 2004). The relation between gut mictobiota such as *B. fragilis* and *E.*

faecalis and colorectal cancer is far less convincing. Although the oncogenic potential of *B. fragilis* and *E. faecalis* is not disputed, the scarcity of epidemiological evidence renders any association hypothetical.

In case of viral agents, while HPV and JCV have oncogenic properties both in cell culture and experimental animals (Butel, 2000), the detection of viral genomes in tumour tissues is inconsistent, which can be attributed to the fact that PCR technique, used for detection of viral DNA in most studies, is subject to contamination. At this point, this precludes a causative role for these viruses in colorectal cancer, and obtaining more credible results mandates employment of combination of in situ methods for detection of viral genome and its products such as *in situ* cytohybridization and immunohistochemistry (Panago et al., 2004).

In case of *S. japonicum*, the growing epidemiological evidence and the unique clinic-pathological features of schistosome-related colorectal cancer point to a reasonably consistent association. However, *S. japonicum* has been classified by IARC as possible and not as definite carcinogen in human leading to colorectal cancer (IARC, 1994). This perhaps reflects the confounding uncertainties presented by epidemiological studies and the lack of experimental evidence. For *S. mansoni* species, it is still a matter of controversy as to whether or not *S. mansoni* infection is an association factor in colorectal cancer development and progression.

Infection-related colorectal carcinogenesis is a complex multistage process that utilizes several mechanisms. For most bacterial species and helminths associated with colorectal cancer, chronic inflammatory response and immunomodulation induced by secretory or structural proteins are the principal mechanisms of carcinogenesis. These involve release of protumorigenic mediators and dysregulation of multiple cellular transcriptional pathways including NF-κB and β–catenin. Others such as *H. pylori* primarily induce production of growth factor resulting disruption of proliferation-antiproliferation pathways. DNA tumour viruses, such as HPV and JCV, primarily target cellular tumour suppressor proteins, thus modulating cell cycle progression (Butel, 2000).

Together, our observations underpin the necessity of epidemiological studies focusing on specific strains such as $CagA^{+}$ H. pylori, *S. gallolyticus*, ETBF, and Mad-1 JCV. In addition, the interaction between various infectious agents in relation to carcinogenesis, as illustrated in the additive effect of *B. fragilis* and *E. faecalis* needs further evaluation. Finally it is likely that more agents, both known and unidentified, have yet to be implicated in human colorectal cancer. In the meantime, study of tumorigenic infectious agents will continue to illuminate molecular oncogenic processes.

6. Acknowledgement

Acknowledgement to Dr. Salwa O. Mekki, Director of Pathology Department, Soba University Hospital, to Ms. Abeer Musa, Lab Technician for preparing the slides, and to the patients who gave us the permission to add their pictures in our chapter.

7. References

Abdulamir, A. S., Hafidh, R. R. & Abu Bakar, F. (2010). Molecular detection, quantification, and isolation of *Streptococcus gallolyticus* bacteria colonizing colorectal tumors:

inflammation-driven potential of carcinogenesis via IL-1, COX-2, and IL-8. *J Exp Clin Cancer Res*, 9, 249.

Abdulamir, A. S., Hafidh, R. R., Mahdi, L. K., Al-jeboori, T. & Abubaker F. (2009) Investigation into the controversial association of *Streptococcus gallolyticus* with colorectal cancer and adenoma. *BMC Cancer*, 9, 403.

Agostini, H. T., Jobes, D. V., Chima, S. C., Ryschkewitsch, C. F. & Stoner, G. L. (1999). Natural and pathogenic variation in the JC virus genome. *Recent Res Dev Virol*, 1, 683–701.

Alazmi, W., Bustamante, M., O'Loughlin, C., Gonzalez, J. & Raskin, J. B. (2006). The association of *Streptococcus bovis* bacteremia and gastrointestinal diseases: a retrospective analysis. *Dig Dis Sci*, 51, 732 - 736.

Avni, A., Haikin, H., Feuchtwanger, M. M., Sacks, M., Naggan, L., Sarov, B. & Sarov, I. (1981). Antibody pattern to human cytomegalovirus in patients with adenocarcinoma of the colon. *Intervirology*, 16, 4, 244–249.

Aydin, A., Karasu, Z., Zeytinoglu, A., Kumanlioglu, K. & Ozacar, T. (1999). Colorectal adenomateous polyps and Helicobacter pylori infection. *Am J Gastroenterol*, 94, 4, 1121–1122.

Baldwin, G. S. & Shulkes, A. (1998). Gastrin, gastrin receptors and colorectal carcinoma. *Gut*, 42, 4, 581–584.

Balish, E. & Warner, T. (2002). *Enterococcus faecalis* induces inflammatory bowel disease in interleukin-10 knockout mice. *Am J Pathol*, 160, 6, 2253–2257.

Ballet, M., Gevigney, G., Gare, J. P., Delahaye, F., Etienne, J. & Delahaye J. P. (1995). Infective endocarditis due to *Streptococcus bovis*. A report of 53 cases. *Eur Heart J*, 16, 12, 1975–1980.

Basset, C., Holton, J., Bazeos, A., Vaira, D. & Bloom, S. (2004). Are *Helicobacter* species and enterotoxigenic *Bacteroides fragilis* involved in inflammatory bowel disease? *Dig Dis Sci*, 49, 9, 1425–1432.

Beeching, N. J., Christmas, T. I., Ellis-Pegler, R. B. & Nicholson, G. I. (1985). *Streptococcus bovis* bacteraemia requires rigorous exclusion of colonic neoplasia and endocarditis. *Q J Med*, 56, 220, 439–450.

Biarc, J., Nguyen, I. S., Pini, A., Gosse, F., Richert, S., Thierse, D., Van Dorsselaer, A., Leize-Wagner, E., Raul, F., Klein, J. P. & Schöller-Guinard, M. (2004). Carcinogenic properties of proteins with pro-inflammatory activity from *Streptococcus infantarius* (formerly *S.bovis*). *Carcinogenesis*, 25, 8, 1477-1484.

Bodaghi, S., Yamanegi, K., Xiao, S. Y., Da Costa, M., Palefsky, J. M. & Zheng, Z. M. (2005). Colorectal papillomavirus infection in patients with colorectal cancer. *Clin Cancer Res*, 11, 8, 2862–2867.

Boguszakova, L., Hirsch, I., Brichacek, B., Faltýn, J., Fric, P., Dvoráková, H. & Vonka, V. (1988). Absence of cytomegalovirus, Epstein-Barr virus, and papillomavirus DNA from adenoma and adenocarcinoma of the colon. *Acta Virol*, 32, 4, 303–308.

Bonnet, M., Guinebretiere, J. M., Kremmer, E., Grunewald, V., Benhamou, E., Contesso, G. & Joab, I. (1999). Detection of Epstein-Barr virus in invasive breast cancers. *J Natl Cancer Inst*, 91, 16, 1376–1381.

Breuer-Katschinski, B., Nemes, K., Marr, A., Rump, B., Leiendecker, B., Breuer, N. & Goebell, H. (1999). *Helicobacter pylori* and the risk of colonic adenomas. Colorectal Adenoma Study Group. *Digestion*, 60, 3, 210–215.

Bulajic, M., Stimec, B., Jesenofsky, R., Kecmanovic, D., Ceranic, M., Kostic, N., Schneider-Brachert, W., Lowenfels, A., Maisonneuve, P. & Löhr, J. M. (2007). *Helicobacter pylori* in colorectal carcinoma tissue. *Cancer Epidemiol Biomarkers Prev*, 16, 3, 631 - 633.

Burns, C.A., McCaughey, R. & Lauter, C. B. (1985). The association of *Streptococcus bovis* fecal carriage and colon neoplasia: possible relationship with polyps and their premalignant potential. *Am J Gastroenterol*, 80, 1, 42–46.

Butel, J. S. (2000). Viral carcinogenesis: revelation of molecular mechanisms and etiology of human disease. *Carcinogenesis*, 21, 3, 405–426.

Buyru, N., Budak, M., Yazici, H. & Dalay, N. (2003). *p53* gene mutations are rare in human papillomavirus-associated colon cancer. *Oncol Rep*, 10, 6, 2089–2092.

Buyru, N., Tezol, A. & Dalay, N. (2006). Coexistence of K-ras mutations and HPV infection in colon cancer. *BMC Cancer*, 6, 115.

Caldarelli-Stefano, R., Boldorini, R., Monga, G., Meraviglia, E., Zorini, E. O. & Ferrante, P. (2000). JC virus in human glial-derived tumors. *Hum Pathol*, 31, 3, 394–395.

Campello, C., Comar, M., Zanotta, N., Minicozzi, A., Rodella, L. & Poli A. (2010). Detection of SV40 in colon cancer: a molecular case-control study from northeast Italy. *J Med Virol*, 82, 7, 1197-1200.

Casini, B., Borgese, L., Del Nonno, F., Galati, G., Izzo, L., Caputo, M., Perrone Donnorso, R., Castelli, M., Risuleo, G. & Visca, P. (2005). Presence and incidence of DNA sequences of human polyomaviruses BKV and JCV in colorectal tumor tissues. *Anticancer Res*, 25, 2A, 1079–1085.

Castro, C. Y., Ostrowski, M. L., Barrios, R., Green, L. K., Popper, H. H., Powell, S., Cagle, P. T. & Ro, J. Y. (2001). Relationship between Epstein-Barr virus and lymphoepithelioma-like carcinoma of the lung: a clinicopathologic study of 6 cases and review of the literature. *Hum Pathol*, 32, 8, 863–872.

Chaturvedi, A. K., Engels, E. A., Gilbert, E. S., Chen, B. E., Storm, H., Lynch, C. F., Hall, P., Langmark, F., Pukkala, E., Kaijser, M., Andersson, M., Fosså, S. D., Joensuu, H., Boice, J. D., Kleinerman, R. A. & Travis, L. B. (2007). Second cancers among 104,760 survivors of cervical cancer: evaluation of long-term risk. *J Natl Cancer Inst*, 99, 21, 1634–1643.

Cheever, A. W., Kamel, I. A., Elwi, A. M., Mosimann, J. E., Danner, R. & Sippel, J. E. (1987). *Schistosoma mansoni* and *S. haematobium* infections in Egypt. III. Extrahepatic pathology. *Am J Trop Med Hyg*, 27, 1, 55-75

Chen, J., Campbell, T. C., Li, J. & Peto, R. (1990). *Diet, Life-style, and Mortality in China. A Study of the Characteristics of 65 Chinese Counties*, Oxford University Press, Oxford.

Cheng, J. Y., Sheu, L. F., Lin, J. C. & Meng, C. L. (1995). Detection of human papillomavirus DNA in colorectal adenomas. *Arch Surg*, 130, 1, 73–76.

Chieffi, P. P. (1992). Interrelationship between schistosomiasis and concomitant diseases. *Mem Inst Oswaldo Cruz*, 87, Suppl 4, 291-296.

Ciccotosto, G. D., McLeish, A., Hardy, K. J. & Shulkes. A. (1995). Expression, processing, and secretion of gastrin in patients with colorectal carcinoma. *Gastroenterology*, 109, 4, 1142–1153

Corredoira, J., Alonson, M. P., Coira, A. & Varela, J. (2008). Association between *Streptococcus infantarius* (formerly *S. bovis* II/1) bacteremia and noncolonic cancer. *J Clin Microbiol*, 46, 4, 1570.

Coykendall, A. L. & Gustafson, K. B. (1985). Deoxyribonucleic acid hybridization among strains of *Streptococcus salivarius* and *Streptococcus bovis*. *Int J Syst Bacteriol*, 35, 3, 274-280.

Curren, R. D., Putman, D. L., Yang, L, L., Haworth, S. R., Lawlor, T. E., Plummer, S. M. & Harris, C. C. (1987). Genotoxicity of fecapentaene-12 in bacterial and mammalian cell assay systems. *Carcinogenesis*, 8, 2, 349-352.

D'Onghia, V., Leoncini, R., Carli, R., Santoro, A., Giglioni, S., Sorbellini, F., Marzocca ,G., Bernini, A., Campagna, S., Marinello, E. & Vannoni, D. (2007). Circulating gastrin and ghrelin levels in patients with colorectal cancer: correlation with tumour stage, Helicobacter pylori infection and BMI. *Biomed Pharmacother*, 61, (2–3), 137–141.

D'Souza, G., Kreimer, A. R., Viscidi, R., Pawlita, M., Fakhry, C., Koch, W. M., Westra, W. H. & Gillison, M. L. (2007). Case-control study of human papillomavirus and oropharyngeal cancer. *N Engl J Med*, 356, 19, 1944–1956.

Darjee, R. & Gibb, A. P. (1993). Serological investigation into the association between *Streptococcus bovis* and colonic cancer. *J Clin Pathol*, 46, 12, 1116–1119.

de Kok, T. M., Pachen, D., van Iersel, M. L., Baeten, C. G., Engels, L. G., ten Hoor, F. & Kleinjans, J.C. (1993). Case-control study on fecapentaene excretion and adenomatous polyps in the colon and rectum. *J Natl Cancer Inst*, 85, 15, 1241–1244.

Del Valle, L., Gordon, J., Assimakopoulou, M., Enam, S., Geddes, J. F., Varakis, J. N., Katsetos, C. D., Croul, S. & Khalili, K. (2001). Detection of JC virus DNA sequences and expression of the viral regulatory protein T-antigen in tumors of the central nervous system. *Cancer Res*, 61, 10, 4287–4293.

Del Valle, L., White, M. K., Enam, S., Piña Oviedo, S., Bromer, M. Q., Thomas, R. M., Parkman, H. P. & Khalili, K. (2005). Detection of JC virus DNA sequences and expression of viral T antigen and agnoprotein in esophageal carcinoma. *Cancer*, 103, 3, 516–527.

Dickinson, C. J. (1995). Relationship of gastrin processing to colon cancer. *Gastroenterology*, 109, 4, 1384–1388

Dimmette, R. M., Elwi, A. M. & Sproate, H. F. (1956). Relationship of schistosomiasis to polyposis and adenocareinoma of large intestine. *Am J Clin Patho*, 26, 3, 266-276

Dubrow, R., Edberg, S., Wikfors, E., Callan, D., Troncale, F., Vender, R., Brand, M. & Yapp, R. (1991). Fecal carriage of *Streptococcus bovis* and colorectal adenomas. *Gastroenterology*, 101, 3, 721–725.

Ellmerich, S., Djouder, N., Scholler, M. & Klein, J. P. (2000b). Production of cytokines by monocytes, epithelial and endothelial cells activated by *Streptococcus bovis*. *Cytokine*, 12, 1, 26-31.

Ellmerich, S., Scholler, M., Duranton, B., Gosse, F., Galluser, M., Klein, J. P. & Raul, F. (2000a). Promotion of intestinal carcinogenesis by *Streptococcus bovis*. *Carcinogenesis,* 21, 4, 753-756.

Enam, S., Del Valle, L., Lara, C., Gan, D. D., Ortiz-Hidalgo, C., Palazzo, J. P. & Khalili K. (2002). Association of human polyomavirus JCV with colon cancer: evidence for interaction of viral T-antigen and beta-catenin. *Cancer Res*, 62, 23, 7093–7101.

EUROGAST Study Group. (1993). An international association between *Helicobacter pylori* infection and gastric cancer. *Lancet*, 341, 8857, 1359 - 1362.

Fina, F., Romain, S., Ouafik, L., Palmari, J., Ben Ayed, F., Benharkat, S., Bonnier, P., Spyratos, F., Foekens, J. A., Rose, C., Buisson, M., Gérard, H., Reymond, M. O., Seigneurin, J. M. & Martin, P. M. (2001). Frequency and genome load of Epstein-Barr virus in 509 breast cancers from different geographical areas. *Br J Cancer*, 84, 6, 783–790.

Fireman, Z., Trost, L., Kopelman, Y., Segal, A. & Sternberg, A. (2000). *Helicobacter pylori*: seroprevalence and colorectal cancer. *Isr Med Assoc J*, 2, 1, 6–9.

Friedrich, I. A., Wormser, G. P. & Gottfried, E. B. (1982a). The association of recent *Streptococcus bovis* bacteremia with colonic neoplasia. Mil Med, 147,7, 584 - 5.

Friedrich, I.A., Wormser, G. P. & Gottfried, E. B. (1982b). The association of remote *Streptococcus bovis* bacteremia with colonic neoplasia. *Am J Gastroenterol,* 77, 2, 82-84.

Fujimori, S., Kishida, T., Kobayashi, T., Sekita, Y., Seo, T., Nagata, K., Tatsuguchi, A., Gudis, K., Yokoi, K., Tanaka, N., Yamashita, K., Tajiri, T., Ohaki, Y. & Sakamoto, C. (2005). Helicobacter pylori infection increases the risk of colorectal adenoma and adenocarcinoma, especially in women. J Gastroenterol, 40, 9, 887–893

Georgopoulos, S. D., Polymeros, D., Triantafyllou, K., Spiliadi, C., Mentis, A., Karamanolis, D. G. & Ladas, S. D. (2006). Hypergastrinemia is associated with increased risk of distal colon adenomas. *Digestion*, 74, 1, 42–46.

Goel, A., Li, M. S., Nagasaka, T., Shin, S. K., Fuerst, F., Ricciardiello, L., Wasserman, L. & Boland CR. (2006). Association of JC virus T-antigen expression with the methylator phenotype in sporadic colorectal cancers. *Gastroenterology,* 130, 7, 1950–1961.

Gold, J. S., Bayar, S. & Salem, R. R. (2004). Association of *Streptococcus bovis* bacteremia with colonic neoplasia and extracolonic malignancy. *Arch Surg*, 139, 7, 760 - 765.

Goodman, J. E., Hofseth, L. J., Hussain, S. P. & Harris, C. C. (2004). Nitric oxide and p53 in cancer-prone chronic inflammation and oxyradical overload disease. *Environ Mol Mutagen*, 44, 1, 3-9.

Grahn, N., Hmani-Aifa, M., Fransen, K., Soderkvist, P. & Monstein, H. J. (2005). Molecular identification of *Helicobacter* DNA present in human colorectal adenocarcinomas by 16S rDNA PCR amplification and pyrosequencing analysis. *J Med Microbiol*, 54, 11, 1031 - 1035.

Grinstein, S., Preciado, M. V., Gattuso, P., Chabay, P. A., Warren, W. H., De Matteo, E. & Gould, V. E. (2002). Demonstration of Epstein-Barr virus in carcinomas of various sites. *Cancer Res*, 62, 17, 4876–4878.

Guo, W., Zheng, W., Li, J. Y., Chen, J. S. & Blot, W. J. (1993). Correlations of colon cancer mortality with dietary factors, serum markers, and schistosomiasis in China. *Nutr Cancer*, 20, 1, 13-20

Hakanson, R., Axelson, J., Ekman, R. & Sundler, F. (1988). Hypergastrinaemia evoked by omeprazole stimulates growth of gastric mucosa but not of pancreas or intestines in hamster, guinea pig and chicken. *Regul Pept*, 23, 1, 105–115.

Hakanson, R., Blom, H., Carlsson, E., Larsson, H., Ryberg, B. & Sundler, F. (1986). Hypergastrinaemia produces trophic effects in stomach but not in pancreas and intestine. *Regul Pept*, 13, (3-4), 225–233.

Han, A. J., Xiong, M., Gu, Y. Y., Lin, S. X. & Xiong, M. (2001). Lymphoepithelioma-like carcinoma of the lung with a better prognosis. A clinicopathologic study of 32 cases. *Am J Clin Pathol*, 115, 6, 841–850.

Hart, H., Neill, W. A. & Norval, M. (1982). Lack of association of cytomegalovirus with adenocarcinoma of the colon. *Gut*, 23, 1, 21–30.

Hartwich J, Konturek SJ, Pierzchalski P, Zuchowicz M, Konturek PC, Bielański W, Marlicz K, Starzyńska T, Ławniczak M. (2001b). Molecular basis of colorectal cancer - role of gastrin and cyclooxygenase-2. *Med Sci Monit*, 7, 6, 1171-1181.

Hartwich, A., Konturek, S. J., Pierzchalski, P., Zuchowicz, M., Labza, H., Konturek, P. C., Karczewska, E., Bielanski, W., Marlicz, K., Starzynska, T., Lawniczak, M. & Hahn, E. G. (2001a). *Helicobacter pylori* infection, gastrin, cyclooxygenase-2, and apoptosis in colorectal cancer. *Int J Colorectal Dis* 16, 4, 202–210.

Hashiro, G. M., Horikami, S. & Loh, P. C. (1979). Cytomegalovirus isolations from cell cultures of human adenocarcinomas of the colon. *Intervirology*, 12, 2, 84–88.

Herrera, L. A., Benitez-Bribiesca, L., Mohar, A. & Ostrosky-Wegman, P. (2005). Role of infectious diseases in human carcinogenesis. *Environ Mol Mutagen*, 45, (2-3), 284-303.

Herrero, I. A., Rouse, M. S., Piper, K. E, Alyaseen, S. A., Steckelberg, J. M. & Patel, R. (2002). Reevaluation of *Streptococcus bovis* endocarditis cases from 1975 to 1985 by 16S ribosomal DNA sequence analysis. *J Clin Microbiol*, 40, 10, 3848–3850.

Hoen, B., Briancon, S., Delahaye, F., Terhé, V., Etienne, J., Bigard, M. A., Canton, P. (1994). Tumors of the colon increase the risk of developing *Streptococcus bovis* endocarditis: case-control study. *Clin Infect* Dis, 19, 2, 361 - 362.

Hope, M.E., Hold, G.L., Kain, R. & El-Omar, E.M. (2005). Sporadic colorectal cancer—role of the commensal microbiota. *FEMS Microbiol Lett*, 244, 1, 1-7.

Hori, R., Murai, Y., Tsuneyama, K., Abdel-Aziz, H. O., Nomoto, K., Takahashi, H., Cheng, C. M., Kuchina, T., Harman, B. V. & Takano, Y. (2005). Detection of JC virus DNA sequences in colorectal cancers in Japan. *Virchows Arch*, 447, 4, 723–730.

Hori, T., Matsumoto, K., Sakaitani, Y., Sato, M. & Morotomi, M. (1998). Effect of dietary deoxycholic acid and cholesterol on fecal steroid concentration and its impact on the colonic crypt cell proliferation in azoxymethane-treated rats. *Cancer Lett*, 124, 1, 79-84.

Huang, E. S. & Roche, J. K. (1978). Cytomegalovirus D.N.A. and adenocarcinoma of the colon: evidence for latent viral infection. *Lancet*, 1, 8071, 957–960.

Huycke, M. M., Abrams, V. & Moore, D. R. (2002). *Enterococcus faecalis* produces extracellular superoxide and hydrogen peroxide that damages colonic epithelial cell DNA. *Carcinogenesis*, 23, 3, 529–536.

IARC (1994). Monograph on the evaluation of carcinogenic risks to humans: Schistosomes, liver flukes and *Helicobacter pylori*. WHO: *International Agency for Research on Cancer* 61, 9–240.

IARC (1997). Monograph on the evaluation of carcinogenic risks to humans: Epstein-Barr Virus and Kaposi's Sarcoma Herpesvirus/Human Herpesvirus 8. WHO: *International Agency for Research on Cancer* 70, 47–374.

Inaba, Y. (1984). A cohort study on the causes of death in an endemic area of schistosomiasis japonica in Japan. *Ann Acad Med Singapore*, 13, 2, 142-148.

Ishii, A., Matsuoka, H., Aji, T., Hayatsu, H., Wataya, Y., Arimoto, S. & Tokuda, H. (1989). Evaluation of the mutagenicity and the tumor-promoting activity of parasite extracts: *Schistosoma japonicum* and *Clonorchis sinensis*. *Mutat Res*, 224, 2, 229-233.

Ishii, A., Matsuoka, H., Aji, T., Ohta, N., Arimoto, S., Wataya, Y. & Hayatsu, H. (1994). Parasite infection and cancer: with special emphasis on *Schistosoma japonicum* infections (Trematoda). A review. *Mutat Res*, 305, 2, 273-281.

Itzkowitz, S. H. & Yio, X. Inflammation and cancer IV. Colorectal cancer in inflammatory bowel disease: the role of inflammation. (2004). *Am J Physiol Gastrointest Liver Physiol*, 287, 1, G7–17

Jones, M., Helliwell, P., Pritchard, C., Tharakan, J. & Mathew, J. (2007). *Helicobacter pylori* in colorectal neoplasms: is there an aetiological relationship? *World J Surg Oncol*, 5, 51.

Jung, W. T., Li, M. S., Goel, A. & Boland, C. R. (2008). JC virus T-antigen expression in sporadic adenomatous polyps of the colon. *Cancer*, 112, 5, 1028–1036.

Kanno, T., Matsuki, T., Oka, M., Utsunomiya, H., Inada, K., Magari, H., Inoue, I., Maekita, T., Ueda, K., Enomoto, S., Iguchi, M., Yanaoka, K., Tamai, H., Akimoto, S., Nomoto, K., Tanaka, R. & Ichinose, M. (2009). Gastric acid reduction leads to an alteration in lower intestinal microflora. *Biochem Biophys Res Commun*, 381, 4, 666–670.

Karpinski, P., Myszka, A., Ramsey, D., Kielan, W. & Sasiadek, M. M. (2011). Detection of viral DNA sequences in sporadic colorectal cancers in relation to CpG island methylation and methylator phenotype. *Tumour Biol*, 32, 4, 653-659.

Kawano, A., Ishikawa, H., Kamano, T., Kanoh, M., Sakamoto, K., Nakamura, T., Otani, T., Sakai, T. & Kono, K. (2010). Significance of fecal deoxycholic Acid concentration for colorectal tumor enlargement. *Asian Pacific J Cancer Prev*, 11, 6, 1541-1546

Kean, J. M., Rao, S., Wang, M. & Garcea, R. L. (2009). Seroepidemiology of Human Polyomaviruses. *PLoS Pathog*, 5, 3, e1000363.

Keenan, J. I., Beaugie, C. R., Jasmann, B., Potter, H. C., Collett, J. A., Frizelle, F. A. (2010). *Helicobacter* species in the human colon. *Colorectal Dis*, 12, 1, 48-53

Kermorgant, S. & Lehy, T. (2001). Glycine-extended gastrin promotes the invasiveness of human colon cancer cells. *Biochem Biophys Res Commun*, 285, 1, 136–141.

Keusch, G. T. (1974). Opportunistic infections in colon carcinoma. *Am J Clin Nutr*, 27, 12, 1481-1485.

Khalili, K., Del Valle, L., Otte, J., Weaver, M. & Gordon, J. (2003a). Human neurotropic polyomavirus, JCV, and its role in carcinogenesis. *Oncogene*, 22, 33, 5181–5191.

Kim, J. H., Park, H. J., Cho, J. S., Lee, K. S., Lee, S. I., Park, I. S., & Kim, C. K. (1999). Relationship of CagA to serum gastrin concentrations and antral G, D cell densities in *Helicobacter pylori* infection. *Yonsei Med J*, 40, 4, 301–306.

Kim, J. M., Cho, S. J., Oh, Y. K., Jung, H. Y., Kim, Y. J. & Kim, N. (2002). Nuclear factor-kappa B activation pathway in intestinal epithelial cells is a major regulator of chemokine gene expression and neutrophil migration induced by *Bacteroides fragilis* enterotoxin. *Clin Exp Immunol*, 130, 1, 59-66

Kim, J. M., Oh, Y.K., Oh, H. B. & Cho, Y. J. (2001). Polarized secretion of CXC chemokines by human intestinal epithelial cells in response to *Bacteroides fragilis* enterotoxin: NF-jB plays a major role in the regulation of IL-8 expression. *Clin Exp Immunol*, 123, 3, 421–427.

Kim, S. C., Tonkonogy, S. L., Karrasch, T., Jobin, C. & Sartor, R. B. (2007). Dual-association of gnotobiotic IL-10-/- mice with 2 nonpathogenic commensal bacteria induces aggressive pancolitis. *Inflamm Bowel Dis*, 13, 12, 1457-1466.

Kim, S. C., Tonkonogy, S.L., Albright, C.A., Tsang, J., Balish, E. J., Braun, J., Huycke, M. M. & Sartor, R. B. (2005). Variable phenotypes of enterocolitis in interleukin 10-deficient mice monoassociated with two different commensal bacteria. *Gastroenterology*, 128, 4, 891–906.

Kirgan, D., Manalo, P., Hall, M. & McGregor, B. (1990). Association of human papillomavirus and colon neoplasms. *Arch Surg*, 125, 7, 862–865.

Klein, R. S., Catalano, M. T., Edberg, S. C., Casey, J. I., Steigbigel, N. H. (1979). *Streptococcus bovis* septicemia and carcinoma of the colon. *Ann Intern Med*, 91, 4, 560 - 562.

Klein, R. S., Recco, R. A., Catalano, M. T., Edberg, S. C., Casey, J. I., Steigbigel, N. H. (1977). Association of *Streptococcus bovis* with carcinoma of the colon. *N Engl J Med*, 297, 15, 800–802.

Koh, T. J., Dockray, G. J., Varro, A., Cahill, R. J., Dangler, C. A., Fox, J. G. & Wang, T. C. (1999). Overexpression of glycine-extended gastrin in transgenic mice results in increased colonic proliferation. *J Clin Invest*, 103, 8, 1119–1126.

Konda, A. & Duffy, M. C. (2008). Surveillance of patients at increased risk of colon cancer: inflammatory bowel disease and other conditions. *Gastroenterol Clin North Am*, 37, 1, 191-213

Koriyama, C., Akiba, S., Iriya, K., Yamaguti, T., Hamada, G. S., Itoh, T., Eizuru, Y., Aikou, T., Watanabe, S., Tsugane, S. & Tokunaga, M. (2001). Epstein-Barr virus-associated gastric carcinoma in Japanese Brazilians and non-Japanese Brazilians in Sao Paulo. *Jpn J Cancer Res*, 92, 9, 911–917.

Koulos, J., Symmans, F., Chumas, J. & Nuovo, G. (1991). Human papillomavirus detection in adenocarcinoma of the anus. *Mod Pathol*, 4, 1, 58–61.

Koutsky, L. (1997). Epidemiology of genital human papillomavirus infection. *Am J Me*, 102, 5A, 3–8.

Kupferwasser, I., Darius, H., Muller, A. M., Mohr-Kahaly, S., Westermeier, T., Oelert, H., Erbel, R. & Meyer, J. (1998). Clinical and morphological characteristics in *Streptococcus bovis* endocarditis: a comparison with other causative microorganisms in 177 cases. *Heart*, 80, 3, 276–280.

Labrecque, L. G., Barnes, D. M., Fentiman, I. S. & Griffin, B. E. (1995). Epstein-Barr virus in epithelial cell tumors: a breast cancer study. *Cancer Res*, 55, 1, 39–45.

Laghi, L., Randolph, A. E., Chauhan, D. P., Marra, G., Major, E. O., Neel, J. V., Boland, C. R. (1999). JC virus DNA is present in the mucosa of the human colon and in colorectal cancers. *Proc Natl Acad Sci U S A*, 96, 13, 7484–7489.

Lee, Y. M., Leu, S. Y., Chiang, H., Fung, C. P. & Liu, W. T. (2001). Human papillomavirus type 18 in colorectal cancer. *J Microbiol Immunol Infect*, 34, 2, 87–91.

Legakis, N., Ioannides, H., Tzannetis, S., Golematis, B. & Papavassiliou, J. (1981). Faecal bacterial flora in patients with colon cancer and control subjects. *Zentralbl Bakteriol Mikrobiol Hyg A*, 251, 1, 54-61

Li, A., Varney, M. L. & Singh, R. K. (2001). Expression of interleukin 8 and its receptors in human colon carcinoma cells with different metastatic potentials. *Clin Cancer Res*, 7, 10, 3298–3304

Limburg, P. J., Stolzenberg-Solomon, R. Z., Colbert, L.H., Perez-Perez, G. I., Blaser, M. J., Taylor, P. R., Virtamo, J. & Albanes, D. (2002). *Helicobacter pylori* seropositivity and colorectal cancer risk: a prospective study of male smokers. *Cancer Epidemiol Biomarkers Prev*, 11, 10, 1095–1099.

Lin, M., Hanai, J. & Gui, L. (1998). Peanut lectin-binding sites and mucins in benign and malignant colorectal tissues associated with schistomatosis. *Histol Histopathol*, 1998, 13, 4, 961-966.

Lin, P. Y., Fung, C. Y., Chang, F. P., Huang, W. S., Chen, W. C., Wang, J. Y. & Chang, D. (2008). Prevalence and genotype identification of human JC virus in colon cancer in Taiwan. *J Med Virol*, 80, 10, 1828–1834.

Lin, Y. L., Chiang, J. K., Lin, S. M. & Tseng, C. E. (2010). *Helicobacter pylori* infection concomitant with metabolic syndrome further increase risk of colorectal adenomas. *World J Gastroenterol*, 16, 30, 3841-3846.

Link, A., Shin, S. K., Nagasaka, T., Balaguer, F., Koi, M., Jung, B., Boland, C. R. & Goel, A. (2009). JC virus mediates invasion and migration in colorectal metastasis. *PLoS One*, 4, 12, e8146.

Liou, J. M., Lin, J. W., Huang, S. P., Lin, J. T. & Wu, M. S. (2006). *Helicobacter pylori* infection is not associated with increased risk of colorectal polyps in Taiwanese. *Int J Cancer*, 119, 8, 1999 - 2000

Little, J., Owen, R. W., Femandez, F., Hawtin, P. G., Hill, M. J., Logan, R. F., Thompson, M. H. & Hardcastle, J. D. (2002). Asymptomatic colorectal neoplasia and fecal characteristics: a case-control study of subjects participating in the Nottingham fecal occult blood screening trial. *Dis Colon Rectum*, 45, 9, 1233-1241.

Liu, H. X., Ding, Y. Q., Li, X. & Yao, K. T. (2003). Investigation of Epstein-Barr virus in Chinese colorectal tumors. *World J Gastroenterol*, 9, 11, 2464-2468.

Liu, H. X., Ding, Y. Q., Sun, Y. O., Liang, L., Yang, Y. F., Qi, Z. L., Liu, J. H. & Xiong, P. X. (2002). Detection of Epstein-Barr virus in human colorectal cancer by in situ hybridization. *Di Yi Jun Yi Da Xue Xue Bao*, 22, 10, 915–917.

Long, X. C., Bahgat, M., Chlichlia, K., Ruppel, A. & Li, Y. L. (2004). Detection of inducible nitric oxide synthase in *Schistosoma japonicum* and *S. mansoni*. *J Helminthol*, 78, 1, 47-50.

Ludlow, J. W. (1993). Interactions between SV40 large-tumor antigen and the growth suppressor proteins *pRB* and *p53*. *FASEB J*, 7, 866–871.

Lundstig, A., Stattin, P., Persson, K., Sasnauskas, K., Viscidi, R. P., Gislefoss, R. E. & Dillner, J. (2007). No excess risk for colorectal cancer among subjects seropositive for the JC polyomavirus. *Int J Cancer*, 121, 5, 1098–1102.

Machida-Montani, A., Sasazuki, S., Inoue, M., Natsukawa, S., Shaura, K., Koizumi, Y., Kasuga, Y., Hanaoka, T. & Tsugane, S. (2007). Atrophic gastritis, Helicobacter pylori, and colorectal cancer risk: a case-control study. *Helicobacter*, 12, 4, 328–332.

Madbouly, K. M., Senagore, A. J., Mukerjee, A., Hussien, A. M., Shehata, M. A., Navine. P., Delaney, C. P. & Fazio, V. W. (2007). Colorectal cancer in a population with endemic *Schistosoma mansoni*: is this an at-risk population?. *Int J Colorectal Dis*, 22, 2, 175-181

Maddocks, O. D., Short, A. J., Donnenberg, M. S., Bader, S. & Harrison, D. J. (2009). Attaching and effacing *Escherichia coli* downregulate DNA mismatch repair protein in vitro and are associated with colorectal adenocarcinomas in humans. *PLoS One*, 4, 5, e5517.

Martin, H. M., Campbell, B. J., Hart, C. A., Mpofu, C., Nayar, M., Singh, R., Englyst, H., Williams, H. F. & Rhodes, J. M. (2004). Enhanced *Escherichia coli* adherence and invasion in Crohn's disease and colon cancer. *Gastroenterology*, 127, 1, 80–93.

Matsuda, K., Masaki, T., Ishii, S., Yamashita, H., Watanabe, T., Nagawa, H., Muto, T., Hirata, Y., Kimura, K. & Kojima, S. (1999). Possible associations of rectal carcinoma with *schistosoma japonicum* infection and membranous nephropathy: a case report with a review. *Jpn J Clin Oncol*, 29, 11, 576-578.

Mayer, D. A. & Fried, B. (2007). The Role of Helminth Infections in Carcinogenesis, In: *Advances in Parasitology*, Vol 65, Muller, R., Rollinson, D., & Hay, S. I., 239-296, Academic Press, London.

McGregor, B., Byrne, P., Kirgan, D., Albright, J., Manalo, P. & Hall, M. (1993). Confirmation of the association of humanpapillomavirus with human colon cancer. *Am J Surg*, 166, 6, 738–740.

McLaughlin-Drubin, M. E. & Munger, K. (2008). Viruses associated with human cancer. *Biochim Biophys Acta*, 1782, 3, 127-150.

Meucci, G., Tatarella, M., Vecchi, M., Ranzi, M. L., Biguzzi, E., Beccari, G., Clerici, E. & de Franchis, R. (1997). High prevalence of *Helicobacter pylori* infection in patients with colonic adenomas and carcinomas. *J Clin Gastroenterol*, 25, 4, 605–607.

Militello, V., Trevisan, M., Squarzon, L., Biasolo, M. A., Rugge, M., Militello, C., Palù, G. & Barzon, L. (2009). Investigation on the presence of polyomavirus, herpesvirus, and papillomavirus sequences in colorectal neoplasms and their association with cancer. *Int J Cancer*, 124, 10, 2501-2503.

Ming-Chai, C., Chang, P. Y., Chuang, C. Y., Chen, Y. J., Wang, F. P., Tang, Y. C. & Chou, S. C. (1981). Colorectal cancer and schistomiasis. *Lancet*, 1, 8227, 971-973.

Ming-Chai, C., Chi-Yuan, C., Pei-Yu, C. & Jen-Chun, H. (1980). Evolution of colorectal cancer in schistosomiasis: transitional mucosal changes adjacent to large intestinal carcinoma in colectomy specimens. *Cancer*, 46, 7, 1661-1675

Ming-Chai, C., Hu, J. C., Chang, P. Y., Chuang, C. Y., Tsao, P. F., Chang, S. H., Wang, F. P., Ch'en, T. L. & Chou, S. C. (1965), Pathogenesis of carcinoma of the colon and rectum in schistosomiasis japonica: a study on 90 cases. *Chin Med J*, 84, 8, 513-525.

Mizuno, S., Morita, Y., Inui, T., Asakawa, A., Ueno, N., Ando, T., Kato, H., Uchida, M., Yoshikawa, T. & Inui, A. (2005) *Helicobacter pylori* infection is associated with colon adenomatous polyps detected by high-resolution colonoscopy. *Int J Cancer*, 117, 6, 1058–1059.

Mohamed, A. R., Al Karawi, M. A. & Yasawy, M. I. (1990). Schistosomal colonic disease. *Gut*, 31,4, ,439-442

Moore, W. E. & Moore, L. H. (1995). Intestinal flora of populations that have a high risk for colon cancer. *Appl Env Microbiol*, 61, 9, 3202–3207.

Moss, S. F., Neugut, A. I., Garbowski, G. C., Wang, S., Treat, M. R. & Forde, K. A. (1995). *Helicobacter pylori* seroprevalence and colorectal neoplasia: evidence against an association. *J Natl Cancer Inst*, 87, 10, 762–763.

Muhlemann, K., Graf, S. & Tauber, M. G. (1999). *Streptococcus bovis* clone causing two episodes of endocarditis 8 years apart. *J Clin Microbiol*, 37, 3, 862–863.

Munoz, N., Bosch, F. X., de Sanjose, S., Herrero, R., Castellsagué, X., Shah, K.mV., Snijders, P. J. & Meijer, C. J. (2003). Epidemiologic classification of human papillomavirus types associated with cervical cancer. *N Engl J Med*, 348, 6, 518–527.

Murray, H. W. & Roberts, R. B. (1978). *Streptococcus bovis* bacteremia and underlying gastrointestinal disease. *Arch Intern Med*, 138, 7, 1097 - 1099.

Newcomb, P. A., Bush, A. C., Stoner, G. L., Lampe, J. W., Potter, J. D. & Bigler, J. (2004). No evidence of an association of JC virus and colon neoplasia. Cancer Epidemiol Biomarkers Prev, 13, 4, 662–666.

Nguyen, I., Biarc, J., Pini, A., Gosse, F., Richert, S., Thierse, D., Van Dorsselaer, A., Leize-Wagner, E., Raul, F., Klein, J. P., Scholler-Guinard, M. (2006). *Streptococcus infantarius* and colonic cancer: Identification and purification of cell wall proteins putatively involved in colorectal inflammation and carcinogenesis in rats. *International Congress Series*, 1289, 257-261.

Niv, Y., Vilkin, A. & Levi, Z. (2010b). Patients with sporadic colorectal cancer or advanced adenomatous polyp have elevated anti-JC virus antibody titer in comparison with healthy controls: a cross-sectional study. *J Clin Gastroenterol*, 44, 7, 489-494.

Niv, Y., Vilkin, A., Brenner, B., Kendel, Y., Morgenstern, S. & Levi, Z. (2010a). hMLH1 promoter methylation and JC virus T antigen presence in the tumor tissue of colorectal cancer Israeli patients of different ethnic groups. *Eur J Gastroenterol Hepatol*, 22, 8, 938-941.

Norfleet, R. G. & Mitchell, R. G. (1993). *Streptococcus bovis* does not selectively colonize colorectal cancer and polyps. *J Clin Gastroenterol*, 17, 1, 25–28.

Nosho, K., Shima, K., Kure, S., Irahara, N., Baba, Y., Chen, L., Kirkner, G. J., Fuchs, C. S. & Ogino, S. (2009). JC virus T-antigen in colorectal cancer is associated with p53 expression and chromosomal instability, independent of CpG island methylator phenotype. *Neoplasia*, 11, 1, 87–95.

Nosho, K., Yamamoto, H., Takahashi, T., Mikami, M., Hizaki, K., Maehata, T., Taniguchi, H., Yamaoka, S., Adachi, Y., Itoh, F., Imai, K. & Shinomura, Y. (2008). Correlation of laterally spreading type and JC virus with methylator phenotype status in colorectal adenoma. *Hum Pathol*, 39, 5, 767–775.

Ogino, S., Nosho, K., Irahara, N., Shima, K., Baba, Y., Kirkner, G. J., Meyerhardt, J. A. & Fuchs, C. S. (2009). Prognostic significance and molecular associations of 18q loss of heterozygosity: a cohort study of microsatellite stable colorectal cancers. *J Clin Oncol*, 27, 27, 4591–4598.

Ohshima, H. & Bartsch, H. (1994). Chronic infections and inflammatory processes as cancer risk factors: possible role of nitric oxide in carcinogenesis. *Mutat Res*, 305, 2, 253-264.

Ojo, O. S., Odesanmi, W. O. & Akinola, O. O. (1991). The surgical pathology of colorectal carcinoma in Nigerians. *Trop Gastroenterol*, 13, 2, 180-184.

Osada, Y., Kumagai, T., Masuda, K., Suzuki, T. & Kanazawa, T. (2005). Mutagenicity evaluation of *Schistosoma* spp. extracts by the umu-test and V79/HGPRT gene mutation assay. *Parasitol Int*, 54, 1, 29-34.

Pagano, J. S., Blaser, M., Buendia, M. A., Damania, B., Khalili, K., Raab-Traub, N. & Roizman, B. (2004). Infectious agents and cancer: criteria for a causal relation. *Semin Cancer Biol*, 14, 6, 453-471

Parkin, D. M. (2006). The global health burden of infection-associated cancers in the year 2002. *Int J Cancer*, 118, 12, 3030–3044.

Parkin, D. M., Arslan, A., Bieber, A., Bouvy, O., Muir, C.S., Owor, R. & Whelan, S. (1986). Cancer Occurrence in Developing Countries, In: *International Agency for Research on Cancer (IARC) Scientific Publication No. 75*, IARC Press, Lyon, France.

Parsonnet, J. (1995). Bacterial infection as a cause of cancer. *Environ Health Perspect*, 103, Suppl 8, 263-268.

Peek, R. M., Jr., Miller, G. G., Tham, K. T., Perez-Perez, G. I., Zhao, X., Atherton, J. C., and Blaser, M. J. (1995). Heightened inflammatory response and cytokine expression in vivo to cagA+ *Helicobacter pylori* strains. *Lab Investig*, 73, 6, 760–770.

Peiffer, L. P., Peters, D. J. & McGarrity, T. J. (1997). Differential effects of deoxycholic acid on proliferation of neoplastic and differentiated colonocytes in vitro. *Dig Dis Sci*, 42, 11, 2234-2240.

Penman, I. D., el-Omar, E., Ardill, J. E., McGregor, J. R., Galloway, D. J., O'Dwyer, P. J., McColl, K. E. (1994). Plasma gastrin concentrations are normal in patients with colorectal neoplasia and unaltered following tumour resection. *Gastroenterology*, 106, 5, 1263–1270.

Perez, L. O., Abba, M. C., Laguens, R. M. & Golijow, C. D. (2005). Analysis of adenocarcinoma of the colon and rectum: detection of human papillomavirus (HPV) DNA by polymerase chain reaction. *Colorectal Dis*, 7, 5, 492–495.

Pergola, V., Di Salvo, G., Habib, G., Avierinos, J. F., Philip, E., Vailloud, J. M., Thuny, F., Casalta, J. P., Ambrosi, P., Lambert, M., Riberi, A., Ferracci, A., Mesana, T., Metras, D., Harle, J. R., Weiller, P. J., Raoult, D. & Luccioni, R. (2001). Comparison of clinical and echocardiographic characteristics of *Streptococcus bovis* endocarditis with that caused by other pathogens. *Am J Cardiol*, 88, 8, 871–875.

Pigrau, C., Lorente, A., Pahissa, A. & Martinez-Vazquez, J. M. (1988) *Streptococcus bovis* bacteremia and digestive system neoplasms. *Scand J Infect Dis*, 20, 4, 459–460.

Plummer, S.M., Grafstrom, R.C., Yang, L. L., Curren, R. D., Linnainmaa, K. & Harris, C. C. (1986). Fecapentaene-12 causes DNA damage and mutations in human cells. *Carcinogenesis*, 7, 9, 1607-1609.

Potter, M. A., Cunliffe, N. A., Smith, M., Miles, R. S., Flapan, A. D. & Dunlop, M. G. (1998). A prospective controlled study of the association of *Streptococcus bovis* with colorectal carcinoma. *J Clin Pathol*, 51, 6, 473 -474.

Prindiville, T. P., Sheikh, R. A., Cohen, S. H., Tang, Y. J., Cantrell, M. C. & Silva, J. Jr. (2000). *Bacteroides fragilis* enterotoxin gene sequences in patients with inflammatory bowel disease. *Emerg Infect Dis*, 6, 2, 171–174.

Qiu, D. C., Hubbard, A. E., Zhong, B., Zhang, Y. & Spear, R. C. (2005). A matched, case control study of the association between *Schistosoma japonicum* and liver and colon cancers, in rural China. *Ann Trop Med Parasitol*, 99, 1, 47-52

Reddy, B. S. & Wynder, E.L. (1977). Metabolic epidemiology of colon cancer: fecal bile acids and neutral sterols in colon cancer patients and patients with adenomas polyps. *Cancer*, 39, 6, 1533-1539.

Renga, M., Brandi, G., Paganelli, G. M., Calabrese, C., Papa, S., Tosti, A., Tomassetti, P., Miglioli, M. & Biasco, G. (1997). Rectal cell proliferation and colon cancer risk in patients with hypergastrinaemia. *Gut*, 41, 3, 330–332.

Rex, D. (2000). Should we colonoscope women with gynecologic cancer? *Am J Gastroenterol*, 95, 3, 812–813.

Reynolds, J. G., Silva, E. & McCormack, W. M. (1983). Association of *Streptococcus bovis* bacteremia with bowel disease. *J Clin Microbiol*, 17, 4, 696–697.

Rhee, K. J., Wu, S., Wu, X., Huso, D. L., Karim, B., Franco, A. A., Rabizadeh, S., Golub, J. E., Mathews, L. E., Shin, J., Sartor, R. B., Golenbock, D., Hamad, A. R., Gan, C. M., Housseau, F. & Sears, C. L. (2009). Induction of persistent colitis by a human commensal, enterotoxigenic *Bacteroides fragilis*, in wild-type C57BL/6 mice. *Infect Immun*, 77, 4, 1708–1718.

Ricciardiello, L., Baglioni, M., Giovannini, C., Pariali, M., Cenacchi, G., Ripalti, A., Landini, M. P., Sawa, H., Nagashima, K., Frisque, R. J., Goel, A., Boland, C. R., Tognon, M., Roda, E. & Bazzoli, F. (2003). Induction of chromosomal instability in colonic cells by the human polyomavirus JC virus. *Cancer Res*, 63, 21, 7256–7262.

Ricciardiello, L., Chang, D. K., Laghi, L., Goel, A., Chang, C. L. & Boland, C. R. (2001). Mad-1 is the exclusive JC virus strain present in the human colon, and its transcriptional control region has a deleted 98-base-pair sequence in colon cancer tissues. *J Virol*, 75, 4, 1996–2001.

Ricciardiello, L., Laghi, L., Ramamirtham, P., Chang, C. L., Chang, D. K., Randolph, A. E. & Boland, C. R. (2000). JC virus DNA sequences are frequently present in the human upper and lower gastrointestinal tract. *Gastroenterology*, 119, 5, 1228–1235.

Robbins, N. & Klein, R. S. (1983). Carcinoma of the colon 2 years after endocarditis due to *Streptococcus bovis*. *Am J Gastroenterol*, 78, 3, 162–163.

Robertson, D. J., Sandler, R. S., Ahnen, D. J., Greenberg, E. R., Mott, L. A., Cole, B. F. & Baron, J. A. (2009). Gastrin, *Helicobacter pylori*, and colorectal adenomas, 7, 2, 163-167.

Rollison, D. E., Helzlsouer, K. J., Lee, J. H., Fulp, W., Clipp, S., Hoffman-Bolton, J. A., Giuliano, A. R., Platz, E. A. & Viscidi, R. P. (2009). Prospective study of JC virus seroreactivity and the development of colorectal cancers and adenomas. *Cancer Epidemiol Biomarkers Prev*, 18, 5, 1515–1523.

Rosin, M. P., Anwar, W. A. & Ward, A. J. (1994). Inflammation, chromosomal instability, and cancer: the schistosomiasis model. *Cancer Res*, 54, Suppl 7, 1929-1933.

Ross, A. G., Bartley, P. B., Sleigh, A. C., Olds, G. R., Li, Y., Williams, G. M. & McManus, D. P. (2002). Schistosomiasis. *N Engl J Med*, 346, 16, 1212-1220.

Ruger, R. & Fleckenstein, B. (1985). Cytomegalovirus DNA in colorectal carcinoma tissues. *Klin Wochenschr*, 63, 9, 405–408.

Ruoff, K. L., Miller, S. I., Garner, C. V., Ferraro, M. J. & Calderwood S. B. (1989). Bacteremia with *Streptococcus bovis* and *Streptococcus salivarius*: clinical correlates of more accurate identification of isolates. *J Clin Microbiol*, 27, 2, 305–308.

Ruoff, K.L., Whiley, R. A. & Beighton, D. (1999). Streptococcus, In: *Manual of Clinical Microbiology*, 7th edn. P. R. Murray, E. J. Baron, M. A. Pfaller, F. C. Tenover, and R. H. Yolken (ed.), 283–296, ASM press, Washington, D.C.

Sanfiloppo, L., Li, C. K., Seth, R., Balwin, T. J., Menozzi, M. G. & Mahida, Y. R. (2000). *Bacteroides fragilis* enterotoxin induces the expression of IL-8 and transforming growth factor beta by human colonic epithelial cells. *Clin Exp Immunol*, 119, 3, 456–463.

Schiffman, M. H., Van Tassell, R. L., Robinson, A., Smith, L., Daniel, J., Hoover, R. N., Weil, R., Rosenthal, J., Nair, P. P., Schwartz, S. (1989). Case-control study colorectal cancer and fecapentaene excretion. *Cancer Res*, 49, 5, 1322–1326.

Schlegel, L., Grimont, F., Ageron, E., Grimont, P. A. & Bouvet, A. (2003). Reappraisal of the taxonomy of the *Streptococcus bovis/Streptococcus equines* complex and related species: description of *Streptococcus gallolyticus* subsp. *gallolyticus* subsp. nov., *S. gallolyticus* subsp. *macedonicus* subsp. nov. and *S. gallolyticus* subsp. *pasteurianus* subsp. nov. *Int J Syst Evol Micribiol*, 53, 3, 631–645.

Sears, C. L., Islam, S., Saha, A., Arjumand, M., Alam, N. H., Faruque, A. S., Salam, M. A., Shin, J., Hecht, D., Weintraub, A., Sack, R. B. & Qadri, F. (2008). Association enterotoxigenic *Bacteroides fragilis* infection with inflammatory diarrhea. *Clin Infect Dis*, 47, 6, 797–803.

Selgrad, M., Koornstra, J. J., Fini, L., Blom, M., Huang, R., Devol, E. B., Boersma-van Ek, W., Dijkstra, G., Verdonk, R. C, de Jong, S., Goel, A., Williams, S. L., Meyer, R. L., Haagsma, E. B., Ricciardiello, L. & Boland, C. R. (2008). JC virus infection in colorectal neoplasia that develops after liver transplantation. *Clin Cancer Res*, 14, 20, 6717–6721.

Shah, K. V. (1996). Polyomaviruses, In: *Fields Virology*, B. N. Fields, D. M. Knipe, P. M. Howley, (Eds), 2027–2043, Lippincott-Raven, Philadelphia, USA.

Shah, K. V., Daniel, R. W., Simons, J. W. & Vogelstein, B. (1992). Investigation of colon cancers for human papillomavirus genomic sequences by polymerase chain reaction. *J Surg Oncol*, 51, 1, 5–7.

Shin, S. K., Li, M. S., Fuerst, F., Hotchkiss, E., Meyer, R., Kim, I. T., Goel, A. & Boland, C. R. (2006). Oncogenic T-antigen of JC virus is present frequently in human gastric cancers. *Cancer,* 107, 3, 481–488.

Shindo, K. (1976). Significance of schistosomiasis japonica in the development of cancer of the large intestine: Report of a case and review of the literature. *Dis Colon Rectum,* 19, 5, 460-469.

Shmuely, H., Passaro, D., Figer, A., Niv, Y., Pitlik, S., Samra, Z., Koren, R. & Yahav, J. (2001). Relationship between *Helicobacter pylori* CagA status and colorectal cancer. *Am J Gastroenterol,* 96, 12, 3406–3410.

Shroyer, K. R., Kim, J. G., Manos, M. M., Greer, C. E., Pearlman, N. W. & Franklin, W. A. (1992). Papillomavirus found in anorectal squamous carcinoma, not in colon adenocarcinoma. *Arch Surg,* 127, 6, 741–744.

Siddheshwar, R. K., Muhammad, K. B., Gray, J. C. & Kelly, S. B. (2001). Seroprevalence of *Helicobacter pylori* in patients with colorectal polyps and colorectal carcinoma. *Am J Gastroenterol,* 96, 1, 84–88.

Singh, P., Velasco, M., Given, R., Varro, A. & Wang T. C. (2000a). Progastrin expression predisposes mice to development of colon carcinomas and adenomas in response to AOM. *Gastroenterology,* 119, 1, 162–171.

Singh, P., Velasco, M., Given, R., Wargovich, M., Varro, A. & Wang, T. C. (2000b). Mice overexpressing progastrin are predisposed for developing aberrant colonic crypt foci in response to AOM. *Am J Physiol Gastrointest Liver Physiol,* 278, 3, G390–399.

Slattery, M. L., Curtin, K., Schaffer, D., Anderson, K. & Samowitz, W. (2002). Associations between family history of colorectal cancer and genetic alterations in tumors. *Int J Cancer,* 97, 6, 823–827.

Soliman, A. S., Bondy, M. L., El-Badawy, S. A., Mokhtar, N., Eissa, S., Bayoumy, S., Seifeldin, I. A., Houlihan, P. S., Lukish, J. R., Watanabe, T., Chan, A. O., Zhu, D., Amos, C. I., Levin, B. & Hamilton, S. R. (2001). Contrasting molecular pathology of colorectal carcinoma in Egyptian and Western patients. *Br J Cancer,* 85, 7, 1037-1046.

Song, L. B., Zhang, X., Zhang, C. Q., Zhang, Y., Pan, Z. Z., Liao, W. T., Li, M. Z. & Zeng, M. S. (2006). Infection of Epstein-Barr virus in colorectal cancer in Chinese. *Ai Zheng,* 25, 11, 1356–1360.

Soylu, A., Ozkara, S., Alis, H., Dolay, K., Kalayci, M., Yasar, N. & Kumbasar, A. B. (2008). Immunohistochemical testing for *Helicobacter Pylori* existence in neoplasms of the colon. *BMC Gastroenterol,* 14, 8, 35.

Steenbergen, R. D., de Wilde, J., Wilting, S. M., Brink, A. A., Snijders, P. J., Meijer, C. J. (2005). HPV-mediated transformation of the anogenital tract. *J Clin Virol,* 2005; 32, 1, S25–33.

Swidsinski, A., Khilkin, M., Kerjaschki, D., Schreiber, S., Ortner, M., Weber, J. & Lochs H. (1998). Association between intraepithelial *Escherichia coli* and colorectal cancer. *Gastroenterology,* 115, 2, 281–286.

Takada, K. (2000). Epstein-Barr virus and gastric carcinoma. *Mol Pathol,* 53, 5, 255–261.

Takeda, H. & Asaka, M. (2005) *Helicobacter pylori* and colorectal neoplasm: a mysterious link? *J Gastroenterol,* 40, 9, 919-920.

Theodoropoulos, G., Panoussopoulos, D., Papaconstantinou, I., Gazouli, M., Perdiki, M., Bramis, J. & Lazaris, A. Ch. (2005). Assessment of JC polyoma virus in colon neoplasms. *Dis Colon Rectum*, 48, 1, 86–91.

Thorburn, C. M., Friedman, G. D., Dickinson, C. J., Vogelman, J. H., Orentreich, N. & Parsonnet, J. (1998). Gastrin and colorectal cancer: a prospective study. *Gastroenterology*, 115, 2, 275–280.

Tjalsma, H., Scholler-Guinard, M., Lasonder, E., Ruers, T. J., Willems, H. L. & Swinkels, D. W. (2006). Profiling the humoral immune response in colon cancer patients: diagnostic antigens from *Streptococcus bovis*. *Int J Cancer*, 119, 9, 2127–2135.

Toprak, N. U., Yagci, A., Gulluoglu, B. M., Akin, M. L., Demirkalem, P., Celenk, T. and Soyletir. G. (2006). A possible role of *Bacteroides fragilis* enterotoxin in the aetiology of colorectal cancer. *Clin Microbiol Infect*, 12, 8, 782–786.

Trakatelli, C., Frydas, S., Hatzistilianou, M., Papadopoulos, E., Simeonidou, I., Founta, A., Paludi, D., Petrarca, C., Castellani, M. L., Papaioannou, N., Salini, V., Conti, P., Kempuraj, D. & Vecchiet, J. (2005). Chemokines as markers for parasiteinduced inflammation and tumors. *Int J Biol Markers*, 20, 4, 197-203

Tripodi, M. F., Adinolfi, L. E., Ragone, E., Durante-Mangoni, E., Fortunato, R., Iarussi, D., Ruggiero, G. & Utili, R. (2004). *Streptococcus bovis* endocarditis and its association with chronic liver disease: an underestimated risk factor. *Clin Infect Dis*, 38, 10, 1394–1400.

Tuazon, C. U., Nash, T., Cheever, A. & Neva, F. (1985). Interaction of *Schistosoma japonicum* with *Salmonellae* and other gram-negative bacteria. *J Infect Dis*, 152, 4, 722-726.

van Riet, E., Hartgers, F. C. & Yazdanbakhsh, M. (2007). Chronic helminth infections induce immunomodulation: consequences and mechanisms. *Immunobiology*, 212, 6, 475-490

Vaska, V. L. & Faoagali, J. L. (2009) *Streptococcus bovis* bacteraemia: identification within organism complex and association with endocarditis and colonic malignancy. *Pathology*, 41, 2, 183-186.

Vennervald, B. J. & Polman, K. (2009). Helminths and malignancy. *Parasite Immunol*, 31, 11, 686-696.

Waku, M., Napolitano, L., Clementini, E., Staniscia, T., Spagnolli, C., Andama, A., Kasiriye, P. & Innocenti, P. (2005). Risk of cancer onset in sub-Saharan Africans affected with chronic gastrointestinal parasitic diseases. *Int J Immunopathol Pharmacol*, 18, 3, 503-511.

Wang, L., Yi, T., Kortylewski, M., Pardoll, D. M., Zeng, D. & Yu, H. (2009). IL-17 can promote tumor growth through an IL-6-Stat3 signaling pathway. *J Exp Med*, 206, 7, 1457–1464

Wang, S., Liu, Z., Wang, L. & Zhang, X. (2009). NF-kappaB signaling pathway, inflammation and colorectal cancer. *Cell Mol Immunol*, 6, 5, 327-334.

Wang, T. C., Koh, T. J., Varro, A., Cahill, R. J., Dangler, C. A., Fox, J. G., Dockray, G. J. (1996). Processing and proliferative effects of human progastrin in transgenic mice. *J Clin Invest*, 98, 8, 1918–1929.

Wang, X. & Huycke, M. M. (2007). Extracellular superoxide production by *Enterococcus faecalis* promotes chromosomal instability in mammalian cells. *Gastroenterology*, 132, 2, 551–561.

Wang, X., Allen, T. D., May, R. J., Lightfoot, S., Houchen, C. W. & Huycke, M. M. (2008). *Enterococcus faecalis* induces aneuploidy and tetraploidy in colonic epithelial cells through a bystander effect. *Cancer Res*, 68, 23, 9909–9917.

Weinberg, D. S., Newschaffer, C. J. & Topham, A. (1999). Risk for colorectal cancer after gynecologic cancer. *Ann Intern Med*, 131, 3, 189–193.

Wexler, H. M. (2007). Bacteroides: the good, the bad, and the nitty-gritty. *Clin Microbiol Rev*, 20, 4, 593–621.

Wiley, D. & Masongsong, E. (2006). Human papillomavirus: the burden of infection. *Obstet Gynecol Surv*, 61, 6, S3–14.

Winters, M. D., Schlinke, T. L., Joyce, W. A., Glore, S. R. & Huycke, M. M. (1998). Prospective case-cohort study of intestinal colonization with enterococci that produce extracellular superoxide and the risk for colorectal adenomas or cancer. *Am J Gastroenterol*, 93, 12, 2491–2500.

Wong, M. P., Chung, L, P., Yuen, S. T., Leung, S. Y., Chan, S. Y., Wang, E. & Fu, K. H. (1995). In situ detection of Epstein-Barr virus in nonsmall cell lung carcinomas. *J Pathol*, 177, 3, 233–240.

Wong, N. A., Herbst, H., Herrmann, K., Kirchner, T., Krajewski, A. S., Moorghen, M., Niedobitek, F., Rooney, N., Shepherd, N. A. & Niedobitek, G. (2003). Epstein-Barr virus infection in colorectal neoplasms associated with inflammatory bowel disease: detection of the virus in lymphomas but not in adenocarcinomas. *J Pathol*, 201, 2, 312–318.

World Health Organization. (2003). The global burden of cancer, In: *World Cancer Report*, B. W. Stewart, P. Kleihues, (ed.), pp. 13, IARC Press, Lyon, France.

Wu, S., Lim, K. C., Huang, J., Saidi, R. F. & Sears, C. L. (1998). *Bacteroides fragilis* enterotoxin cleaves the zonula adherens protein, E-cadherin. *Proc Natl Acad Sci*, 95, 25, 14979–14984.

Wu, S., Morin, P. J., Mauyo, D. & Sears, C. (2003). *Bacteroides fragilis* enterotoxin induces *c-myc* expression and cellular proliferation. *Gastroenterology*, 124, 2, 392–400.

Wu, S., Rhee, K. J., Albesiano, E., Rabizadeh, S., Wu, X., Yen, H. R., Huso, D. L., Brancati, F. L., Wick, E., McAllister, F., Housseau, F., Pardoll, D. M. & Sears, C. L. (2009). A human colonic commensal promotes colon tumorigenesis via activation of T helper type 17 T cell responses. *Nat Med*, 15, 9, 1016–1022.

Xu, Z. & Su, D. (1984). *Schistosoma japonicum* and colorectal cancer: an epidemiological study in the People's Republic of China. *Int J Cancer*, 34, 3, 315-318.

Yu, X. R., Chen, P. H., Xu, J. Y., Xiao, S., Shan, Z. J. & Zhu, S. J. (1991). Histological classification of schistosomal egg induced polyps of colon and their clinical significance. An analysis of 272 cases. *Chin Med J(Engl)* 104, 1, 64-70

Yuen, S. T., Chung, L. P., Leung, S. Y., Luk, I. S., Chan, S. Y. & Ho, J. (1994). In situ detection of Epstein-Barr virus in gastric and colorectal adenocarcinomas. *Am J Surg Pathol*, 18, 11, 1158–1163.

Zalata, K. R., Nasif, W. A., Ming, S. C., Lotfy, M., Nada, N. A., El-Hak, N. G. & Leech, S. H. (2005). *p53*, *Bcl-2* and *C-myc* expressions in colorectal carcinoma associated with schistosomiasis in Egypt. *Cell Oncol*, 27, 4, 245-253

Zarkin, B. A., Lillemoe, K. D., Cameron, J. L., Effron, P. N., Magnuson, T. H. & Pitt, H. A. (1990). The triad of *Streptococcus bovis* bacteremia, colonic pathology, and liver disease. *Ann Surg*, 211, 6, 786 - 791

Zhang, R., Takahashi, S., Orita, S., Yoshida, A., Maruyama, H., Shirai, T. & Ohta, N. (1998). *p53* gene mutations in rectal cancer associated with schistosomiasis japonica in Chinese patients. *Cancer Lett*, 131, 2, 215-221.

Zhao, E. S. (1981). Cancer of the colon and schistosomiasis. *J R Soc Med*, 74, 9, 645.

Zhao, Y. S., Wang, F., Chang, D., Han, B. & You, D. Y. (2008). Meta-analysis of different test indicators: *Helicobacter pylori* infection and the risk of colorectal cancer. *Int J Colorectal Dis*, 23, 9, 875-882.

Zumkeller, N., Brenner, H., Chang-Claude, J., Hoffmeister, M., Nieters, A., Rothenbacher, D. (2007). *Helicobacter pylori* infection, interleukin-1 gene polymorphisms and the risk of colorectal cancer: evidence from a case-control study in Germany. *Eur J Cancer*, 43, 8, 1283–1289.

Zumkeller, N., Brenner, H., Zwahlen, M. & Rothenbacher, D. (2006). *Helicobacter pylori* infection and colorectal cancer risk: a meta-analysis. *Helicobacter*, 11, 2, 75 - 80.

17

Streptococcus bovis/gallolyticus Induce the Development of Colorectal Cancer

A.S. Abdulamir[1,2], R.R. Hafidh[1,3] and F. Abu Bakar[1]
[1]*Institute of Bioscience, University Putra Malaysia, Serdang, Selangor,*
[2]*Microbiology Department, College of Medicine, Alnahrain University PO, Baghdad,*
[3]*Microbiology Department, College of Medicine, Baghdad University,*
[1]*Malaysia*
[2,3]*Iraq*

1. Introduction

The role, of microbial agents and the infection of the intestinal mucosa in the carcinogenesis, or the development of colorectal cancer (CRC) is one of the hot topics in the field of CRC where much research has been done. However, this topic has long been underestimated by most of the related books. This chapter is intended to cover the relationship of CRC development with bacteria implicated in the development of CRC such as *S. bovis, S. gallolyticus, S. equines, S. infantarius, E .coli, C. difficile*...etc. However, *S. gallolyticus* and *S. bovis* will be discussed thoroughly in this chapter as they are considered the prototype for intestinal microorganisms related to CRC and colorectal premalignant lesions.

Studying CRC association with infection of intestinal mucosa is not complete without studying the underlying mechanisms. There is compelling evidence that CRC is largely affected by the status of intestinal bioflora. CRC has been found to be affected by certain microbial agents that have particular characteristics capable of inducing dysplastic changes in intestinal mucosa. However, the underlying mechanisms of the association of implicated infective agents with CRC development are yet not clear. In addition, the role of oncogenic factors, cell growth factors, and pro-inflammatory cytokines in the association of bacterial infection in intestinal mucosa with CRC has not yet been clarified well. Therefore, the current chapter attempts to scrutinize the nature and the underlying mechanisms of the association of infective agents represented by *S. bovis/gallolyticus* with CRC. Nevertheless, the association of *S. bovis/gallolyticus* with CRC is still under controversy regarding whether the bacterial infection of intestine, along with associated bacteremia/endocarditis, is a consequence or the etiological factor of CRC. Hence, this chapter also attempts to explore the facts available in the field to assess which scenario is more favorable for the association of *S. bovis/gallolyticus* with CRC namely, the consequence or the etiology scenario.

One of the bacterial agents that have been most associated with cancer is *Streptococcus bovis* (*S. bovis*). *S. bovis* has been shown to be important in human health because 25 to 80% of patients with *S. bovis* bacteremia had also colorectal tumor, and the incidence of association of colonic neoplasia with *S. bovis* endocarditis was shown to be 18 to 62% (Gupta et al., 2009; Kok et al., 2007; Leport et al., 1987; Malkin et al., 2008; Reynolds et al., 1983; Wilson et al.,

1981; Zarkin et al., 1990). Later, it was shown that a new species resembling *S. bovis* is actually most implicated in CRC development; *S. bovis* infecting human intestine has been named as *S. gallolyticus* (Osawa et al., 1995). More precisely, *S. bovis* biotype I and II/2 isolates were shown to be *S. gallolyticus* (Devriese et al., 1998). Accordingly, *S. bovis* biotype I was replaced by *S. gallolyticus* subspecies *gallolyticus* and biotype II/2 was replaced by *S. gallolyticus* subspecies *pasterianus* and *S. gallolyticus* subspecies *macedonicus* (Schlegel et al., 2003). *S. gallolyticus* subspecies *gallolyticus*, rather than other related taxa, have been found to be constantly associated with underlying colorectal cancer.

2. The association of colorectal cancer with *S. bovis/gallolyticus* bacteremia/endocarditis

S. bovis, has long been linked to the development of CRC. However, the extent, nature, and basis of this association are still not completely understood. *S. bovis/gallolyticus* became important in human health since it was shown that 25 to 80% of patients who presented *S. bovis/gallolyticus* bacteremia had also a colorectal tumor and the incidence of association of colonic neoplasia with *S. bovis/gallolyticus* endocaditis was shown to be 18 to 62% (Gupta et al., 2009; Kok et al., 2007; Leport et al., 1987; Malkin et al., 2008; Murray & Roberts, 1978; Reynolds et al., 1983; Wilson et al., 1981; Zarkin et al., 1990). The knowledge that there is an association between endocarditis from *S. bovis/gallolyticus* and carcinoma of the colon has important clinical implications (Boleij et al., 2009a; Kok et al., 2007). The majority of the studies that found clues on the association of *S. bovis/gallolyticus* with CRC was in Europe and North America. Actually, it is true that the association of *S. bovis/gallolyticus* bacteremia with colorectal cancer has been found variable among different geographical and ethnic groups (Boleij et al., 2009a), but this association is not restricted to certain geographical region. A recent study done in Malaysia found that 48.6% of *S. bovis* isolates was found in patients with colonic polyps, adenocarcinomas, inflammatory bowel diseases. It was also found that colorectal cancer incidence was 24.7%, adenocarinomas accounting for 51% with the highest incidence in the sigmoid part of the colon(Al-Jashamy et al., 2010). This study indicates a strong relationship between *S. bovis/gallolyticus* and colonic premalignant as well as malignant lesions in a geographical region that was considered of low incidence for CRC cases associated with bacterial infections. Moreover, an epidemiological study conducted in Hong Kong on *S. bovis* bacteremia and its relation to colorectal cancer, confirmed the association of *S. bovis/gallolyticus* with CRC and found that *S. bovis* biotype II/2 is the dominant in Hong Kong rather than biotype I (*S. gallolyticus*) which is dominant in Western countries (Lee et al., 2003).

Thorough studies on *S. bovis* have shown that associations between *S. bovis* bacteraemia and carcinoma of the colon and infective endocarditis were biotype-specific. It was shown that there is 94% association between *S. bovis* biotype I bacteraemia and infective endocarditis and 71% association between *S. bovis* biotype I bacteraemia and colonic carcinoma. On the other hand, it is only 18% association between *S. bovis* biotype II bacteraemia and infective endocarditis and 17% association between *S. bovis* biotype II bacteraemia and colonic carcinoma (Murray & Baron, 2007). Following the description of *S. gallolyticus*, Devriese team used whole-cell protein analysis to show that all six bacterial isolates studied, which were derived from patients with endocarditis and identified by conventional techniques as *S. bovis*, were in fact *S. gallolyticus*. Therefore, they suggested that *S. gallolyticus* is more likely to be involved in human infections than is *S. bovis* (Devriese et al., 1998).

The underlying mechanisms for the association of CRC with *S. bovis/gallolyticus* bacteremia/endocarditis have been obscure for a long time. The possible reason behind that, maybe, *S. bovis/gallolyticus* is a member of intestinal flora in 2.5 to 15% of individuals which usually make scientists counteract any malicious role of this bacteria (Burns et al., 1985; Murray & Roberts, 1978). It was conceived in the beginning that the ulceration of neoplastic lesions might form a pathway for the microorganism to enter the bloodstream (Gupta et al., 2009). However, the latter scenario of bacterial access into the circulation does not explain the cases of patients with infectious endocarditis and non-ulcerated colonic polyps (Cutait et al., 1988). Furthermore, colonic neoplasia may arise years after the presentation of the condition of bacterial bacteremia or infectious endocarditis (Fagundes et al., 2000; Zarkin et al., 1990). For this reason, patients with infectious endocarditis and normal colonoscopy may be included in the group who present risk for developing colonic cancer because of the late appearance of such lesions after the infectious episode *of S. bovis/gallolyticus* (Fagundes et al., 2000). Moreover, in supporting the second scenario, it has been shown that the relative risk of developing infectious endocarditis from *S. bovis/gallolyticus* in the presence of carcinoma of the colon is merely 3 to 6% (Bisno & 12.ed. New York: , 1991) while 60 to 75% of patients with endocarditis by *S. bovis/gallolyticus* simultaneously present malignant gastrointestinal disease that was not previously diagnosed (Grinberg et al., 1990).

3. The association of premalignant colorectal lesions with *S. bovis/gallolyticus*

There is a high incidence of colorectal cancer in individuals with polyps; about 90% of preinvasive neoplastic lesions of the colorectum are polyps or polyp precursors, namely aberrant crypt foci (Nielsen et al., 2007). Neoplastic polyps are often referred to more specifically as adenomas or adenomatous polyps (Srivastava et al., 2001). Adenomatous polyps are considered as good and few surrogate end point markers for colorectal cancer (Kelly et al., 1989; Nielsen et al., 2007).

It would be of interest to substantiate any relationship between bacterial colonic carriage, colonic polyps and the type of polyp and its malignant potential (Boleij et al., 2009a; Schlegel et al., 2003). Contrary to the more commonly reported association between *S. bovis/gallolyticus* bacteremia and colorectal cancer, a link to pre-neoplastic adenomatous polyps was less frequently reported (Burns et al., 1985; Ellmerich et al., 2000a). Nevertheless, the relationship between colorectal bacterial infection and the progressive development of malignant disease in pre-neoplastic adenomatous polyps was supported by recent reports (Abdulamir et al., 2009; Kahveci et al., 2010; Murinello et al., 2006). Interestingly, benign lesions (diverticulosis, inflammatory bowel disease, cecal volvulus, perirectal abscess hemorrhoids, benign polyps) were found to be mildly associated with intestinal bacterial infections such as *S. bovis/gallolyticus* while a strong relationship between more malignant diseases of the colon (cancer and neoplastic polyps) and *S. bovis/gallolyticus* was found (Abdulamir et al., 2009; Burns et al., 1985; Klein et al., 1979; Nielsen et al., 2007; Reynolds et al., 1983; Smaali et al., 2008). It was also revealed that *S. bovis/gallolyticus* septicemia and/or endocarditis is selectively related to the presence of villous or tubulovillous adenomas in the large intestine (Fagundes et al., 2000; Smaali et al., 2008). In fact, Villous and tubulovillous adenomas, which have risk of malignant transformation about 15-25%, were found to be associated with *S. bovis/gallolyticus* bacteria more often than other types of adenomas (Bond, 2005). For example, Hoen team performed a case-control study on subjects underwent colonoscopy comparing between patients with *S. bovis/gallolyticus* endocarditis and sex- and age- matched unaffected patients. This study showed that colonic adenomatous polyps were present in twice as many cases as controls (15 of 32 *vs* 15 of 64), and colorectal cancer was present approximately 3 times as often (3 of 32 *vs* 2 of 64) (Hoen et al., 1994). However, surprisingly, another study (Devis et al., 1989) found that the association between *S. bovis/gallolyticus* and adenoma was more evident than that with colorectal cancer; they reported that 36% of positive blood cultures of *S. bovis/gallolyticus* were found in proliferative lesions (15% of cancers and 21% of adenomas). A recent study (Abdulamir et al., 2009) supported this concept showing that the level of *S. bovis/gallolyticus* IgG antibodies in adenoma patients is much higher than in both colorectal cancer patients and control subjects. However, other reports did not reveal the same thing. (Burns et al., 1985) stated that the incidence of *S. bovis/gallolyticus* carriage in all colons with polyps was intermediary between normal colons and colons with carcinoma although the difference did not achieve statistical significance.

Regarding the fecal carriage of *S. bovis/gallolyticus*, (Burns et al., 1985) demonstrated that highly premalignant polyps were found to be more often associated with *S. bovis/gallolyticus* carriage than were benign polyps. A clue for the active role of intestinal bacteria in the development of CRC, *S. bovis/gallolyticus* endocarditis, rather than other members of group D Streptococcus, showed special predilection to colonic lesions. It was found that of 77 infections with group D Streptococcus endocarditis, colonic polyps and colonic carcinoma were significantly more frequent in the *S. bovis/gallolyticus* group (67 and 18%) respectively than in the Enterococcus group (21 and 2%) respectively (Leport et al., 1987). This indicates that certain bacteria have role in the etiology of CRC development from premalignant poly lesions.

The remarkable association between adenomatous polyps and *S. bovis/gallolyticus* seems to be of importance due to the compelling evidence that colon cancer progresses from normal tissue to adenoma and then to carcinoma through an accumulation of genetic alterations (Baron & Sandler, 2000). Although ulceration of the neoplastic lesion might form a pathway for the *S. bovis/gallolyticus* to enter the bloodstream (Gupta et al., 2009), the association of *S. bovis/gallolyticus* bacteremia with non-ulcerated colonic polyps indicates an etiological/promoter role of these bacteria in polyps progression (Cutait et al., 1988; Konda & Duffy, 2008). The possibility of *S. bovis/gallolyticus* to act as a promoter for the preneoplastic lesions is worthy to be considered. A remarkable study supported this hypothesis using rats treated with *S. bovis* wall extracted antigens (WEA), rats treated with a chemical carcinogen, rats treated with both WEA and chemical carcinogen, and untreated rats. All groups of rats did not develop hyperplastic colonic crypts except for the group treated with both WEA and the chemical carcinogen; about 50 % rats of this group developed neoplastic lesions (Ellmerich et al., 2000a). This indicated that *S. bovis* bacteria might exert their pathological activity in the colonic mucosa only when preneoplastic lesions are established. Another model supporting the promoter effect of *S. bovis/gallolyticus*, H. pylori infection and subsequent inflammation seem most likely to be promoters in the multistep development of carcinoma (from chronic gastritis to atrophy, intestinal metaplasia, dysplasia, and, ultimately, cancer) rather than the causative agents (Leung, 2006). Therefore, the association of *S. bovis/gallolyticus* in etiology and/or acceleration of the transformation of aberrant crypts to adenoma and to cancer is now being reconsidered.

Accordingly, the knowledge of association of colorectal adenoma with *S. bovis/gallolyticus* has important clinical implications. If the lesion can be discovered at an early stage, curative resection may become possible (Waisberg et al., 2002). Thus, bacteremia due to *S. bovis/gallolyticus* should prompt rigorous investigation to exclude both endocarditis and tumors of the large bowel (Beeching et al., 1985; Konda & Duffy, 2008). Therefore, it was concluded that the discovery of a malignant or premalignant proliferative lesion in one third of the cases justifies the exploration of the colon by barium enema and/or colonoscopy in the case of *S. bovis/gallolyticus* septicemia (Beeching et al., 1985; Konda & Duffy, 2008). This would empirically aid for the early detection of adenoma in the gastrointestinal tract before its progression to cancer.

4. The proposed mechanisms for the development of colorectal cancer by *S. bovis/gallolyticus*

Chronic inflammation is associated with malignant changes. Host genetic polymorphisms of the adaptive and innate immune response play an important role in bacteria-induced cancer formation (El-Omar, 2006; Hou et al., 2007; Karin & Greten, 2005). Therefore, studying the immunological responses to chronic bacterial infections is likely to yield important clues on both the mechanisms of persistent infection and the relationship between inflammation and cancer formation (Ernst et al., 2006; Monack et al., 2004). Clinical studies have shown that the use of non-steroidal anti-inflammatory drugs is associated with a reduced risk of gastric cancer (Dai & Wang, 2006). However, bacteria implicated in carcinogenesis, like *S. bovis/gallolyticus*, might use several mechanisms for carcinogenesis such as the colonization of epithelial surfaces and the use of virulence factors to chronically affect host cell cycle control, apoptosis, cell junction integrity or cell polarity ((Vogelmann & Amieva, 2007).

4.1 Clues for etiological role

The big question is whether bacteria play an etiological role in the carcinoma of colon or it is merely marker of the disease. There are many clues collectively provide evidence for the etiological role of bacteria in colon cancer development. The striking association between bacteremia caused by *S. bovis* biotype I and both colonic neoplasia (71%) and bacterial endocarditis (94%), rather than bacteremia caused by closely related organisms such as *S. bovis* variant and *S. salivarius*, suggests the possibility of specific bacterium-host interactions (Ruoff et al., 1989). Moreover, the appearance of new colonic lesions 2-4 after the incidence of *S. bovis/gallolyticus* bacteremia/endocarditis, provides more evidence that *S. bovis/gallolyticus* is not merely a consequence of the tumor lesion (Wentling et al., 2006). In terms of pathogenesis, as *S. bovis/gallolyticus* is a transient normal flora in the gut, researchers have postulated that the increased bacterial load of *S. bovis/gallolyticus* in colon might be responsible for its association with colon cancer. Several studies have shown that increased stool carriage of *S. bovis/gallolyticus* is particularly found in patients with inflammatory bowel diseases or malignant/premalignant lesions of the colon while *S. bovis/gallolyticus* bacteria were rarely isolated from normal subjects (Teitelbaum & Triantafyllopoulou, 2006). Another clue supporting the etiological role of *S. bovis/gallolyticus*, patients diagnosed with colon cancer have only 3-6% chance to develop *S. bovis/gallolyticus* endocarditis (zur Hausen, 2006), which is far lower than the percentage of the detection of colorectal cancer in patients with *S. bovis/gallolyticus* bacteremia/endocarditis, which his more than 70%.

4.2 Mechanisms of the proposed etiological role of *S. bovis/gallolyticus* in the development of colorectal cancer

4.2.1 Selective adherence to intestinal tumor cells

Some bacteria such as *S. bovis/gallolyticus* are frequent colonizers of the intestinal tract, which can also cause endocarditis. However, their ability to adhere to and colonize host tissues is largely unknown. It was found that *S. bovis/gallolyticus* bacteria possess collagen-binding proteins and pili that are responsible for adhesion to colorectal mucosa as well as to endocardium (Sillanpaa et al., 2009). On the other hand, another study (Boleij et al., 2009b) found a histone-like protein A on the surface of *S. bovis/gallolyticus* able to bind heparan sulfate proteoglycans at the colon tumor cell surface during the first stages of infection; this cell surface protein in *S. gallolyticus* acts as one of the main heparin-binding proteins that is largely responsible for bacteria selective adhesive potential as well as entry to the blood circulation. Another study assessing 17 endocarditis-derived human isolates, identified 15 *S. gallolyticus* subspecies *gallolyticus*, one *S. gallolyticus* subspecies *pasteurianus* (biotype II/2) and one *S. infantarius* subspecies *coli* (biotype II/1) for their in vitro adherence to components of the extracellular matrix; this study provided evidence that *S. gallolyticus* subspecies *gallolyticus* bacteria possess very efficient adherence characteristics to the host extracellular matrix; this bacteria showed powerful adherence to collagen type I and type IV, fibrinogen, collagen type V, and fibronectin (Sillanpaa et al., 2008). These adherence merits render these bacteria successful colonizers in both intestinal and cardiac tissues which might explain the association between *S. bovis/gallolyticus* endocarditis and intestinal lesions.

4.2.2 Changing the intestinal bacterial flora and alterations in the local vascular attributes

Increased incidence of hepatic dysfunction has been reported in patients with bacterial infectious endocarditis (Fagundes et al., 2000). It has been speculated that *S. bovis/gallolyticus* affects portal circulation through bacterial translocation, thereby determining hepatic alterations. Modifications in the hepatic secretion of bile salts and the production of immunoglobulins contribute towards increasing the participation of S. bovis/gallolyticus in abnormal changes in the bacterial flora of the colonic lumen which might then promote carcinogenesis of the intestinal mucosa (Beeching et al., 1985; Gupta et al., 2009).

It has been suggested that alterations in local conditions and disruption of capillary channels at the site of neoplasm allowed S. bovis/gallolyticus to proliferate and gain entry into blood stream (Biarc et al., 2004; Ellmerich et al., 2000a; Nguyen et al., 2006). The local action of cytokines or of chemical mediators able to promote vasodilatation and the enhancement of capillary permeability, may support the bacterial entry at tumor sites, and increase bacterial adherence to various cells (Biarc et al., 2004; Ellmerich et al., 2000b).

4.2.3 Promoting/propagating effect on preneoplastic lesions and inflammation-driven carcinogenesis

A series of interesting experiments was conducted for investigating the role of *S. bovis/gallolyticus* in the initiation and development of colorectal cancer. Chemical carcinomas were induced by giving adult rats intraperitonial injections of azoxymethane (15 mg/kg body weight) once per week for 2 weeks. Fifteen days (week 4) after the last injection of the carcinogen, the rats received, by gavage twice per week during 5 weeks, either *S. bovis* (10^{10} bacteria) or wall-extracted antigens (WEAs) (100 µg). One week after the last gavage (week 10), it was found that administration of either *S. bovis* or its antigens promoted the progression of preneoplastic lesions into neoplastic lesions through the increased formation of hyperproliferative aberrant colonic crypts, which enhanced the expression of proliferation markers and increased the production of IL-8 in the colonic mucosa (Biarc et al., 2004; Ellmerich et al., 2000b). Therefore, this study suggests that *S. bovis/gallolyticus* bacteria act as potential promoters of early preneoplastic lesions in the colon of rats, and their cell wall proteins are more potent inducers of neoplastic transformation than the intact bacteria. This study also revealed that the development of colonic adenomas increased remarkably in 50% of the tested rats and the expression level of proliferation markers, the polyamine content and proliferating cell nuclear antigen was also increased (Biarc et al., 2004; Ellmerich et al., 2000a; Nguyen et al., 2006). This provided extra evidence that *S. bovis/gallolyticus* acts more likely as promoter/propagator of colorectal carcinoma rather than just a consequence of the tumor lesion. These studies might suggest that bacteria, in general, are often not capable to induce cancer without the presence of other predisposing factors for carcinogenesis. In this regard, it was conceived that the transformation process of colorectal tumors associated with *S. bovis/gallolyticus* is more likely accompanied with long-lasting bacterial promoting/propagating effect along with chronic inflammation status in intestinal mucosa. This conclusion was supported by Balkwill et al. stating that tumor formation might require independent mutations in oncogenic signaling pathways in addition to chronic inflammatory conditions which are needed to promote transformation process (Balkwill et al., 2005).

In vitro experiments showed that the binding of *S. bovis* wall extracted antigens to various cell lines including human colonic cancer cells (Caco-2) stimulated the production of inflammatory cytokines by those cells (Biarc et al., 2004; Nguyen et al., 2006). Earlier it was found that the production of inflammatory cytokines in response to *S. bovis/gallolyticus*, such as TNF-α, IL-1ß and IL-6, and the chemokine IL-8, were found to contribute to the normal defense mechanisms of the host (Ellmerich et al., 2000b; Travers & Rosen, 1997) leading to the formation of nitric oxide and free radicals such as superoxide, peroxynitrites, hydroxyl radicals as well as alkylperoxy radicals (Nguyen et al., 2006; Ohshima & Bartsch, 1994). Owing to their potent mutagenicity, all these molecular species can contribute to the neoplastic processes by modifying cellular DNA. On the other hand, in the colonic mucosa, the production of angiogenic factors, such as IL-8, triggered by *S. bovis/gallolyticus* antigens may also favor the progression of colon carcinogenesis (Eisma et al., 1999; Ellmerich et al., 2000b; Norrby, 1996). This resembles *H. pylori* infection for the development of chronic inflammation in the gastric mucosa (Dixon et al., 1996); therefore, it seems that chronic infection and subsequent chronic inflammation are responsible for the maintenance and development of pre-existing neoplastic lesions (Shacter & Weitzman, 2002).

Moreover, it was found that WEAs of *S. bovis* induced *in vitro* overexpression of cyclooxygenase-2 (COX-2) (Biarc et al., 2004; Nguyen et al., 2006). COX-2, via prostaglandins, promotes cellular proliferation and angiogenesis and inhibits apoptosis, thus acting as a promoter in the cancer pathway (Tafte & Ruoff, 2007). It is noteworthy to mention that non-steroidal anti-inflammatory drugs (NSAIDS) were found to decrease the relative risk of gastrointestinal carcinomas and their main target was found to be cyclooxygenase 2 (COX-2) that is over-expressed in up to 85% of colorectal adenocarcinomas (Kargman et al., 1995). Moreover, (Haqqani et al., 2000) revealed that the activation of leukocytes by *S. bovis/gallolyticus* was found to release various other inflammatory mediators (NO, free radicals, peroxynitriles, etc.) which could interfere directly or indirectly with the cell proliferation process. A recent study conducted by our team, *S. gallolyticus* has shown a specific association with colorectal cancer and colorectal adenoma when compared with the more dominant intestinal bacteria, *B. fragilis*. This provided evidence for a possible important role of *S. gallolyticus* in the carcinogenesis of colorectal cancer from pre-malignant polyps. In addition, it was also found that NF-κB and IL-8 rather than other transformation factors p21, p27 and p53 act as important mediators for the *S. gallolyticus*-associated transformation of adenoma to carcinoma (Abdulamir et al., 2009). Moreover, it was concluded that NF-κB exerts most probably a promoting carcinogenic effect and IL-8 exerts mainly an angiogenic-based propagating effect on colorectal mucosal cells (Abdulamir et al., 2009). In addition, a more recent study done by our team showed a direct and active role of *S. bovis/gallolyticus* in colorectal cancer development through inflammation-based sequel of tumor development or propagation via IL-1, COX-2, and IL-8 (Abdulamir et al., 2010). By these studies, a strong relationship was shown to be evident between the proinflammatory potential of *S. bovis/gallolyticus* bacteria and their carcinogenic properties confirming the linkage between inflammation and colon carcinogenesis.

In the presence of WEAs proteins of *S. bovis/gallolyticus*, Caco-2 cells exhibited enhanced phosphorylation of 3 classes of mitogen activated protein kinases (MAPKs) (Biarc et al., 2004). Several reports showed that MAPKs activation stimulates cells to undergo DNA synthesis and cellular uncontrolled proliferation (Hirata et al., 2001; Ihler, 1996; Smith & Lawson, 2001). Therefore *S. bovis/gallolyticus* proteins could promote cell proliferation by triggering MAPKs which might increase the incidence of cell transformation and the rate of genetic mutations. Furthermore MAPKs, particularly p38 MAPK, can induce COX-2 which is an important factor in tumorogenesis (Lasa et al., 2002; Wang & Dubois, 2010) and up-regulate the expression of NFkB which is considered the central link between inflammation and carcinogenesis (Karin & Greten, 2005). Accordingly, the pro-inflammatory potential of *S. bovis/gallolyticus* proteins and their pro-carcinogenic properties as well as the chronic inflammation and the leucocytic recruitment driven by *S. bovis/gallolyticus* provide strong evidence on the possible causal link between *S. bovis/gallolyticus* inflammation and colonic carcinogenesis. Therefore, the above data support the hypothesis that colonic bacteria can contribute to cancer development particularly via chronic infection/inflammation where bacterial components may interfere with cell function for long time (Biarc et al., 2004; Wang & Dubois, 2010).

5. Selective colonization of *S. bovis/gallolyticus* in colorectal mucosa

The association of bacteria with colorectal cancer has always been described through the incidence of *S. bovis/gallolyticus* bacteremia and/or endocarditis (Leport et al., 1987; Murray & Roberts, 1978; Reynolds et al., 1983; Wilson et al., 1981; Zarkin et al., 1990). On the other hand, little bacteriological research has been done on elucidating the colonization of *S. bovis/gallolyticus* in tumor lesions of colorectal cancer in order to confirm or refute, on solid bases, the direct link between colorectal cancer and *S. bovis/gallolyticus* (Norfleet & Mitchell, 1993; Potter et al., 1998). A recent study of by our team was conducted to assess the colonization of *S. bovis/gallolyticus* bacteria in colon by detecting *S. bovis/gallolyticus* DNA in colorectal cancer tumors using advanced molecular assays (Abdulamir et al., 2010). In Abdulamir et al. study, *S. bovis/gallolyticus*-specific primers and probes were used in PCR and in situ hybridization (ISH) assays, respectively, to detect *S. bovis/gallolyticus* DNA from feces, tumor mucosal surfaces, and from the inside of tumor lesions. In addition, bacteriological isolation of *S. bovis/gallolyticus* was conducted to isolate *S. bovis/gallolyticus* cells from feces, tumor mucosal surfaces, and from the inside of tumor lesions. In this study, *S. bovis/gallolyticus* was successfully isolated, via bacteriological assays, from tumorous and non-tumorous tissues, of colorectal cancer patients with bacteremia, 20.5% and 17.3%, and of colorectal cancer patients without bacteremia, 12.8% and 11.5%, respectively while only 2% of control tissues revealed colonization of *S. bovis/gallolyticus*.

On the other hand, the positive detection of *S. bovis/gallolyticus* DNA, via PCR, in tumorous and non-tumorous tissues of colorectal cancer patients with bacteremia, 48.7 and 35.9%, and without bacteremia, 32.7 and 23%, respectively, was remarkably higher than that in control tissues, 4%. And the positive detection of *S. bovis/gallolyticus* DNA, via ISH, in tumorous and non-tumorous tissues of colorectal cancer patients with bacteremia, 46.1 and 30.7%, and without bacteremia 28.8 and 17.3%, respectively was remarkably higher than that in control tissues, 2%. In addition, by using absolute quantitative PCR for *S. bovis/gallolyticus* DNA, the *S. bovis/gallolyticus* count, in terms of copy number (CN), in tumorous and non-tumorous tissues of colorectal cancer patients with bacteremia, 2.96-4.72 and 1.29-2.81 $\log_{10}$ CN/g, respectively, and colorectal cancer patients without bacteremia, 2.16-2.92 and 0.67-2.07 $\log_{10}$ CN/g, respectively, showed significantly higher level of colonization in tumorous than in non-tumorous tissues and in colorectal cancer patients with bacteremia than in colorectal cancer patients without bacteremia. Accordingly, this study provided several new observations. First, *S. bovis/gallolyticus* colonizes selectively tumorous tissues of colorectal cancer patients rather than normal mucosal tissues. Second, the colonization of *S. bovis/gallolyticus* is mainly found inside tumor lesions rather than on mucosal surfaces of tumors. Third, the titer of the colonizing *S. bovis/gallolyticus* bacteria in colorectal cancer patients with bacteremia/endocarditis was much higher than in patients without bacteremia/endocarditis; this explains why some colorectal cancer patients develop concomitant bacteremia of *S. bovis/endocarditis* while others do not. Actually, the newly discovered selective colonization of *S. bovis/gallolyticus* explains the conclusions of an earlier report (Tjalsma et al., 2006) stating that colonic lesions provide a suitable microenvironment for *S. bovis/gallolyticus* colonization resulting in silent tumor-associated infections that only become apparent when cancer patients become immunocompromised, as in bacteraemia, or have coincidental cardiac valve lesions and develop endocarditis.

6. Using *S. bovis/gallolyticus* in the early detection of colorectal tumors

For a long time, it has been conceived that there is a need to establish a good screening test for colonic cancer patients, particularly a test which could detect early lesions. It has been suggested that the presence of antibodies to certain bacterial antigens or the presence of certain bacterial antigens in the bloodstream may act as markers for carcinogenesis of the colon (Beeching et al., 1985; Potter et al., 1998). The serology-based detection of colorectal cancer has advantage on other tests such as fecal occult blood which is neither sensitive nor specific or carcinoembryonic antigen which is regularly detectable in only advanced diseases (Tafte & Ruoff, 2007). Darjee and Gibb stated that it might be possible to develop a test to screen patients for the presence of colonic cancer by measuring IgG antibody titer of *S. bovis/gallolyticus* (Darjee & Gibb, 1993). Hence, since the association between slow evolving bacterial inflammation and colorectal cancer takes long time, it is prudent to seek specifically for IgG antibodies. Furthermore, IgG antibodies reflect an image of the past and the chronic presence of *S. bovis/gallolyticus* antigens in the circulation.

Some studies showed the possibility of constructing a serology test for the successful detection of colonic cancer based on the detection of antibody to *S. bovis/gallolyticus* or *Enterococcus faecalis* (Abdulamir et al., 2009; Groves, 1997). Therefore, a simple ELISA test with no more than 2 ml of patient's blood might be a good candidate for screening high risk individuals for the presence of premalignant neoplastic polyps, adenomas, and cancers. However, some other studies of antibody response to *S. bovis/gallolyticus* and other streptococci have found that antibody is detectable in endocarditis but not in either clinically insignificant bacteremias (Burnie et al., 1987), or colonic cancers ((Kaplan et al., 1983) by using immunoblotting, immunoflourescence and other techniques. In a recent study of our team (Abdulamir et al., 2009), the serum level of IgG antibodies against *S. gallolyticus* subspecies *gallolyticus* antigens adsorbed on solid phase of ELISA was found to be significantly higher in colorectal cancer patients than in control subjects. This is in full agreement with the study of (Darjee & Gibb, 1993) who showed that patients with colonic cancer had higher median IgG antibody titers to *S. bovis* and *E. faecalis* preparations than did the control samples. Accordingly, the applicability of using ELISA as a cheap and effective assay for the early detection of colorectal cancer using IgG antibodies against *S. bovis/gallolyticus* has been tested and proven (Abdulamir et al., 2009). Therefore, the early detection of colorectal cancer using simple means of testing opens doors to monitor high risk groups of colorectal cancer more efficiently.

7. Conclusions

Colorectal tumors, adenoma or carcinoma, are associated remarkably with bacterial infections of intestine. The manifestation of this association is usually observed as concurrent bacteremia or endocarditis of *S. bovis/gallolyticus*. The association of *S. bovis/gallolyticus* bacteria with colorectal cancer is more likely etiological in nature rather than a consequence of the disease. The proposed etiological role of *S. bovis/gallolyticus* in the development of colorectal cancer might be attributed to many factors including selective adhesion potential of *S. bovis/gallolyticus* to tumor tissues, the selective colonization of *S. bovis/gallolyticus* inside tumor tissues, the suitable microenvironment of tumors for *S. bovis/gallolyticus* proliferation, the local disruption of tumor tissues and capillaries which allow the entry of *S. bovis/gallolyticus* into blood circulation leading to bacteremia and endocarditis, and the bacterially-induced cytokines and transcriptional factors, such as IL-1, IFN-γ, IL-8, and NFkB, which induce and propagate the chronic inflammatory environment which promote/propagate premaligant intestinal lesions to malignant ones. This is a very important role of *S. bovis/gallolyticus* in the carcinogenesis of colorectal tissues since the majority of cases of colorectal cancer are sporadic cancers arising through the transformation of normal colorectal tissues to premalignant lesions, adenomas, and finally to malignant tissues. Besides, the early detection of colorectal adenomas or carcinomas via detection of *S. bovis/gallolyticus* DNA or their specific IgG antibodies might be of high value in screening the high risk groups for colorectal cancer. More in-depth research is needed to exploit the association of bacteria with colorectal cancer in terms of early diagnosis of the disease as well as understanding the bacterial carcinogenic potential to determine the appropriate means to prevent and/or treat bacterially-associated cancers.

8. References

Abdulamir, A.S., Hafidh, R.R., Bakar, F.A., (2010). Molecular detection, quantification, and isolation of Streptococcus gallolyticus bacteria colonizing colorectal tumors: inflammation-driven potential of carcinogenesis via IL-1, COX-2, and IL-8. *Mol Cancer*, Vol. 9, No. pp. 249, 1476-4598 (Electronic)1476-4598 (Linking)

Abdulamir, A.S., Hafidh, R.R., Mahdi, L.K., Al-jeboori, T., Abubaker, F., (2009). Investigation into the controversial association of Streptococcus gallolyticus with colorectal cancer and adenoma. *BMC Cancer*, Vol. 9, No. pp. 403, 1471-2407 (Electronic) 1471-2407 (Linking)

Al-Jashamy, K., Murad, A., Zeehaida, M., Rohaini, M., Hasnan, J., (2010). Prevalence of colorectal cancer associated with Streptococcus bovis among inflammatory bowel and chronic gastrointestinal tract disease patients. *Asian Pac J Cancer Prev*, Vol. 11, No. 6, pp. 1765-1768, 1513-7368 (Print) 1513-7368 (Linking)

Balkwill, F., Charles, K.A., Mantovani, A., (2005). Smoldering and polarized inflammation in the initiation and promotion of malignant disease. *Cancer Cell*, Vol. 7, No. 3, pp. 211-217, 1535-6108 (Print) 1535-6108 (Linking)

Baron, J.A., Sandler, R.S., (2000). Nonsteroidal anti-inflammatory drugs and cancer prevention. *Annu Rev Med*, Vol. 51, No. pp. 511-523, 0066-4219 (Print) 0066-4219 (Linking)

Beeching, N.J., Christmas, T.I., Ellis-Pegler, R.B., Nicholson, G.I., (1985). Streptococcus bovis bacteraemia requires rigorous exclusion of colonic neoplasia and endocarditis. *Q J Med*, Vol. 56, No. 220, pp. 439-450, 0033-5622 (Print) 0033-5622 (Linking)

Biarc, J., Nguyen, I.S., Pini, A., Gosse, F., Richert, S., Thierse, D., Van Dorsselaer, A., Leize-Wagner, E., Raul, F., Klein, J.P., Scholler-Guinard, M., (2004). Carcinogenic properties of proteins with pro-inflammatory activity from Streptococcus infantarius (formerly S.bovis). *Carcinogenesis*, Vol. 25, No. 8, pp. 1477-1484, 0143-3334 (Print) 0143-3334 (Linking)

Bisno, A., 12.ed. New York:, (1991). Streptococcal infection. In: *Harrison's principles of internal medicine.* Harrison, T., Stone, R.s (Eds.), pp. 563-569, McGraw-Hill, New York.

Boleij, A., Schaeps, R.M., de Kleijn, S., Hermans, P.W., Glaser, P., Pancholi, V., Swinkels, D.W., Tjalsma, H., (2009b). Surface-exposed histone-like protein a modulates adherence of Streptococcus gallolyticus to colon adenocarcinoma cells. *Infect Immun*, Vol. 77, No. 12, pp. 5519-5527, 1098-5522 (Electronic) 0019-9567 (Linking)

Boleij, A., Schaeps, R.M., Tjalsma, H., (2009a). Association between Streptococcus bovis and colon cancer. *J Clin Microbiol*, Vol. 47, No. 2, pp. 516, 1098-660X (Electronic) 0095-1137 (Linking)

Bond, J.H., (2005). Colon polyps and cancer. *Endoscopy*, Vol. 37, No. 3, pp. 208-212, 0013-726X (Print) 0013-726X (Linking)

Burnie, J.P., Holland, M., Matthews, R.C., Lees, W., (1987). Role of immunoblotting in the diagnosis of culture negative and enterococcal endocarditis. *J Clin Pathol*, Vol. 40, No. 10, pp. 1149-1158, 0021-9746 (Print) 0021-9746 (Linking)

Burns, C.A., McCaughey, R., Lauter, C.B., (1985). The association of Streptococcus bovis fecal carriage and colon neoplasia: possible relationship with polyps and their premalignant potential. *Am J Gastroenterol*, Vol. 80, No. 1, pp. 42-46, 0002-9270 (Print) 0002-9270 (Linking)

Cutait, R., Mansur, A., Habr-Gama, A., (1988). Endocardite por Streptococcus bovis e pólipos de cólon. *Rev Bras Coloproctol*, Vol. 8, No. pp. 109-110,

Dai, Y., Wang, W.H., (2006). Non-steroidal anti-inflammatory drugs in prevention of gastric cancer. *World J Gastroenterol*, Vol. 12, No. 18, pp. 2884-2889, 1007-9327 (Print) 1007-9327 (Linking)

Darjee, R., Gibb, A.P., (1993). Serological investigation into the association between Streptococcus bovis and colonic cancer. *J Clin Pathol*, Vol. 46, No. 12, pp. 1116-1119, 0021-9746 (Print) 0021-9746 (Linking)

Devis, A., Dony, A., De Boelpaepe, F., Verhulst, C., Serste, J.P., (1989). [Streptococcus bovis septicemia and colonic cancer]. *Acta Chir Belg*, Vol. 89, No. 1, pp. 58-60, 0001-5458 (Print) 0001-5458 (Linking)

Devriese, L.A., Vandamme, P., Pot, B., Vanrobaeys, M., Kersters, K., Haesebrouck, F., (1998). Differentiation between Streptococcus gallolyticus strains of human clinical and veterinary origins and Streptococcus bovis strains from the intestinal tracts of ruminants. *J Clin Microbiol*, Vol. 36, No. 12, pp. 3520-3523, 0095-1137 (Print) 0095-1137 (Linking)

Dixon, M.F., Genta, R.M., Yardley, J.H., Correa, P., (1996). Classification and grading of gastritis. The updated Sydney System. International Workshop on the Histopathology of Gastritis, Houston 1994. *Am J Surg Pathol*, Vol. 20, No. 10, pp. 1161-1181, 0147-5185 (Print) 0147-5185 (Linking)

Eisma, R.J., Spiro, J.D., Kreutzer, D.L., (1999). Role of angiogenic factors: coexpression of interleukin-8 and vascular endothelial growth factor in patients with head and neck squamous carcinoma. *Laryngoscope*, Vol. 109, No. 5, pp. 687-693, 0023-852X (Print) 0023-852X (Linking)

El-Omar, E.M., (2006). Role of host genes in sporadic gastric cancer. *Best Pract Res Clin Gastroenterol*, Vol. 20, No. 4, pp. 675-686, 1521-6918 (Print) 1521-6918 (Linking)

Ellmerich, S., Djouder, N., Scholler, M., Klein, J.P., (2000b). Production of cytokines by monocytes, epithelial and endothelial cells activated by Streptococcus bovis. *Cytokine*, Vol. 12, No. 1, pp. 26-31, 1043-4666 (Print) 1043-4666 (Linking)

Ellmerich, S., Scholler, M., Duranton, B., Gosse, F., Galluser, M., Klein, J.P., Raul, F., (2000a). Promotion of intestinal carcinogenesis by Streptococcus bovis. *Carcinogenesis*, Vol. 21, No. 4, pp. 753-756, 0143-3334 (Print) 0143-3334 (Linking)

Ernst, P.B., Peura, D.A., Crowe, S.E., (2006). The translation of Helicobacter pylori basic research to patient care. *Gastroenterology*, Vol. 130, No. 1, pp. 188-206; quiz 212-183, 0016-5085 (Print) 0016-5085 (Linking)

Fagundes, J., Noujain, H., Coy, C., Ayrizono, M., Góes, J., Martinuzzo, W., (2000). Associação entre endocardite bacteriana e neoplasias - relato de 4 casos. *Rev Bras Coloproctol*, Vol. 20, No. pp. 95-99,

Grinberg, M., Mansur, A., Ferreira, D., Bellotti, G., Pileggi, F., (1990). Endocardite por Streptococcus bovis e neoplasias de cólon e reto. *Arq Bras Cardiol*, Vol. 67, No. pp. 265-269,

Groves, C., (1997). Case presentation. *The Jhon Hokins Microbiology Newsletter*, Vol. 16, No. pp. 42-44,

Gupta, A., Madani, R., Mukhtar, H., (2009). Streptococcus bovis endocarditis; a silent sign for colonic tumour. *Colorectal Dis*, Vol., No. pp., 1463-1318 (Electronic) 1462-8910 (Linking)

Haqqani, A.S., Sandhu, J.K., Birnboim, H.C., (2000). Expression of interleukin-8 promotes neutrophil infiltration and genetic instability in mutatect tumors. *Neoplasia*, Vol. 2, No. 6, pp. 561-568, 1522-8002 (Print) 1476-5586 (Linking)

Hirata, Y., Maeda, S., Mitsuno, Y., Akanuma, M., Yamaji, Y., Ogura, K., Yoshida, H., Shiratori, Y., Omata, M., (2001). Helicobacter pylori activates the cyclin D1 gene through mitogen-activated protein kinase pathway in gastric cancer cells. *Infect Immun*, Vol. 69, No. 6, pp. 3965-3971, 0019-9567 (Print) 0019-9567 (Linking)

Hoen, B., Briancon, S., Delahaye, F., Terhe, V., Etienne, J., Bigard, M.A., Canton, P., (1994). Tumors of the colon increase the risk of developing Streptococcus bovis endocarditis: case-control study. *Clin Infect Dis*, Vol. 19, No. 2, pp. 361-362, 1058-4838 (Print) 1058-4838 (Linking)

Hou, L., El-Omar, E.M., Chen, J., Grillo, P., Rabkin, C.S., Baccarelli, A., Yeager, M., Chanock, S.J., Zatonski, W., Sobin, L.H., Lissowska, J., Fraumeni, J.F., Jr., Chow, W.H., (2007). Polymorphisms in Th1-type cell-mediated response genes and risk of gastric cancer. *Carcinogenesis*, Vol. 28, No. 1, pp. 118-123, 0143-3334 (Print) 0143-3334 (Linking)

Ihler, G.M., (1996). Bartonella bacilliformis: dangerous pathogen slowly emerging from deep background. *FEMS Microbiol Lett*, Vol. 144, No. 1, pp. 1-11, 0378-1097 (Print) 0378-1097 (Linking)

Kahveci, A., Ari, E., Arikan, H., Koc, M., Tuglular, S., Ozener, C., (2010). Streptococcus bovis bacteremia related to colon adenoma in a chronic hemodialysis patient. *Hemodial Int*, Vol. 14, No. 1, pp. 91-93, 1542-4758 (Electronic) 1492-7535 (Linking)

Kaplan, M.H., Chmel, H., Stephens, A., Hsieh, H.C., Tenenbaum, M.J., Rothenberg, I.R., Joachim, G.R., (1983). Humoral reactions in human endocarditis due to Streptococcus bovis: evidence for a common S bovis antigen. *J Infect Dis*, Vol. 148, No. 2, pp. 266-274, 0022-1899 (Print) 0022-1899 (Linking)

Kargman, S.L., O'Neill, G.P., Vickers, P.J., Evans, J.F., Mancini, J.A., Jothy, S., (1995). Expression of prostaglandin G/H synthase-1 and -2 protein in human colon cancer. *Cancer Res*, Vol. 55, No. 12, pp. 2556-2559, 0008-5472 (Print) 0008-5472 (Linking)

Karin, M., Greten, F.R., (2005). NF-kappaB: linking inflammation and immunity to cancer development and progression. *Nat Rev Immunol*, Vol. 5, No. 10, pp. 749-759, 1474-1733 (Print) 1474-1733 (Linking)

Kelly, C., Evans, P., Bergmeier, L., Lee, S.F., Progulske-Fox, A., Harris, A.C., Aitken, A., Bleiweis, A.S., Lehner, T., (1989). Sequence analysis of the cloned streptococcal cell surface antigen I/II. *FEBS Lett*, Vol. 258, No. 1, pp. 127-132, 0014-5793 (Print) 0014-5793 (Linking)

Klein, R.S., Catalano, M.T., Edberg, S.C., Casey, J.I., Steigbigel, N.H., (1979). Streptococcus bovis septicemia and carcinoma of the colon. *Ann Intern Med*, Vol. 91, No. 4, pp. 560-562, 0003-4819 (Print) 0003-4819 (Linking)

Kok, H., Jureen, R., Soon, C.Y., Tey, B.H., (2007). Colon cancer presenting as Streptococcus gallolyticus infective endocarditis. *Singapore Med J*, Vol. 48, No. 2, pp. e43-45, 0037-5675 (Print) 0037-5675 (Linking)

Konda, A., Duffy, M.C., (2008). Surveillance of patients at increased risk of colon cancer: inflammatory bowel disease and other conditions. *Gastroenterol Clin North Am*, Vol. 37, No. 1, pp. 191-213, viii, 0889-8553 (Print) 0889-8553 (Linking)

Lasa, M., Abraham, S.M., Boucheron, C., Saklatvala, J., Clark, A.R., (2002). Dexamethasone causes sustained expression of mitogen-activated protein kinase (MAPK) phosphatase 1 and phosphatase-mediated inhibition of MAPK p38. *Mol Cell Biol*, Vol. 22, No. 22, pp. 7802-7811, 0270-7306 (Print) 0270-7306 (Linking)

Lee, R.A., Woo, P.C., To, A.P., Lau, S.K., Wong, S.S., Yuen, K.Y., (2003). Geographical difference of disease association in Streptococcus bovis bacteraemia. *J Med Microbiol*, Vol. 52, No. Pt 10, pp. 903-908, 0022-2615 (Print) 0022-2615 (Linking)

Leport, C., Bure, A., Leport, J., Vilde, J.L., (1987). Incidence of colonic lesions in Streptococcus bovis and enterococcal endocarditis. *Lancet*, Vol. 1, No. 8535, pp. 748, 0140-6736 (Print) 0140-6736 (Linking)

Leung, W.K., (2006). Helicobacter pylori and gastric neoplasia. *Contrib Microbiol*, Vol. 13, No. pp. 66-80, 1420-9519 (Print) 1420-9519 (Linking)

Malkin, J., Kimmitt, P.T., Ou, H.Y., Bhasker, P.S., Khare, M., Deng, Z., Stephenson, I., Sosnowski, A.W., Perera, N., Rajakumar, K., (2008). Identification of Streptococcus gallolyticus subsp. macedonicus as the etiological agent in a case of culture-negative multivalve infective endocarditis by 16S rDNA PCR analysis of resected valvular tissue. *J Heart Valve Dis*, Vol. 17, No. 5, pp. 589-592, 0966-8519 (Print) 0966-8519 (Linking)

Monack, D.M., Mueller, A., Falkow, S., (2004). Persistent bacterial infections: the interface of the pathogen and the host immune system. *Nat Rev Microbiol*, Vol. 2, No. 9, pp. 747-765, 1740-1526 (Print) 1740-1526 (Linking)

Murinello, A., Mendonca, P., Ho, C., Traverse, P., Peres, H., RioTinto, R., Morbey, A., Campos, C., Lazoro, A., Milheiro, A., Arias, M., Oliveira, J., Braz, S., (2006). Streptococcus gallolyticus bacteremia assoaiced with colonic adenmatous polyps. *GE-J-Port Gastrentrol* Vol. 13, No. pp. 152-156,

Murray, H.W., Roberts, R.B., (1978). Streptococcus bovis bacteremia and underlying gastrointestinal disease. *Arch Intern Med*, Vol. 138, No. 7, pp. 1097-1099, 0003-9926 (Print) 0003-9926 (Linking)

Murray, P.R., Baron, E.J., (2007). *Manual of clinical microbiology* (9th). ASM Press, 1555813712 (set) 9781555813710 (set) Washington, D.C.

Nguyen, I., Biarc, J., Pini, A., Gosse, F., Richert, S., Thierse, D., Van Dorsselaer, A., Leize-Wagner, E., Raul, F., Klein, J., Scholler-Guinard, M., (2006). Streptococcus infantarius and colonic cancer: Identification and purification of cell wall proteins putatively involved in colorectal inflammation and carcinogenesis in rats. *International Congress Series* Vol., No. pp. 257- 261,

Nielsen, S.D., Christensen, J.J., Laerkeborg, A., Haunso, S., Knudsen, J.D., (2007). [Molecular-biological methods of diagnosing colon-related Streptococcus bovis endocarditis]. *Ugeskr Laeger*, Vol. 169, No. 7, pp. 610-611, 1603-6824 (Electronic) 0041-5782 (Linking)

Norfleet, R.G., Mitchell, P.D., (1993). Streptococcus bovis does not selectively colonize colorectal cancer and polyps. *J Clin Gastroenterol*, Vol. 17, No. 1, pp. 25-28, 0192-0790 (Print) 0192-0790 (Linking)

Norrby, K., (1996). Interleukin-8 and de novo mammalian angiogenesis. *Cell Prolif*, Vol. 29, No. 6, pp. 315-323, 0960-7722 (Print) 0960-7722 (Linking)

Ohshima, H., Bartsch, H., (1994). Chronic infections and inflammatory processes as cancer risk factors: possible role of nitric oxide in carcinogenesis. *Mutat Res*, Vol. 305, No. 2, pp. 253-264, 0027-5107 (Print) 0027-5107 (Linking)

Osawa, R., Fujisawa, T., LI., S., (1995). Streptococcus gallolyticus sp. nov.: gallate degrading organisms formerly assigned to Streptococcus bovis. *Syst. Appl. Microbiol.*, Vol. 18, No. pp. 74-78,

Potter, M.A., Cunliffe, N.A., Smith, M., Miles, R.S., Flapan, A.D., Dunlop, M.G., (1998). A prospective controlled study of the association of Streptococcus bovis with colorectal carcinoma. *J Clin Pathol*, Vol. 51, No. 6, pp. 473-474, 0021-9746 (Print) 0021-9746 (Linking)

Reynolds, J.G., Silva, E., McCormack, W.M., (1983). Association of Streptococcus bovis bacteremia with bowel disease. *J Clin Microbiol*, Vol. 17, No. 4, pp. 696-697, 0095-1137 (Print) 0095-1137 (Linking)

Ruoff, K.L., Miller, S.I., Garner, C.V., Ferraro, M.J., Calderwood, S.B., (1989). Bacteremia with Streptococcus bovis and Streptococcus salivarius: clinical correlates of more accurate identification of isolates. *J Clin Microbiol*, Vol. 27, No. 2, pp. 305-308, 0095-1137 (Print) 0095-1137 (Linking)

Schlegel, L., Grimont, F., Ageron, E., Grimont, P.A., Bouvet, A., (2003). Reappraisal of the taxonomy of the Streptococcus bovis/Streptococcus equinus complex and related species: description of Streptococcus gallolyticus subsp. gallolyticus subsp. nov., S. gallolyticus subsp. macedonicus subsp. nov. and S. gallolyticus subsp. pasteurianus subsp. nov. *Int J Syst Evol Microbiol*, Vol. 53, No. Pt 3, pp. 631-645, 1466-5026 (Print) 1466-5026 (Linking)

Shacter, E., Weitzman, S.A., (2002). Chronic inflammation and cancer. *Oncology (Williston Park)*, Vol. 16, No. 2, pp. 217-226, 229; discussion 230-212, 0890-9091 (Print) 0890-9091 (Linking)

Sillanpaa, J., Nallapareddy, S.R., Qin, X., Singh, K.V., Muzny, D.M., Kovar, C.L., Nazareth, L.V., Gibbs, R.A., Ferraro, M.J., Steckelberg, J.M., Weinstock, G.M., Murray, B.E., (2009). A collagen-binding adhesin, Acb, and ten other putative MSCRAMM and pilus family proteins of Streptococcus gallolyticus subsp. gallolyticus (Streptococcus bovis Group, biotype I). *J Bacteriol*, Vol. 191, No. 21, pp. 6643-6653, 1098-5530 (Electronic) 0021-9193 (Linking)

Sillanpaa, J., Nallapareddy, S.R., Singh, K.V., Ferraro, M.J., Murray, B.E., (2008). Adherence characteristics of endocarditis-derived Streptococcus gallolyticus ssp. gallolyticus (Streptococcus bovis biotype I) isolates to host extracellular matrix proteins. *FEMS Microbiol Lett*, Vol. 289, No. 1, pp. 104-109, 0378-1097 (Print) 0378-1097 (Linking)

Smaali, I., Bachraoui, K., Joulek, A., Selmi, K., Boujnah, M.R., (2008). [Infectious endocarditis secondary to streptococcus bovis revealing adenomatous polyposis coli]. *Tunis Med*, Vol. 86, No. 7, pp. 723-724, 0041-4131 (Print) 0041-4131 (Linking)

Smith, D.G., Lawson, G.H., (2001). Lawsonia intracellularis: getting inside the pathogenesis of proliferative enteropathy. *Vet Microbiol*, Vol. 82, No. 4, pp. 331-345, 0378-1135 (Print) 0378-1135 (Linking)

Srivastava, S., Verma, M., Henson, D.E., (2001). Biomarkers for early detection of colon cancer. *Clin Cancer Res*, Vol. 7, No. 5, pp. 1118-1126, 1078-0432 (Print) 1078-0432 (Linking)

Tafte, L., Ruoff, K., (2007). Streptococcus bovis: Answers and Questions. *Clin microbial newslett*, Vol. 29, No. pp. 49-55,

Teitelbaum, J.E., Triantafyllopoulou, M., (2006). Inflammatory bowel disease and Streptococcus bovis. *Dig Dis Sci*, Vol. 51, No. 8, pp. 1439-1442, 0163-2116 (Print) 0163-2116 (Linking)

Tjalsma, H., Scholler-Guinard, M., Lasonder, E., Ruers, T.J., Willems, H.L., Swinkels, D.W., (2006). Profiling the humoral immune response in colon cancer patients: diagnostic antigens from Streptococcus bovis. *Int J Cancer*, Vol. 119, No. 9, pp. 2127-2135, 0020-7136 (Print) 0020-7136 (Linking)

Travers, P., Rosen, F.S., 1997. Immuno biology bookshelf the comprehensive resource on CD-ROM. Current Biology; Garland Pub., [London ; San Francisco] [New York], pp. 1 CD-ROM.

Vogelmann, R., Amieva, M.R., (2007). The role of bacterial pathogens in cancer. *Curr Opin Microbiol*, Vol. 10, No. 1, pp. 76-81, 1369-5274 (Print) 1369-5274 (Linking)

Waisberg, J., Matheus Cde, O., Pimenta, J., (2002). Infectious endocarditis from Streptococcus bovis associated with colonic carcinoma: case report and literature review. *Arq Gastroenterol*, Vol. 39, No. 3, pp. 177-180, 0004-2803 (Print) 0004-2803 (Linking)

Wang, D., Dubois, R.N., (2010). The role of COX-2 in intestinal inflammation and colorectal cancer. *Oncogene*, Vol. 29, No. 6, pp. 781-788, 1476-5594 (Electronic) 0950-9232 (Linking)

Wentling, G.K., Metzger, P.P., Dozois, E.J., Chua, H.K., Krishna, M., (2006). Unusual bacterial infections and colorectal carcinoma--Streptococcus bovis and Clostridium septicum: report of three cases. *Dis Colon Rectum*, Vol. 49, No. 8, pp. 1223-1227, 0012-3706 (Print) 0012-3706 (Linking)

Wilson, W.R., Thompson, R.L., Wilkowske, C.J., Washington, J.A., 2nd, Giuliani, E.R., Geraci, J.E., (1981). Short-term therapy for streptococcal infective endocarditis. Combined intramuscular administration of penicillin and streptomycin. *JAMA*, Vol. 245, No. 4, pp. 360-363, 0098-7484 (Print) 0098-7484 (Linking)

Zarkin, B.A., Lillemoe, K.D., Cameron, J.L., Effron, P.N., Magnuson, T.H., Pitt, H.A., (1990). The triad of Streptococcus bovis bacteremia, colonic pathology, and liver disease. *Ann Surg*, Vol. 211, No. 6, pp. 786-791; discussion 791-782, 0003-4932 (Print) 0003-4932 (Linking)

zur Hausen, H., (2006). Streptococcus bovis: causal or incidental involvement in cancer of the colon? *Int J Cancer*, Vol. 119, No. 9, pp. xi-xii, 0020-7136 (Print) 0020-7136 (Linking)

18

Intestinal Host-Microbiome Interactions

Harold Tjalsma and Annemarie Boleij
Department of Laboratory Medicine, Nijmegen Institute for Infection, Inflammation and Immunity (N4i) & Radboud University Centre for Oncology (RUCO) of the Radboud University Nijmegen Medical Centre, The Netherlands

1. Introduction

A human body contains at least tenfold more bacteria cells than human cells and the most abundant and diverse microbial community (also known as microbiota or microbiome) resides in the large intestine (colon). It is estimated that this colonic microbiome is composed of ~10^{14} bacterial cells, comprising >10^3 species (Dethlefsen *et al.*, 2006; Qin *et al.*, 2010). Intestinal microbiomes differ from individual to individual but remain relatively stable during adult life (Green *et al.*, 2006; Arumugam *et al.*, 2011). The resident microbiome provides the host with core functions that are essential for digestion of food and control of intestinal epithelial homeostasis. Conversely, an increasing body of evidence supports a relationship between infective agents and human colorectal cancer (CRC) by production of DNA damaging metabolites or toxins, and the induction of cell proliferation and pro-carcinogenesis pathways by a subpopulation of the intestinal microbiota. It could be speculated that the intrinsic intestinal microbiome of a certain individual may contain an unfavorable number of disease-inducing bacteria. On the long term, their activities may override the health-promoting activities of the commensal bacterial population. On the other hand, the dramatic physiological alterations that result from colon carcinogenesis itself (Hirayama *et al.*, 2009) disturbs the local intestinal microenvironment and causes (local) shifts in the microbiota composition and provides a portal of infection for certain opportunistic pathogens. The latter phenomenon could explain why some uncommon bacterial infections are often associated with CRC. In this chapter we will discuss the mechanisms by which intestinal bacteria may drive the initiation and progression of sporadic CRC, but also the driving forces of intestinal carcinogenesis on local microbial dysbiosis and the consequences thereof will be reviewed.

2. Intestinal microbiome

The colonic epithelium is the first line of defense against enteric antigens and bacteria. In a healthy colon, the epithelial barrier regulates uptake of nutrients and limits uptake of potential toxic substances and infectious agents (Chichlowski & Hale, 2008). Goblet cells are specialized epithelial cells within the mucosa that produce a viscous mucus layer that covers the intestinal epithelium (Heazlewood *et al.*, 2008). This mucus layer is thick and consists of an inner firmly attached layer, that excludes bacteria from direct contact with the underlying mucosa, and an outer loose mucus layer that mainly functions as lubricant (Atuma *et al.*, 2001). Bacterial colonization of the gastrointestinal tract occurs during the first two years of life. After this period, the microbiota composition is rather stable throughout adulthood (Dethlefsen *et al.*, 2006). Nevertheless, it is likely that the colonic microbiota transiently respond to dietary intake and host physiology (Thompson-Chagoyan *et al.*, 2007). The inter-individual microbiomes differ consistently, however, it is thought that these different marked microbiota may perform similar functions, and genetically complement their host with crucial physiological functions that are not provided by the human genome itself (Candela *et al.* 2010; Gill *et al.*, 2006; Neish, 2009; O'Hara & Shanahan, 2006; Xu *et al.*, 2007). Intestinal microbiome-specific metabolic functions increase energy yield and storage from diet, regulate fat storage and generate essential vitamins, which are primarily due to the fermentation of indigestible dietary polysaccharides (Neish, 2009). It has been shown that mucosa-associated bacteria differ from the community recovered from feces, but are rather uniformly distributed throughout the colon (Green *et al.*, 2006; Macfarlane *et al.*, 2004; Zoetendal *et al.*, 2002). This mucosa-adherent population is less prone to physiological effects, such as dietary changes (Sonnenburg *et al.*, 2004), and prohibits colonization of intruding pathogens (Stecher & Hardt, 2008). Malfunctioning of the host epithelial defense mechanisms, increases the risk for bacterial infection and intestinal inflammation, as seen in patients with inflammatory bowel disease (IBD). Intestinal disease can also be directly triggered by enteropathogenic pathogens, like *Shigella*, *Citrobacter* and *Salmonella* species, that avail of virulence mechanisms that allows them to outcompete the commensal mucosa-associated bacterial population and to breach the mucosal barrier and intestinal innate immune system (Stecher *et al.*, 2007).

3. Bacterial promotion of CRC

The genetic background of the host together with dietary intake, influences the microbial composition in the gut. However progression of CRC itself also influences the gut barrier and micro-environment in the intestine. This dynamic interplay between environment, genetic and microbial influences makes it hard to dissect the exact contribution of the microbiota in the development and progression of CRC. In the next paragraphs, the mechanisms by which the intestinal microbiota could contribute to CRC are further discussed. The significance of the intestinal microbiome on the development of CRC is probably best illustrated by the fact that patients with IBD, which originates from an altered host response to a normal intestinal bacterial population (Round & Mazmanian, 2009), have a high predisposition for CRC (Macfarlane *et al.*, 2005).

3.1 Promotion of tumorigenesis

The effect of intestinal bacteria on CRC development has been studied in the intestinal neoplasia mouse model (*Apc*$^{min/+}$). This mutant mouse strain carries a heterozygous mutation in the *APC* locus (Moser *et al.*, 1990), meaning that only a single hit in the wild-type allele results in adenoma formation. Studies with germ-free *Apc*$^{min/+}$ mice revealed that the formation of adenomas was strongly reduced by as much as 50%, compared to mice bred under conventional conditions (Dove *et al.*, 1997; Moser *et al.*, 1990; Su *et al.*, 1992). When such mice were exposed to enterotoxigenic *Bacteroides fragilis* (ETBF), tumors developed more rapidly, whereas mice colonized with non-toxigenic *Bacteroides fragilis*

(NTBF) showed no increased tumor formation compared to conventional mice (Housseau & Sears, 2010).
These data clearly show that the intestinal microbial population has a strong promoting effect on tumor progression in mice that have a genetic predisposition for developing intestinal adenomas and that certain species within the intestinal microbiota contribute more than average to this process.

3.2 Stimulation of TLR signaling

A balanced immune stimulation to commensal and pathogenic bacteria is crucial for a healthy intestinal tract. Toll-like receptors (TLRs) are proteins that activate immune responses towards potentially harmful pathogens upon sensing of pathogenic substances, such as cell wall components. However, chronic overstimulation of these responses may be detrimental by leading to the initiation and progression of CRC (Fukata & Abreu, 2007).
A direct impact of bacteria on the development of CRC through the TLR5/MyD88 pathway was demonstrated in germ-free and gnotobiotic mice. These animal experiments revealed that *MyD88*$^{-/-}$ knock-out mice that were treated with the carcinogen azoxymethane (AOM) failed to develop colorectal tumors when these mice were subjected to bacteria. In contrast, control mice rapidly developed CRC upon bacterial colonization of their intestinal tract. These results implicate that TLR/MyD88 signaling is a prerequisite for the development of CRC (Uronis *et al.*, 2009). In addition, it was shown that tumors in *Apc*$^{min/+}$ *MyD88*$^{-/-}$ mice were significantly smaller than those found in *Apc*$^{min/+}$ mice (Rakoff-Nahoum & Medzhitov, 2007). Another study showed that *TLR4*$^{-/-}$ mice were partly protected against the development of neoplasia by tumor-inducing chemical agents (Killeen *et al.*, 2009). Additional evidence was presented that TLR4 signaling can promote colon carcinogenesis by stimulating tumor infiltration of Th17 cells (T-helper cell subset that produces IL-17) through the increased production of pro-inflammatory signals (Su *et al.*, 2010). It can be envisaged that bacterial TLR4 ligands, such as LPS, play an important role in this increased chemotactic activity of tumor cells (Scanlan *et al.*, 2008). Importantly, Th17 cells have directly been implicated in the pathogenesis of Enterotoxigenic *Bacteroides fragilis*-induced CRC (Housseau & Sears, 2010; Wu *et al.*, 2009). Thus, although TLR signaling is important for the effective clearance of harmful pathogens and can mediate anti-tumor cell responses, chronic TLR activation may tip the delicate balance towards tumor-promoting activities (Rakoff-Nahoum & Medzhitov, 2009).
Altogether, the above mentioned studies indicate that chronic bacterial stimulation of inflammatory pathways at malignant sites promotes, and may even be a prerequisite for, intestinal tumor development.

3.3 Upregulation of COX-2

Cyclooxygenase-2 (COX-2) is one of the key players in the progression of CRC. The expression of COX-2 is highly elevated in colonic tumors and correlated with disease stage and stimulates cell proliferation and pro-inflammatory pathways by the production of prostaglandins (Menter *et al.*, 2010). Human intervention studies have clearly shown that the usage of Non-Steroidal Anti-Inflammatory Drugs (NSAIDS) can reduce CRC risk by as much as 75% (Eaden *et al.*, 2000; Labayle *et al.*, 1991; Thun *et al.*, 1991). Evidence for bacterial involvement in the upregulation of COX-2 during CRC development was gained through animal and *in vitro* studies. First, superoxide radicals produced by *Enterococcus faecalis* were shown to upregulate the expression of COX-2 in hybrid hamster cells containing human chromosomes, as well as in macrophages (Wang & Huycke, 2007). Furthermore, macrophages that were pre-treated with a COX-2 inhibitor and subsequently exposed to *E. faecalis* totally inhibited the induction of chromosome instability (CIN) in these hybrid hamster cells. Second, an animal study published by Ellmerich *et al.* (2000b) indicated that *Streptococcus bovis* biotype II.1 (*Streptococcus infantarius*) could also play a role in the progression of CRC through induction of the COX-2 pathway. These investigators employed a rat model in which pre-treatment with azoxymethane (AOM) induced pre-neoplastic aberrant crypt foci (ACF). When such rats were co-exposed to *S. infantarius* or cell wall antigens from this bacterium, the number of ACF increased drastically and also adenomas were found, whereas the latter were totally absent in the control mice treated with AOM alone. In addition, the production of the pro-inflammatory cytokine IL-8 in the mucosa of rats exposed to *S. infantarius* was increased. This finding is in accordance with *in vitro* studies on epithelial Caco-2 cells that release both IL-8 and PGE2 upon incubation with *S. infantarius* (Biarc *et al.*, 2004). Moreover, Abdulamir *et al.* (2010) have recently shown that increased COX-2 and IL-8 expression was associated with the presence of *Streptococcus gallolyticus* (*S. bovis* biotype I) in human colon tumor tissue. However, IL-8 expression was not increased in non-malignant tissue that contained *S. gallolyticus.* Together these studies indicate that COX-2 induction is associated with both tumor development and exposure to bacterial stimulants.

3.4 Toxin-induced promotion of cell proliferation

Enterotoxigenic *Bacteroides fragilis* (ETBF) has been implicated in the promotion of CRC through inflammatory pathways. *B. fragilis* is a normal inhabitant of the gastrointestinal tract, but its enterotoxigenic form is only present in approximately 20% of the healthy population (Sears, 2009). ETBF produces the *B. fragilis* toxin that degrades E-cadherin in epithelial cells, which causes β-catenin to migrate towards the nucleus where it can activate cell proliferation pathways (Wu *et al.*, 2003). Consequently, *APC*$^{min/+}$ mice colonized with ETBF were shown to suffer from increased tumor burden compared to control mice colonized with non-toxigenic *B. fragilis* (NTBF) strains (Housseau & Sears, 2010; Wu *et al.*, 2009). Importantly, Wu *et al* (2009). showed that this increased tumor burden was mediated through the increased expression of STAT3 that leads to a Th17 response. Importantly, increased tumor formation could be blocked by anti-IL17 therapy. These experiments clearly show that induction of a STAT3/Th17-dependent pathway for inflammation, leads to inflammation-induced cancer by ETBF in a mouse model. Since ETBF is a quite common bacterium in the gastro-intestinal tract, this finding could have major implications for the role of these bacteria in the development of CRC in the human population. This idea is further corroborated by the fact that patients with CRC have indeed increased carriage rates of ETBF compared to NTBF (Toprak *et al.*, 2006). It should be realized that this mechanism of tumor induction could also be associated with other toxigenic intestinal bacterial strains.

3.5 Toxin-induced DNA damage

Certain *E. coli* strains can induce increased mutation rates in eukaryotic cells as demonstrated by Cuevas-Ramos and colleagues (2010). Their experiments showed that *E. coli* strains harboring the *pks* island caused DNA damage in human epithelial cells and in an *ex vivo* mouse intestinal model by the induction of single strand breaks and activation of DNA damage signaling pathways. The *pks* gene cluster codes for nonribosomal peptide synthetases and polyketide synthetases (pks) that synthesize a genotoxin named Colibactin. The *pks* island is commonly present in about 34% of commensal *E. coli* isolates. Upon infection of epithelial cells with physiological concentrations of *pks*$^+$ strains, initial DNA damage occurred. Furthermore, it was shown that cells continued to proliferate in the presence of DNA damage after *E. coli* infection, resulting in an increased mutation frequency (Cuevas-Ramos *et al.*, 2010). These studies suggest that *pks*$^+$ strains of *E. coli* could be involved in the initiation and progression of CRC. As, *E. coli* is generally regarded as a normal commensal inhabitant of the gastro-intestinal tract, Bronowski and co-workers investigated the differences between *E. coli* strains collected from healthy individuals and CRC patients (Bronowski *et al.*, 2008). These experiments showed that a subset of *E. coli* strains recovered from CRC tissue shared pathogenicity islands, encoding an alfa haemolysin and a cytotoxic necrotizing factor, with uropathogenic *E. coli* strains. This suggests that besides Colibactin production, other virulence characteristics may also mediate the tumor promoting capacity of *E. coli pks*$^+$ strains.

3.6 Metabolite-induced DNA damage

Sulfate reducing bacteria use sulfate as energy source by converting it to sulfide and hydrogen sulfide (H_2S) in the human colon. The genotoxic potential of H_2S is in part mediated by oxidative free radicals, which results in increased levels of DNA damage in cultured epithelial cells (Attene-Ramos *et al.*, 2006; Attene-Ramos *et al.*, 2007; Attene-Ramos *et al.*, 2010). Furthermore, exposure to H_2S may disrupt the balance between apoptosis, proliferation and differentiation (Cai *et al.*, 2010; Deplancke & Gaskins, 2003). Interestingly, also COX-2 was shown to be upregulated in epithelial cells after H_2S treatment at physiological concentrations, probably through generation of reactive oxygen species (Attene-Ramos *et al.*, 2010). Increased fecal H_2S concentration was implicated as a risk factor for the development of colonic neoplasia in a clinical study (Kanazawa *et al.*, 1996). Whether these increased H_2S levels originates from increased activity of sulfate reducing bacteria and/or reduced epithelial capacity to degrade H_2S remains to be investigated.

E. faecalis was also found to produce extracellular superoxide in colonic tissue of rats, which is the result of dysfunctional microbial respiration (Huycke *et al.*, 2002). These rats produced up to 25-fold increased concentrations of hydroxylated aromatic metabolites in urine than rats colonized with a closely-related strain. Importantly, superoxide can be converted to hydrogen peroxide, which has the potential to diffuse into epithelial cells and cause DNA damage. In an *in vitro* setup, it was shown that the formation of DNA adducts by *E. faecalis* was mediated by activated COX-2 expression in macrophages that in turn promoted DNA damage in epithelial target cells (Wang & Huycke, 2007; Wang *et al.*, 2008). Since COX-2 induction has a clear clinical association with CRC, this might indicate that superoxide-producing bacteria have a contributing role in disease development. This notion is further underscored by the finding that *E. faecalis* fecal carriage was increased in CRC patients, whereas the number of butyrate producing bacteria was decreased (Balamurugan *et al.*, 2008). However, no clinical evidence has been presented that associates superoxide producing enterococci with adenomas or CRC (Winters *et al.*, 1998). This clearly indicates that, although the *in vitro* data and animal studies strongly suggest that oxygen radicals from bacterial origin could play an important role in CRC initiation or progression, the

clinical impact of these findings remains to be properly examined in well-designed clinical studies (Huycke & Gaskins, 2004).
Bacteroides species produce fecapentaenes that are potent mutagens that have been shown to alkylate DNA, which leads to mutagenic adducts. Some evidence points towards a mechanism in which oxygen radicals cause oxidative damage to DNA (Hinzman *et al.*, 1987; Povey *et al.*, 1991; Shioya *et al.*, 1989). Fecapentaenes appear in relatively high concentrations in human feces, however, no significant differences in fecapentaene levels were found in feces from CRC patients and controls (Schiffman *et al.*, 1989). In view of their mutagenic potential, however, fecapentaenes should be regarded as possible bacterial inducers of CRC (de Kok & van Maanen, 2000). For instance, their detrimental effects may locally contribute to the accumulation of mutations in epithelial cells, which is not directly reflected by the increased levels in fecal material.

3.7 Induction of pro-carcinogenic pathways

Some evidence exists that certain intestinal bacteria can also directly induce host epithelial pathways that make cells more susceptible to DNA damage by carcinogenic substances. Maddocks *et al.* (2009) have shown that enteropathogenic *E. coli* can down-regulate mismatch repair genes in colon epithelial cells. It may be envisaged that this impaired expression can lead to a net increased mutation rate upon co-exposure to genotoxic dietary compounds. This study accentuates that bacteria can directly interfere with gene expression in epithelial cells which, under certain conditions, may lead to increased carcinogenesis rates.

4. CRC microbiome

The preceding paragraphs describe the potential mechanisms by which bacteria can play a role in the initiation and progression of CRC. In the following paragraphs, the effects of colonic malignancies on the (local) microbial composition are discussed. It is evident that the dramatic physiological and metabolic alterations that result from colon carcinogenesis itself (Hirayama et al., 2009) will locally disturb the intestinal environment. Consequently, this will cause (local) shifts in microbiota composition as the altered tumor metabolites and intestinal physiology will recruit a bacterial population with a competitive advantage in this specific microenvironment. This is exemplified by the fact that infections with certain opportunistic intestinal pathogens have been associated with CRC for many years (see Section 5). Thus pre-malignant sites seem to constitute a preferred niche for a subset of intestinal bacteria and facilitate their outgrowth and eventually entry into the human body. Importantly, local outgrowth of harmful bacteria could also accelerate tumor progression after disease has been initiated by other factors.
The effect of colonic tumors on the microbiome composition has been investigated by several studies. First, Scanlan *et al.* (2008) investigated the bacterial diversity in healthy, polypectomized patients with increased risk for CRC and CRC patients. These studies showed a significant increased diversity of the *Clostridium leptum* and coccoides subgroups in the CRC patients compared to a healthy control group. Importantly, metabonomic faecal water analysis was able to distinguish CRC and polypectomized patients from healthy individuals, which is indicative for an altered metabolic activity of the intestinal microbiota

in these patients. In another study by Maddocks *et al.* (2009) it was shown that the mucosa of adenomas and carcinomas contained increased numbers of *E. coli* compared to colonic mucosa from healthy controls. It was speculated that certain surface antigens on tumor cells, which display homology to surface antigens of fetal origin, may be responsible for the binding of *E. coli* and thus local recruitment of these bacterial strains (Martin *et al.*, 2004; Maddocks *et al.*, 2009; Swidsinski *et al.*, 1998). A similar relation has been described for the opportunistic pathogen *Streptococcus bovis*. This bacterium is thought to selectively colonize malignant and pre-malignant colonic sites by which it can cause systemic infections in susceptible individuals (see Section 5). Some contradicting results on actual *S. bovis* colonization of tumor tissue have, however, been reported. Conventional culturing techniques to determine the carriage rate of *S. bovis* in adenoma, carcinoma and healthy biopsies did not provide clear evidence for the selective colonization of adenomas or carcinomas by this bacterium (Norfleet & Mitchell, 1993; Potter et al., 1998). More recently, Abdulamir and co-workers showed the presence of *Streptococcus gallolyticus* (*S. bovis* biotype I) DNA in carcinoma and adenoma tissue via polymerase chain reaction (PCR)-based techniques, which are more sensitive than conventional culturing techniques. DNA from *S. gallolyticus* was detected in about 50% of the tumor biopsies and in 35% of off- tumor tissue samples from the same patients. Strikingly, however, *S. gallolyticus* DNA was only found in <5% of the colonic tissue samples of healthy control subjects (Abdulamir *et al.*, 2010). More recently, several studies have assessed the bacterial communities in healthy, adenoma and CRC tissue by deep 16S ribosomal DNA sequencing approaches. Shen and colleagues compared the bacterial composition in normal tissue samples from adenoma patients and from individuals without colon abnormalities. The data showed increased levels of proteobacteria and decreased bacteroidetes species in off- tumor tissue samples from adenoma patients (Shen *et al.*, 2010). Interestingly, Sobhani *et al.* (2011) reported that the abundance of Bacteroides was significantly increased in tumor and normal tissue of cancer patients compared to healthy controls. More importantly, the abundance of Bacteroides was higher in tumor tissue of cancer patients than adjacent off-tumor tissue, which was paralleled by an increased IL-17/CD3 immune cell infiltration in the malignant tissues. Another recent study by Marchesi *et al.* (2011), compared differences in healthy and cancerous tissue within cancer patients and found that tumor tissue was overrepresented by species of the genera *Coriobacteridae, Roseburia, Fusobacterium* and *Faecalibacterium* that are generally regarded as gut commensals with probiotic features. On the contrary, this study found decreased colonization of *Enterobacteriaceae,* such as *Citrobacter, Shigella, Cronobacter,* and *Salmonella* in adjacent off- tumor mucosa from the same investigated patients.

The development of colorectal tumors is schematically depicted from left to right. Initiation of carcinogenesis is a process in which many factors are involved. As discussed in this Chapter, certain bacterial pathogens, bacterial toxins, or bacterial toxic metabolites (**1**) may contribute to the initiation and progression of CRC by causing DNA damage, induction of COX-2/IL-8, TLR signalling and/or cell proliferation pathways (**2**). Consequently, the altered metabolic profile of colon tumor cells and/or differentially expression of bacterial receptor molecules on tumor cells (**3**) creates a new niche that recruits a different bacterial population (**4**) of which certain opportunistic pathogens can eventually breach the bowel wall and cause a systemic bacterial infection (**5**). The latter group of bacteria may play an important signalling function for the early detection of CRC by serological assays.

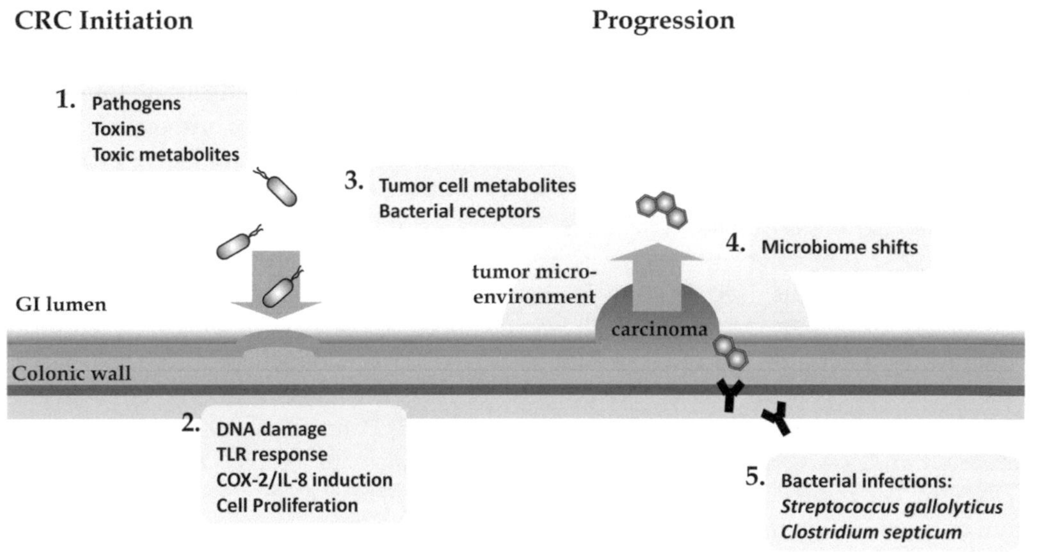

Fig. 1. Host-Microbiome interactions during CRC

5. CRC-associated bacterial infections

5.1 Streptococcus bovis

The most extensively studied bacterium that has a well-appreciated association with CRC concerns *Streptococcus bovis*. McCoy and Mason first reported such a case in 1951 (McCoy & Mason, 1951). In the 1970's this association was re-discovered by Hoppes and Lerner, who reported that 64% of the *S. bovis* endocarditis cases had gastrointestinal disease (Hoppes & Lerner, 1974). A few years later, Klein *et al.* (1977) reported an increased incidence of CRC in patients with *S. bovis* endocarditis. These investigators additionally discovered that fecal carriage of *S. bovis* in CRC patients was increased about 5-fold compared to healthy controls. At the time, these findings led to the recommendation to perform colonic evaluation in patients that were diagnosed with an *S. bovis* infection. Over the years, many studies have confirmed the association between *S. bovis* infection and CRC. In these studies, the prevalence of *S. bovis* infection with underlying CRC ranged from 10 - 100% (median 60%) for patients that underwent colonic evaluation (Boleij *et al.*, 2011b).

5.1.1 Streptococcus bovis biotypes

Based on phenotypic diversity, *S. bovis* was previously divided into three biotypes I, II.1 and II.2. Of these biotypes, biotype I is most often associated with endocarditis, while biotype II is mostly found in cases of bacteremia or liver disease. Strikingly, the association between *S. bovis* biotype I infection and CRC (21- 71%) is much higher then that of *S. bovis* biotype II (11-30%) (Corredoira *et al.*, 2008; Corredoira *et al.*, 2005; Giannitsioti *et al.*, 2007; Herrero *et al.*, 2002; Jean *et al.*, 2004; Lee *et al.*, 2003; Ruoff *et al.*, 1989; Vaska & Faoagali, 2009)(Beck *et al.*, 2008; Tripodi *et al.*, 2004). In fact, the reported incidences of carcinomas and adenomas in *S. bovis* biotype II infected patients are within the range for the normal asymptomatic population (0.3% for carcinomas / 10-25% for adenomas), whereas the rates for *S. bovis* biotype I were significantly increased (Lieberman & Smith, 1991; Lieberman *et al.*, 2000; Spier *et al.*, 2010). The distinct association of these different *S. bovis* biotypes with CRC may have accounted for the wide range of association percentages that have been reported over the years in literature. More importantly, because most studies have not discriminated between *S. bovis* biotypes the association between *S. bovis* biotype I and CRC may have structurally been underestimated. It is important to note that Schlegel *et al.* (2003) suggested renaming *S. bovis* biotype I into *S. gallolyticus* subsp. *gallolyticus*, *S. bovis* biotype II/1 into *S. infantarius* subsp. *coli* or *S. infantarius* subsp. *infantarius* and to rename *S. bovis* biotype II/2 into *S. gallolyticus* subsp. *pasteurianus*. This new nomenclature should be used to better discriminate between the different *S. bovis* subspecies of which *S. gallolyticus* is the only species with an unambiguous association with CRC (Boleij *et al.*, 2011b).

5.1.2 Streptococcus gallolyticus

Recently, some striking differences between *S. bovis* biotypes were revealed that could explain their different association rates with CRC. First of all, *S. gallolyticus* seems to contain distinguished mechanisms to adherence to extracellular matrix (ECM) structures like collagen and fibrinogen (Ellmerich *et al.*, 2000a; Sillanpaa *et al.*, 2008; Sillanpaa *et al.*, 2009). Interestingly, (pre-)malignant colonic sites are characterized by displaced collagen of the lamina propria (Galbavy *et al.*, 2002; Yantiss *et al.*, 2001), through which specifically *S. gallolyticus* may colonize these sites. Besides the ECM components, also other structures at the epithelial surface may play a role in the initial adhesion to enterocytes. For example, Henry-Stanley *et al.* (2003) reported binding of *S. bovis* strains to heparan sulfate proteoglycans, which may be mediated by surface-associated HlpA (Boleij *et al.*, 2009). In an *in vitro* trans-well model containing a differentiated intestinal monolayer, the paracellular translocation efficiency of *S. gallolyticus* was shown to be significantly higher than that of other *S. bovis* biotypes. This could mean that this bacterium has an advantage over other *S. bovis* subspecies to cross an intestinal epithelium, which possibly only occurs at (pre-)malignant sites with reduced barrier function (Boleij *et al.*, 2011a). Recent data suggested that *S. gallolyticus* does not induce a strong pro-inflammatory IL-8 response in epithelial cells in contrast to other *S. bovis* strains, which may be a possibly mechanism by which *S. gallolyticus* stays rather invisible for macrophages in the lamina propria. Furthermore, Hirota *et al.* (1995) discovered that *S. gallolyticus* isolates from endocarditis patients, express human sialyl Lewis^x antigens on their cell surface unlike other fecal isolates. Mimicking human sialyl antigens, which are naturally present on monocytes and granulocutes, could therefore be a second mechanism of *S. gallolyticus* to remain unnoticed by the human innate immune system. Moreover, sialyl Lewis^x antigens could make these bacteria more efficient in binding to endothelial cells and invasion into the circulatory system (Hirota *et al.*, 1996). Finally, *S. gallolyticus* was shown to have superior efficiency to form biofilms on collagen I and IV surfaces (Boleij *et al.*, 2011a; Sillanpaa *et al.*, 2008). The latter finding could explain the increased incidence of *S. gallolyticus* as causative agent in infective endocarditis. Based on the current state-of-the-literature (July 2011), the following events in CRC-associated *S. gallolyticus* endocarditis can be envisaged **i)** *S. gallolyticus* specifically adheres to (pre-)malignant colonic sites for instance via binding to displaced collagen of the lamina propria or other tumor cell specific adherence factors; **ii)** *S. gallolyticus* may promote tumor progression by induction of the COX-2 pathway; **iii)** *S. gallolyticus* takes advantage of the distorted structure of the colonic epithelium at (pre-)malignant sites to pass the colonic wall; **iv)** *S. gallolyticus* stays relatively invisible for the innate immune system and can reach the blood stream; **v)** *S. gallolyticus* can cause a secondary infection at sites with high exposure of collagens, such as present at damaged heart values. It should be noted, however, that many of these data were obtained by *in vitro* studies and that it remains to be determined how this relates to the *in vivo* situation.

5.2 Clostridium septicum

In addition to *S. gallolyticus* endocarditis, also *Clostridium septicum* infections have been clinically associated with sporadic CRC (Chew & Lubowski, 2001; Mirza *et al.*, 2009). *C. septicum* is not considered to be part of the normal intestinal microbiota and is a rare cause of bacteremia (<1% of all cases). Hermsen *et al.* (2008) investigated 320 cases of *C. septicum* infections, 42% of which had a gastrointestinal origin. Malignant disease was present in 30-50% of these cases. The underlying mechanism of this association is not known, but it has been speculated that the hypoxic and acidic environment of the tumor specifically favor germination of *C. septicum* spores that enter the gastrointestinal tract via contaminated food (Dylewski & Luterman). A direct involvement of *C. septicum* in the development of CRC has thus far not been investigated, but it is hypothesized that *C. septicum* infections are primarily a consequence of CRC itself. Also *Clostridium perfringens* and *Clostridium butyricum* have been described in relation with CRC (Cabrera *et al.*, 1965; Rathbun, 1968). However, these strains are much less virulent than *C. septicum* and their association with CRC is less evident. Although infections with *C. septicum* are rare, underlying malignancy should be suspected and also in these cases full bowel examination could eventually save patients' lives.

5.3 Helicobacter pylori

Helicobacter pylori has been classified as gastric cancer-causing infective agent by the International Agency for Research on Cancer (IARC) in 1994. Most *H. pylori* strains, however, are non-invasive organism and exist in a non-adherent extracellular mucous environment. A small number of strains adheres to gastric epithelial cells, which most likely involves a number of different surface receptors (Wilkinson *et al.*, 1998). The presence of the pathogenicity island, expressing the cytotoxins VacA and CagA, is an important virulence determinant in these strains (Ekstrom *et al.*, 2001; Huang *et al.*, 2003; Crabtree *et al.*, 1994; Kuipers *et al.*, 1995). It is thought that long-term exposure to these toxins induces gastric inflammation that can eventually lead to gastric carcinomas (Higashi *et al.*, 2002; Fox, 2002). A meta-analysis conducted in 2006 by Zumkeller *et al.* indicated also a slightly increased risk for CRC (factor 1.4) in individuals with a *H. pylori* infection (Zumkeller *et al.*, 2006). Another study showed that CagA status was associated with a significantly increased risk (factor >10) for CRC among hospitalized patients that were *H. pylori* seropositive (Shmuely *et al.*, 2001). Notably, this study again underscores the importance of proper microbiological classification and characterization of cancer-associated infectious agents, since not all *Helicobacter* strains may be associated with CRC. Like has been the case for *S. bovis*, lack of proper distinction between *H. pylori* subspecies could have biased or even underestimated a possible association of this bacterium with this disease (Erdman *et al.*, 2003a,b).

6. CRC Microbiome-based Immunoassays

The occurrence of specific CRC-associated bacterial infections, as discussed in the previous section, paves the way for the development of novel diagnostic tools. In this respect, it is important to realize that *S. gallolyticus* infections occur without clinical symptoms due to its mild virulence (Haimowitz *et al.*, 2005). Clinical manifestation of *S. gallolyticus* infections in otherwise compromised patients (*e.g.* damaged heart valves), may very well only represent the tip of the iceberg of all infections with this bacterium in individuals with (pre-)malignant colonic lesions. This notion has been the incentive to investigate whether a humoral immune response to sub-clinical *S. gallolyticus* infections could aid in the early detection of CRC. Notably, as infectious agents in general induce a more pronounced immune response compared to tumor "self" antigens, CRC-associated bacterial antigens could be instrumental in the immunodiagnosis of this disease (Tjalsma, 2011). Furthermore, several features of circulating antibodies make these attractive targets in diagnostic medicine: **i)** they reflect a molecular imprint of disease-related antigens from all around the human body, **ii)** although an antigen may be present only briefly, the corresponding antibody response is likely to be persistent, **iii)** the half-life of antibodies is about 15 days which minimizes daily fluctuations, **iv)** antibodies are highly stable compared to many other serum proteins making serum-handling protocols less stringent, **v)** the amplification cascade governed by the humoral immune system causes a surplus of circulating antibodies after appearance of the cognate (low-abundance) antigen. Several studies have shown that serum antibody levels against *S. bovis/S. gallolyticus* antigens could discriminate CRC cases from healthy controls (Abdulamir *et al.*, 2009; Darjee & Gibb, 1993; Tjalsma *et al.*, 2006). Interestingly, the humoral immune response to ribosomal protein (Rp) L7/L12 from *S. gallolyticus* was found to be higher in early CRC compared to late CRC stages, whereas this was not paralleled by increased antibody production to endotoxin, an intrinsic cell wall component of the majority of intestinal bacteria (Boleij *et al.*, 2010). This implies that the immune response to RpL7/L12 is not a general phenomenon induced by the loss of colonic barrier function. Furthermore, this observation could point to a temporal relationship between *S. gallolyticus* and CRC, suggesting that late stage tumors may change in such a way that bacterial survival in the tumor microenvironment is diminished. The possibility that disease progression may drive bacteria out of the cancerous tissue is similar to what has been reported for *H. pylori* during gastric cancer progression (Corfield *et al.*, 2000; Kang *et al.*, 2006). A relationship of *S. bovis* with early stages of CRC is underscored by a vast amount of case studies showing that its infection was associated with pre-malignant adenomas. These cases would have remained undiscovered if these patients did not present with an active *S. bovis* infection. Future research should be aimed at development of more specific *S. gallolyticus*-based serological assays to investigate the clinical utility of such tests for the early detection of CRC (Tjalsma *et al.*, 2006, 2008; Tjalsma, 2010). Furthermore, as CRC is a highly heterogeneous disease that is probably accompanied by even more heterogeneous microbiome shifts, accurate diagnosis based on biomarkers from a single bacterial species on the population level is highly unlikely. Therefore, future research should also be aimed at the identification of additional tumor-associated intestinal bacteria that may never have been found to cause clinical infections but do induce a humoral immune response. Furthermore, as discussed in Section 3 of this Chapter, certain mucosa-associated bacteria may be involved in CRC initiation or progression. Invasiveness of these pathogens or exposure to their antigens may elicit IgG responses that are valuable for CRC risk assessment. These individuals may not directly need bowel examination, but could be enrolled in a more strict monitoring program.

7. Conclusions

The development of CRC is a multistep process that may take over 20 years to progress from an adenoma into an advanced carcinoma. The fact that the intestinal microbiome plays an important role in this process is clearly shown by the inflammatory effects of intestinal bacteria, which are essential to develop disease in animal models. Furthermore, accumulating evidence suggests that bacterial production of toxins, toxic metabolites and the direct influences on pro-carcinogenic pathways in host epithelial cells are contributing factors that promote the accumulation of mutations that may eventually lead to carcinomas. However, still many questions remain to be answered. For example, our knowledge on the on the impact of CRC on the local intestinal microbiota and *vice versa*, is still in its infancy. Future research should focus on the detailed mapping of the microbiota in close proximity of early adenomas and carcinomas. These local changes in microbiota may for instance provide clues in the understanding why only 10% of the adenomas progress into carcinomas. Such knowledge could give us new leads for cancer diagnosis, for example by using signaling bacteria, such as *S. gallolyticus* that benefit from the altered tumor environment, as diagnostic targets. Furthermore, this knowledge could provide leads for the selective removal of high-risk bacterial populations by health promoting species, as a new strategy in CRC prevention. Altogether, this Chapter points out that the colonic microbiota should be regarded as an important factor in intestinal carcinogenesis. Further research in this field is crucial to fully understand the etiology of CRC and has a high potential to lead to new diagnostic tools and therapeutic interventions.

8. Acknowledgements

We thank Albert Bolhuis, Dorine Swinkels, Bas Dutilh, Carla Muytjens, Guus Kortman, Ikuko Kato, Julian Marchesi, Philippe Glaser, Rian Roelofs, Shaynoor Dramsi & Wilbert Peters for inspiring discussions. Work in our laboratory was supported by the Dutch Cancer Society (KWF; project KUN 2006-3591) and the Dutch Digestive Diseases Foundation (MLDS; project WO10-53). Correspondence to: Harold Tjalsma, Department of Laboratory Medicine (LGEM 830), Radboud University Nijmegen Medical Centre, P.O. Box 9101, 6500 HB, Nijmegen, The Netherlands; H.Tjalsma@labgk.umcn.nl.

9. References

Abdulamir, A. S., Hafidh, R. R., Mahdi, L. K., Al-jeboori, T. & Abubaker, F. (2009). Investigation into the controversial association of Streptococcus gallolyticus with colorectal cancer and adenoma. *BMC Cancer* 9, 403.

Abdulamir, A. S., Hafidh, R. R. & Abu Bakar, F. (2010). Molecular detection, quantification, and isolation of Streptococcus gallolyticus bacteria colonizing colorectal tumors: inflammation-driven potential of carcinogenesis via IL-1, COX-2, and IL-8. *Mol Cancer* 9, 249.

Arumugam, M., Raes, J., Pelletier, E., Le Paslier, D., Yamada, T., Mende, D.R., Fernandes, G.R., Tap, J., Bruls, T., Batto, J.M., Bertalan, M., Borruel, N., Casellas, F., Fernandez, L., Gautier, L., Hansen, T., Hattori, M., Hayashi, T., Kleerebezem, M., Kurokawa, K., Leclerc, M., Levenez, F., Manichanh, C., Nielsen, H.B., Nielsen, T., Pons, N., Poulain, J., Qin, J., Sicheritz-Ponten, T., Tims, S., Torrents, D., Ugarte, E., Zoetendal, E.G., Wang, J., Guarner, F., Pedersen, O., de Vos, W.M., Brunak, S., & Doré, J. (2011) Enterotypes of the human gut microbiome. *Nature* 473, 174-80.

Attene-Ramos, M. S., Wagner, E. D., Plewa, M. J. & Gaskins, H. R. (2006). Evidence that hydrogen sulfide is a genotoxic agent. *Mol Cancer Res* 4, 9-14.

Attene-Ramos, M. S., Wagner, E. D., Gaskins, H. R. & Plewa, M. J. (2007). Hydrogen sulfide induces direct radical-associated DNA damage. *Mol Cancer Res* 5, 455-459.

Attene-Ramos, M. S., Nava, G. M., Muellner, M. G., Wagner, E. D., Plewa, M. J. & Gaskins, H. R. (2010). DNA damage and toxicogenomic analyses of hydrogen sulfide in human intestinal epithelial FHs 74 Int cells. *Environ Mol Mutagen* 51, 304-314.

Atuma, C., Strugala, V., Allen, A. & Holm, L. (2001). The adherent gastrointestinal mucus gel layer: thickness and physical state in vivo. *Am J Physiol* 280, G922-929.

Balamurugan, R., Rajendiran, E., George, S., Samuel, G. V. & Ramakrishna, B. S. (2008). Real-time polymerase chain reaction quantification of specific butyrate-producing bacteria, Desulfovibrio and Enterococcus faecalis in the feces of patients with colorectal cancer. *J Gastroenterol Hepatol* 23, 1298-1303.

Biarc, J., Nguyen, I. S., Pini, A. & other authors (2004). Carcinogenic properties of proteins with pro-inflammatory activity from Streptococcus infantarius (formerly S. bovis). *Carcinogenesis* 25, 1477-1484.

Boleij, A., Schaeps, R. M. J., de Kleijn, S., Hermans, P. W., Glaser, P., Pancholi, V., Swinkels, D. W. & Tjalsma, H. (2009). Surface-exposed Histone-like protein A modulates adherence of Streptococcus gallolyticus to colon adenocarcinoma cells. *Infec Immun* 77, 5519-5527.

Boleij, A., Roelofs, R., Schaeps, R. M., Schulin, T., Glaser, P., Swinkels, D. W., Kato, I. & Tjalsma, H. (2010). Increased exposure to bacterial antigen RpL7/L12 in early stage colorectal cancer patients. *Cancer* 116, 4014-4022.

Boleij, A., Muytjens, C. M. J., Bukhari, S. I., Cayet, N., Glaser, P., Hermans, P. W., Swinkels, D. W., Bolhuis, A. & Tjalsma, H. (2011a). Novel clues on the specific association of Streptococcus gallolyticus subsp gallolyticus with colorectal cancer. *J Infect Dis* 203, 1101-1109.

Boleij, A., van Gelder, M.M.H.J., Swinkels, D. W., & Tjalsma, H. (2011b). Clinical Importance of Streptococcus gallolyticus infections among colorectal cancer patients: systematic review and meta-analysis. *Clin Infect Dis,* in press.

Bronowski, C., Smith, S. L., Yokota, K., Corkill, J. E., Martin, H. M., Campbell, B. J., Rhodes, J. M., Hart, C. A. & Winstanley, C. (2008). A subset of mucosa-associated Escherichia coli isolates from patients with colon cancer, but not Crohn's disease, share pathogenicity islands with urinary pathogenic E. coli. *Microbiology* 154, 571-583.

Cabrera, A., Tsukada, Y. & Pickren, J. W. (1965). Clostridial Gas Gangrene and Septicemia in Malignant Disease. *Cancer* 18, 800-806.

Cai, W. J., Wang, M. J., Ju, L. H., Wang, C. & Zhu, Y. C. (2010). Hydrogen sulfide induces human colon cancer cell proliferation: role of Akt, ERK and p21. *Cell Biol Int* 34, 565-572.

Candela, M., Maccaferri, S., Turroni, S., Carnevali, P. & Brigidi, P. (2010) Functional intestinal microbiome, new frontiers in prebiotic design. *Int Journal Food Microbiol* 140, 93-101.

Chew, S. S. & Lubowski, D. Z. (2001). Clostridium septicum and malignancy. *ANZ journal of surgery* 71, 647-649.

Chichlowski, M. & Hale, L. P. (2008). Bacterial-mucosal interactions in inflammatory bowel disease: an alliance gone bad. *Am J Physiol Gastrointest Liver Physiol* 295, G1139-1149.

Corfield, A. P., Myerscough, N., Longman, R., Sylvester, P., Arul, S. & Pignatelli, M. (2000). Mucins and mucosal protection in the gastrointestinal tract: new prospects for mucins in the pathology of gastrointestinal disease. *Gut* 47, 589-594.

Corredoira, J., Alonso, M. P., & Coira, A (2008). Characteristics of Streptococcus bovis endocarditis and its differences with Streptococcus viridans endocarditis. *Eur J Clin Microbiol Infect Dis* 27, 285-291.

Corredoira, J. C., Alonso, M. P., & Garcia, J. F. (2005). Clinical characteristics and significance of Streptococcus salivarius bacteremia and Streptococcus bovis bacteremia: a prospective 16-year study. *Eur J Clin Microbiol Infect Dis* 24, 250-255.

Crabtree, J. E., Farmery, S. M., Lindley, I. J., Figura, N., Peichl, P. & Tompkins, D. S. (1994). CagA/cytotoxic strains of Helicobacter pylori and interleukin-8 in gastric epithelial cell lines. *J Clin Pathol* 47, 945-950.

Cuevas-Ramos, G., Petit, C. R., Marcq, I., Boury, M., Oswald, E. & Nougayrede, J. P. (2010). Escherichia coli induces DNA damage in vivo and triggers genomic instability in mammalian cells. *Proc Nat AcadSci USA* 107, 11537-11542.

Darjee, R. & Gibb, A. P. (1993). Serological investigation into the association between Streptococcus bovis and colonic cancer. *J Clin Pathol* 46, 1116-1119.

de Kok, T. M. & van Maanen, J. M. (2000). Evaluation of fecal mutagenicity and colorectal cancer risk. *Mutation Res* 463, 53-101.

Deplancke, B. & Gaskins, H. R. (2003). Hydrogen sulfide induces serum-independent cell cycle entry in nontransformed rat intestinal epithelial cells. *FASEB J* 17, 1310-1312.

Dethlefsen, L., Eckburg, P. B., Bik, E. M. & Relman, D. A. (2006). Assembly of the human intestinal microbiota. *Trends Ecol Evol*, 21, 517-523.

Dove, W. F., Clipson, L., Gould, K. A., Luongo, C., Marshall, D. J., Moser, A. R., Newton, M. A. & Jacoby, R. F. (1997). Intestinal neoplasia in the ApcMin mouse: independence from the microbial and natural killer (beige locus) status. *Cancer Res* 57, 812-814.

Dylewski, J. & Luterman, L. Septic arthritis and Clostridium septicum: a clue to colon cancer. *Cmaj* 182, 1446-1447.

Eaden, J., Abrams, K., Ekbom, A., Jackson, E. & Mayberry, J. (2000). Colorectal cancer prevention in ulcerative colitis: a case-control study. *Alimen Pharmacol Therapeutics* 14, 145-153.

Ekstrom, A. M., Held, M., Hansson, L. E., Engstrand, L. & Nyren, O. (2001). Helicobacter pylori in gastric cancer established by CagA immunoblot as a marker of past infection. *Gastroenterology* 121, 784-791.

Ellmerich, S., Djouder, N., Scholler, M. & Klein, J. P. (2000a). Production of cytokines by monocytes, epithelial and endothelial cells activated by Streptococcus bovis. *Cytokine* 12, 26-31.

Ellmerich, S., Scholler, M., Duranton, B., Gosse, F., Galluser, M., Klein, J. P. & Raul, F. (2000b). Promotion of intestinal carcinogenesis by Streptococcus bovis. *Carcinogenesis* 21, 753-756.

Erdman, S. E., Poutahidis, T., Tomczak, M., Rogers, A. B., Cormier, K., Plank, B., Horwitz, B. H. & Fox, J. G. (2003a). CD4+ CD25+ regulatory T lymphocytes inhibit microbially induced colon cancer in Rag2-deficient mice. *Am J Pathol* 162, 691-702.

Erdman, S. E., Rao, V. P., Poutahidis, T. & other authors (2003b). CD4(+)CD25(+) regulatory lymphocytes require interleukin 10 to interrupt colon carcinogenesis in mice. *Cancer Res* 63, 6042-6050.

Fox, J. G. (2002). The non-H pylori helicobacters: their expanding role in gastrointestinal and systemic diseases. *Gut* 50, 273-283.

Fukata, M. & Abreu, M. T. (2007). TLR4 signalling in the intestine in health and disease. *Biochem Soc Trans* 35, 1473-1478.

Galbavy, S., Lukac, L., Porubsky, J., Cerna, M., Labuda, M., Kmet'ova, J., Papincak, J., Durdik, S. & Jakubovsky, J. (2002). Collagen type IV in epithelial tumours of colon. *Acta Histochem* 104, 331-334.

Giannitsioti, E., Chirouze, C., Bouvet, A. & other authors (2007). Characteristics and regional variations of group D streptococcal endocarditis in France. *Clin Microbiol Infect* 13, 770-776.

Gill, S. R., Pop, M., Deboy, R. T. & other authors (2006). Metagenomic analysis of the human distal gut microbiome. *Science (New York, NY* 312, 1355 1359.

Green, G. L., Brostoff, J., Hudspith, B. & other authors (2006). Molecular characterization of the bacteria adherent to human colorectal mucosa. *J Appl Microbiol* 100, 460-469.

Haimowitz, M. D., Hernandez, L. A. & Herron, R. M., Jr. (2005). A blood donor with bacteraemia. *Lancet* 365, 1596.

Heazlewood, C. K., Cook, M. C., Eri, R. & other authors (2008). Aberrant mucin assembly in mice causes endoplasmic reticulum stress and spontaneous inflammation resembling ulcerative colitis. *PLoS Med* 5, e54.

Henry-Stanley, M. J., Hess, D. J., Erickson, E. A., Garni, R. M. & Wells, C. L. (2003). Role of heparan sulfate in interactions of Listeria monocytogenes with enterocytes. *Med Microbiol Immunol* 192, 107-115.

Hermsen, J. L., Schurr, M. J., Kudsk, K. A. & Faucher, L. D. (2008). Phenotyping Clostridium septicum infection: a surgeon's infectious disease. *J Surgical Res* 148, 67-76.

Herrero, I. A., Rouse, M. S., Piper, K. E., Alyaseen, S. A., Steckelberg, J. M. & Patel, R. (2002). Reevaluation of Streptococcus bovis endocarditis cases from 1975 to 1985 by 16S ribosomal DNA sequence analysis. *J Clin Microbiol* 40, 3848-3850.

Higashi, H., Tsutsumi, R., Fujita, A., Yamazaki, S., Asaka, M., Azuma, T. & Hatakeyama, M. (2002). Biological activity of the Helicobacter pylori virulence factor CagA is determined by variation in the tyrosine phosphorylation sites. *Proc Nat Acad Sci USA* 99, 14428-14433.

Hinzman, M. J., Novotny, C., Ullah, A. & Shamsuddin, A. M. (1987). Fecal mutagen fecapentaene-12 damages mammalian colon epithelial DNA. *Carcinogenesis* 8, 1475-1479.

Hirayama, A., Kami, K., Sugimoto, M., Sugawara, M., Toki, N., Onozuka, H., Kinoshita, T., Saito, N., Ochiai, A., Tomita, M., Esumi, H., & Soga, T. (2009). Quantitative metabolome profiling of colon and stomach cancer microenvironment by capillary electrophoresis time-of-flight mass spectrometry. *Cancer Res* 69: 4918-25.

Hirota, K., Kanitani, H., Nemoto, K., Ono, T. & Miyake, Y. (1995). Cross-reactivity between human sialyl Lewis(x) oligosaccharide and common causative oral bacteria of infective endocarditis. *FEMS Immun Med Microbiol* 12, 159-164.

Hirota, K., Osawa, R., Nemoto, K., Ono, T. & Miyake, Y. (1996). Highly expressed human sialyl Lewis antigen on cell surface of streptococcus gallolyticus. *Lancet* 347, 760.

Homann, N., Tillonen, J. & Salaspuro, M. (2000). Microbially produced acetaldehyde from ethanol may increase the risk of colon cancer via folate deficiency. *Int J Cancer* 86, 169-173.

Hoppes, W. L. & Lerner, P. I. (1974). Nonenterococcal group-D streptococcal endocarditis caused by Streptococcus bovis. *Annals Int Med* 81, 588-593.

Housseau, F. & Sears, C. L. (2010). Enterotoxigenic Bacteroides fragilis (ETBF)-mediated colitis in Min (Apc+/-) mice: a human commensal-based murine model of colon carcinogenesis. *Cell Cycle* 9, 3-5.

Huang, J. Q., Zheng, G. F., Sumanac, K., Irvine, E. J. & Hunt, R. H. (2003). Meta-analysis of the relationship between cagA seropositivity and gastric cancer. *Gastroenterology* 125, 1636-1644.

Huycke, M. M., Abrams, V. & Moore, D. R. (2002). Enterococcus faecalis produces extracellular superoxide and hydrogen peroxide that damages colonic epithelial cell DNA. *Carcinogenesis* 23, 529-536.

Huycke, M. M. & Gaskins, H. R. (2004). Commensal bacteria, redox stress, and colorectal cancer: mechanisms and models. *Exp Biol Med* 229, 586-597.

Itzkowitz, S. H. & Yio, X. (2004). Inflammation and cancer IV. Colorectal cancer in inflammatory bowel disease: the role of inflammation. *Am J Physiology* 287, G7-17.

Jean, S. S., Teng, L. J., Hsueh, P. R., Ho, S. W. & Luh, K. T. (2004). Bacteremic Streptococcus bovis infections at a university hospital, 1992-2001. *J Formosan Med Ass* 103, 118-123.

Jemal, A., Siegel, R., Ward, E., Hao, Y. P., Xu, J. Q. & Thun, M. J. (2009). Cancer Statistics, 2009. *CA-Cancer J Clin* 59, 225-249.

Kanazawa, K., Konishi, F., Mitsuoka, T., Terada, A., Itoh, K., Narushima, S., Kumemura, M. & Kimura, H. (1996). Factors influencing the development of sigmoid colon cancer. Bacteriologic and biochemical studies. *Cancer* 77, 1701-1706.

Kang, H. Y., Kim, N., Park, Y. S., Hwang, J. H., Kim, J. W., Jeong, S. H., Lee, D. H., Jung, H. C. & Song, I. S. (2006). Progression of atrophic gastritis and intestinal metaplasia drives Helicobacter pylori out of the gastric mucosa. *Dig Dis Sci* 51, 2310-2315.

Killeen, S. D., Wang, J. H., Andrews, E. J. & Redmond, H. P. (2009). Bacterial endotoxin enhances colorectal cancer cell adhesion and invasion through TLR-4 and NF-kappaB-dependent activation of the urokinase plasminogen activator system. *Br J Cancer* 100, 1589-1602.

Klein, R. S., Recco, R. A., Catalano, M. T., Edberg, S. C., Casey, J. I. & Steigbigel, N. H. (1977). Association of Streptococcus bovis with carcinoma of the colon. *New Engl J Med* 297, 800-802.

Knasmuller, S., Steinkellner, H., Hirschl, A. M., Rabot, S., Nobis, E. C. & Kassie, F. (2001). Impact of bacteria in dairy products and of the intestinal microflora on the genotoxic and carcinogenic effects of heterocyclic aromatic amines. *Mutation Res* 480-481, 129-138.

Kuipers, E. J., Perez-Perez, G. I., Meuwissen, S. G. & Blaser, M. J. (1995). Helicobacter pylori and atrophic gastritis: importance of the cagA status. *J Nat Cancer Inst* 87, 1777-1780.

Labayle, D., Fischer, D., Vielh, P., Drouhin, F., Pariente, A., Bories, C., Duhamel, O., Trousset, M. & Attali, P. (1991). Sulindac causes regression of rectal polyps in familial adenomatous polyposis. *Gastroenterology* 101, 635-639.

Lee, R. A., Woo, P. C., To, A. P., Lau, S. K., Wong, S. S. & Yuen, K. Y. (2003). Geographical difference of disease association in Streptococcus bovis bacteraemia. *JMed Microbiol* 52, 903-908.

Lieberman, D. A. & Smith, F. W. (1991). Screening for colon malignancy with colonoscopy. *Am J Gastroenterol* 86, 946-951.

Lieberman, D. A., Weiss, D. G., Bond, J. H., Ahnen, D. J., Garewal, H. & Chejfec, G. (2000). Use of colonoscopy to screen asymptomatic adults for colorectal cancer. Veterans Affairs Cooperative Study Group 380. *New Engl J Med* 343, 162-168.

Macfarlane, S., Furrie, E., Cummings, J. H. & Macfarlane, G. T. (2004). Chemotaxonomic analysis of bacterial populations colonizing the rectal mucosa in patients with ulcerative colitis. *Clin Infect Dis* 38, 1690-1699.

Macfarlane, S., Furrie, E., Kennedy, A., Cummings, J. H. & Macfarlane, G. T. (2005). Mucosal bacteria in ulcerative colitis. *Brit J Nutr* 93 Suppl 1, S67-72.

Maddocks, O. D., Short, A. J., Donnenberg, M. S., Bader, S. & Harrison, D. J. (2009). Attaching and effacing Escherichia coli downregulate DNA mismatch repair protein in vitro and are associated with colorectal adenocarcinomas in humans. *PloS One* 4, e5517.

Marchesi, J. R., Dutilh, B. E., Hall, N., Peters, W. H. M., Roelofs, R., Boleij, A. & Tjalsma, H. (2011). Towards the human colorectal cancer microbiome. *PloS One* 6:e20447.

Martin, H. M., Campbell, B. J., Hart, C. A., Mpofu, C., Nayar, M., Singh, R., Englyst, H., Williams, H. F. & Rhodes, J. M. (2004). Enhanced Escherichia coli adherence and invasion in Crohn's disease and colon cancer. *Gastroenterology* 127, 80-93.

McCoy, W. & Mason, J. M. (1951). Enterococcal endocarditis associated with carcinoma of the sigmoid; report of a case. *J Med Ass Alab* 21, 162-166.

Menter, D. G., Schilsky, R. L. & DuBois, R. N. (2010). Cyclooxygenase-2 and cancer treatment: understanding the risk should be worth the reward. *Clin Cancer Res* 16, 1384-1390.

Mirza, N. N., McCloud, J. M. & Cheetham, M. J. (2009). Clostridium septicum sepsis and colorectal cancer - a reminder. *World J Surg Oncol* 7, 73.

Moser, A. R., Pitot, H. C. & Dove, W. F. (1990). A dominant mutation that predisposes to multiple intestinal neoplasia in the mouse. *Science* 247, 322-324.

Neish, A. S. (2009). Microbes in gastrointestinal health and disease. *Gastroenterology* 136, 65-80.

O'Hara, A. M. & Shanahan, F. (2006). The gut flora as a forgotten organ. *EMBO reports* 7, 688-693.

Povey, A. C., Schiffman, M., Taffe, B. G. & Harris, C. C. (1991). Laboratory and epidemiologic studies of fecapentaenes. *Mutation Res* 259, 387-397.

Qin, J., Li, R., Raes, J., Arumugam, M., Burgdorf, K.S., Manichanh, C., Nielsen, T., Pons, N., Levenez, F., Yamada, T., Mende, D.R., Li, J., Xu, J., Li, S., Li, D., Cao, J., Wang, B., Liang, H., Zheng, H., Xie, Y., Tap, J., Lepage, P., Bertalan, M., Batto, J.M., Hansen, T., Le Paslier, D., Linneberg, A., Nielsen, H.B., Pelletier, E., Renault, P., Sicheritz-Ponten, T., Turner, K., Zhu, H., Yu, C., Li, S., Jian, M., Zhou, Y., Li, Y., Zhang, X., Li, S., Qin, N., Yang, H., Wang, J., Brunak, S., Doré, J., Guarner, F., Kristiansen, K., Pedersen, O., Parkhill, J., Weissenbach, J., (2010). A human gut microbial gene catalogue established by metagenomic sequencing. *Nature* 464, 59-65.

Rakoff-Nahoum, S. & Medzhitov, R. (2007). Regulation of spontaneous intestinal tumorigenesis through the adaptor protein MyD88. *Science* 317, 124-127.

Rakoff-Nahoum, S. & Medzhitov, R. (2009). Toll-like receptors and cancer. *Nat Rev Cancer* 9, 57-63.

Rathbun, H. K. (1968). Clostridial bacteremia without hemolysis. *Arch Int Medicine* 122, 496-501.

Round, J. L. & Mazmanian, S. K. (2009). The gut microbiota shapes intestinal immune responses during health and disease. *Nat Rev Immunol* 9, 313-323.

Ruoff, K. L., Miller, S. I., Garner, C. V., Ferraro, M. J. & Calderwood, S. B. (1989). Bacteremia with Streptococcus bovis and Streptococcus salivarius: clinical correlates of more accurate identification of isolates. *J Clin Microbiol* 27, 305-308.

Rutter, M., Saunders, B., Wilkinson, K. & other authors (2004). Severity of inflammation is a risk factor for colorectal neoplasia in ulcerative colitis. *Gastroenterology* 126, 451-459.

Scanlan, P. D., Shanahan, F., Clune, Y., Collins, J. K., O'Sullivan, G. C., O'Riordan, M., Holmes, E., Wang, Y. & Marchesi, J. R. (2008). Culture-independent analysis of the gut microbiota in colorectal cancer and polyposis. *Environl Microbiol* 10, 789-798.

Schiffman, M. H., Van Tassell, R. L., Robinson, A. & other authors (1989). Case-control study of colorectal cancer and fecapentaene excretion. *Cancer Res* 49, 1322-1326.

Sears, C. L. (2009). Enterotoxigenic Bacteroides fragilis: a rogue among symbiotes. *Clin Microbiol Rev* 22, 349-369.

Sellon, R. K., Tonkonogy, S., Schultz, M., Dieleman, L. A., Grenther, W., Balish, E., Rennick, D. M. & Sartor, R. B. (1998). Resident enteric bacteria are necessary for development of spontaneous colitis and immune system activation in interleukin-10-deficient mice. *Infect Immun* 66, 5224-5231.

Shen, X. J., Rawls, J. F., Randall, T. & other authors (2010). Molecular characterization of mucosal adherent bacteria and associations with colorectal adenomas. *Gut Microbes* 1, 138-147.

Shioya, M., Wakabayashi, K., Yamashita, K., Nagao, M. & Sugimura, T. (1989). Formation of 8-hydroxydeoxyguanosine in DNA treated with fecapentaene-12 and -14. *Mutation Res* 225, 91-94.

Shmuely, H., Passaro, D., Figer, A., Niv, Y., Pitlik, S., Samra, Z., Koren, R. & Yahav, J. (2001). Relationship between Helicobacter pylori CagA status and colorectal cancer. *Am J Gastroenter* 96, 3406-3410.

Sillanpaa, J., Nallapareddy, S. R., Singh, K. V., Ferraro, M. J. & Murray, B. E. (2008). Adherence characteristics of endocarditis-derived Streptococcus gallolyticus ssp. gallolyticus (Streptococcus bovis biotype I) isolates to host extracellular matrix proteins. *FEMS Microbiology Lett* 289, 104-109.

Sillanpaa, J., Nallapareddy, S. R., Qin, X. & other authors (2009). A collagen-binding adhesin, Acb, and 10 other putative MSCRAMM and pilus family proteins of Streptococcus gallolyticus subsp. gallolyticus (S. bovis biotype I). *J Bact* 191, 6643-6653.

Sobhani, I., Tap, J., Roudot-Thoraval, F., Roperch, J. P., Letulle, S., Langella, P., Corthier, G., Tran Van Nhieu, J. & Furet, J. P. (2011). Microbial dysbiosis in colorectal cancer (CRC) patients. *PloS One* 6, e16393.

Sonnenburg, J. L., Angenent, L. T. & Gordon, J. I. (2004). Getting a grip on things: how do communities of bacterial symbionts become established in our intestine? *Nature immunol* 5, 569-573.

Spier, B. J., Walker, A. J., Cornett, D. D., Pfau, P. R., Halberg, R. B. & Said, A. (2010). Screening colonoscopy and detection of neoplasia in asymptomatic, average-risk, solid organ transplant recipients: case-control study. *Transpl Int* 23, 1233-1238.

Stecher, B., Robbiani, R., Walker, A. W. & other authors (2007). Salmonella enterica serovar typhimurium exploits inflammation to compete with the intestinal microbiota. *PLoS Biol* 5, 2177-2189.

Stecher, B. & Hardt, W. D. (2008). The role of microbiota in infectious disease. *Trends Microbiol* 16, 107-114.

Su, L. K., Kinzler, K. W., Vogelstein, B., Preisinger, A. C., Moser, A. R., Luongo, C., Gould, K. A. & Dove, W. F. (1992). Multiple intestinal neoplasia caused by a mutation in the murine homolog of the APC gene. *Science* 256, 668-670.

Su, X., Ye, J., Hsueh, E. C., Zhang, Y., Hoft, D. F. & Peng, G. (2010). Tumor microenvironments direct the recruitment and expansion of human Th17 cells. *J Immunol* 184, 1630-1641.

Swidsinski, A., Khilkin, M., Kerjaschki, D., Schreiber, S., Ortner, M., Weber, J. & Lochs, H. (1998). Association between intraepithelial Escherichia coli and colorectal cancer. *Gastroenterology* 115, 281-286.

Takada, H., Hirooka, T., Hiramatsu, Y. & Yamamoto, M. (1982). Effect of beta-glucuronidase inhibitor on azoxymethane-induced colonic carcinogenesis in rats. *Cancer Res* 42, 331-334.

Thompson-Chagoyan, O. C., Maldonado, J. & Gil, A. (2007). Colonization and impact of disease and other factors on intestinal microbiota. *Dig Dis Sci* 52, 2069-2077.

Thun, M. J., Namboodiri, M. M. & Heath, C. W., Jr. (1991). Aspirin use and reduced risk of fatal colon cancer. *The New Engl J Medicine* 325, 1593-1596.

Tjalsma, H., Scholler-Guinard, M., Lasonder, E., Ruers, T. J., Willems, H. L. & Swinkels, D. W. (2006). Profiling the humoral immune response in colon cancer patients: diagnostic antigens from Streptococcus bovis. *Int J Cancer* 119, 2127-2135.

Tjalsma, H., Schaeps, R. M. & Swinkels, D. W. (2008). Immunoproteomics: From biomarker discovery to diagnostic applications. *Proteomics Clin Appl* 2, 167-180.

Tjalsma, H. (2010). Identification of biomarkers for colorectal cancer through proteomics-based approaches. *Exp Rev Proteomics* 7, 879-895.

Tjalsma, H. (2011).Hybrid multiplex assays for the early detection of colorectal cancer: a perspective. *Clin Lab Int* 35, 10-12.

Toprak, N. U., Yagci, A., Gulluoglu, B. M., Akin, M. L., Demirkalem, P., Celenk, T. & Soyletir, G. (2006). A possible role of Bacteroides fragilis enterotoxin in the aetiology of colorectal cancer. *Clin Microbiol Infect* 12, 782-786.

Uronis, J. M., Muhlbauer, M., Herfarth, H. H., Rubinas, T. C., Jones, G. S. & Jobin, C. (2009). Modulation of the intestinal microbiota alters colitis-associated colorectal cancer susceptibility. *PloS One* 4, e6026.

Vaska, V. L. & Faoagali, J. L. (2009). Streptococcus bovis bacteraemia: identification within organism complex and association with endocarditis and colonic malignancy. *Pathology* 41, 183-186.

Wang, X. & Huycke, M. M. (2007). Extracellular superoxide production by Enterococcus faecalis promotes chromosomal instability in mammalian cells. *Gastroenterology* 132, 551-561.

Wang, X., Allen, T. D., May, R. J., Lightfoot, S., Houchen, C. W. & Huycke, M. M. (2008). Enterococcus faecalis induces aneuploidy and tetraploidy in colonic epithelial cells through a bystander effect. *Cancer Res* 68, 9909-9917.

Wilkinson, S. M., Uhl, J. R., Kline, B. C. & Cockerill, F. R., 3rd (1998). Assessment of invasion frequencies of cultured HEp-2 cells by clinical isolates of Helicobacter pylori using an acridine orange assay. *J Clin Pathol* 51, 127-133.

Winters, M. D., Schlinke, T. L., Joyce, W. A., Glore, S. R. & Huycke, M. M. (1998). Prospective case-cohort study of intestinal colonization with enterococci that produce extracellular superoxide and the risk for colorectal adenomas or cancer. *Am J Gastroenterol* 93, 2491-2500.

Wu, S., Morin, P. J., Maouyo, D. & Sears, C. L. (2003). Bacteroides fragilis enterotoxin induces c-Myc expression and cellular proliferation. *Gastroenterology* 124, 392-400.

Wu, S., Rhee, K. J., Albesiano, E. & other authors (2009). A human colonic commensal promotes colon tumorigenesis via activation of T helper type 17 T cell responses. *Nature medicine* 15, 1016-1022.

Xu, J., Mahowald, M. A., Ley, R. E. & other authors (2007). Evolution of symbiotic bacteria in the distal human intestine. *PLoS Biology* 5, e156.

Yantiss, R. K., Goldman, H. & Odze, R. D. (2001). Hyperplastic polyp with epithelial misplacement (inverted hyperplastic polyp): a clinicopathologic and immunohistochemical study of 19 cases. *Mod Pathol* 14, 869-875.

Zoetendal, E. G., von Wright, A., Vilpponen-Salmela, T., Ben-Amor, K., Akkermans, A. D. & de Vos, W. M. (2002). Mucosa-associated bacteria in the human gastrointestinal tract are uniformly distributed along the colon and differ from the community recovered from feces. *Appl Environ Microbiol* 68, 3401-3407.

Zumkeller, N., Brenner, H., Zwahlen, M. & Rothenbacher, D. (2006). Helicobacter pylori infection and colorectal cancer risk: a meta-analysis. *Helicobacter* 11, 75-80.

Part 5

Study Reports

19

Tumor Infiltrating Lymphocytes as Prognostic Factor of Early Recurrence and Poor Prognosis of Colorectal Cancer After Radical Surgical Treatment

Vaclav Liska[1], Ondrej Daum[2], Petr Novak[1], Vladislav Treska[1], Ondrej Vycital[1], Jan Bruha[1], Pavel Pitule[1] and Lubos Holubec[3]
[1]*Department of Surgery,*
[2]*Institute of Pathology,*
[3]*Department of Oncology, Charles University Prague, Medical School and Teaching Hospital Pilsen, Czech Republic*

1. Introduction

Sixty percent of patients with colorectal cancer (CRC) are afflicted with distant metastases (liver or lung metastatic process) or a local relapse of malignancy (Bird et al., 2006). The possibilities of surgical and oncological treatment of this disease offer us a large spectrum of treatments including the combination of surgical procedures and consecutive oncological treatments. In the case of radical surgical therapy we can consider the curative access. The main medical problem of CRC is the high rate of recurrences after radically performed surgical therapy. The operability of recurrence is only about 30% in the case of local relapse and 20% in the case of distant metastases (Coleman et al., 2008; Kobayashi et al., 2007). The second dominant problem is the early recurrence of CRC after radical surgical treatment, when the patients undergo a difficult and exhausting procedure with a high risk of perioperative complications without any significant differences in overall survival against modern palliative therapy (Van den Eynde & Hendlisz, 2009).

Contemporary clinical and histopathological prognostic factors (staging, grading, etc.) used for the detection of patients with a high risk of relapse and a short overall survival rate and for the indication of adjuvant oncological treatment after radical surgery are not sufficient. Tumor infiltrating lymphocytes (TIL) were described as a good prognostic factor for patients with a high risk of relapse. They are critical indicators of efficient antitumor immunological response. Their number, type and morphology of TIL cells determine resulting tumor prognosis (Atreya & Neurath, 2008; Galon et al., 2006). They could be connected also with the suppression of micrometastatical disease after radical surgery (Gajewski et al., 2006; Pages et al., 2005). We can recognize either the type of immune cells or distinguish their morphological aspects (infiltration of any part of tumor or surrounding of tumor or tributary lymph nodes) (Talmadge et al., 2007).

We detail only short overview of their types and function. We recommend the readers with deeper interest in these problems to find comprehensive reviews in the cited papers (Jochems et al., 2011; Ohtani 2007). From this view we find CD8+ and CD4+ T lymphocytes (Fig. 1a & Fig. 1b), natural killer cells (Fig. 1c), dendritic cells (Fig. 1d), macrophages, etc. The exact function of these cells is under current discussion. We only know that they play main role in controlling tumor development and growth. CD8+ T lymphocytes within cancer cell nests of colorectal cancer have significant impact on the survival of patients. They contain the cytolytic enzyme granzyme-B. In case of increased proliferating activity of CD8+ T lymphocytes we observe their activated and cytotoxic phenotype that is significantly associated with the absence of early metastatic events (vascular emboli, lymphatic invasion or perineural invasion of tumor cells) and with a decreased rate of cancer recurrence (Atreya & Neurath, 2008, Pages et al., 2010). A high density of memory T lymphocytes within colorectal cancer tissue was more frequently observed in patients without early detectable signs of metastatic events and was associated with both improved disease free interval (DFI) and prolonged overall survival (OS) (Galon et al., 2006; Pages et al., 2005).

Natural killer cells (NK cells) mediate an effective lysis of cancer cells but the mechanism of detection of cancer cells is different from CD8+ T lymphocytes (Cooper et al., 2009). NK cells are mainly involved in the innate immune response and do not recognize specific tumor associated antigen on the surface of cancer cells as CD8+ T lymphocytes. NK cells lyse the cancer cells that are opsonized by surface antibody. NK cells also respond to other signals as cytokines produced by antigen presenting cells, which allow them to mediate early host responses against pathogen (Moretta et al., 2006). Decreased preoperative number of NK cells was associated with increased frequency of postoperative recurrence of colorectal cancer (Atreya & Neurath, 2008; Cooper et al., 2001). Their crucial role in the elimination of haematological malignancies, primary and secondary tumors has been recognized (Lucas et al., 2007; Ljunggren & Malmberg, 2007, Stojanovic & Cerwenka, 2011). In the last year there are some signs that NK-cells have the capacity for memory-like responses, a property that was previously thought to be limited to adaptive immunity, but in this view the discussion still continues (Cooper et al., 2009).

Dendritic cells are considered to be most potent antigen presenting cells. They play key role in activation, stimulation and recruitment of T lymphocytes. They can also induce antigen-specific unresponsiveness or immune tolerance. Immature dendritic cells enter tumor tissue, uptake and process its antigens. Then after they migrate to lymph nodes, undergo maturation and interact with T-lymphocytes that are able to recognize presented antigen and so T-lymphocytes play effector role of this tumor-specific immunity (Atreya & Neurath, 2008; Pages et al., 2005; Sandel et al., 2005; Steinman et al., 2003).

Macrophages are important producers of different factors that have function during tumor progression and also during tumor progression control. Their function is not fully understand, but it was described that the number of tumor infiltrating macrophages correlates with overall survival of colorectal cancer patients (Atreya & Neurath, 2008; Pollard, 2004; Forssell et al., 2007). It seems that several types of tumor infiltrating macrophages influence the balance between pro- and anti-tumor properties of immune system (Forssell et al., 2007).

From the morphologic view we can observe TIL in the specific portions of tumor and so we detect lymphocytic infiltration intratumoral (ITL – intratumoral lymphocytes) (Fig.

2a),intrastromal (ISL - intrastromal lymphocytes) (Fig. 2b), peritumoral (PTL - peritumoral lymphocytes) (Fig. 2c) and Crohn-like reaction (Crohn-like PTL)(Fig. 2d). We can also describe reactive histological changes in tributary lymph nodes (LN reactions). It means follicular hyperplasia (LN-FH) (Fig. 3a.), sinus histiocytosis (LN-SH) (Fig. 3b.) and the presence of granulomas (LN-GR) (Fig. 3c) (Ogino et al, 2009; Pages et al., 2005).

The aim of this study was to analyze the relationship of contemporary clinical and histopathological factors and TIL to determine patients with a high risk of poor overall survival and tendency to early recurrence of malignancy with shortened disease free interval (DFI) after radical surgery for CRC.

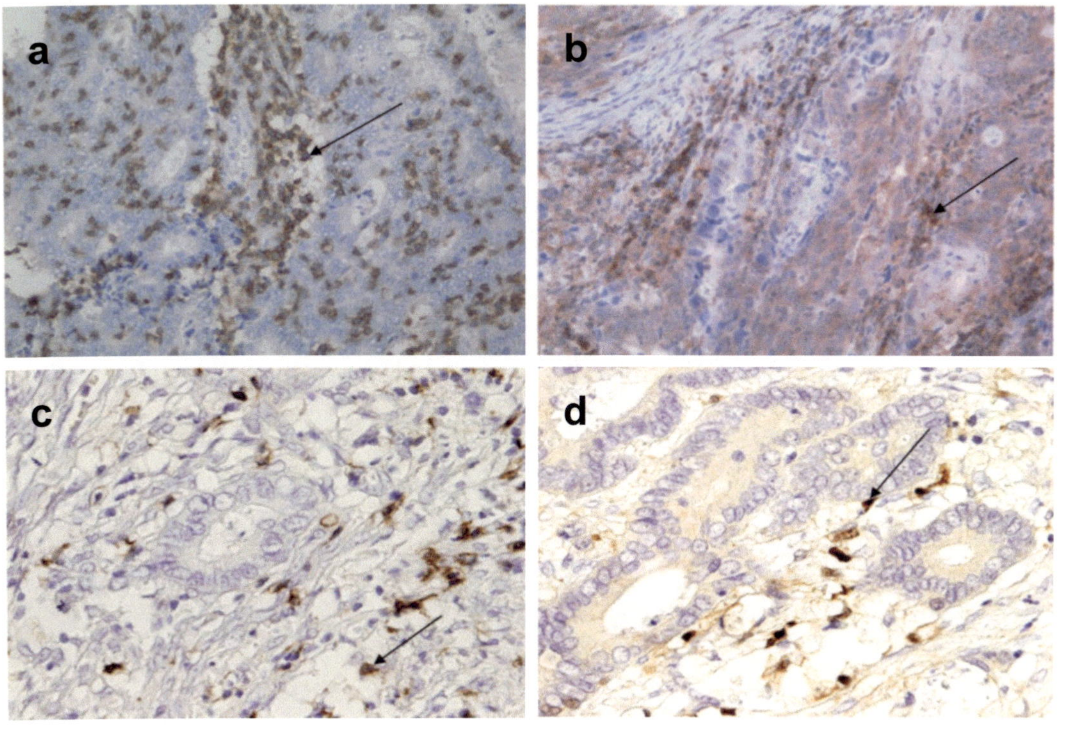

Fig. 1. Examples of tumor infiltration by immune cells: a) CD8+ T lymphocytes; b) CD4+ T lymphocytes; c) Natural killer cell (CD 57 staining) and d) Dendritic cells (S 100 staining).

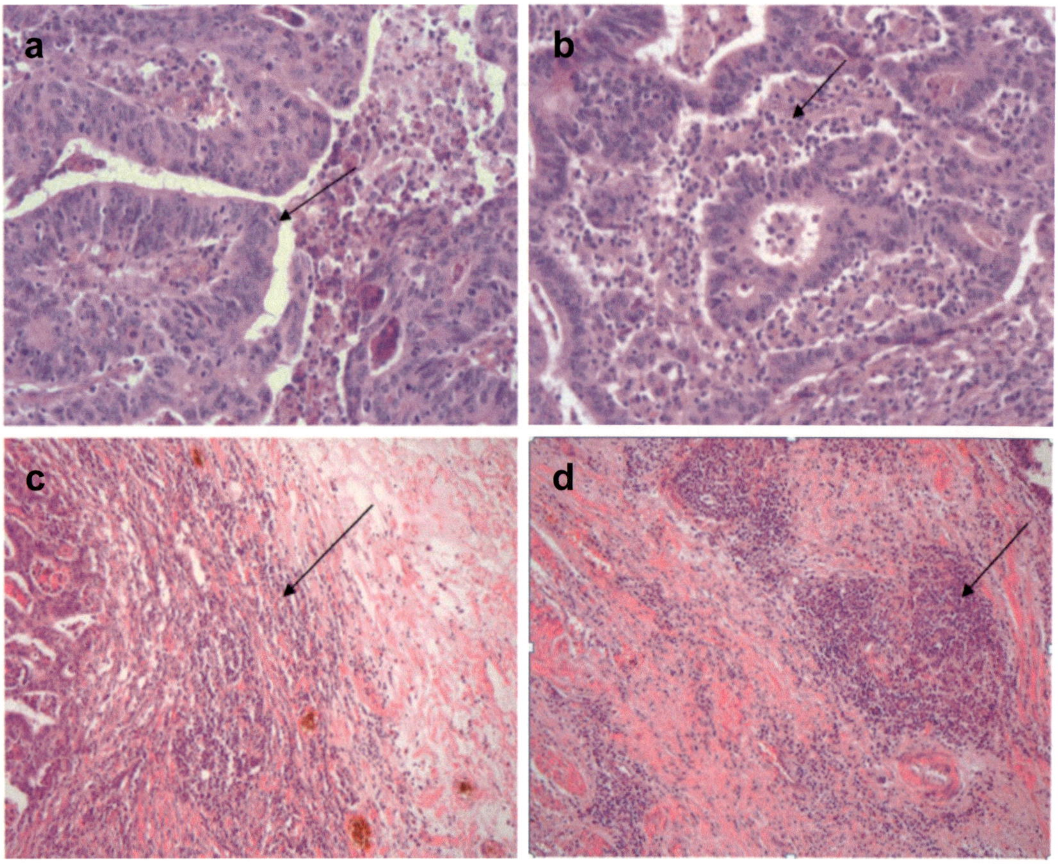

Fig. 2. Different localisation of TIL within the tumor tissue: a) intratumoral lymphocytes; b) intrastromal lymphocytes; c) peritumoral lymphocytes and d) Crohn-like peritumoral lymphocytes. All sections stained with hematoxylin-eosin.

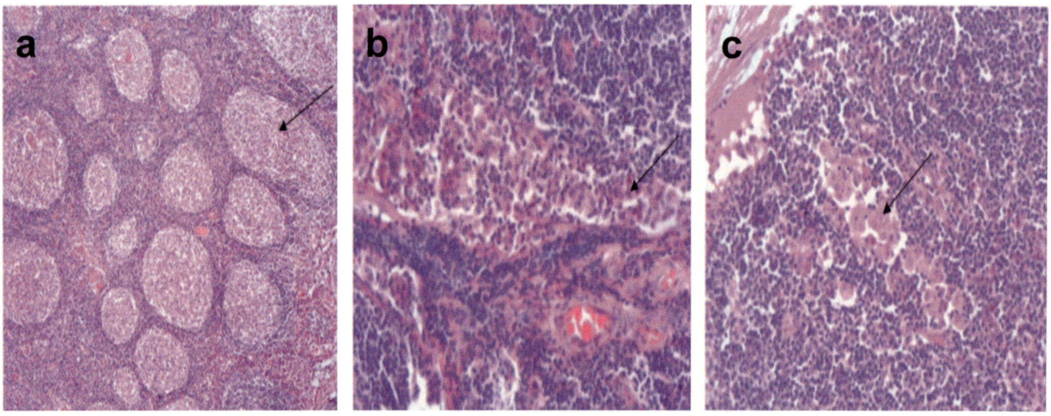

Fig. 3. Reactive histological changes in tributary lymph nodes: a) follicular hyperplasia; b) sinus histiocytosis and c) presence of granulomas. All sections stained with hematoxylin-eosin.

2. Methods

We analyzed 150 patients who underwent radical surgical procedure for CRC between the years 2004-2007 at the Department of Surgery, Medical School and Teaching Hospital in Pilsen, Charles University in Prague. We selected only patients who were operated on electively – our aim was to decrease the risk of inflammation that is often connected with the acute operation of CRC and does not depend on the immune reaction against a tumor but could be evoked by the distension of the bowel. We also excluded patients who had risk of understaging (for example low number of analysed lymph nodes) and patients with a synchronous metastatic process. The inclusion standard was also the entire follow-up of patients during the whole postoperative period to increase the number of patients with a diagnosed early recurrence of CRC.

The following clinical parameters were statistically analysed in relation to the disease free interval (DFI) and the overall survival (OS): staging, grading, preoperative leukocytosis, type of surgical procedure (radical vs. palliative), postoperative complications and postoperative oncological treatment.

2.1 Histology

We examined three different sections of each tumor and also sections of all found lymph nodes. Tissue for light microscopy was fixed in 4% formaldehyde and embedded in paraffin using routine procedures. Five micrometer-thick sections were cut from the tissue blocks and stained with hematoxylin-eosin.

The type and grade of all tumors were determined according to WHO 2000 guidelines. The stage of tumors was established according to UICC 2002 guidelines. We evaluated endovascular (VI), endolymphatic (LI) and perineural infiltration (PI) by cancer cells (0 – none, 1 – yes). Lymphocytic infiltration was detected as intratumoral (ITL – intratumoral lymphocytes), intrastromal (ISL – intrastromal lymphocytes), peritumoral (PTL – peritumoral lymphocytes) and Crohn-like reaction (Crohn-like PTL), and scaled as none (0), mild (1), moderate (2) and severe (3). Reactive histological changes in lymph nodes (LN reactions) were detected as follicular hyperplasia (LN-FH), sinus histiocytosis (LN-SH) and the presence of granulomas (LN-GR), and all these parameters were quantified in the same manner as lymphocytic infiltration.

2.2 Immunohistochemistry

For immunohistochemical investigations the following primary antibodies were used: CD4 (clone 4B12, 1:50, Vector Laboratories, Burlingame, CA, USA) and CD8 (clone C8/144B, 1:50, Dako, Glostrup, Denmark). Microwave pretreatment was used in both cases. The primary antibodies were visualized using the supersensitive streptavidin-biotin-peroxidase complex (Biogenex, San Ramon, CA). Appropriate positive and negative control slides were employed. The density of intratumoral infiltration by lymphocytes was evaluated in five High power microscopical fields (HPF) and expressed as the number of immunopositive cells per HPF.

2.3 Statistical evaluation

Statistical analysis was processed by the statistical software Statistica 9.0. The mean, median, standard deviation (SD), minimum, maximum, quartiles, frequencies and other basic statistical measurements were computed in given groups and subgroups of patients corresponding to studied clinical and histopathological parameters.

The relationships between the variables were described by Spearman rank correlation coefficients.
The analyses of Overall survival (OS) and Disease free interval (DFI) were performed by Kaplan-Meier´s survival functions. The influence of given covariates (clinical and histopathological factors) was tested by the Log-Rank test and Wilcoxon test. The Cox regression hazard model, hazard ratio (HR) and 95% confidence interval (CI) for HR were computed for the evaluation of given clinical and histopathological factors to OS or DFI. Multivariate analysis was performed by the use of classification and regression trees (CART). The Cox regression hazard model (stepwise regression) was applied to find the predictors in CART.

3. Results

The statistical analysis of the studied cohort of patients after surgical treatment for colorectal cancer demonstrated an acceptable distribution of basic statistical description parameters (gender ratio 93:57 (male vs. female)). 1, 3 and 5 years overall survival was 92.2%, 76.5% and 70.2% and 1, 3 and 5 year DFI was 85.3%, 64.3% and 49.4%.
The Spearman rank correlation coefficient did not prove any stronger correlation than a moderate correlation at endolymphatic invasion (LI) and lymph node infiltration by metastatic process (Spearman rank correlation coefficient 0.56, p<0,05). All the other studied factors were independent factors or factors with a low correlation.
Statistical analysis proved lymph node infiltration by metastatic process as statistically significant for the prognosis of overall survival (p<0.05) and N2 status of lymph nodes increased the risk of shorter overall survival 9.3x (Fig. 4.).

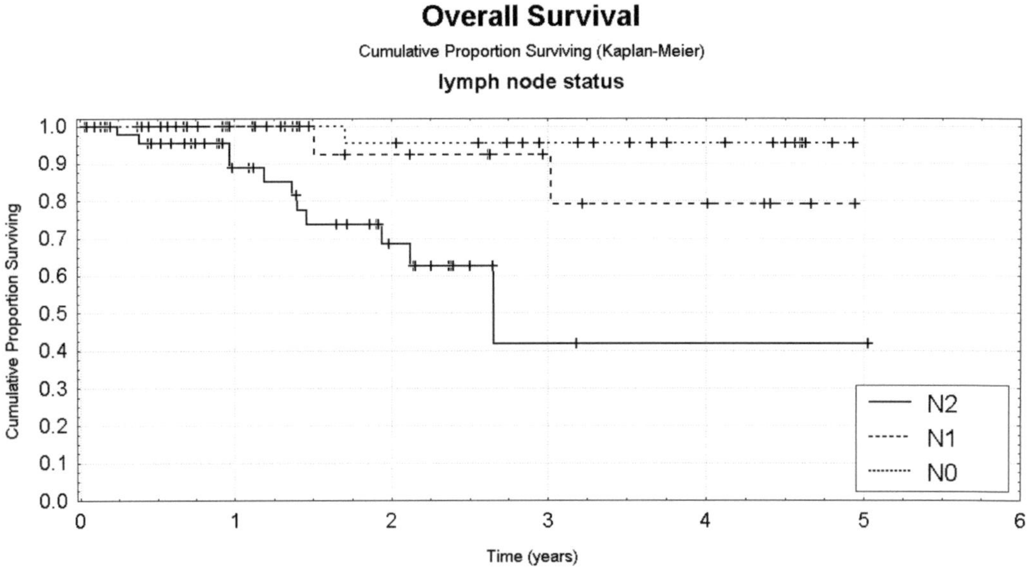

Fig. 4. Statistical analysis proved the lymph node infiltration by a metastatic process as statistically significant for the prognosis of overall survival (p<0.05), and the N2 status of lymph nodes increased the risk of a shorter overall survival 9.3x.

Endovascular infiltration (VI) was proved as a negative prognostic factor of shorter overall survival (Fig.5.). Patients with positive histopathological findings of VI have 3.1x increased risk for shorter overall survival. The presence of peritumoral lymphocytes (PTL) (Fig.6.) and of Crohn-like PTL (Fig.7.) was proved as a positive prognostic factor of OS. Patients with a positive histopathological finding of PTL and Crohn-like PTL have a decreased risk for shorter overall survival (2.3x and 2.3x respectively). Lymph node follicular hyperplasia (LN-FH) was verified as a positive prognostic factor for longer overall survival (Fig.8.). The statistical significance of LN-FH increased also with the raised density of infiltration. LN-FH positivity decreased the risk of shorter overall survival 3.3times.
The severity of CD8+ lymphocytic infiltration was proved by the Cox regression hazard model as a positive prognostic factor enlarging overall survival (cut off 30 cells/HPF). The severity of CD4+ lymphocytic infiltration was proved as a significant factor for the prognosis of overall survival (cut off 4cells/HPF) with 2.5x increased hazard ratio in patients over the cut off (Fig.9.). Statistical analysis did not confirm the statistical significance of CD8/CD4 ratio.

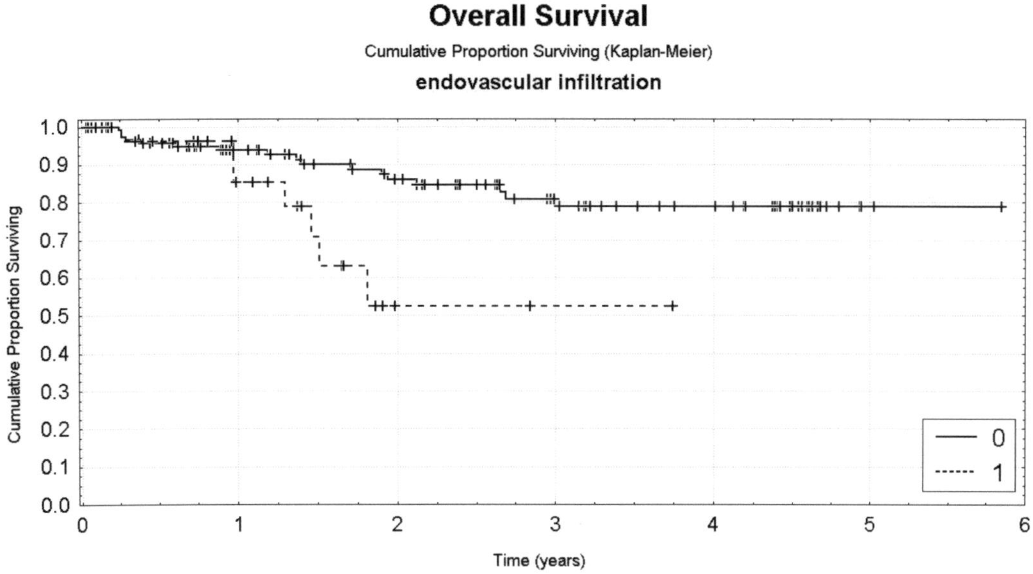

Fig. 5. Endovascular infiltration by cancer cells (VI) was proved as a statistically significant factor for the prognosis of overall survival ($p<0.05$). The patients with a positive histopathological finding of VI have 3.1x higher risk ratio for shorter overall survival.

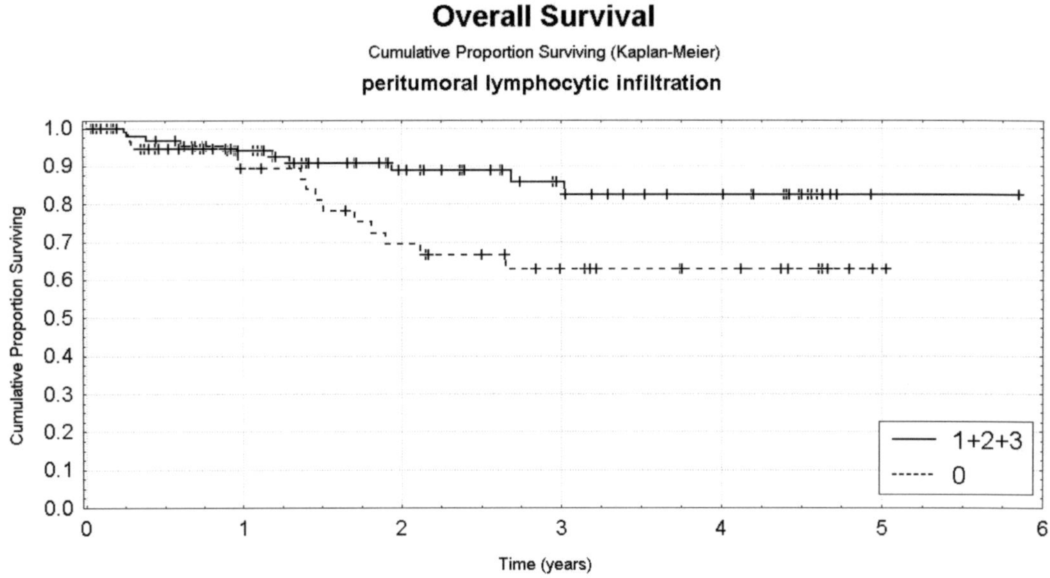

Fig. 6. Presence of peritumoral lymphocytes (PTL) was proved as a statistically significant positive factor for the prognosis of overall survival ($p<0.05$). The patients with a positive histopathological finding of PTL have 2.3x lower risk ratio for a shorter overall survival.

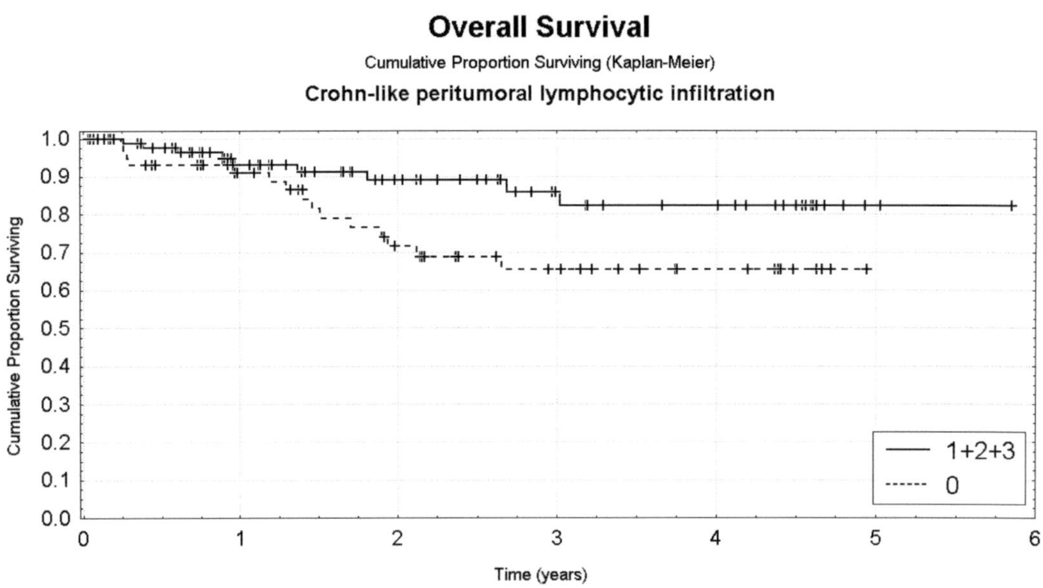

Fig. 7. Presence of Crohn-like PTL was proved as a statistically significant positive factor for the prognosis of overall survival ($p<0.05$). The patients with a positive histopathological finding of PTL have 2.3x lower risk ratio for a shorter overall survival.

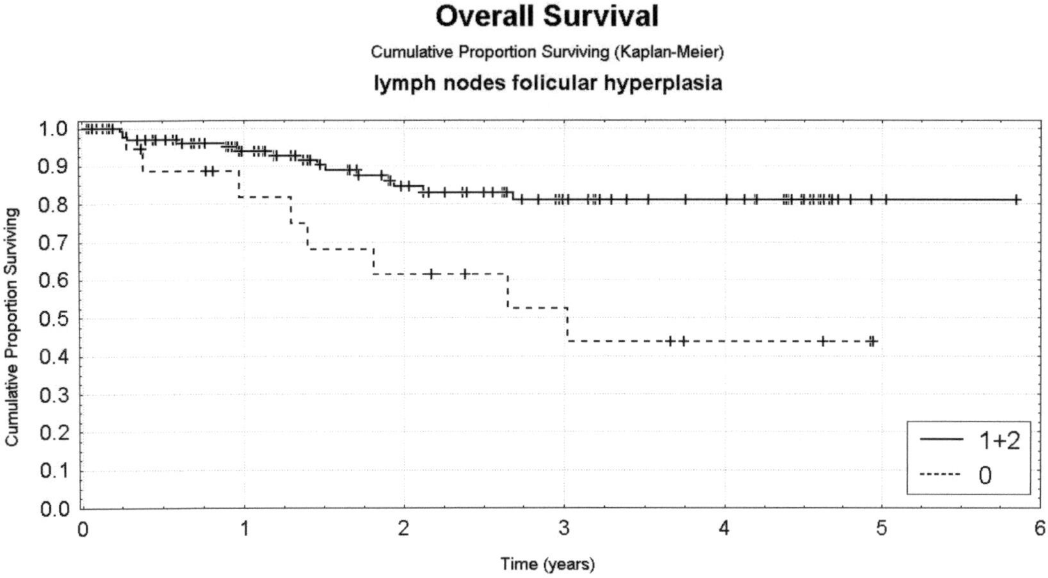

Fig. 8. Lymph node follicular hyperplasia (LN-FH) was verified as a positive prognostic factor for a longer overall survival ($p<0.05$). The statistical significance of LN-FH increased also with the raised density of infiltration. LN-FH positivity decreased the risk of a shorter overall survival 3.3x.

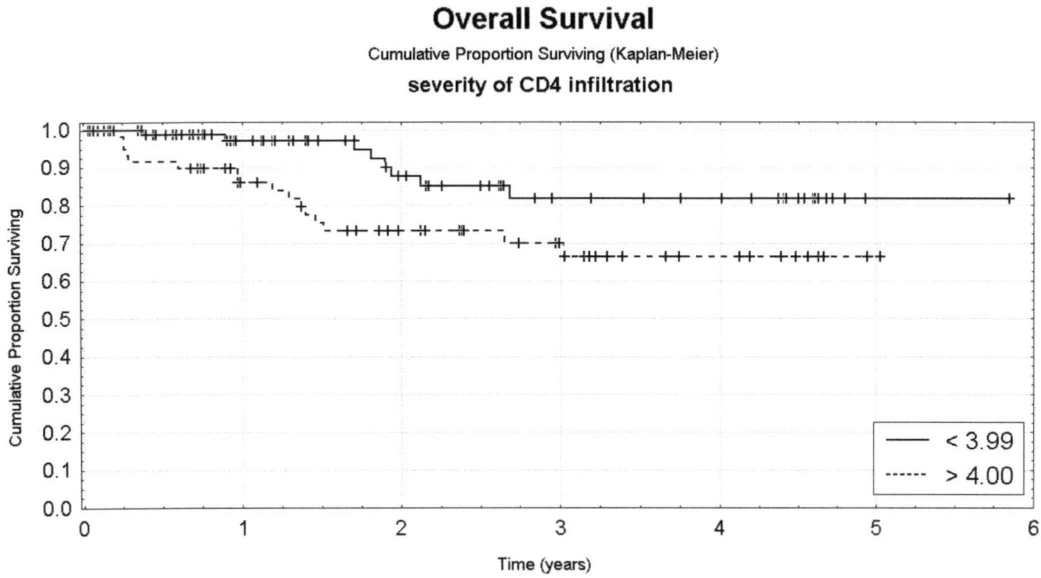

Fig. 9. Severity of CD4+ lymphocytic intratumoral infiltration was proved as a significant factor for the prognosis of overall survival (cut off 4cells/HPF) with a 2.5x increased hazard ratio in patients over the cut off ($p<0.05$).

The Multivariate Cox Regression Hazard Model proved the combination of the severity of lymph node infiltration by metastatic process and LN-FH as the best prognostic factors for the prediction of the risk of shorter overall survival. This situation is demonstrated in the Classification and Regression Tree (CART)($p<0.05$) (Fig.10.). All other studied parameters were not proved as statistically significant for the prognosis of overall survival.

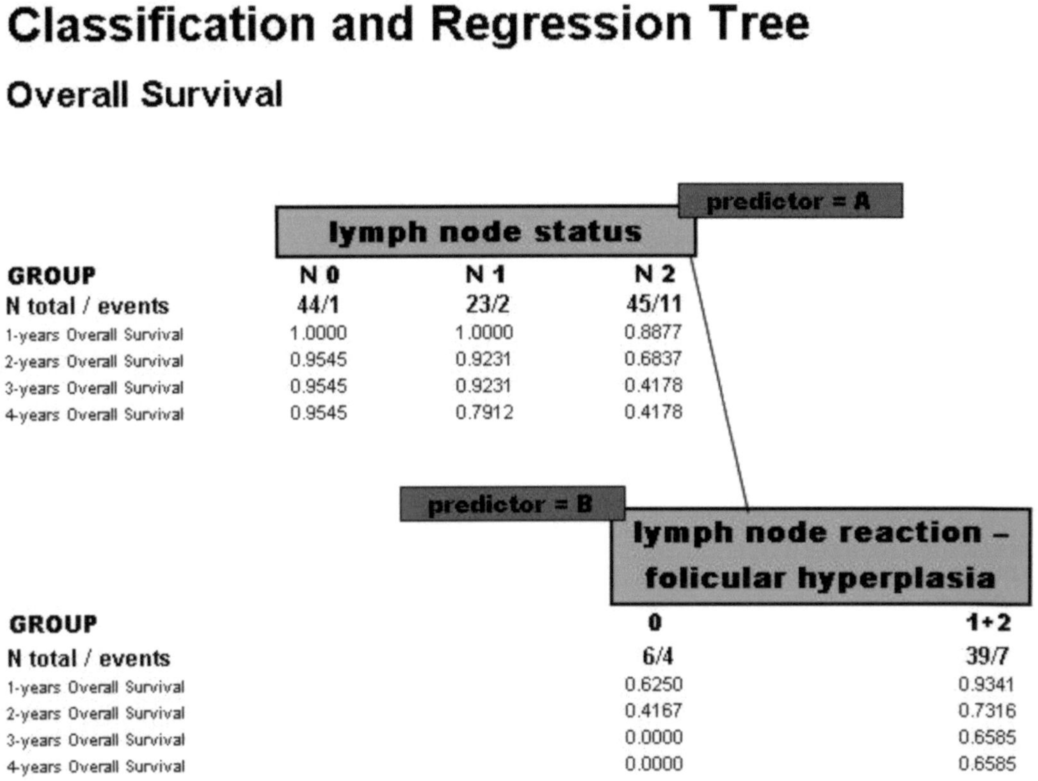

Fig. 10. Multivariate Cox Regression Hazard Model proved the combination of the severity of lymph node infiltration by a metastatic process and LN-FH as the best prognostic factors for the prediction of risk of a shorter overall survival ($p<0.05$). This situation is demonstrated in the Classification and Regression Tree (CART).

Perineural infiltration (PI) was proved as a negative prognostic factor of an earlier recurrence (Fig.11.). Patients with a positive histopathological finding of PI have 3.8x increased risk for shorter DFI.

The severity of CD8+ lymphocytic infiltration was proved by the Cox regression hazard model as a positive prognostic factor enlarging DFI (cut off 30cells/HPF) (Fig.12.). Patients over the cut off have 2.2x increased risk of an early recurrence. The severity of CD4+ lymphocytic infiltration was not proved as a significant factor for the prognosis of DFI. Statistical analysis did not confirm the statistical significance of the CD8/CD4 ratio.

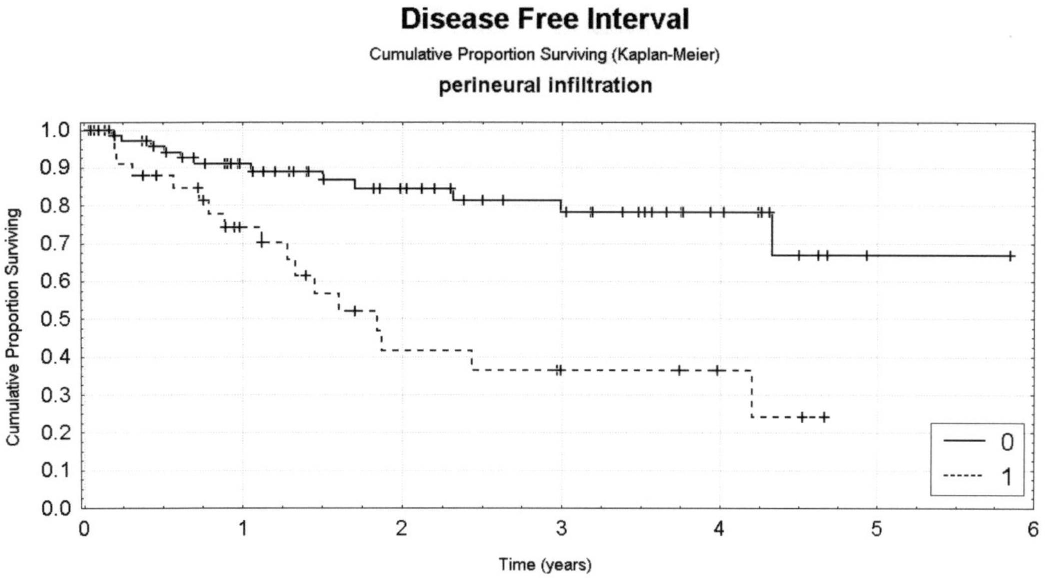

Fig. 11. Perineural infiltration (PI) was proved as a negative prognostic factor of an earlier recurrence ($p<0.05$). Patients with a positive histopathological finding of PI have a 3.8x increased risk for shorter DFI.

Statistical analysis proved lymph node infiltration by a metastatic process as statistically significant for the prognosis of DFI and N2 status of lymph nodes increased the risk of shorter DFI 5x (Fig. 13.).

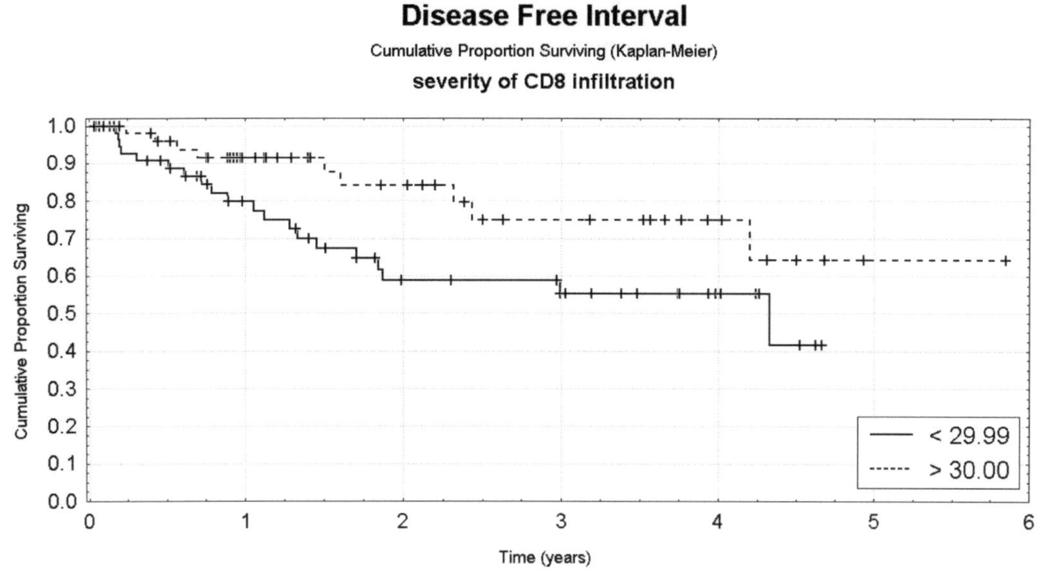

Fig. 12. Severity of CD8+ lymphocytic intratumoral infiltration was proved as a positive prognostic factor enlarging DFI (cut off 30 cells/HPF) by the Cox regression hazard model ($p<0.05$). Patients over the cut off have a 2.2x increased risk of an early recurrence.

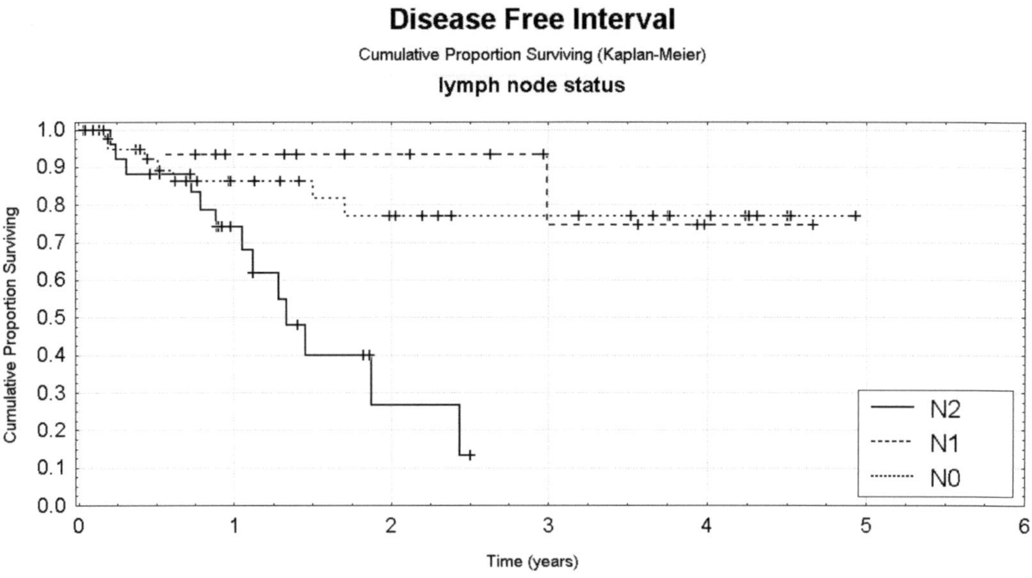

Fig. 13. Statistical analysis proved lymph node infiltration by a metastatic process as statistically significant for the prognosis of DFI, and a N2 status of lymph nodes 5x increased the risk of a shorter DFI ($p<0.05$).

The Multivariate Cox Regression Hazard Model proved the combination of the severity of the lymph node infiltration by a metastatic process and the severity of CD8 positivity of infiltrating lymphocytes as the best prognostic factors for the prediction of risk of early recurrence ($p<0.05$). This situation is demonstrated in the Classification and Regression Tree (CART) (Fig. 14). All other studied parameters were not proved as statistically significant for the prognosis of DFI.

4. Discussion

The role of the adaptive immunological response in controlling the growth and relapse of CRC remains controversial and contemporary studies have not answered all the questions about the prognosis of patients after radical surgical treatment of CRC (Galon et al., 2006; Ohtani, 2007; Van den Eynde & Hendlisz, 2009). We analysed our large cohort of patients of CRC with consideration to detect the negative and also positive prognostic factors of early recurrence of the disease and the poor overall survival after radical surgery. It was stimulated by the unsatisfactory situation and some dilemmas in the indication of surgical and oncological treatment, when early recurrence depreciates our effort to radical surgery with a high risk of complications and the long time of the decreased quality of life of our patients.

In the presented clinico-pathological study we demonstrated that lymph node infiltration by a metastatic process, N2 status of lymph nodes, VI, and extent of CD4+ lymphocytic intratumoral infiltration as negative prognostic factors of OS. In contrary PTL, Crohn-like PTL, LN-FH, and severity of CD8+ lymphocytic intratumoral infiltration were proved as positive prognostic factors of the overall survival.

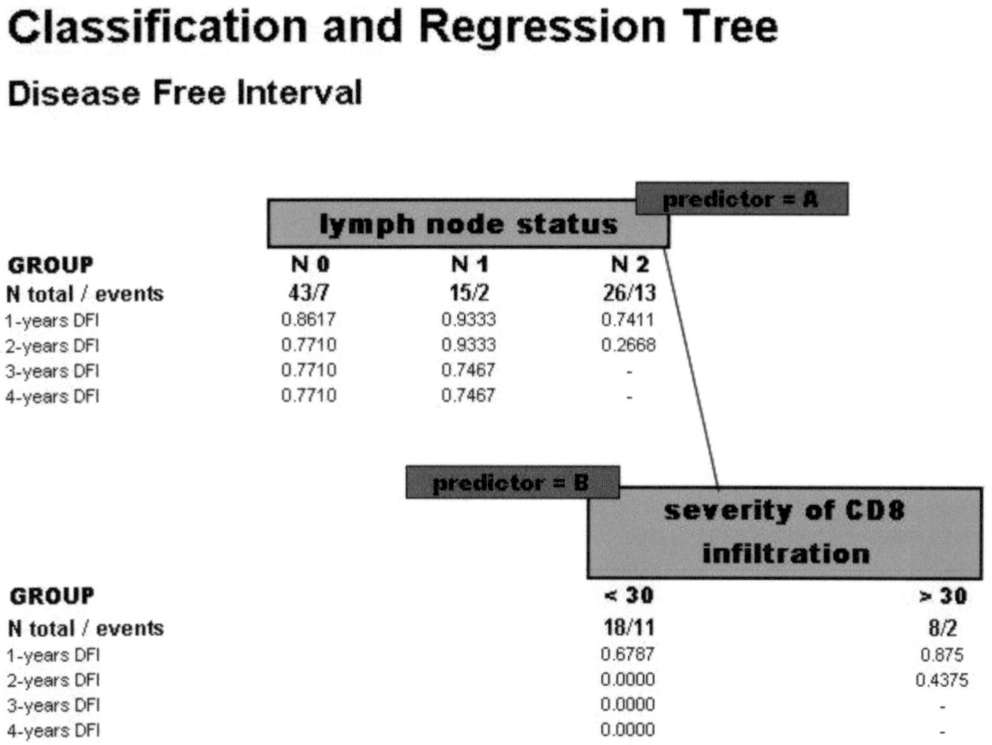

Fig. 14. Multivariate Cox Regression Hazard Model proved the combination of the severity of lymph node infiltration by a metastatic process and the severity of CD8 positivity as the best prognostic factors for the prediction of risk of an early recurrence ($p<0.05$). This situation is demonstrated in the Classification and Regression Tree (CART).

The combination of the severity of the lymph node infiltration by a metastatic process and LN-FH were proved as the best prognostic factors for the prediction of risk of a shorter overall survival by the Multivariate Cox Regression Hazard Model.

We also demonstrated PI, lymph node metastatic infiltration and the N2 status of lymph nodes as negative prognostic factors of an earlier recurrence, and the severity of CD8+ lymphocytic intratumoral infiltration as a positive prognostic factor enlarging DFI. The combination of the severity of the lymph node infiltration by a metastatic process and the severity of CD8+ lymphocytic intratumoral infiltration were proved as the best prognostic factors for the prediction of the risk of an early recurrence by the Multivariate Cox Regression Hazard Model.

Our results support the hypothesis that the adaptive immunological response in tumor tissue and its reaction in regional lymph nodes can influence the behavior of CRC and so affect the prognosis of patients (Atreya & Neurath, 2008; Galon et al., 2006). CD4 and CD8 positivity of ITL was demonstrated as a key histopathological sign of tumor-specific immune response that could reflect the contemporary clinical situation and a tendency to relapse (CD4+) or the larger overall survival (CD8+) (Chiba et al. 2004; Koch et al., 2006, Pages et al., 2010).

We assessed several types of tumor infiltrating lymphocytes and clearly identified their relationships to relapse and the overall survival as positive or negative prognostic factors in contrary to previous publications that evaluated only the infiltration of the tumor but not the quality and type of infiltration (Ogino et al., 2009).
Tumor infiltration by lymphocytes seems to be a promising prognostic factor reflecting the risk of patients to early recurrence or poor overall survival. Future work has to be focused on the molecular-biological background of tumor infiltration by lymphocytes to understand their pathophysiological functions (Pages et al., 2005, Zbar, 2004).

5. Conclusion

Tumor infiltrating lymphocytes seem to be promising prognostic factors that could find their use in colorectal surgery and consecutive oncological treatment as an indicator of the type or combinations of therapies reflecting the risk of patients to early recurrence or poor overall survival. The TIL status corresponds to immune control of cancer progression.

6. Acknowledgment

This article was supported by research project MSM 0021620819 (Replacement of and support to some vital organs) and grant IGA MZ CR 10230 and IGA MZ CR 12025 and specific students research grant of Charles University SVV-2011- 262 806.

7. References

Atreya, I., & Neurath, M. F. (2008). Immune cells in colorectal cancer: prognostic relevance and therapeutic strategies. *Expert Review of Anticancer Therapy,* Vol.8, No.4, (April 2008), pp. 561-572, ISSN 1473-7140

Bird, N. C., Mangnall, D., & Majeed, A. W. (2006). Biology of colorectal liver metastases: a review. *Journal of Surgical Oncology,* Vol.94, No.1, (July 2006), pp. 68-80, ISSN 0022-4790

Chiba, T., Ohtani, H., Mizoi, T., Naito, Y., Sato, E., Nagura, H., Ohuchi, A., Ohuchi, K., Shiiba, K., Kurokawa, Y. & Satomi, S. (2004). Intraepithelial CD8+ T-cell-count becomes a prognostic factor after a longer follow-up period in human colorectal carcinoma: possible association with suppression of micrometastasis. *British Journal of Cancer,* Vol.91, No.9, (November 2004), pp. 1711-1717, ISSN 0007-0920

Coleman, M. P., Quaresma, M., Berrino, F., Lutz, J. M., De Angelis, R., Capocaccia, R., Baili, P., Rachet, B., Gatta, G., Hakulinen, T., Micheli, A., Sant, M., Weir, H. K., Elwood, J. M., Tsukuma, H., Koifman, S., Silva, E., Francisci, S., Santaquilani, M., Verdecchia, A., Storm, H. H., Young, J. L. & CONCORD Working Group. (2008). Cancer survival in five continents: a worldwide population-based study (CONCORD). *The Lancet Oncology,* Vol.9, No.8, (August 2008), pp. 730-756, ISSN 1470-2045

Cooper, M. A., Fehniger, T. A., & Caligiuri, M. A. (2001). The biology of human natural killer - cell subsets. *Trends in Immunology,* Vol.22, No.11, (November 2001), pp. 633-640, ISSN 1471-4906

Cooper, M. A., Colonna, M., & Yokoyama, W. M. (2009). Hidden talents of natural killers: NK cells in innate and adaptive immunity. *Embo reports,* Vol.10, No.10, (October 2009), pp. 1103-1110, ISSN 1469-221X

Forssell, J., Oberg, A., Henriksson, M. L., Stenling, R., Jung, A., & Palmquist, R. (2007). High macrophage infiltration along the tumor front correlates with improved survival in colon cancer. *Clinical Cancer research*, Vol.1, No.13, (March 2007), pp. 1472-1479, ISSN 1078-0432.

Gajewski, T. F., Meng, Y., Harlin, H. (2006). Immune suppression in the tumor microenvironment. *Journal of Immunotherapy*, Vol.29, No.3, (May-June 2006), pp. 233-240, ISSN 1524-9557

Galon, J., Costes, A., Sanchez-Cabo, F., Kirilovsky, A., Mlecnik, B., Lagorce-Pagès, C., Tosolini, M., Camus, M., Berger, A., Wind, P., Zinzindohoué, F., Bruneval, P., Cugnenc, P. H., Trajanoski, Z., Fridman, W. H. & Pagès, F. (2006). Type, density, and location of immune cells within human colorectal tumors predict clinical outcome. *Science*, Vol.313, No.5795, (September 2006), pp. 1960-1964, ISSN 0036-8075

Jochems C, Schlom J. (2011). Tumor-infiltrating immune cells and prognosis: the potential link between conventional cancer therapy and immunity. *Exp Biol Med (Maywood).* Vol. 236, No.5 (May 2011), pp. 567-79, ISSN 1535-3702

Kobayashi, H., Mochizuki, H., Sugihara, K., Sugihara, K., Morita, T., Kotake, K., Teramoto, T., Kameoka, S., Saito, Y., Takahashi, K., Hase, K., Oya, M., Maeda, K., Hirai, T., Kameyama, M., Shirouzu, K. & Muto T. (2007). Characteristics of recurrence and surveillance tools after curative resection for colorectal cancer: a multicenter study. *Surgery*, Vol.141, No.1, (January 2007), pp. 67-75, ISSN 0039-6060

Koch, M., & Beckhove, P. (2006). Op den Winkel J et al. Tumor infiltrating T lymphocytes in colorectal cancer: Tumor-selective activation and cytotoxic activity in situ. *Annals of Surgery*, Vol.244, No.6, (December 2006), pp. 986-992, ISSN 0003-4932

Ljunggren, H.G., & Malmberg, K.J. (2007). Prospects for the use of NK cells in immunotherapy of human cancer. *Nature Reviews. Immunology*, Vol.7, No.5, (May 2007), pp. 329-339, ISSN 1474-1733

Lucas, M., Schachterle, W., Oberle, K., Aichele, P., & Diefenbach, A. (2007). Dendritic cells prime natural killer cells by trans-presenting interleukin 15. *Immunity*, Vol.26, No.4, (April 2007), pp. 503-517, ISSN 1074-7613

Moretta, L., Ferlazzo, G., Bottino, C., Vitale, M., Pende, D., Mingari M. C., & Moretta, A. (2006). Effector and regulatory events during natural killer-dendritic cell interaction. *Immunological Reviews*, Vol.214, No.1, (December 2006), pp. 219-228, ISSN 0105-2896

Ogino, S., Nosho, K., Iraha, N., Meyerhardt, J. A., & Baba, Y. (2009). Lymphocytic reaction to colorectal cancer is associated with longer survival, independent of lymph node count, microsatellite instability, and CpG island methylation phenotype. *Clinical Cancer Research*, Vol. 15, No. 20, (October 2009), pp. 6412-6420, ISSN 1078-0432

Ohtani, H. (2007). Focus on TILs: prognostic significance of tumor infiltrating lymphocytes in human colorectal cancer, *Cancer immunity*, Vol. 7, (February 2007), pp. 4, ISSN 1424-9634

Pagès, F., Berger, A., Camus, M., Costes, A., Molidor, R., Mlecnik, B., Kirilovsky, A., Nilsson, M., Damotte, D., Meatchi, T., Bruneval, P., Cugnenc, P. H., Trajanoski, Z., Fridman, W. H., & Galon, J. (2005). Effector memory T cells, early metastasis, and survival in colorectal cancer. *The New England Journal of Medicine*, Vol.353, No.25, (December 2005), pp. 2654-2666, ISSN 0028-4793

Pagès, F., Galon, J., Die-Nosjeanu, M. C., Tartour, E., & Sautes-Fridman, C. (2010). Immune infiltration in human tumors: a prognostic factor that should not be ignored. *Oncogene*, Vol.29, No.8, (February 2010), pp. 1093-1102, ISSN 0950-9232

Pollard, J. W. (2004). Tumor-educated macrophages promote tumour progression and metastasis. *Nature Reviews. Cancer*, Vol.4, No.1, (January 2004), pp. 71-78, ISSN 1474-175X

Sandel, M. H., Dadabayev, A. R., Menon, A. G., Morreau, H., Melief, C. J., Offringa, R., van der Burg, S. H., Janssen-van Rhijn, C. M., Ensink, N. G. , Tollenaar, R. A., van de Velde, C. J., & Kuppen, P. J. (2005). Prognostic value of tumor-infiltrating dendritic cells in colorectal cancer: role of maturation status and intratumoral localization. *Clinical Cancer Research*, Vol.11, No.7, (April 2005), pp. 2576-2582, ISSN 1078-0432

Steinman, R. M., Hawiger, D., & Nussenzweig, M. C. (2003). Tolerogenic dendritic cells. *Annual review of immunology*, Vol.21, pp. 685-711, ISSN 0732-0582

Stojanovic, A., & Cerwenka, A. (2011). Natural Killer cells and solid tumors. In: *Journal of Innate Immunity*, 10.6.2011, Available from: <http://content.karger.com/produktedb/produkte.asp?doi=325465>.

Talmadge, J. E., Donkor, M., & Scholar, E. (2007). Inflammatory cell infiltration of tumors: Jekyll or Hyde. *Cancer and Metastasis Reviews*. Vol.26, No.3-4, (December 2007), pp. 373-400, ISSN 0167-7659

Van den Eynde, M., & Hendlisz, A. (2009) Treatment of colorectal liver metastases: a review. *Reviews on Recent Clinical Trials,*, Vol.4, No.1, (January 2009), pp. 56-62, ISSN 1574-8871

Zbar, A. P. (2004) The immunology of colorectal cancer. *Surgical Oncology*, Vol.13, No.2-3, (August-November 2004), pp. 45-53, ISSN 0960-7404

20

Fluorescent Biomarker in Colorectal Cancer

E. Kirilova[1], I. Kalnina[1], G. Kirilov[1] and G. Gorbenko[2]
[1]*Daugavpils University, Daugavpils,*
[2]*N. Karazin University of National Academy of Sciences, Kharkov,*
[1]*Latvia*
[2]*Ukraine*

1. Introduction

Patients with gastrointestinal cancer exhibit a poorly functioning immune system that is characterized, in part, by decreases in T-lymphocyte proliferation (Greenstein, et al., 1991; Milasiene et al., 2007) and reduced $CD4^{+}$:$CD8^{+}$ ratios (Arista et al., 1994; Franciosi et al., 2002). In different pathologies (including these and other types of cancers), membrane damage in immune cells (and other cell types) often evolves as a consequence of alterations that are induced in cell-associated lipids and proteins in the affected patients (Gryzunov and Dobretsov, 1994, 1998; Rolinsky et al., 2007). It is now widely accepted that the dynamics (actual rate of occurrence - not only incidence) of these changes, along with the types of alterations in structure(s) of the immune system cells' lipids/proteins themselves, play a critical role in the maintenance of the immune status of any given organism (Lakowicz, 2000).
As a result of the potential importance of changes in the structural integrity of cells of the immune system, it is important for clinicians to receive information on the biophysical status of these cells via quick, reliable, reproducible methods. In this regard, fluorescent probes have shown to be excellent tools for use in such protocols (Lakowicz, 2000, 2006). The work reported here, which built upon earlier findings reported by our laboratories, investigated the possibility of using the fluorescent probe ABM (an amine derivative of benzanthrone) for the detection of structural/functional alterations in blood plasma albumin and among immunocompetent cells in patients with select types of pathologies, i.e,. cancers. Such an analysis has a great potential for use not only for helping to comprehend mechanisms of immunomodulation associated with the induction/progression of malignancies, but might also have the potential to serve as a very important prognostic indicator of long-term survival among patients with such pathologies.
In the work reported here, ABM fluorescence intensity in blood plasma and following combination with cell suspensions from colorectal cancer patients was examined in the context of the host's immunological parameters and state of cancer progression. For study patients with colorectal cancer were examined: 1) 1 day before and 10 days after their surgical treatment (Stages II-III) (Kalnina et al., 2009); 2) as disease worsened (Stages IIa, IIIb, IV) (Kalnina et al., 2010b); 3) advanced cancer patients, they were divided into two groups in accordance of its survival rate (0-6 months and > 24 months) (Kalnina et al., 2011).
Apart from the aforementioned potential benefits from these types of studies to clinicians in general, this type of research is very important in Latvia itself. This is because, in the context

of oncological diseases seen among the Latvian population (as recently as in 2006), colorectal cancers rank third in incidence, only surpassed by lung cancers and urogenital tumors.

2. ABM: Distribution and spectral characteristics in cells and blood plasma

A new fluorescent probe, a derivative of 3-aminobenzanthrone (ABM) at the Daugavpils University, Daugavpils, Latvia.

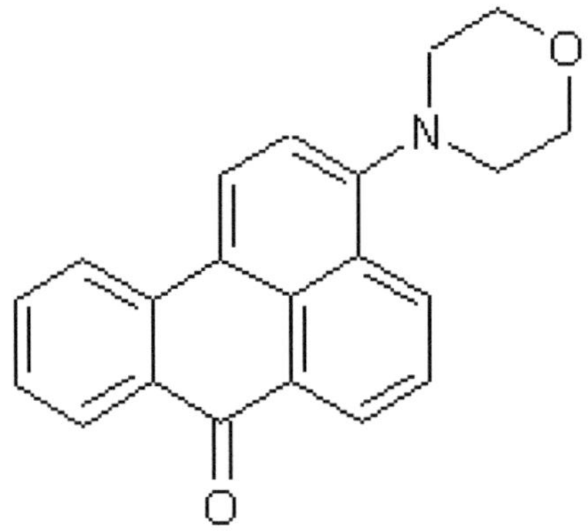

Fig. 1.Chemical Structure of probe ABM

Synthesis and properties of probe ABM were described in (Kalnina et al., 2004, 2007, 2009, 2010a; Kirilova et al., 2008).

3. ABM binding with blood plasma albumin

3.1 ABM binding with blood plasma albumin before and after surgical treatment

In the colorectal cancer patients, the ABM emission spectra maximum (i.e., at 650 nm)—after combination with the patients' blood plasma—was not altered in comparison to that seen with the plasma from the healthy control volunteers. In contrast, with respect to fluorescence intensity, before their individual surgical treatments, the average ABM intensity in the patients' blood plasma was decreased compared to that seen with the samples from the healthy donors. Specifically, the fluorescence associated with samples from the colorectal cancer group (Figure 2) were decreased by 23.0%. At 10 days after their operations, the average ABM fluorescence intensity in the samples from the colorectal cancer group were decreased further by 13.9%.

The average intensity values of the plasma samples from the cancer patients were significantly ($P < 0.05$) different from the control volunteers' average value. Whether these observations tracked actual changes in the levels of plasma albumin were also investigated. The results (data not shown) indicate that plasma albumin concentrations (μg/μL) pre-surgery in the patient group (71.73 ± 1.34) were below those in the plasma of the health controls (83.41 ± 1.16). This meant that the pre-surgery values for albumin only indicated levels in colorectal group samples that were ≈ 14% below control, while the samples' fluorescence intensity was correspondingly lower than the control value by 23.0% . The plasma albumin concentrations after surgery seemed to be insignificantly impacted. Specifically, these value was in colorectal cancer patients samples 68.48 ± 1.78 (in μg/μL, mean ± SD).

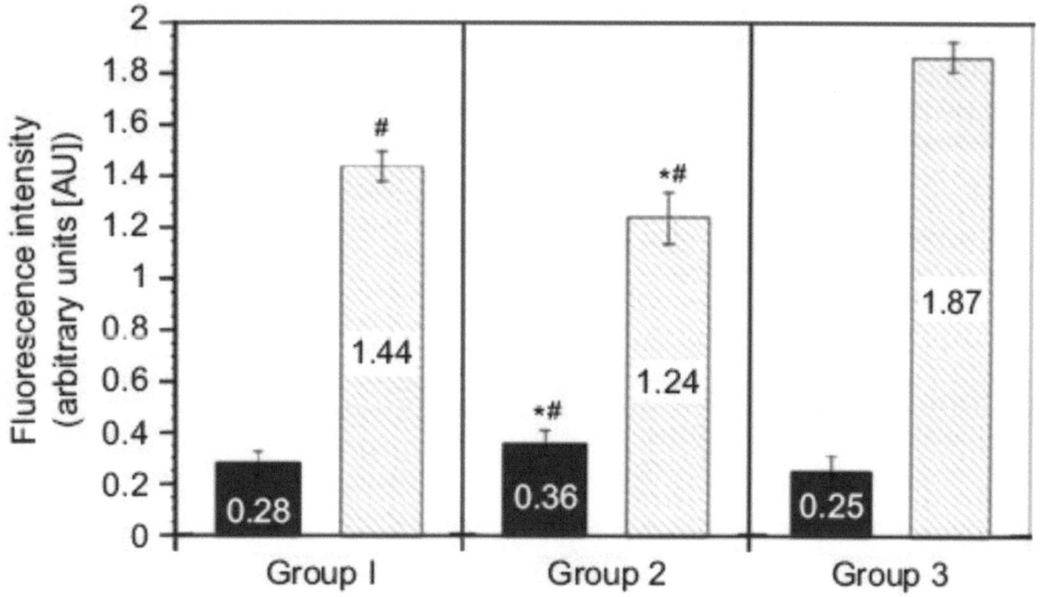

Fig. 2. ABM fluorescence intensity in lymphocytes and in plasma from "Colorectal group" patients. Colorectal cancer patients only (Stage II–III) (n = 10). Group number in figure is used to reflect from whom/when samples were isolated [i.e., Group 1: pre-surgery; Group 2: post-surgery; and Group 3: from healthy donors (control group; n = 14)]. Solid bar in each set: ABM fluorescence in lymphocytes; hatched bar in each set: ABM fluorescence in plasma. All intensity values are shown in AU (arbitrary units; mean ± SE). At $P < 0.05$, *value significantly different from pre-surgical value and/or #significantly different from control group value.

It is of interest to note that while the post-surgery albumin values in these patients samples were ≈18% below control levels, their corresponding fluorescence intensity were now even more depressed relative to that of the controls by ≈ 34%. These results strongly suggest that the noted changes in ABM fluorescence post-surgery in the cancer patients were most likely attributable to some change in the protein(s) themselves rather than due to post-surgery complications (i.e., bleeding or other mechanisms affecting blood volume/composition). To ascertain whether these results (different ABM spectral characteristics) could be explained, in part, by altered structural characteristics of the plasma albumin in the cancer patients, the average binding constant (*K*a) values were determined using the Klotz graphical method. These analyses revealed that the average *K*a values for the pre-surgery samples from the colorectal patient group decreased strongly from the respective constant associated with the control group (i.e., 1.0 X 10^5 M−1, colorectal cancer group; 1.8 X 10^5 M−1, healthy control group). These values represent decrements of from 28% to 45% in the binding of ABM to albumin in the plasma of these patients; the reason for the decrement remains to be fully determined. Interestingly, even though the fluorescence intensity values decreased further for the patients following their surgical procedures, the average *K*a values for the samples from the patients increased relative to corresponding preoperative values (i.e., 1.3 X 10^5 M−1).

3.2 ABM binding with blood plasma albumin as a function of stage

The average ABM fluorescence intensity in patient's blood plasma was decreased compared to that seen with healthy donors. Specifically, the fluorescence intensity associated with samples from colorectal cancer patients (Table 1) was decreased by 23% (average value of 1.44 fluorescence units for those at Stage IIA-IIIB) and 42% (average value of 1.09 units for those at Stage IV) relative for the healthy controls(an average value of 1.87 units).

Group	Stage	F (PI)[a]
1	IIA-IIIB	#*1.44±0.12
2	IV	*1.09±0.11
3	Controls	1.87±0.13

[a]F (PI) = fluorescence intensity in blood plasma; Values shown are in mean (± SE).
Value (p<0.05) significantly different from that of * control or # Group 2 patients.

Table 1. Spectral characteristics of ABM in blood plasma of colorectal cancer patients

3.3 ABM spectral characteristics in blood plasma of advanced cancer patients

The average ABM fluorescence intensity in the patients (Group 1 and Group 2) blood plasma was decreased (i.e., by 37.4% and 24.1%, respectively) as compared to that seen in healthy donors (Table 2). In Group 2 average intensity significantly (p<0.05) differs from Group 1 value and also control group value by 10.6 % and 31.7 %, respectively. Total albumin (TA) concentration in Group 1 and Group 2 patients was decreased (relative to control value) by 23.5% and 16.1%, respectively. Effective albumin (EA) concentration was decreased by 40.0% and 27.7%, respectively. The lowest value EA/TA in these patients plasma reached 0.61 (Group 1), and 0.66 (Group 2); (donor group 0.79-0.81).

Group	Survival rate (months)	F (PI)	EA	TA	EA/TA
1	0-6	1.17 ± 0.14	39.0 + 1.1	63,80 + 1.02	0,61
2	> 24	1.42 ± 0.09	47.0 + 1.2	70,80 + 1.14	0,66
Control		1.87 ± 0.13	65.0 + 1.3	83,4 + 1.16	0,78
P<0.05 between groups		1-2, 1-3, 2-3	1-2, 1-3, 2-3	1-2, 1-3, 2-3	

F (PI) = fluorescence intensity in blood plasma;. Values shown are in mean (± SE).
EA- "healthy" albumin equivalent in patients plasma, g/L
TA- total albumin concentration, g/L
EA/TA- reserve of albumin binding capacity

Table 2. Spectral parameters and binding sites čaracteristics of ABM in blood plasma of advanced cancer patients

4. ABM binding with lymphocytes

4.1 ABM binding with lymphocytes before and after surgical treatment

In the colorectal cancer patients, the ABM emission spectra maximum (i.e., at 650 nm) after combination with the patients' lymphocytes (as with their plasma) was not altered in comparison to that seen with the cells from the healthy control volunteers. Surprisingly, the average ABM fluorescence intensity value noted from colorectal patients group was actually 12.0% greater than the control level (Figure 3); however, even with this increase, the value was not significantly different from the average control value. In contrast to what was observed with the plasma samples, the average ABM fluorescence intensity values noted with the cells from patients at 10 days after their operations were greater than the values seen with the control volunteers' cells by 44%. In comparison to the pre-operative values, these average ABM fluorescence intensity values at 10 days after the patients' operations had increased by 28.6%.

COLORECTAL CANCER PATIENTS (Stage II-III) (n=10)					
	$CD16^+$%	[a]$CD16^+$	$CD4^+$:$CD8^+$	$CD38^+$%	Lymphocytes (%)
[b]1	‡15.95±2.18	‡314.18±39.27	‡1.27±0.10	‡3.40±1.20	28.00±1.30
2	*‡7.93±1.43	*‡144.75±22.44	*‡1.50±0.13	*‡12.70±3.40	*‡23.50±2.20
3(Controls)	12.50±1.10	389.00±24.11	1.88±0.16	24.60±1.60	28.00±1.30

[a] Values shown are in terms of absolute numbers (mean ± SE).
[b] Indicates when or from whom samples were isolated: (1) before surgical treatment; (2) after surgical treatment; and (3) healthy donors (control group; n=14).
* Value significantly different from pre-surgical value ($P<0.05$); ‡significantly different from control group value ($P<0.05$).

Table 3. Peripheral blood lymphocyte subpopulation counts in the distinct subsets of the study's cancer patients.

4.2 ABM binding with lymphocytes as a function of stage

In general, among the gastrointestinal cancer patients examined here, the ABM emission spectra maximum (i.e., at 650 nm) after combination of the probe with the patients' lymphocytes was not altered in comparison to that seen with the cells from the healthy control volunteers (spectral data not shown). The ABM fluorescence intensity in the samples from colorectal patient group in Stages IIA-IIIB was not significantly different from the average control value (0.28 vs. 0.25 fluorescence units, respectively; Fig.3). In contrast, there was a significant reduction in ths parameter among the cells from the cancer patients in Stage IV (a decrease of 44%; (0.14 vs. 0.25 units).

4.3 ABM spectral characteristics in lymphocytes of advanced cancer patients

The ABM fluorescence intensity in the samples from advanced cancer patients (Group 1) was not different from the average value (0.25 vs. 0.25) fluorescence units, respectively: (Table 4). In contrast, there was a significant increase in this parameter among the cells from the cancer patients Group 2 as compared with Group 1 (by 80.8%) and healthy donors (by 112%) (0.25 vs. 0.52 units).

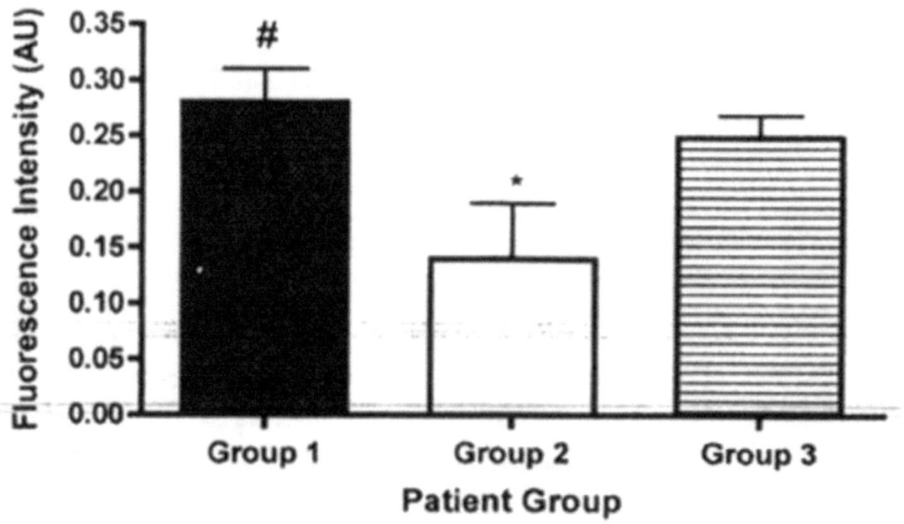

Fig. 3. ABM fluorescence intensity in lymphocytes from colorectal cancer patients as a function of stage. 1) Stage IIA-IIIB (black fill); 20 Stage IV (clear fill); 3) healthy donors (control group; stripped fill). All values are shown as mean (-+SE). At $p < 0.05$, values significantly different from that of "control patients, Group 2 patients.

5. Lymphocyte count and subpopulations

5.1 Lymphocytes count and subpopulations before and after surgical treatment

The absolute number of CD3+ cells and CD16+ natural killer cells; the relative percentages of all lymphocytes, CD16+ and CD38+ cells; as well as the CD4+:CD8+ ratio in the blood samples of the healthy volunteers and of the cancer patients, before and after each underwent their operations, were determined. The results among the patients in the "colorectal" group (Table 3) indicate that, before surgery, the numbers of CD16+ cells, the relative percentage of CD38+ cells, and the CD4+:CD8+ ratio were each significantly decreased (i.e., by 19.2%, 86.2%, and 32.4%, respectively) as compared to corresponding control subject values. Somewhat unexpectedly, relative percentages of CD16+ cells in this group were actually significantly greater (by 27.6%)—and the relative percentage of lymphocytes no different—than in the blood of the control volunteers. Within this same group, after surgery, the number and percentages of CD16+ cells, as well as the percentages of all lymphocytes, were each significantly reduced (i.e., by 53.9%, 50.3%, and 16.1%, respectively) relative to corresponding pre-surgery levels. Again, the relative percentage of CD38+ cells and the CD4+:CD8+ ratio increased (by 27.4% and 18.1%, respectively) compared to pre-surgical values, but again did not reach control levels (i.e., still were 48.4 and 20.2% lower, respectively).

5.2 Lymphocytes count and subpopulations as a function of stage

On the other hand, there were significant changes in the relative percentages of $CD4^+$ cells at almost every stage in both cancer groups (Fig. 4). Among colorectal cancer patients, the percentages of $CD4^+$ cells decreased 25.5 and 38.3% from control levels as the stages progressed (actual values: 28.6%, Stage IIA-IIIB; 23.7%, Stage IV; and, 38.4%, controls). Patients with Stage IV colorectal cancer yielded any statistically significant shift from control subject levels of CD8+ cells (an increase of ≈38%, i.e., shift from 19.5% to 26.9%).

The levels of lymphocytes (both total and the $CD4^+$ and $CD8^+$ sub-populations) in the blood samples of the cancer patients and healthy volunteers were also assessed here. The results show that among the patients in both cancer groups, the relative percentages of lymphocytes were moreover not significantly altered relative to the control levels irrespective of disease stage (Figures 4 and 5). Of all the patients, only those in Stage IV had lower blood lymphocyte levels that approached or reached statistical significance. Among the Stage IV colorectal cancer patients, levels were decreased 18.5% (a shift from 28.0% [control] down to ≈22.8%);

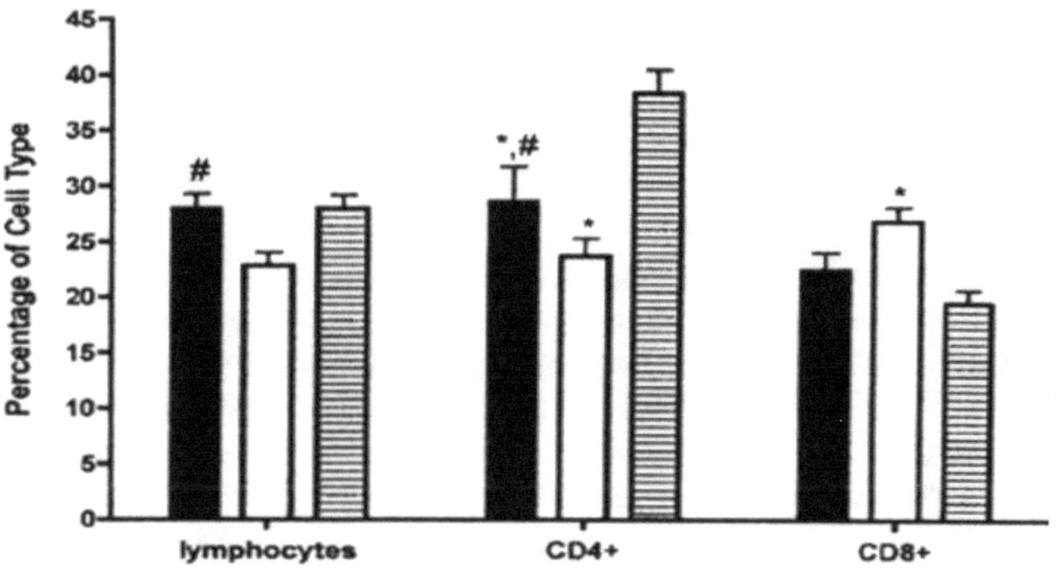

Fig. 4. Lymphocyte counts (as percentage %) and T-lymphocyte subpopulation Levels (as % of all lymphocytes present) in cancer patients as a function of stage. 1) Stage IIA-IIIB (black fill); 2) Stage IV (clear fill); 3) healthy donors (control group; striped fill).

Because shifts in $CD4^+$:$CD8^+$ ratios are often used as indices of altered host immune status, these values were also calculated from the patients' blood samples. The results show that among the colorectal cancer patients (Fig 5.), the $CD4^+$:$CD8^+$ ratios were all significantly lower than those for the healthy control subjects and became significantly further lower as the stage worsened. Specifically, the ratios dropped to 1.27 and 0.88 (shifts of 32.4% and 53.2%) at Stages IIA-IIIB and IV, respectively, from the 1.88 value for the controls.

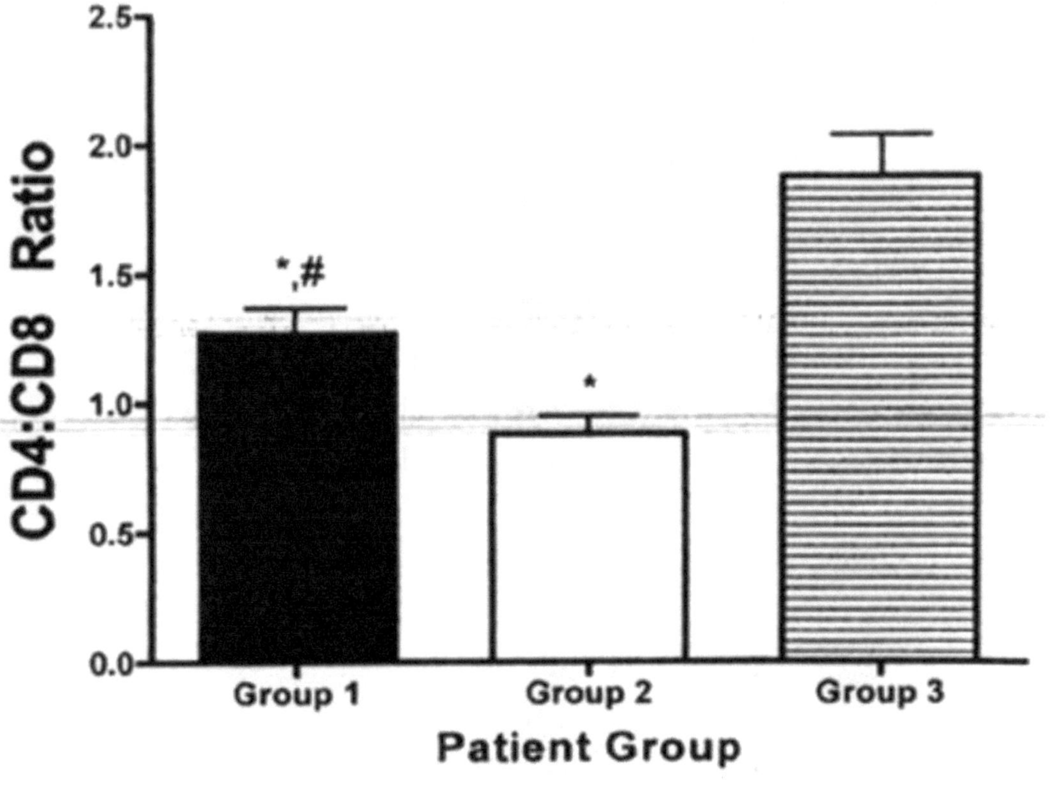

Fig. 5. T-lymphocyte subpopulation ratios in cancer patients as a function of stage.
1) Stage IIA- IIIB (black fill); 2) Stage IV (clear fill); 3) healthy donors (control group; striped fill).

5.3 Lymphocytes count and subpopulations in advanced cancer patients

Among the patients in both advanced cancer groups, the relative number of lymphocytes were significantly decreased (i.e.by 52.6% and 39.6%, respectively) as compared to corresponding control values. It is necessary to note that relative number of lymphocytes in Group 2 is significantly higher than in the Group 1 patients, but lower than the control value (see Table 4). In patients with advanced cancer and metastases there is reduction in both numbers of lymphocytes and proportions of CD4+/CD8+ T-lymphocytes which are thought to play an important role in cell-mediated immunity. The results indicate that in Group 1 and Group 2 patients the ratio CD4+/CD8+ was significantly reduced (i.e. by 58.5% and 47.9%, respectively) relative to corresponding control level. Actual values of Group 1 and Group 2 - 0.78, 0.98, respectively from the 1.88 control value. It is of interest to note that in Group 2 this parameter stay significantly higher as compared with results in Group 1, but did not reached control value.

Group	Survival rate, months	F(Ly), a.u.	Ly (%)	CD4+(%)	CD8+(%)	CD4+/CD8+
1	0-6	0,25±0,03	13,31±1,16	20,93±1,13	27,00±1,39	0,78±0,09
2	>24	0,53±0,11	16,95±1,18	26,14±1,32	26,70±1,31	0,98±0,08
3 Control		0,25±0,03	28,00±1,30	38,40±2,10	19,50±1,20	1,88±0,16
p<0.05, between groups		1-2;2-3	1-2;1-3;2-3	1-2;1-3;2-3	1-3;2-3	1-2;1-3;2-3

F(Ly) - fluorescence intensity in lymphocytes
Values shown are in mean (±SE)

Table 4. ABM fluorescence intensity in lymphocytes. Peripheral blood lymphocytes subpopulation counts in advanced cancer patients

6. Examination of relationship between ABM fluorescence and blood lymphocyte profiles

Pre-operation, in the colorectal patient group, the ABM fluorescence intensity was found to correlate with the relative number of CD38+ cells (r = +0.956). After the operations, both the CD4+:CD8+ ratio and relative number of CD38+ cells in patients blood was observed to be increased.

In colorectal cancer group, the ABM fluorescence intensity in blood plasma and the lymphocytes was found to correlate with $CD4^+$:$CD8^+$ ratios (in all stages of cancer) and the percentage (%) of lymphocytes/ subtypes in their blood. The degree of any relationship between cancer progression/staging, lymphocyte levels, and fluorescence among the lymphocytes was less obvious. Specifically, in terms of disease progression, cell levels and fluorescence intensity weakly tracked together (i.e., r = +0.512) for the colorectal patients. . With respect to associations between the plasma albumin fluorescence measurements and each of the individual lymphocyte-associated endpoints measured (except for cell fluorescence itself), many of the same patterns as noted above were evident. Once again, in terms of disease progression, although cell levels and albumin fluorescence intensity weakly tracked together (i.e., r = +0.513) among the colorectal patients.

In both groups of advanced cancer the ABM fluorescence intensity in blood plasma and lymphocytes was found to correlate to with CD4+/CD8+ ratios. In advanced cancer groups (in contrast to other groups) there is direct (not inverse) correlation between lymphocytes count and ABM fluorescence intensity. There seemed to be a good relationship between total lymphocyte (and subpopulation) levels and ABM fluorescence in both groups of patients. There is also good associations between the plasma albumin fluorescence measurements and each of the individual lymphocyte/albumin associated endpoints measured "effective" and total albumin concentration, reserve of albumin binding capacity.

7. Discussion

The novel fluorescent probe ABM (an amino derivative of benzanthrone) localizes deep within the phospholipids bilayer of lymphocytes membrane. Thus, in studies with lymphocytes, it can be concluded that changes in the spectral parameters of ABM (i.e., shifts in magnitude of fluorescence or actual wavelength associated with normal maximal fluorescence [i.e., *F*max]) could reflect modifications in one/ more interdependent (i.e., inter-related) properties of the cells. These could include the lymphocytes' (1) outer membrane physicochemical state, (2) membrane microviscosity,
(3) proliferative activity, (4) lipid metabolism, and/or (5) phenotypical profile. As seen in the studies mentioned here, while the noted changes in the studied parameters (i.e., fluorescence behavior) could be useful in reflecting alterations in lymphocytes of the cancer patients in each subgroup (at both pre- and post-surgical stages), they may also ultimately be of use as potential indicators of alteration in cellular immunity in these individuals. Follow-up studies are underway to see whether this concept can be validated. We also sought to ascertain whether shifts in ABM binding with plasma albumin could potentially be utilized as a part of an overall preliminary immunodiagnostic screening test in cancer patients. The choice to examine albumin, among the myriad of constituents in plasma, is that this protein is practically the single source of ABM binding and subsequent fluorescence in plasma (Gryzunov and Dobretsov, 1994, 1998). Our earlier studies showed that within plasma, albumin is nearly alone in binding with ABM with a very high level of selectivity (Kalnina et al., 1996, 2004, 2007). The distribution of ABM fluorescence (intensity) within fractions of human plasma was seen to be albumin >>> globulins >> non-specific binding by other components (i.e., 90%, ≈ 5%, < 1%, respectively). These widely disparate binding results were confirmed in studies wherein exogenous globulin was added to plasma samples and there was no shift in fluorescence intensity or *F*max. Clearly, only significant shifts in albumin levels or alterations/ conformational changes in albumin itself seemed to have a major impact on these ABM fluorescence endpoints. In the present study, the differences in total albumin concentrations, **pre- and post-surgery**, among the cancer patients in each group did not seem to correlate well with the relative changes in ABM fluorescence (relative to values in control subjects' plasma). This apparent "extra diminution" in fluorescence strongly suggested that there was either a novel competition for probe by other substances in the patients' plasma or that the albumin in these patients had undergone modification(s) that affected its ability to bind ABM. The fact there were substantive changes in binding constant (*K*a) values lends support to the latter viewpoint. However, this finding in and of itself does not outright preclude the possibility of the former event having occurred as well.These shifts in ABM binding constants in the plasma samples from the cancer patients, as noted earlier, could be due to a generic decreased binding by/conformational changes in their albumin molecules. Structural or functional alterations of albumin could be manifest as "shifts" away from normal "main" binding sites with high affinity for the probe to other binding sites with far lower affinities and specificities. Such shifts would be in agreement with the observations of Togashi and Ryder (2006) that albumin molecules are known to contain different binding sites (i.e., classes) for various probes. As Petitpas et al. (2001b, 2003) noted, albumin normally carries a variety of endogenous ligands like nonesterified fatty acids, bilirubin, and thyroxine; however, this protein can also bind an impressive array of drug molecules, including warfarin, ibuprofen, and indomethacin, as well as their metabolites (Petitpas et al., 2001a). It seems very likely

that patients in the groups in the present study had ingested painkillers (both prescribed and retail) during the course of their disease; thus, a presence of these drugs/ metabolites on their albumin could have contributed to the noted shifts in ABM fluorescence /*Ka* values. Our future studies will endeavor to recruit non-cancer patients with a "similar" history of painkiller intake in order to ascertain whether this was a main reason underlying our observations (regarding the albumin outcomes) or if there is something more inherently unique to the patient's cancer-bearing status that influenced the measured endpoints. This second standpoint is not without foundation. In oncopathology, the blood plasma content of two important unsaturated fatty acids (i.e., oleic acid and arachidonic acid) is increased, and these natural constituents also increasingly occupy binding sites on albumin (Gryzunov and Dobretsov, 1994, 1998). Both are observed to occupy binding sites distributed across the protein that happen to also be bound by medium or long-chain saturated fatty acids. The resulting restrictions imparted on the binding configurations of the protein would then account for shifts in the binding affinities at the primary sites between polyunsaturated fatty acids and their saturated or mono-unsaturated counterparts (Petitpas et al., 2001). It remains to be determined whether these alterations in fatty acid composition/binding also result in conformational changes in the albumin that impact upon ABM binding to its major (high selectivity) binding sites. As noted earlier, changes in fluorescence parameters of the cancer patients' lymphocytes could be reflective of changes in one/more inherent characteristics of their cells. In these studies, at least two, that is, proliferative activity and phenotypical character, could readily, albeit indirectly, be evaluated by examining changes in lymphocyte populations (i.e., their numbers) themselves. While the flow cytometry studies did indicate significant changes in lymphocyte (and subpopulation) levels among the cancer patients, unfortunately, the studies failed to yield overall lymphocyte (or subtype) population patterns that paralleled the concurrent changes in ABM fluorescence (i.e., Table 1 vs. Figure 2, example of this "lack of comparativeness"). Among all the subpopulation endpoints reported, only those of "CD38+%" and the "CD4+:CD8+ ratios" approached reflecting trends seen with the patients' fluorescence measurements. Specifically, the pre-surgery levels of each of these cytometric values were "maximally" reduced relative to the control subjects' values; post-surgery, these two values were increased, but in contrast to the fluorescence levels, these values did not reattain (or surpass) counterpart control levels. In light of the cancer patients' post-surgical (1) persistent lower numbers of lymphocytes (both total and within subclasses) and (2) fluorescence values that were uniformly significantly greater than in control subjects' cells, we surmise some factor(s) about these patients' lymphocytes (i.e., some undefined phenotypical characteristics) can cause amplification of the ABM fluorescent response. The fact that this "disconnect" between these two parameters is most predominant during the post-operative period strongly suggests that these as yet-undefined modifying factors in the cancer patients might be related to their general immune response to the surgical procedure. Our future studies will need to recruit non-cancer patients with a "similar" history of surgical intervention/protocols (such as among patients suffering enterocolitis, undergoing local biopsies for non-cancer disorders, etc.) to ascertain whether the surgical procedure itself was a main reason for our observations (regarding the "disconnect") or whether, as with the albumin findings, there is something more inherently unique to a cancer-bearing status that influenced the measured endpoints. As expected, the CD4+:CD8+ ratios were seen to be increased in the cancer patients after they had undergone their respective operation. This would be expected as it is well accepted that CD4+ helper cells stimulate and CD8+ (suppressor and cytotoxic) cells inhibit the immune response during the healing process. While that explanation for any potential changes in the phenotypic characteristics of these patients' lymphocytes is somewhat straightforward, what is less clear is the basis for the post-surgical increase in CD38+% values and why, to begin with, they are lower than in the control groups. This is because, most often, increased levels of CD38+ cells are associated with patients suffering with lymphocytic leukemias than with the solid tumors (such as those associated with gastrointestinal cancers (Kalnina et al., 2009). In general, CD38 is expressed primarily on B-lymphocytes and T-lymphocytes, as well as stem/germ cells, the CD38 ligand is an ADP-ribosyl cyclase enzyme that regulates the activation and growth of these lymphoid (as well as myeloid) cells . The data in the current study clearly show no evidence of any B-lymphocyte-based leukemia (Kalnina et al., 2009) (i.e., CD16+ cell levels were lower in patients' pre- and post-surgery blood samples than in controls) among the cancer patients. Thus, we conclude that the increase in CD38+ cell levels is more probably due to an increased presence of CD38+ T-lymphocytes. We conclude from our findings that the increase in CD38+ cell levels post-surgery was not likely due to absolute increases in T-lymphocytes, but in their activities. Such an outcome would be in keeping with the changes in the fluorescence values for these lymphocytes. For this premise to be valid, apart from showing that there are increases in relative levels of CD38-bearing T-lymphocytes due to activation during the post-surgery healing process, there still needs to be an explanation as to why these cells' levels were initially lower in the patients than in the controls. One potential explanation is in the biology of the tumors themselves, that is, they are solid tumors of the gastrointestinal system that impact on a wide variety of local cell types, including the endothelium. This particular cell type in the gut is of interest here in that there appears to be a critical relationship among endothelial cells, CD38 expression, and activation of T-lymphocytes (i.e., CD4+CD45RA+ cells. It is plausible that normal interactions between T-lymphocytes and endothelium are likely "interrupted" simply as a result of changes in accessibility (secondary to alterations in gut architecture as tumor grew). A lack of lymphocyte- endothelium interactions could help explain why there was a diminution in CD38+ cell levels before surgery; during the post-surgery recovery, angiogenic processes (i.e., during microvasculature repair/reformation at wound site) would allow for an increase in these particular cell–cell interactions—in particular, with a population of endothelial cells in very active states during the reparative processes. Future histopathology studies using biopsied samples from the gastrointestinal tracts of patients with cancers and those that underwent biopsies for non-cancer-based reasons (see earlier comments) should be useful in allowing us to verify the degree of these hypothesized cell–cell interactions. Apart from potential changes in lymphocyte-endothelium interactions as contributing factors for the reductions (vs. controls) in CD38+ cell levels—and their "recoveries" after surgical removal of the tumor—in the cancer patients, there are other possible reasons for these two observations. Among these, specifically, is the fact that patients with colorectal/gastrointestinal cancers (especially those at more advanced stages) tend to have significant levels of circulating interleukin (IL)-4 . This is critical in that it has been shown, at least with B-lymphocytes, that exposure of these cells to IL-4 reduced the amount of CD38 antigen on and in these cells; no evidence was obtained for accelerated breakdown, shedding, or internalization of CD38 molecules, or for the accumulation of CD38 molecules in the cell interior, due to IL-4 (Kalnina et al., 2009). In our ongoing studies, we will analyze patients' blood samples for IL-4 both pre- and post-surgery to see whether its levels reflect the observed changes in the CD38+ lymphocytes and their fluorescence responses (indicative of phenotypic changes likely related to activation) in the presence of ABM. The results of the ABM studies presented here show that, as might be expected, the presence of solid tumors and surgical interventions can affect the functional activity of lymphocytes. These results are in agreement with previously- performed investigations to characterize the outer cell membrane of lymphocytes of cancer patients, patients with autoimmune disease (i.e., rheumatoid arthritis), and workers who had been contaminated during the clean up at Chernobyl (Kalnina et al., 2004, 2010a, Zvagule, 2010). Likewise, the observed changes in the ABM spectral parameters in blood plasma are probably coupled with alterations in cellular mechanisms of immune regulation in the patients here. Ongoing studies are seeking to answer this very question.

The studies here showed that spectral characteristics (fluorescence intensity) differed among the various patient sub-groups. These findings suggest likely physical (structural) and functional alterations in the patients' cells were a **function of cancer stage.** It is known that ABM fluorescence intensity can change in accordance with environment polarity and, consequently, in relation to plasma membrane microviscosity (that in turn correlates with cell lipid metabolism). There are various pathological states (i.e., cancer) in which the lipid composition and specific fatty acid content in lymphocyte membranes and blood plasma are disturbed (Kalofoutis et al., 1996). For example, colorectal cancer patients have abnormal plasma and erythrocyte fatty acid levels, as well as of their polyunsaturated metabolites (Robinson et al., 2001). Ultimately, in lymphocytes, because membrane physicochemical status and cell lipid metabolism play pivotal roles in signal transduction pathway(s) activities important in maintaining cell function (Kim et al., 1999), it would not be unexpected that disturbances in these parameters could result in altered immunocompetence in hosts with these affected cells. Fluorescence intensity of ABM in lymphocytes suspension tended to decrease with progression of cancer. Shifts in magnitude of ABM fluorescence could reflect modifications in one/more interdependent properties of cells (Kalnina et al., 2007). As seen in the studies mentioned here, at least two parameters are responsible for this phenomenon. In this studies, at least two, that is proliferative activity and phenotypical character could readily, albeit indirectly, be evaluated by examining changes in lymphocytes populations (ie., their numbers) themselves. While the flow cytometry studirs did indicate significant changes in lymphocytes (and sunpopulations) levels among the cancer patients, unfortunately, the studies failed to yield overall lymphocyte (or subtipe) population patterns that paralleled the concurrent changes in ABM fluorescence example of this "lack of comparativeness"). The studie of Milasiene (Milasiene et al., 2007) also suggest that immunosuppression covers many aspects of the complex immune system, and therefore, we have many unexpected findings.

The studies here also revealed significant changes in ABM fluorescence associated with the plasma (re: albumin) of the cancer patients. The choise to examine albumin, among the myriad of constituents in plasma, is that this protein is practically the single source of ABM binding and subsequent fluorescence in plasma. We know form earlier studies that plasma albumin binds ABM with a very high selectivity (Kalnina et al., 1996, 2004, 2007, 2009, 2010b, Zvagule et al., 2010) and that only very significant shifts in plasma albumin levels or structural changes in albumin itself seemed to impact on ABM fluorescence. In the previous study (Kalnina et al., 2009) the differences in total albumin concentrations in patients groups did not seem to correlate well with the relative changes in ABM fluorescence (relative to values of control subjects plasma). The fluorescent method reveal the "effective" concentration of albumin (equivalent of "healthy" albumin in blood plasma). The total concentration of albumin is conservative. In general, serious alterations in plasma albumin levels are often reflective of poor outcomes in cancer patients (Seve et al., 2007). As noted above, the changes in patient plasma albumin levels (≈14-18% below control) were far less than the recorded shifts in ABM intensities and it seemed these measures were "picking up" changes beyond those that could solely be attributed to a change in total albumin status. The additional 'binding shifts' seen with the cancer patients' plasma samples could be due, in part, to decreased binding by/conformational changes in their albumin. There are several ways in which tumor-and/or treatment-associated agents can bind to albumin and cause allosteric modifications that lead to structure and function changes: (1) tumor cells release a variety of bioactive proteins/peptide fragments - sequestration by carrier proteins (like albumin) protect these materials from clearance (and amplify their circulating levels; Kazmierczak et al., 2006); (2) plasma content of select key unsaturated fatty acids (i.e., oleic and arachidonic acids) is increased - these then increasingly occupy binding sites on albumin (Gryzunov and Dobretsov, 1994, 1998; Petitpas et al., 2001b); and, (3) an array of drugs, e.g., ibuprofen, indomethacin, etc. (and their metabolites) commonly ingested by cancer patients readily bind with albumin (Petitpas et al., 2001a, 2003). As was the case with lymphocytes, the shifts in cancer patient plasma ABM fluorescence intensity were related to disease stage. While moderate alterations in albumin-ABM signals were already noted at early (Stages II) phases of cancer, the effects were amplified as cancer evolved to Stages III-IV. It is likely that as cancer progressed, the levels of pathological/pharmacological metabolites in the patient's blood increased and their albumin could not ultimately bind them all. One consequent structural/functional alteration induced in the albumin could be a shift in ABM binding away from normal primary high affinity sites to others with lower affinities/specificities. Such shifts would be in agreement with the observations of Togashi and Ryder (2006) and Rolinski et al. (2007) who noted that albumin molecules contained different binding sites (i.e., classes) that differed in affinity, quantum yield, and degrees of polarization (i.e., higher mobility of bound probe and increased accessibility by water) for ABM and various other probes. The results of the current investigation also seemed to reflect what was predicted to occur based upon electron spin resonance (ESR) spectroscopy studies that measured structural and functional changes in serum albumin of patients with other cancers (Kazmierczak et al., 2006). Specifically, analyses of ESR spectra (using spin probes) revealed substantial differences in spectrum variables when samples from patients were compared with those from healthy hosts. For example, the increasing width of the spectral line in samples from the cancer patients indicated an alteration in albumin conformation that limited the movement of the spin probe at a binding site, as well as changes in the albumin capacity to bind spin probe, polarity of spin probe binding site, and probe mobility (Kazmierczak et al., 2006). While increased binding of tumor-/treatment-associated agents (leading to the sequelea outlined above) could be a means by which changes in albumin-ABM fluorescence evolved here, there are other means by which the albumin ability to bind the probe may have been altered. While we demonstrated here there were changes in ABM fluorescence after inter-actions with lymphocytes (and plasma albumin) obtained from gastrointestinal cancer patients, another major question that needed addressing was whether there were actual biologic/immunologic modifications associated with these alterations. As noted earlier, changes in fluorescence parameters of patient lymphocytes could reflect changes in one/more inherent characteristics of these cells, including their phenotypical character. While the flow cytometry studies identified significant alterations in lymphocyte (and sub-populations) levels among all the cancer patients, variations in total lymphocyte levels never *clearly and consistently* paralleled the corresponding changes in ABM fluorescence for the gastric cancer subjects. In contrast, there seemed to be a good relationship between these endpoints in the colorectal patients. For now, it remains unclear why there should be a divergence in these patterns based on the cancer type itself.

The observed changes in ABM intensity in the lymphocytes might be useful to reflect current $CD4^+$ and/or $CD8^+$ status in the pacients. In this regard, the same (as above) disease-related differences in the relationships were apparent between changes in ABM fluorescence and those in $CD4^+$ levels in the patients. The noted shifts in $CD4^+$ levels were expected; cancer- related $CD4^+$ cell deficiency is a frequent finding in digestive system cancer patients (Franciosi et al, 2002). In our previous investigations, $CD4^+$:$CD8^+$ ratios tended to parallel ABM fluorescence levels (i.e., lowest among patients who manifested decreased fluorescence in their lymphocyte suspensions (Kalnina et al, 2007, 2009, 2010a,2010b). In those earlier studies, $CD4^+$:$CD8^+$ ratios gradually decreased as $CD8^+$ levels increased with progression of cancer stage (Wang et al., 2004; Kalnina et al., 2007). In the studies here, the shifts seem to depend more on decreases in $CD4^+$ levels as each disease became metastatic. These outcomes would be in keeping with the studies by Tancini et al. (1990) and (McMillan et al. (1997) that indicated that decreases in $CD4^+$:$CD8^+$ ratios in gastric cancer patients mainly depended on increases in $CD8^+$ T-cytotoxic cells in patients with early stage disease whereas it was due to decreases in $CD4^+$ T-helper cells in those with metastases (later stage disease). Thus, at least clearly for colorectal cancer patients, our results suggest that measures of ABM fluorescence intensity values for lymphocytes (and to a lesser extent, for plasma albumin) could potentially be used in clinical immunological screenings (instead of more expensive routine tests) to provide a snapshot of immune status in these cancer patients. Whether the utility of these measures could/would extend to human disease states remains to be determined.

8. Conclusion

Fluorescence behaviour of ABM could be useful to reflecting alterations in lymphocytes in each subgroup and they may ultimately be of use as potential indicators of alterations in cellular immunity in individuals. We also sought to ascertain whether shifts in ABM binding with plasma albumin could be potentially utilized as part of an overall preliminary immunodiagnostic screening test in cancer patients. Taken together it would appear that progression of cancer is associated with changes of immune function and more specifically a reduction in absolute number of CD4 + T-lymphocytes and either an increase or not change in the absolute count of CD8+ T-lynphocytes. Study suggests that higher number of absolute lymphocytes count and ratio CD4+: CD8+ have beneficial effect on overall survival of patients with advanced tumor. Overall survival depends also on quantitative parameters of cellular immunity of cancer patients. Thus, immune status of the immune system of patients with advanced tumor before treatment is important for its survival. The immunosuppression and metastatic spread are interconnected. The low plasma albumin level also were identified as bad independent marker of prognosis. Fluorescent based method is pertinent to pathway profiling, target validation, and clinical diagnosis, prediction of therapeutic effacy, and monitoring of treatment outcomes. ABM fluorescence intensity values for plasma albumin and lymphocytes (as reflection of their functional activity) might be useful tool in the evolution of the immune status of pacients. Taken together, all the results showed that measures of ABM spectral characteristics could potentially be a useful tool to estimate the immune status of gastrointestinal patients. Compared to many commonly used diagnostic protocols, this fluorescence based method is less expensive and not very time consumming, technically simple and 100 times more sensitive than standard absorbance based methods.

9. Acknowledgments

This work was supported by European Structural Funds, Project Nr. 2009/0205/1!DP/1.1.1.2.0/09/APIA/VIAA/152

10. References

Arista, M, Callopoli, A., Franceschi, L., Santini, A., Schiratti, M., Conti, L., Fillippo, F., and Gandolfo, G. M. 1994. Flow cytometric study of lymphocytes subsets in patients at different stages of colorectal carcinoma. *Dis. Colon Rectum* 37:S30-34.

Duncan, D. B. 1970. Query multiple comparison methods for comparison methods for comparing regression coefficient. *Biometrics* 26:141-143.

Franciosi, C., Bravo, A., Romano, F., Fumagalli L., Cerea, K., Conti, M., Rovelli, F., and Uggeri, F. Immunodeficiency in radically operable gastric cancer patients. 2002. *Hepato-gastroenterology* 49:857-859.

Greenstein, A., Pecht, M., Kaver, I., Trainin, N., and Braf, Z. 1991. Characterization of peripheral blood T-cell subpopulation of bladder cancer patients. *Urol. Res.* 19: 219-222.

Gryzunov, Y. A., and Dobretsov, G. E. (Eds.). 1994. *Plasma Albumin in Clinical Medicine*. Moscow: Irius Publishers.

Gryzunov, Y.A., and Dobretsov, G.E. (Eds) . 1998. *Plasma Albumin in Clinical Medicine* (Book2). Moscow: GEOTAR

Kalnina, I., and Meirovics, I. 1999. A new fluorescent probe, ABM: Properties and application in clinical diagnostics. *J. Fluorescence* 9:27-32.

Kalnina, I., Bruvere, R., Gabruseva , N., Zvagule, T., Heisele, O., Volrate, A., Feldmane, G., and Meirovics, I. 2004. Phenotypical characteristics of leukocytes of Chernobyl clean-up workers from Latvia: Use of fluorescent probe ABM. *Biol. Memb.* 21:72-78.

Kalnina, I., Klimkane, L., Kirilova, E., Toma, M. M., Kizane, G., and Meirovics, I. 2007. Fluorescent probe ABM for screening gastrointestinal patient's immune state. *J. Fluoresccence* 17:619-625.

Kalnina, I., Bruvere, R., Zvagule, T., Gabruseva, N., Klimkane, L., Kirilova, E., Meirovics, I., and Kizane, G. 2010a. Fluorescent probe ABM and estimation of immune state in patients with different pathologies. *J. Florescence* 20::9-17.

Kalnina, I., Kirilova, E., Klimkane, L., and Kirilov, G. 2009. Altered characteristics of albumin in blood of gastrointestinal cancer patients: Correlation with changes in lymphocytes populations. *J. Immunotoxicol.* 6:293-300.

Kalnina, I., Kurjane. N., Kirilova, E., Klimkane, L., Kirilov, G., Zvagule, T. 2010b. Correlation of altered plasma albumin characteristics and lymphocyte populations to tomor stage in gastrointestinal cancer patients. *Cancer Biomarkers* 7(2): 91-99.

Kalnina I., Kirilova E., Klimkane L., Kirilov G., Gorbenko G. 2011. Fluorescent biomarker in gastrointestinal and advanced tumor. 2 nd Intrernational Conference on Cancer Immunotherapy and Immunomonitoring (CITIM 2011) ; May 2-5, Budapest, Hungary, p.82.

Kalofoutis, A., Nicolaidou-Politis, V., and Bouloukos, A. 1996. Significance of lymphocyte fatty acid changes in renal failure. *Nephron* 73: 704-706.

Kazmierczak, S. C, Gurachevsky, A., Matthes, G., and Muravsky, V. 2006. Electron spin resonance spectroscopy of serum albumin: A novel new test for cancer diagnosis and monitoring. *Clin. Chem.* 52:2129-2134.

Kim, C. W., Choi, S. H., Chung, E. I., Lee, M. J., Byun, E. K., Ryu, M. N., and Bang Y. I. 1999. Alterations of signal transducing molecules and phenotypical characteristics in peripheral blood lymphocytes from gastric carcinoma patients. *Pathology* 67:123-128.

Kirilova, E. M., Kalnina, I., Kirilov G. 2008. Spectroscopic study of benzanthrone 3-N-derivatives as new hydrophobic fluorescent probes for biomolecules. *J. Fluorescence* 18: 645-648.

Lakowicz, J. R. (Ed.) 2000. *Protein Fluorescence. Vol. 6.* New York: Plenum Press.

Lakowicz J.R. Principles of fluorescence spectroscopy (3rd ed.) Springler Verlag. New York, 2006.

McMillan, D. C., Fyffe, G. D, Wotherspoon, H. A, Cooke, T. G, and McArdle, C. S. 1997. Prospective study of circulating T-lymphocyte subpopulations and disease progression in colorectal cancer. *Dis. Colon Rectum* 40:1068-1071.

Milasiene, V., Stratilatovas, E., and Norkiene, V. 2007. The importance of T-lymphocyte subsets on overall survival of colorectal and gastric cancer patients. *Medicina (Kaunas)* 43:548-554.

Petitpas, I., Bhattacharya, A. A., Twine, S., East, M., and Curry, S. 2001a. Crystal structure analysis of warfarin binding to human serum albumin: Anatomy of drug site I. *J. Biol. Chem.* 276:22804-22809.

Petitpas, I., Grune T., Bhattacharya, A., and Curry, S. 2001b. Crystal structures of human serum albumin complexed with monounsaturated and polyunsaturated fatty acids. *J. Mol. Biol.* 314:955-960.

Petitpas, I., Petersen, C. E., Ha, C. E., Bhattacharya, A. A., Zunszain, P. A., Ghuman, J., Bhagavan, N. V., and Curry, S. 2003. Structural basis of albumin-thyroxine interactions and familial dysalbuminemic hyperthyroxinemia. *Proc. Natl. Acad. Sci. USA* 100:6440-6445.

Robinson L. E., Clandinin M. T., and Field C. I. 2001. R3230 AC Rat mammary tumor and dietary long-chain (n=3) fatty acids change immune cell composition and function during mitogen activation. *J. Nutr.* 131:2001-2027.

Rolinski, O. J., Martin, A., and Birch, D. J. 2007. Human serum albumin and quercetin interactions monitored by time resolved fluorescence evidence of enhanced discrete rotamer conformations. *J. Biomed. Optics* 12:34013.1-34013.7.

Seve, P., Ray-Coquard, I., Trillet-Lenoir, V., Sawyer, M., Hanson, J., Brousolle, C., Negrier, S., Dumontet, C., and Mackey J. R. 2007. Low serum levels and liver metastasis are powerful prognostic markers for survival in patients with carcinomas of unknown primary site. *Cancer* 109:2623-2624.

Tancini, G., Barni, S., Rescaldani, R., Fiorelli, G., Vivani, S., and Lissoni, P. 1990. Analysis of T-helper and suppressor lymphocyte subsets in relation to the clinical stage of solid neoplasma *Oncology* 47:381-384.

Togashi, D. M., and Ryder, A. G. 2006. Time-resolved fluorescence studies on bovine albumin denaturation process. *J. Fluorescence* 16:153-160.

Wang, X. X., Su W. L., and Zhu, W. X. 2004. Correlation of the changes of T-lymphocyte phenotype to tumor stage and operative pattern of gastric cancer. *Al Zhena* 23:1065-1068.

Zvagule T., Kalnina, I., Kurjane, N., Bruvere, R., Gabruseva, N., and Skesters, A. 2010. Long-term effects of low doses of ionizing radiation on Chernobyl clean-up workers from Latvia. *Intern. J. Low Rad.* 7(1) : 20-31.